ETHNIC KNOWLEDGE AND PERSPECTIVES OF MEDICINAL PLANTS

VOLUME 1

Curative Properties and Treatment Strategies

Ethnic Knowledge and Perspectives of Medicinal Plants, 2-volume set
Hardback ISBN: 978-1-77491-231-7
Ebook ISBN: 978-1-00335-315-7

Volume 1: Curative Properties and Treatment Strategies
Hardback ISBN: 978-1-77491-227-0
Ebook ISBN: 978-1-00335-298-3

Volume 2: Nutritional and Dietary Benefits
Hardback ISBN: 978-1-77491-229-4
Ebook ISBN: 978-1-00335-308-9

ETHNIC KNOWLEDGE AND PERSPECTIVES OF MEDICINAL PLANTS

VOLUME 1

Curative Properties and Treatment Strategies

Edited by

Münir Öztürk, PhD

Kandikere R. Sridhar, PhD

Maryam Sarwat, PhD

Volkan Altay, PhD

Francisco Martín Huerta-Martínez, PhD

AAP | APPLE ACADEMIC PRESS

First edition published 2024

Apple Academic Press Inc.
1265 Goldenrod Circle, NE,
Palm Bay, FL 32905 USA

760 Laurentian Drive, Unit 19,
Burlington, ON L7N 0A4, CANADA

CRC Press
2385 NW Executive Center Drive,
Suite 320, Boca Raton FL 33431

4 Park Square, Milton Park,
Abingdon, Oxon, OX14 4RN UK

Library and Archives Canada Cataloguing in Publication

Title: Ethnic knowledge and perspectives of medicinal plants / edited by Münir Öztürk, PhD, Kandikere Ramaiah Sridhar, PhD, Maryam Sarwat, PhD, Volkan Altay, PhD, Francisco Martín Huerta-Martínez, PhD.
Names: Öztürk, Münir A. (Münir Ahmet), editor.
Description: First edition. | Includes bibliographical references and indexes. | Contents: Volume 1. Curative properties and treatment strategies
Identifiers: Canadiana (print) 20230224628 | Canadiana (ebook) 20230224644 | ISBN 9781774912317 (set) | ISBN 9781774912270 (v. 1 ; hardcover) | ISBN 9781774912287 (v. 1 ; paperback) | ISBN 9781003352983 (v. 1 ; ebook)
Subjects: LCSH: Medicinal plants. | LCSH: Medicine, Ayurvedic. | LCSH: Traditional medicine. | LCSH: Biodiversity. | LCSH: Nutrition.
Classification: LCC QK99.A1 E84 2023 | DDC 581.6/34—dc23

Library of Congress Cataloging-in-Publication Data

CIP data on file with US Library of Congress

ISBN: 978-1-77491-227-0 (hbk)
ISBN: 978-1-77491-228-7 (pbk)
ISBN: 978-1-00335-298-3 (ebk)

About the Editors

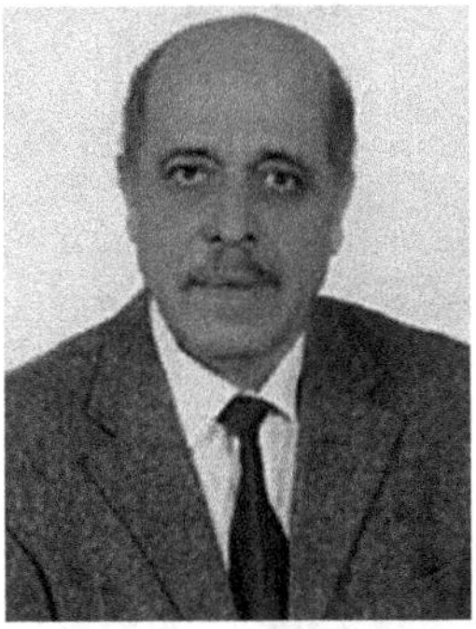

Münir Öztürk, PhD, DSc, has served at Ege University Izmir, Turkiye, for 50 years in various positions. He has received fellowships from the Alexander von Humboldt Foundation, the Japanese Society for Promotion of Science, and the National Science Foundation (USA). Dr. Öztürk has served as Chairman of the Botany Department and Founding Director of the Centre for Environmental Studies at Ege University, Izmir, Turkiye. He was also a Consultant Fellow at the Faculty of Forestry at Universiti Putra Malaysia, Malaysia, and a Distinguished Visiting Scientist at the International Center for Chemical and Biological Sciences (ICCBS) at Karachi University, Pakistan. His fields of scientific interest are plant ecophysiology, medicinal and aromatic plants, conservation of plant diversity, biosaline agriculture and crops, pollution, and biomonitoring. He has published 50 books, 80 book chapters, and 200 papers in journals with significant impact factors. Dr. Öztürk holds PhD and DSc degrees from Ege University, Turkiye.

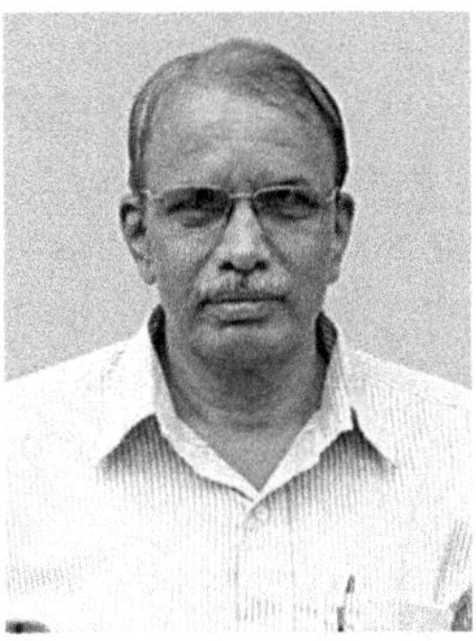

Kandikere R. Sridhar, PhD, is Adjunct Professor in the Department of Biosciences, Mangalore University, and Yenepoya (Deemed to be University), both in Konaje, India. His main area of research is the diversity and ecology of fungi of the Western Ghats, mangroves and marine habitats. He was a NSERC postdoctoral fellow/visiting professor at Mount Allison University, Canada; Helmholtz Centre for Environmental Research–UFZ and Martin Luther University, Germany; and Center of Biology, University of Minho, Portugal. He was a recipient of The Shome Memorial Award (2004) and a Lifetime Achievement Awardee (2019), given by the Mycological Society of India, of which he was Vice-President (2013) and President (2018). He was named a Fellow of the Indian Mycological Society, Kolkata, India (2014), and Distinguished Asian

Mycologist (2015) and Outstanding Leader in Education and Research from the Association of Agricultural Technology of Southeast Asia (2016). He was also a University Grants Commission Basic Scientific Research Faculty Fellow (2014–2017). He is among the world top 2% scientists in the field of mycology (2020–2021), as assessed by Stanford University, the Alper-Doger Scientific Index, and Elsevier. He has over 450 publications and eight edited books to his credit.

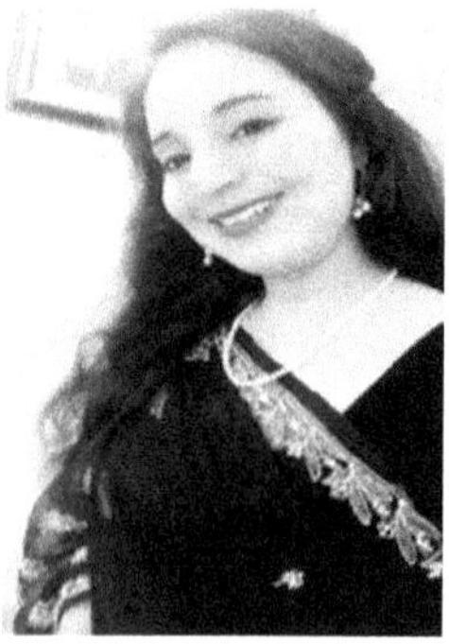

Maryam Sarwat, PhD, is Associate Professor at Amity University, Noida, India. Dr. Sarwat has published over 44 papers in international journals and five books with Springer Nature, Elsevier, and King Abdul Aziz University Press. She has three books (with Elsevier and Taylor and Francis) in progress. Her cumulative impact factor is 152 with 2400 total citations, an h-index of 20, and an i-10 index of 28. She has received a Scientist of the Year award from the National Environment Science Academy (NESA), India. Dr. Sarwat has served as a guest editor of the special issue for Current Pharmaceutical Design (impact factor 3.2) and Seminars in Cell and Development Biology (impact factor 7.7). She is a reviewer and editorial board member of more than 10 international journals. She completed her PhD at Jamia Hamdard University and did her postdoctoral research at the International Centre for Genetic Engineering and Biotechnology (ICGEB), India.

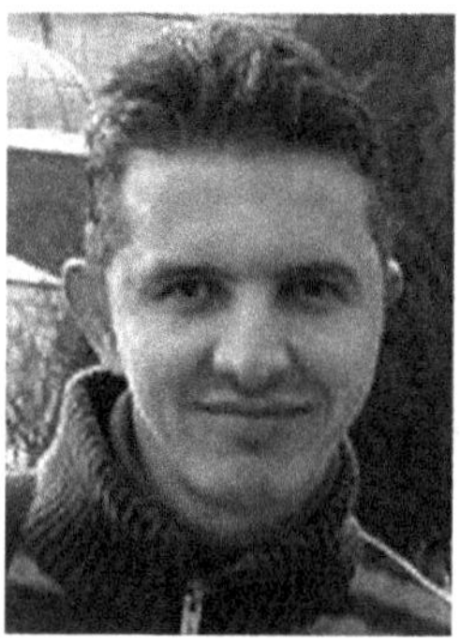

Volkan Altay, PhD, DSc, is a Full Professor in the Biology Department, Faculty of Science and Arts, at Hatay Mustafa Kemal University, Turkiye. His fields of interest are plant ecology, vegetation ecology, taxonomy, biodiversity, biomonitoring and pollution ecology, and sustainable use of medicinal plant resources. He holds a proven track record of nearly 100 publications in highly reputed professional journals. He has also published four books, nearly 45 research articles in impact factor journals, more than 40 book chapters and reviews, and more than 70 international and national congress reports. He received his PhD in 2009.

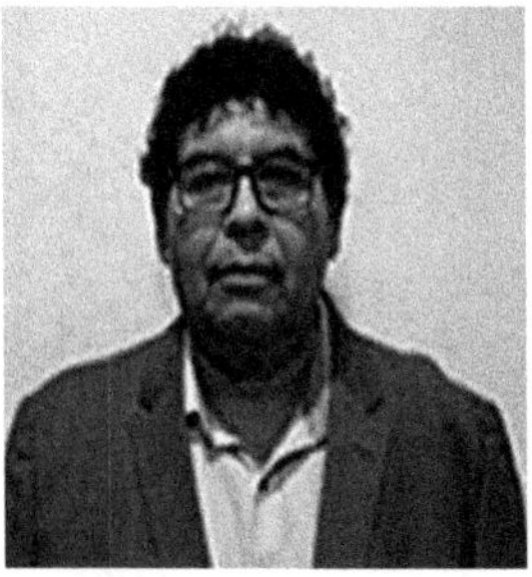

Francisco Martín Huerta-Martínez, PhD, is a Biologist and Professor in the Biological and Environmental Division at the University of Guadalajara, Mexico. He has over 32 years of experience in the Applied Ecology Department, where he teaches and does research on ecology. He has administration experience from his role as Chief at the Applied Ecology Department from 2004 to 2007, as the Academic Coordinator of the bachelor's program in biology from 2007 to 2009, and as Coordinator at a doctorate program from 2015 to 2018. His research interests are plant ecology, plant biodiversity and conservation, biotic interactions, ethnobotany, forest ecology, and biological invasions. He has published research papers in prestigious peer-reviewed journals and one international book. Dr. Huerta-Martínez has supervised PhD, MSc, and undergraduate theses. From 2004 to 2010 and from 2018 to now, he has been a member of the National System of Researchers in Mexico. Currently, he is a member of the Ecological Society of America (ESA) and has participated in several of its annual meetings. Dr. Huerta-Martínez earned his MSc (with a specialty in Botany) from Colegio de Postgraduados in Mexico State in 1995 and his PhD (with a specialty in Botany) at the same institution in 2003.

Contents

Contributors

Jamal Akhtar
Central Council for Research in Unani Medicine, Janakpuri, New Delhi, India

Kestur N. Amruthesh
Department of Studies in Botany, University of Mysore, Manasagangotri, Mysore, Karnataka, India

Aytekin A. Asgerova
Azerbaijan State Agrarian University, Ganja, Azerbaijan

Rajendra Awasthi
Department of Pharmaceutics, Amity Institute of Pharmacy, Amity University Uttar Pradesh, Noida, Uttar Pradesh, India

Lekha Bhagtaney
Caius Laboratory for Interdisciplinary Research, St. Xavier's College (Autonomous), Mumbai, India

Ram Kumar Bhakat
Ecology and Taxonomy Laboratory, Department of Botany and Forestry, Vidyasagar University, Midnapore, West Bengal, India

Sinchita Biswas
Department of Microbiology, West Bengal State University, Berunanpukuria, Malikapur, Barasat, West Bengal, India

Neerupma Dhiman
Department of Pharmaceutics, Amity Institute of Pharmacy, Amity University Uttar Pradesh, Noida, Uttar Pradesh, India

Mysore R. Gangadhar
Department Studies in Anthropology, University of Mysore, Manasagangotri, Mysore, Karnataka, India

Meenakshi Gupta
Amity Institute of Pharmacy, Amity University, Noida, Uttar Pradesh, India

Asmar E. Huseynova
Baku State University, Baku AZ, Azerbaijan

Irada M. Huseynova
Institute of Molecular Biology & Biotechnologies, Azerbaijan National Academy of Sciences, 2A Matbuat Avenue, Baku AZ, Azerbaijan

Sayyara J. Ibadullayeva
Institute of Botany, Azerbaijan National Academy of Sciences, Baku, Azerbaijan

Pradeep Kumar K.
Department of Shalakya Tantra, Yenepoya Ayurveda Medical College and Hospital, Yenepoya (Deemed to be University), Derlakatte, Mangalore, Karnataka, India

Neha Kathuria
Amity Institute of Biotechnology, Amity University Uttar Pradesh, Noida, India

Kakekochi Keshavachandra
Department of Botany, Alva's College, Moodbidre, Karnataka, India

Mohammad Afsar Khan
Molecular Cancer Genetics & Translational Research Lab, Section of Genetics, Department of Zoology, Aligarh Muslim University, Aligarh, India

Giriraj T. Kulkarni
Gokaraju Rangaraju College of Pharmacy, Hyderabad, Telangana, India

K. K. Sampath Kumara
Department of Studies in Biotechnology, University of Mysore, Manasagangothri, Mysore, Karnataka, India

Siddaramaiah Lokesh
Department Studies in Anthropology, University of Mysore, Manasagangotri, Mysore, Karnataka, India

Shivannegowda Mahadevakumar
Department Studies in Botany, University of Mysore, Manasagangotri, Mysore, Karnataka, India

Afig T. Mammadov
Genetic Resources Institute, Azerbaijan National Academy of Sciences, Baku, Azerbaijan

Bendaravaadi R. Manjunatha
Department Studies in Anthropology, University of Mysore, Manasagangotri, Mysore, Karnataka, India

Francisco Martín Huerta Martínez
Applied Ecology Department, University Center for Biological and Agricultural Sciences, University of Guadalajara, Zapopan, Jal, Mexico

Kuppuru M. Marulasiddaswamy
Department of Studies in Biotechnology, University of Mysore, Manasagangotri, Mysore, Karnataka, India

Bettadapura R. Meghavarshinigowda
Department of Studies in Botany, University of Mysore, Manasagangotri, Mysore, Karnataka, India

Abhijit Mitra
Department of Marine Science, University of Calcutta, Kolkata, India

Arijit Mondal
Department of Microbiology, West Bengal State University, Berunanpukuria, Malikapur, Barasat, West Bengal, India

Souvik Nath
Department of Microbiology, West Bengal State University, Berunanpukuria, Malikapur, Barasat, West Bengal, India

Tanveer Naved
Amity Institute of Pharmacy, Amity University, Noida, Uttar Pradesh, India

Bettadapura R. Nuthan
Department of Studies in Microbiology, University of Mysore, Manasagangotri, Karnataka, India

Mundamoole Pavithra
Department of Biosciences, Mangalore University, Mangalagangotri, Mangalore, Karnataka, India

Ashwini Prabhu
Yenepoya Research Centre, Yenepoya (Deemed to be University), Mangalore, Karnataka, India

Priya Pradeep
Department of Roganidana, Yenepoya Ayurveda Medical College and Hospital, Yenepoya (Deemed to be University), Mangalore, Karnataka, India

H. S. Prakash
Department of Studies in Biotechnology, University of Mysore, Mysore, Karnataka, India

Prosenjit Pramanick
Department of Oceanography, Techno India University, West Bengal, Kolkata, India

Devaraju Rakshith
Department of Microbiology, Yuvaraja's College, University of Mysore, Mysore, Karnataka, India

Shazia Rashid
Amity Institute of Biotechnology, Amity University Uttar Pradesh, Noida, India

Tirthankar Saha
Department of Microbiology, West Bengal State University, Berunanpukuria, Malikapur, Barasat, West Bengal, India

Sajida
Yenepoya Research Centre, Yenepoya (Deemed to be University), Mangalore, Karnataka, India

Chandagalu R. Santhosh
Department of Studies in Microbiology, University of Mysore, Mysore, Karnataka, India

Maryam Sarwat
Amity Institute of Pharmacy, Amity University, Noida, Uttar Pradesh, India

Sreedharamurthy Satish
Department of Studies in Microbiology, University of Mysore, Manasagangotri, Mysore, Karnataka

Purvi Saxena
Amity Institute of Pharmacy, Amity University, Noida, Uttar Pradesh, India

Tapti Sengupta
Department of Microbiology, West Bengal State University, Malikapur, Barasat, West Bengal, India

Uday Kumar Sen
Ecology and Taxonomy Laboratory, Department of Botany and Forestry, Vidyasagar University, Midnapore, West Bengal, India

Archana Sharma
Amity Institute of Pharmacy, Amity University, Noida, Uttar Pradesh, India

Bhagya B. Sharma
Centre for Environmental Studies, Yenepoya (Deemed to be University), Derlakatte, Mangalore, Karnataka, India

Bhupesh Sharma
Department of Pharmaceutics, Amity Institute of Pharmacy, Amity University Uttar Pradesh, Noida, Uttar Pradesh, India

S. Shishupala
Department of Microbiology, Davangere University, Shivagangothri, Davangere, Karnataka, India

Hifzur R. Siddique
Molecular Cancer Genetics & Translational Research Lab, Section of Genetics, Department of Zoology, Aligarh Muslim University, Aligarh, India

Kandikere R. Sridhar
Department of Biosciences, Mangalore University, Mangalore, Karnataka, India
Centre for Environmental Studies, Yenepoya (Deemed to be University), Mangalore, Karnataka, India

Venkateshu Srinivas
Department Studies in History, University of Mysore, Manasagangotri, Mysore, Karnataka, India

Sajida Sumaiya
Amity Institute of Pharmacy, Amity University, Noida, Uttar Pradesh, India
School of Unani Medical Education and Research, Jamia Hamdard, New Delhi, India

Priya Sundarrajan
Department of Life Science and Biochemsitry, St. Xavier's College (Autonomous), Mumbai, India

Shruti Tyagi
Department of Pharmaceutics, Amity Institute of Pharmacy, Amity University Uttar Pradesh, Noida, Uttar Pradesh, India

Sufia Zaman
Department of Oceanography, Techno India University, West Bengal, Kolkata, India

Abbreviations

ACA	acetoxychavicol acetate
ACF	aberrant crypt foci
AD	Alzheimer's disease
ADHD	attention deficit hyperactivity disorder
AFI	*Aurantii Fructus Immaturus*
AHH	hydrocarbon hydroxylase
AKP	*Arjuna Ksheera Paka*
ALI	acute lung injury
APCs	antigen-presenting cells
APML	acute promyelocytic leukemia
APW	Appraisal Project Work
ARDS	acute respiratory distress syndrome
ATP	targeting adenosine triphosphate
AYUSH	Ayurveda, Yoga & Naturopathy, Unani, Siddha & Homeopathy
BRM	*Brahma rasayana*
BZYQT	Bu-Zhong-Yi-Qi-Tang
CAIA	collagen antibody-induced arthritis
CAM	crassulacean acid metabolism
CAT	catalase
CBD	Convention on Biological Diversity
CC	*Cinnamomum cassia*
CDRI	Central Drug Research Institute
CHF	congestive heart failure
CHM	*Chyavanaprash*
CIA	collagen-induced arthritis
CJ	*Cymbopogon jwarancusa*
CK-MB	creatine-kinase-MB
CLRs	C-type lectin receptors
CNS	central nervous system
COPD	chronic obstructive pulmonary disease
CoVs	Coronaviruses
COX	cyclooxygenase
CRP	C-reactive protein
CSIR	Council of Scientific and Industrial Research

CTL	cytotoxic T lymphocytes
CTRI	Clinical Trial Registry of India
CVD	cardiovascular disease
CW	*Commiphora wightii*
CZ	*Cinnamomum zeylanicum*
DAR	*Divya Amvatari Ras*
DCs	dendritic cells
DFC	Direct Financial Cooperation
DMBA	7,12-Dimethylbenz[a]anthracene
EBM	evidence-based medicine
ECM	extracellular matrix
EEOS	ethanol-extract of *Ocimum sanctum*
EGCG	epigallocatechin gallate
EGFR	epithelial growth factor receptor
EMT	epithelial-mesenchymal transition
ER	endoplasmic reticulum
ESR	erythrocyte sedimentation rate
FOSHU	Foods for Specific Health Use
FUFOSE	Functional Food Science in Europe
FZQJ	*Fuzheng Qinggjie* granules
GGt	gamma-glutamyltransferase
GLC	Guliu capsule
GMP	good manufacturing practices
GOT	glutamic oxaloacetic transaminase
GTG	*Guggulutiktaka ghritam*
HBV	hepatitis B virus
HCC	hepatocellular carcinoma
HCV	hepatitis C virus
HDL	high-density lipoprotein
HGF	hepatocellular growth factor
HPV	human papillomavirus
ICMR	Indian Council of Medical Research
IgG	immunoglobulin G
IgM	immunoglobulin M
IMPCL	Indian Medicine Pharmaceutical Company Limited
ISSC-MAP	International Standard for Sustainable Wild Collection of Medicinal Plants
ITS	internal transcribed spacer
LDH	lactate dehydrogenase

LDL	low-density lipoprotein
LPS	liposaccharides
LPS	lipopolysaccharides
MAP	microtubule-associated protein
MDA	malondialdehyde
MDSC	myeloid-derived suppressor cell
MIF	migration inhibitory factor
MKD	*Mauktikyukta kamdudha*
MPP	*Mauktikyukta praval panchamruta*
MS	metabolic syndrome
MVL	*Maha vallathy leghiyam*
NCDs	noncommunicable diseases
NIV	National Institute of Virology
NKs	natural killer cells
NLRs	NOD-like receptors
NMVL	Neeradi muthu vallathy leghiyam
nrDNA	ribosomal DNA
nrDNA-ITS	ribosomal DNA internal transcribed spacer
NS	*Nardostachys jatamansi*
PAH	pulmonary arterial hypertension
PBR	People Biodiversity Register
PD	Parkinson's disease
PLIM	Pharmacopoeial Laboratory of Indian Medicines
QCI	Quality Council of India
QOL	quality of life
RdRp	RNA-dependent RNA polymerase
RIG	retinoic acid-inducible gene
ROS	reactive oxygen species
RSV	resveratrol
SAC	S-allyl-cysteine
SBD	*Suvarnabhasmdi*
SBP	*Swarna bindu prashana*
SL	*Saussurea lappa*
SL	Semecarpus Lehyam
SOD	superoxide dismutase
STIP	The Science, Technology and Innovation Policy
TCM	Traditional Chinese Medicine
TCRs	T-cell receptors
TLRs	toll-like receptors

TME	tumor microenvironment
TNF	tumor necrosis factor
TSG	tumor suppressor genes
UV	use value
VBL	vinblastine
WHO	World Health Organization
XBJ	*Xuebijing*
XQLD	*Xiaoqinglong decoction*
8-oHdG	8-hydroxy-2'-deoxyguanosine

Acknowledgment

The editors are highly indebted to the contributing authors for collaborating with us. Our special thanks go to the staff of AAP for their continuous help during the publication of this volume.

Preface

Pollution, industrialization, commercial activities, urbanization, globalization followed by the changes in ways of food production and consumption have strongly affected the diet of human beings. Chronic diseases like diabetes, cardiac failure, and obesity pose a great threat, both economically as well as healthwise, particularly to industrializing countries and economies. The simplification of our dietary habits is associated with increased availability of cheap agricultural products that end up causing agrobiodiversity erosion. These incidents lead to nutrient deficiencies and overconsumption of energy.

Different types of diseases are causing death and disability all over the globe. Most healthy food systems depend on locally available food along with traditional food cultures. Biodiversity conservation and nutrition are linked to different international bodies. Globalization of food production with its supply poses serious challenge to human health and well-being. Although hunger levels have decreased, energy consumption per capita has gone up. We, as humans, generally consume nutritionally and functionally rich and healthy foods of plant origin, but due to simplification, this healthy consumption is getting reduced. Nearly two billion humans suffer from micronutrient deficiencies, and almost 800 million still face the problem of insufficient diet that provides energy. Almost everyone in this world has inadequate access to biodiversity products. The latter can easily improve dietary options, as stressed by Ozturk, Hakeem, Ashraf, and Ahmad (2018) in their book *Global Perspectives on Underutilized Crops*. They have stressed on the fact that neglected and underutilized species and local varieties deserve higher priority in research and evaluation.

Ozturk, Egamberdieva, and Milica (2020) have stressed the fact in their edited volume *Biodiversity and Biomedicine: Our Future* that our rich biodiversity is of great significance for the health and diversity of nutritional diets. The quantitative indicators of biodiversity and diets need to be combined with nutrition and health outcomes. Any loss in the traditional systems will make it difficult to recreate them. Therefore, compilation, timely documentation, and dissemination of eroding knowledge of biodiversity with the use of food culture are a must for promoting positive actions.

Biodiversity makes up most of what is consumed by humans. It is the source of several medicines that provide key components for a healthy environment along with sustainable livelihoods. Any kind of ecosystem degradation, simplification of diets, species loss, and loss of knowledge of them will expose humans to new health challenges. The contribution of biodiversity to dietary quality as well as food security plays an important role for its sustainable use. We get essential energy, lipids, proteins, vitamins, and minerals from many plant and animal foods. Some of the locally important crops have been neglected and are underutilized worldwide. Their contributions to our nutrition and health change from one to another. To avoid small essential nutrient deficiencies in our food, we need to increase the variety of foods that we consume. Many components of our biodiversity that are hardly used are rich in nutrients. In fact, both cultivated and wild species are important for our economy and for small-scale farmers.

In traditional systems, indigenous foods form part of rich knowledge systems. Poor households all over the world live in countries with rich biodiversity; therefore, conservation and biodiversity are interdependent. When we link biodiversity with the health of living beings, it means growth in a positive manner. Today, the data on food composition stresses on the contributions that biodiversity makes toward nutrient availability. Unfortunately, such data is scant or not available for a multitude of species. In dietary diversity, highest priority needs to be given to analysis of food function, composition, digestibility, and safety precautions. Such studies at the local, national, and regional levels are a must for the promotion of dietary diversity. All this will be possible only through the transfer and sharing of information with successful experiences in defending and enhancing the use of plant diversity for dietary diversity.

This volume is volume 1 of the two-volume *Ethnic Knowledge and Perspectives of Medicinal Plants*. It provides detailed information on the curative properties and treatment strategies of traditional medicinal plants, while also emphasizing the link between biodiversity, human nutrition, and food security. This book includes 20 chapters from different countries.

Chapter 1 addresses information about South America, one of the most biodiverse regions in the world. In the last four or five decades, the elements that are part of the diets of modern societies in urban centers have undergone drastic changes, which have generated a state of alert in the quality of life of Mexicans, putting them as one of the countries with the highest rate of obesity, hypertension, diabetes mellitus and of course now, the number of deaths due to COVID-19.

Chapter 2 deals with traditional medicinal plants as bioresource and health security. The chapter plans to shed light on the medicinal plants and indigenous knowledge that has allowed human species to thrive on the natural ecosystem in the Indian subcontinent.

Chapter 3 is devoted to the ethnic use of wild medicinal plants in the flora of the Karabagh region in Azerbaijan. Ethnic knowledge on medicinal flora and application by the tribals is presented in Chapter 4. This documentation of the use of medicinal plant diversity based on tribal folklore serves as valuable baseline data toward conservation, further research, and possible commercialization.

Chapter 5 deals with the ethnomedicinal flora in the sacred groves of Jhargram of West Bengal. This study has identified and documented traditional uses of medicinal plant species used in indigenous medicine or drugs. Some of these medicinal plant species are dwindling owing to overexploitation as well as injudicious utilization.

Chapter 6 presents data on the indigenous medicinal knowledge of the common medicinal plants of coastal Karnataka. The majority of the plants recorded are climbers. Their applications are mainly documented according to use as home remedies, and there is an urgent need to optimise their use through modern investigation methods.

The genus *Phyllanthus* - A rich source of pharmacologically active compounds useful in traditional and modern medicine has been evaluated in Chapter 7. The chapter discusses the use of different *Phyllanthus* species in the traditional and modern medicinal system. In Chapter 8, unique traditional approach to addressing human health issues by *Ocimum sanctum* has been compiled. The traditional sweet rasgulla, a nutritionally and medicinally valued health food which has immense potential in sweet industries, has also been discussed.

Chapter 9 covers studies on the ethnomedicinal and current applications of *Azadirachta indica*. Analysis of genome, transcriptome, and metabolosome of neem has strengthened its precise applications. Ethnomedicinal uses, bioactive compounds, biopesticide potential, and biotechnological applications of neem have been discussed.

In Chapter 10, plant-based medicinal attributes in India are discussed with information on the ethnic knowledge of the application of plant species toward treating several human ailments across the Indian subcontinent.

The recently emerged pandemic due to the novel Coronavirus (2019-nCoV), its threats, and resulting mass mortalities worldwide has been evaluated in Chapter 11. Viral isolates have recently been available and the world is fighting to find a vaccine. International spread through travellers and community spread of the infection poses a challenge. The primary causing factors for this zoonotic disease include anthropogenic stress, food habits and irresponsible laboratory ethics. Some herbal concoctions could be used to combat the side effects and associated symptoms in COVID-19 patients.

In Chapter 12, the principle of Ayurveda is discussed. Ayurveda is based on the complete physical, psychological and spiritual well-being of an individual making it best suited for the treatment of lifestyle disorders. The alternative medicines use herbs, organic matter, and minerals while the preparation of herbal drugs includes the use of medicinal plants only. Today, in some places, Ayurvedic and herbal drugs are considered the first choice of treatment because of the increased side effects of modern medicines and the high mortality rate due to lifestyle diseases.

The multi-targeting efficacy and therapeutic effects of Ayurveda and Chinese medicine: An integrated approach for cancer treatment and management has been presented at length in Chapter 13. This chapter presents the efficacy of Ayurvedic and Chinese herbal medicine in combating different cancers, either alone or in combination with other therapies.

Chapter 14 is titled *Immunomodulatory Compounds Derived from Medicinal Plants as Promising Therapeutics for Cancer*. The chapter discusses various immunomodulatory plant metabolites that could be developed into cancer immunotherapeutics based on their potential pre-clinical and clinical leads. The key signaling pathways that are targeted by these immunomodulatory compounds are also elaborated.

Chapter 15 evaluates the contribution of the Indian traditional medicine in cancer treatment. In this chapter, the Indian traditional system of medicines has been explored for its role in the treatment and management of cancer. The chapter also highlights current research focused on understanding their molecular mechanisms to impart wider acceptability for their use in treatment.

A comprehensive review on the medicinal properties of Dawa-ul-kurkum and its ingredients against liver ailments in the light of ancient wisdom and modern research has been pooled up in Chapter 16. This chapter summarizes the information on the pharmacology and clinical research of individual ingredients of DuK as accessed through scientific journals and classical Unani literature. We have also tried to focus on the numerous possibilities for using DuK as an alternate therapy, alone or in combination with other medications.

Herbal Medicines for the Treatment of Neurodegenerative Disorders are presented in Chapter 17. This article highlights various neurodegenerative disorders, current therapies, and their limitations. Special emphasis has been given to the use of herbal medicines, which can overcome the drawbacks associated with synthetic drugs in the management of neurodegenerative disorders.

Ethnomedicinal practices and the role of Ayurveda in the management of oral health and hygiene are discussed in Chapter 18. Globally, oral diseases are most prevalent and require primary health care services as a part of public health concern. The use of ethnophytotherapeutic remedies for routine oral care and to treat or cure oral ailments have a long recorded history. The present review provides an overview of the database of plant species used toward oral health and hygiene.

Chapter 19 discusses the ethnomedicinal applications of 100 wild mushrooms of the Indian subcontinent. In addition to nutrition, several wild or ethnomedicinal mushrooms are used by many tribals for medicinal, nutraceutical, and health promotion purposes. Tribal knowledge on medicinal mushrooms is one of the main phases of authenticating their pharmaceutical values. This review sheds light on the use of 100 wild mushrooms (belong to 61 genera) for medicinal or health care purposes by the ethnic groups mainly from the northern region of India. Among the 12 states of the Indian Subcontinent, the highest number of ethnomedicinal mushrooms appear in Jammu and Kashmir (42 spp.), followed by Uttar Pradesh (36 spp.), and West Bengal (20 spp.).

Information on ethnomedicinal significance of epiphytic orchids and their fungal endophytes is included in Chapter 20. This chapter encompasses the distribution and ethnomedicinal significance of epiphytic orchids distributed mainly in the Asian region. Bioactive principles of orchids and their activity have been documented along with endophytic fungal diversity of selected orchid species as baseline data.

For thousands of years, the components of our biodiversity have been taken from one place to another to be used outside their region of origin. In recent years, these resources have been over-exploited. The immediate focus should be on the protection of indigenous, genetic, and biological resources against biopiracy. The convention on biological diversity from 1992 legally binds over 150 countries as parties declaring that they have sovereign rights to exploit their resources. At present, indigenous people are the most marginalized ones all over the world. These people have the worst health indicators. Their knowledge is fast dwindling because of pressures from other human beings, but they keep on maintaining their culture and language. These people are like live libraries with rich knowledge about their ecosystems, indigenous medicines, and foods.

We must inform these people and others about the impact of medicinal plants. Trade should work toward their co-operation for implementing measures toward upgrading conservation. The countries of origin should work hard toward the rights of their genetic resources. They should be guaranteed the benefits for the use of such resources on the basis of equal sharing and protection. Much is still to be done. Hopefully, this book will help highlight the importance of awareness and conservation of our biodiversity for their health and nutritional aspects.

—Editors

PART I

Ethnomedicine and Health Security

CHAPTER 1

Traditional Use of Biodiversity for Nutrition and Health in the Americas: A Case Study from Mexico

FRANCISCO MARTÍN HUERTA MARTÍNEZ

Applied Ecology Department, University Center for Biological and Agricultural Sciences, University of Guadalajara. Zapopan, Jalisco, Mexico

ABSTRACT

This chapter does not pretend to be a review of everything that is written about the traditional uses of plants and animals by the peoples of America (that seems to be impossible) but it does address information about this continent. It is in this continent where the domestication of several plants and animals was done and which are currently an important part of the diet since the time world began. Such is the case of corn, beans, pumpkins, potatoes, chili, and others. This domestication process began nearly 10,000 years back in the region called Mesoamerica, particularly in the south-central part of Mexico. The use of species has several forms, which depend on the degree of intervention by humans. These forms are wild, tolerated, sponsored, cultivated, and domesticated, including plants and animals in this management gradient. These degrees of interaction between humans and their biotic resources (mainly plants and animals, but including microorganisms and fungi), dates from prehispanic times. In many rural regions of Mexico, where native cultures still exist and have their traditional knowledge, this knowledge persists despite the efforts of the conquest by the Spanish, who

Ethnic Knowledge and Perspectives of Medicinal Plants, Volume 1: Curative Properties and Treatment Strategies. Munir Ozturk, Kandikere R. Sridhar, Maryam Sarwat, Volkan Altay, & Francisco Martín Huerta-Martínez (Eds.)

destroyed much of the legacy after 1521, the year the Aztec empire fell. The use of medicinal plants represents one of the best examples of this traditional knowledge, and even though much of the material was destroyed, it was possible to rescue very important documents, such as the *Libellus de medicinalibus indorum herbis*, which shows the degree of progress that the Aztecs had on medicinal plants and the development of a whole classification system based on uses and appearance. In addition to medicinal uses, the large number of species are consumed as part of traditional diets of Mexico. However, in the last four or five decades, the elements that are part of the diets of modern societies in urban centers have undergone drastic changes, generating a state of alert for Mexicans life quality, which has the highest rate of obesity, hypertension, diabetes mellitus, and, of course now, many deaths from COVID-19.

1.1 INTRODUCTION

America as a continent is one of the most diverse regions. There are seven countries located in America that belong to the list of megadiverse countries in the world (17 in total). This big region possesses the largest rainforest of the world (the Amazons, but not the most unique), and an important number of rivers, lakes, and wetlands. In the Americas (North, Central, South, and Caribbean region), 122,000 species are registered, representing 51% of the world's amphibians, 41% of birds, 35% each of the mammals and reptiles, and 29% of the seed plants. Also, this region contains more than 5000 species, which is 1/3 of the global fish fauna. Joly (2018) has pointed out that "conservatively, 33 percent of the plant taxa consumed by the humans are distributed in this region, but the Americas is not important only in biodiversity terms, it is home to the 15 percent of global languages."

Research carried out by various authors has revealed important information that among the world regions with oldest remains supporting evidence on the origin of agriculture, are the Fertile Crescent in the West Asia and Mesoamerica, especially in the central part of Mexico (Casas and Caballero, 1995). It is estimated that, in the fertile crescent, agriculture started nearly 11,000 years back, but this may have taken place in Mesoamerica 9000 or 10,000 years ago. Mesoamerica is a region that ranges from central Mexico to northwestern Costa Rica and Peru, Bolivia, Ecuador, Chile, and northern Argentina, forming the Andean region and they are particularly relevant for their antiquity and richness of domesticated species. Recently, several authors have proposed that the Amazon region and the northeastern United

States as probable centers of origin of domestication processes. At present, people believe that agriculture started as a gradual process; however, we have no information on why and how it was accepted as the main form of subsistence, which is still an open question (Mexicanist, 2021). The main theories suggest that it was sought to have access to resources or to ensure their availability.

Mexico is a diverse country according to the number of plant and animal species found and many of them are used as food, so, there are levels of management in each of these species. Not only plants but animals also are resources that are collected from the wild and used. In Mexico, there are about 500 wild species considered as "*quelites*" that grow without cultivation during the rainy season. They are not related to species and some are small with soft and flexible stems, others are with tall and hard stems in the form of shrubs. In general, the leaves, branches, fruits, and flowers are used as vegetables. Other resources are gathered and protected in situ. Other groups of resources are enhanced, they can grow in wild, but generally, people grow them by increasing the population density or removing competitors or pests. Finally, a vast group of resources that are native to Mexico or Mesoamerica and that are under intensive cultivation such as *Agave tequilana* (agave azul del tequila), *Theobroma cacao* (cacao), and the cultivation of *Opuntia* spp. (nopal or prickly pear). In Mesoamerica, several crops have been domesticated, for example, maize (FAO, 1999).

In Mexico, there are a great number of resources with a different use; aside from food, ceremonial, or beverages, the most important use is the medicinal uses of flora and fauna. This type of use has its origin in ancient societies before the conqueror's arrival in America. There is a detailed catalog of medicinal flora written in 1552 named *The Libellus de medicinalibus indorum herbis*, which is a compilation of plants and remedies used by native ancient Mexicans.

The Mexica (the original group of the Aztec culture) divided the plants in different ways, emphasizing the form of growth; thus, we can find that they referred to woody plants (*quahuitl*), shrubs (*quaquauhtzin*), and herbs (*xihuitl*), but there were also other ways to group them, for example, edible vegetables (*quilitl*), ornamental or sought after for their flowers (*xochitl*) and the already mentioned medicinal ones (*patli*). Hunter and gathering of wild species of flora and fauna have been an important subsistence form for inhabitants from semiarid lands of central Mexico since prehispanic times. In these habitats, the mean annual precipitation ranges between 400 and 600 mm, and the temperature ranges from 18 to 22°C (Huerta-Martínez et al., 2020). Water scarcity limits the development of traditional agriculture. The survival of these people has been possible because they have generated a broad knowledge about natural resources they possess and their uses, which, in modern times, is called "traditional science."

1.2 BIODIVERSITY AND NATURAL HISTORY OF AMERICAS

Joly (2018) stated that the American Continent is the world's longest land portion from north to south with a distance of 14,000 km from northernmost to the southernmost point. The American continent comprises 36 countries. There are two biogeographical provinces or biogeographical units: Nearctic (from middle Mexico to the northern portion) and Neotropic (from the middle of Mexico to the southern part of the continent) (Van Vuuren et al., 2006). This region comprises all climatic types and includes a large number of global freshwater ecosystems with several distinctive and irreplaceable species and approximately 20% of worlds identified key biodiversity areas, 26% terrestrial biodiversity conservation hotspots, and three of the six longest coral reefs in the world. The top 18 key marine biodiversity conservation hotspots namely the Gulf of California (the northwest portion of Mexico) and Western Caribbean (Southwest portion of Mexico) are found here (ISC, 2019). The Patagonia, Amazons, and Pacific Northwest are some of the most extensive wilderness areas that are found in this region, and the richest tropical alpine areas together with the tropical wet forests in the world, such as Paramo and Amazonian forests are found here.

The world's 7 of the 17 megadiverse countries in the American continent are located here along with the largest rainforest (the Amazons, but not the most unique). Joly (2018) has described that nearly 29% of the seed plants, 35% of the mammals 35% of the reptiles, 41% of birds, and 51% of amphibians are distributed in the Americas. Almost 33% of the plants used by humans are found here; it is a culturally and socioeconomically diverse region, being home to 15% of the global languages. The population of natives is over 66 million. Their cultures continue in all the subregions and the cultural diversity of these native people and homegrown communities provides tremendous knowledge and understanding for use and management of biological diversity. The estimate is that 40% of the global capacity of natural products comes from this area and all these are essential as food and for water as well as energy security together with other services. The value of ecosystem services reaches USD 24.3 trillion, but biological diversity along with the ecosystem services dependent on the biological diversity face strong pressure and are threatened. Nearly 65% of these services have gone down but 21% are declining very fast. The status of a quarter of the 14,000 species from different groups is nearing extinction and this risk may go up to 40% among the Caribbean the endemics, which is affecting the ecosystem services associated with the provision and protection of human services. The Millennium Ecosystem Assessment (2005) has already marked the health of our planet's ecosystems as yellow.

The efforts to complete botanical inventories has increased globally but the availability of information in extensive databases and the possibility of exchanging it between researchers from different countries have generated wide and close knowledge of the completeness for different regions, America is no exception. The first comprehensive paper on the native vascular flora of the Americas has been published by Ulloa-Ulloa et al. (2017) as per Pyšek et al. (2019). It included 124,993 species belonging to 6227 genera and 355 families. They have reported that in the North American part, 51,241 species with 42,941 endemics have been noted. In the South America, 82,052 species with 73,552 endemics have been recorded. The number shared between the two continents is around 8300 species. Nearly 33,161 species are distributed in Brazil, which shows most diverse flora, 23,104 species occur in Colombia and 22,969 in Mexico (Fig. 1.1). For North and South America, the number of naturalized alien plant species varies. Van Kleunen et al. (2019) have recorded 6569 from North America and 1961 from South America. During the next 20 years, higher numbers of naturalized plant taxa are awaited for the emerging South American economies, particularly in Brazil and Argentina. This has been emphasized by Pyšek et al. (2019) according to the predictions of global trade dynamics together with climate change.

1.3 CENTERS OF ORIGIN OF AGRICULTURE AND DOMESTICATION OF CROPS

The regions with oldest remains of cultivated plants have been identified with the help of archaeologists, probably for being the centers of origin of agriculture; however, there are several authors and disciplines (botany, archeology, anthropology, and ecology), which have developed important investigations to know how, why, and where the activities that gave rise to

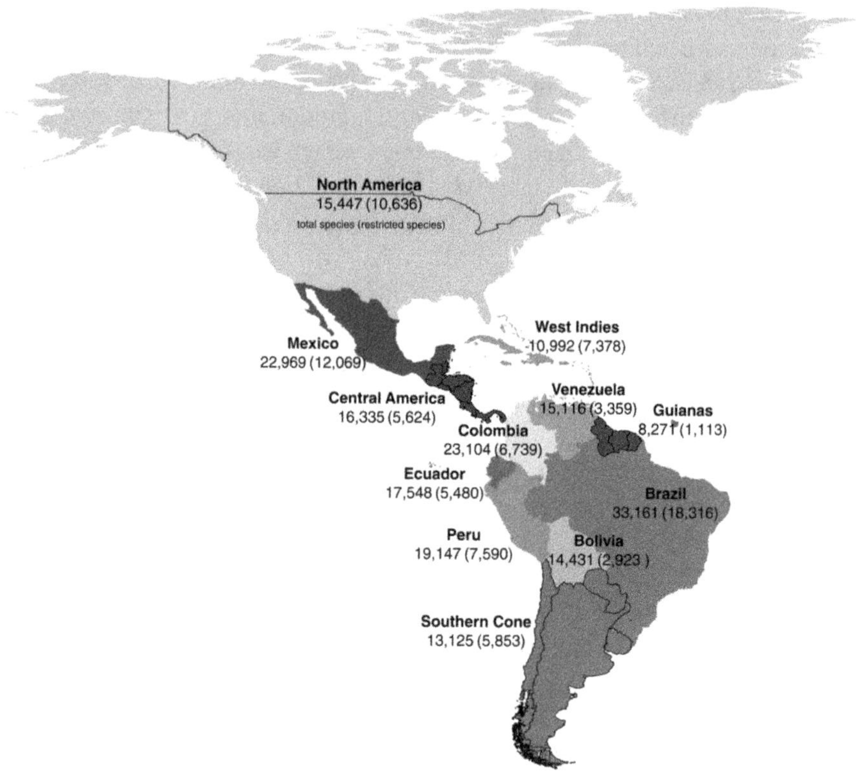
North America
15,447 (10,636)
total species (restricted species)
Mexico
22,969 (12,069)
West Indies
10,992 (7,378)
Central America
16,335 (5,624)
Venezuela
15,116 (3,359)
Guianas
8,271 (1,113)
Colombia
23,104 (6,739)
Ecuador
17,548 (5,480)
Brazil
33,161 (18,316)
Peru
19,147 (7,590)
Bolivia
14,431 (2,923)
Southern Cone
13,125 (5,853)

FIGURE 1.1 The 12 geographical areas from the Americas, representing the 12 data sets used to calculate the plant-data, the numbers are total number of vascular plant species, and the species numbers restricted to that area (in brackets).

Source: Reprinted with permission from Ulloa-Ulloa et al., *Science* **2017,** *358*, 1614–1617.

what we now call cultivation or agriculture proper in America have started. The extensive works that investigate these are Efraim Hernández Xolocotzi (1913–1991), Jack Rodney Harlan (1917–1998), Richard Stockton MacNeish (1918–2001), Kent Vaughn Flannery (who is 87 years old), Robert Bye Boettler (still working at Universidad Nacional Autónoma de México), and in the last decades, Alejandro Casas and a vast group of collaborators from Mexico. The Fertile Crescent from the Middle East and Mesoamerica, especially the central part of Mexico, are regarded by these authors among the regions of the world with the oldest remains. These works support evidence about the origin of agriculture (Casas and Caballero, 1995). Domestication processes are also ancient in China, Southeast Asia, and India, as well as in the Abyssinian plateau region and the equatorial strip of Africa (Hawkes, 1983; Vavilov,

1992; Harlan, 2005). Agriculture may have started nearly 11,000 years back in the Fertile Crescent but in Mesoamerica, this could have happened 9000 or 10,000 years back. In Mesoamerica (a region that ranges from southern Mexico to northwestern Costa Rica) and the Andean region of Peru, Bolivia, Ecuador, Chile, and northern Argentina are particularly relevant for their antiquity and richness of domesticated species. Recently, several authors have proposed that the Amazon region and northeastern United States are probable centers of origin of domestication processes. According to Smith (2011), southcentral Andes, Mexico, and most recently, eastern North America are identified as the independent centers of domestication and agricultural origin. The material recovered from upland caves can reflect a transition to a farming life taken up by the societies living in more sedentary settlements in river valleys. MacNeish (1967) stated that there are two types of incipient agricultural practices, namely (1) barranca horticulture where small human groups settled in caves located in ravines, where they took advantage of the runoff from the rain that reached the lower part of the ravines, that is, the planting of individual hardy cultivars in the barrancas near the cave sites, this type is represented by cultivated squash or pumpkin (*Cucurbita pepo*) and (2) hydro-horticulture, which means that individual domesticates (avocado trees and chili plants) were planted beside springs or along the flanks of the Rio Salado where they received a steady year-round supply of water.

Although the oldest recorded agricultural practices are estimated at 11,000 years (approximately) (MacNeish, 1992; Harris, 1996; Zohary and Hopf, 1993), domestication of both ecosystems and populations is a living process that continues till today (Casas et al., 2007). Casas and Caballero (1995) have pointed out that agricultural adoption followed a gradual process. It has risen independently in the mentioned sites; however, there are still many questions like how and why agriculture was adopted for human subsistence, the main theories suggest that it was to ensure their spatial and temporal availability and sought because of the access to resources (Casas et al, 2016a).

In Mesoamerica, agriculture and gathering of animals and plants show a long history of coexistence. The investigations carried out around the sites occupied by humans during the prehistoric periods reveal hunting and gathering were predominant activities nearly 8500 years back in Mesoamerica. After this epoch, agriculture became very important. Just during the period before the Spanish conquest, cultivated plants covered almost 80% of the indigenous subsistence (Mexicanist, 2021). Currently, this subsistence among the Mexican rural populations is still based on agriculture mainly on seasonal crops like corn, beans, and chili as their basic food items. Nearly 15% of their diets are still obtained by hunting and gathering of wild animals and plants (Mexicanist, 2021). This collection and consumption relationship represents the beginning of a domestication gradient that goes through different stages, which is called incipient management and it includes those resources that are collected directly from the field for consumption for what is called on-site management, which can be in three different ways: (1) tolerance, (2) enhancement, and (3) protection (Blancas et al., 2010).

We can also talk about this gradient of management over natural resources, for plants and animals (Fig. 1.2), *escamoles* (Fig. 1.2a), which are larval stages of ants (*Liometopum apiculatum*) that are extracted from the nests to prepare them as food in various regions of Mexico, and their cost can reach USD 10.5 per kilogram. G*usano de maguey* (maguey worm) (Fig. 1.2b) is the common name of two lepidopteran larvae (*Aegiale hesperiaris*, the white maguey worm, and *Comadia redtenbacheri, el metchikuil,* or red maguey worm). It is obtained from the center of the maguey after the rainy season, so the extraction of about three or four animals (not more) is obtained which makes a small plate of maguey worms as appetizers, and costs around 120 Mexican pesos (USD 6.00). In Mexico, there are around 500 wild plant species known as *quelites* that grow wild during the rainy season (Fig. 1.2c), and are not necessarily taxonomically related species. Some are characterized by having small, soft, and flexible stems, others are shrubs with tall stems and hard, and in general, the leaves, branches, fruits or flowers are used as vegetables. Some of the most commonly consumed species are verdolaga (*Portulaca oleracea*), epazote (*Dysphania ambrosioides*), huauzontle (*Chenopodium berlandieri*), hoja santa (*Piper auritum*), papalo (*Porophyllum ruderale*), quintonil or bledo (*Amaranthus* spp.), chepil (*Crotalaria longirostrata*) quelite de frijol (*Phaseolus coccineus*), romerito (*Suaeda edulis*), chaya (*Cnidosculus cotinifolius*) lengua de vaca (*Rumex mexcanus*) among many more.

Other resources are gathered and protected in situ. *Dactylopius coccus* (cochineal) is a Hemiptera sessile parasitic insect living on *Opuntia ficus-indica,* which produces a red dye known as carmine. This originated from South America, but its disjuncted distribution suggests that it was introduced to Mesoamerica by sea. During the Aztec empire, it was used as a tribute and was the second Mexican exported product during the Spanish domination just after silver (Rodríguez et al., 2001) (Fig. 1.2d). Traditional nondistilled alcoholic beverage pulque is a fermentation product of the aguamiel sap (AM) extracted from different maguey species like *Agave atrovensis* and *Agave americana.* The material collected is transported for fermentation in large open barrels (Escalante et al., 2008). These days this beverage is produced and consumed mainly in the central states of Mexico. The background idea is used as a dietary supplement and risk-buffering food in ancient Teotihuacan (150 B.C. to A.D. 650) (Correa-Ascencio et al., 2014) (Fig. 1.2e). Other groups of resources are enhanced as they can grow wild, but generally, people help them to grow increasing the population density or removing competitor or pests. Here we can find *Physalis ixocarpa* (tomatillo milpero) (Fig. 1.2f), which is a Solanaceae but it is not the same species for red tomatoes (*Solanum lycopersicum*) that is named as jitomate. Other resources from this same category are *Stenocereus queretaroensis* (pitayas) and *Spondias purpurea* (ciruela amarilla), which grow in the wild but are tolerated and enhanced by people to eat their fruits in the dry season of the year (Figs 1.2g and 1.2h, respectively). Finally, a vast group of resources that are native to Mexico or Mesoamerica and are subjected to intensive cultivation include *A. tequilana* (agave azul del tequila), a well-managed plant in the area as the wild individuals are thought to have disappeared, which is the species tequila is made of. Tequila is an emblematic alcoholic beverage of Jalisco, Mexico (Fig. 1.2i); other Mesoamerican resource intensively cultivated is the base of chocolate (*T. cacao*) (Fig. 1.2j), and in ancient times the seeds were used as coins. Finally, several species of *Opuntia* (prickly pear) are cultivated for consumption as vegetables or their fruits (Fig. 1.2k). This group of species is considered as not completely domesticated since there is a high rate of hybridization.

According to the Mexicanist (2021), for cultivation of a wild species we have to change the genetic setup. This comes from the natural selection processes and can be used by us under the conditions managed by humans. Such a manipulation is done mainly through an artificial selection, aiming at designing and creating organisms that can satisfy human requirements and will grow in manmade environments, which is precisely known as the domestication process. As such, agriculture is a productive process where both cultivation and domestication are involved (Casas and Caballero, 1995).

1.4 MESOAMERICA—EVIDENCE OF ORIGIN OF AGRICULTURE

Mesoamerica is regarded as one of the important plant domestication centers in the world. It covers roughly the central portion extending to the south of Mexico and part of central America. A long cultural history coexists with highly diverse plant ecology that could be one possible explanation for this. Almost 30,000 flowering plant species in Mexico coexist with over 60 indigenous ethnic groups. The latter currently use and manage over 5000 plant species maintaining different forms of interaction with these. Mesoamerica can be regarded as a living laboratory of plant domestication (Mexicanist, 2021).

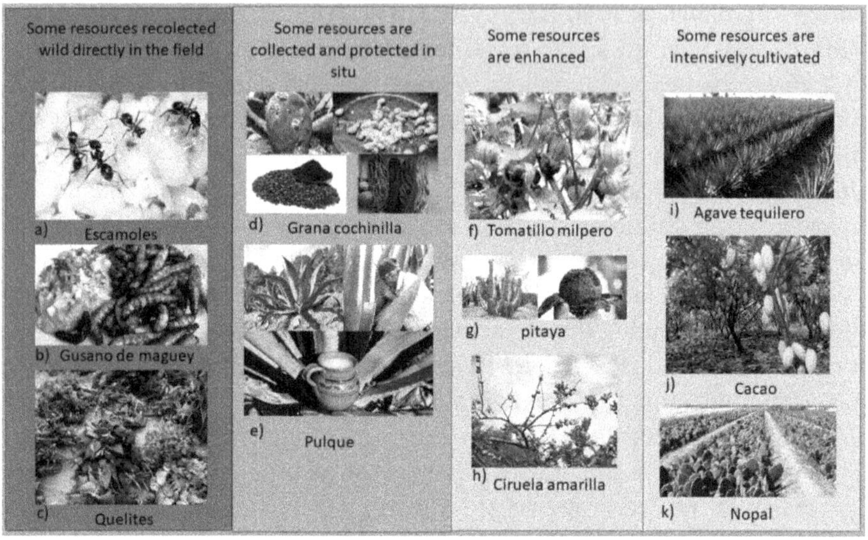
Some resources recolected wild directly in the field
Some resources are collected and protected in situ
Some resources are enhanced
Some resources are intensively cultivated
a) Escamoles
b) Gusano de maguey
c) Quelites
d) Grana cochinilla
e) Pulque
f) Tomatillo milpero
g) pitaya
h) Ciruela amarilla
i) Agave tequilero
j) Cacao
k) Nopal

FIGURE 1.2 The gradient of management over natural resources in Mexico. From left to right, the first column contains resources gathered wild and used seasonally (escamoles, gusano de maguey (maguey worm), and quelites); the second column comprises resources gathered in the field but protected by human (grana cochinilla or cochineal, Pulque); the third column contains enhanced species (tomatillo milpero, pitayas, and ciruela amarilla; Fourth column are highly managed species (agave azul del tequila, cacao, and prickly pear.

Source: Photo: Martin Huerta, Self elaboration.

Full details of the Mesoamerican prehistory are present in the literature published during the archeological investigations in Sierra de Tamaulipas and Tehuacan Valley by MacNeish and in Guilá Naquitz, Oaxaca by Flannery (1986). Smith and MacNeish stress that in the former first evidence of morphological changes in plants, determined by human manipulation, are found in chupandría (*Cyrtocarpa procera*), avocado (*P. americana*), and chili (*Capsicum annum*) in 8000 years (BP) strata. Flannery has found the most ancient evidence of guajes domestication (*Lagenaria siceraria*) in strata of about 9000 years BP in Guilá Naquitz (Mexicanist, 2021). The domesticated *C. pepo* records are the oldest archaeological records in Mexico and these come from the central valley of Oaxaca (10,000 BP), Tehuacán (7900 BP), and the Ocampo caves in Tamaulipas (6300 BP) (Casas et al. 2016a). In the United States, the oldest records date back to only 5000 and 380T0 BP (Smith, 2001, 2006). According to Smith and Yarnell (2009), corn cultivation could have happened about two thousand years later. It is important to state that agricultural production in the Americas is based on the biodiverse American tropics and montane regions.

In Mexico, maize and beans—most often common bean and squash, top the list among the important food crops that are domesticated (Kwak et al. 2009). The wild relative of these crops are distributed in Mexico and neighboring regions. Both archaeological and genetic evidences point to Mexico as a center of domestication of beans, maize, and squash which are often cultivated there in traditional cropping systems called milpa. In other Latin American countries, these complement each other agronomically (Fig. 1.3). Maize was domesticated from *Zea mays* subsp. *parviglumis* or teosinte as its closest wild relative (Doebley, 2004), perhaps somewhere "in a region around the Balsas River basin in Mexico, as per the genetic information" (Matsuoka et al., 2002). Guilá Naquitz cave is the incipient maize domestication area for being the oldest archaeological remains in the south of Balsas basin (Piperno and Flannery, 2001; Kwak et al. 2009), which include the 8000–10,000 years old squash (*C. pepo*) seeds (Smith, 1997). The question now is if common bean was domesticated in the same area as maize (Delgado Salinas et al., 1988). These conclusions are also supported by Kinder et al (2017), who argue that three requirements must be met to infer that there is an interaction between plants and humans: "(1) when a plant appears and it is confined to the archaeological site; (2) when it appears to have had a strong association with ancient and modern indigenous groups; and (3) when it might be at the edge of or beyond its normal range." Sometimes people refer to milpa to the maize plant, but the most popular meaning is the polyculture that comprises more than one species.

One of the questions that was tried to answer is how and why the agricultural activity began, what were the motivations of human groups to start this process that represented a radical change in all existing groups in their way of life. Spengler III (2020) consigned that following large periods of research on the origin of agriculture, general acceptance is that the process was not the result of conscious selection. In my opinion, the academic community is ready to accept the evolution under cultivation and focus on the effects of intense human herbivory on plant communities in mid-Holocene. The evolution of agriculture-type seed dispersal-based mutualism in primates has been developing for at least 40 million years" (Spengler III, 2020).

1.5 HUMAN-BIOTA RELATIONSHIPS IN THE AMERICAS

The American continent has been home to important cultures. The misnamed "discovery of America" was not a discovery, because they were lands that were already populated by the Aztecs, Mexicans, Mayas, or Incas, which are all the great cultures. They had developed a vast knowledge in the fields of science, arts, astronomy, architecture, agriculture, and the domestication of species at a higher level. The ancestral cultures of America were polytheistic, but their daily activity and lifestyle were deeply linked to knowledge and respect for natural resources and the land that sustained them. The Maya god of rain Chac, Tlaloc among the Aztecs, the Quetzal bird for Aztecs, Inti the sun for the Incas, the Moon for the Mapuches, and all over the Andean region, we read about the Pachamama or the mother Earth. We should feel for nature as it is the origin of our life, consequently they did take care of all living beings and their symbolic foods" (Masson-Salaue, 2019).

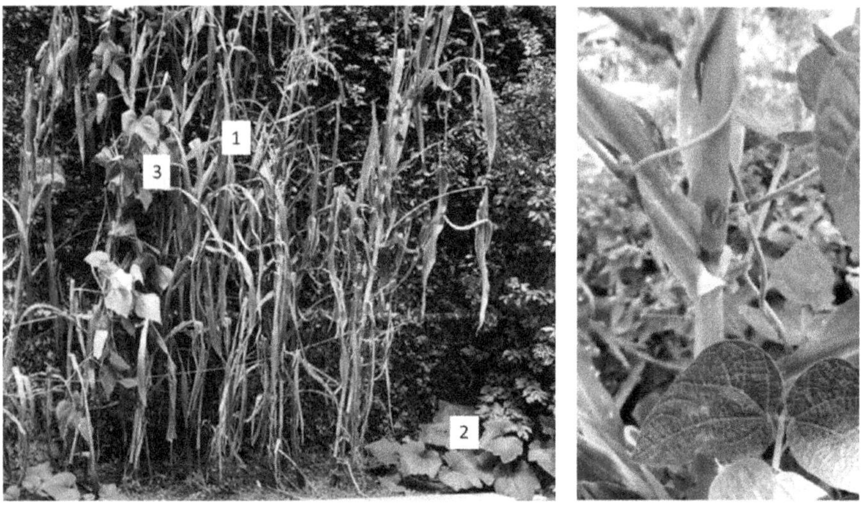

(a) (b)

FIGURE 1.3 Cropping system called milpa (**a**): **1**: maize (*Zea mays*), **2**: squash (*Cucurbita* spp.), and **3**: beans (*Phaseolus vulgaris*); (**b**): bean growing entangled in the corn plant.

Source: Photos: Cecilia Arevalo Cerna.

The arrival of the conquerors in 1492 destroyed much of the knowledge that the ancestral cultures of America had developed. What is still conserved is the great biological diversity and part of the prehispanic traditions, among which the foods that use natural resources originating from these lands and that is currently part of their diet. Ancient cultures in Mesoamerica fed on many plants and animal species, for example, as Castillo et al. (2020) have pointed out that nearly 20,000 plants and almost 2500 animal species served as the potential foods in ancestral diets (Paoletti, 2005). To cover the protein sources in Mesoamerica, we see insects, mammals, reptiles, amphibians, fishes, and leguminous species were consumed with some domesticated and nondomesticated plants as sources of carbohydrates, fats, vitamins, and minerals (Sahagún, 2006). Insects are a diverse group of animals with extended use as food in many countries, for example, in African countries, South and East Asia, and in South and Central America, more than 2000 different species are consumed (Nyberg et al., 2020), in addition to the number of leafy vegetables species which is nearly 500 (Bye and Linares, 2000). Several crop species have been domesticated here and it is the center of origin, diversity, and domestication of maize. These grow along with crops and as such are not considered as domesticates but rather as subjects of incipient or indirect artificial selection (Castillo et al., 2020). A highly beneficial polyculture or milpa provides products every year and brings down biodiversity loss risk, is nutritionally complex, and is highly sustainable compared to intensive crops" (Altieri et al., 2011).

The region of Mexico basin is abundant in nonagricultural food resources. Only few other regions in America share this feature. The fishing, bird-hunting, salt production, turtle capturing, collecting different animal species even at the larvae stage, along with algae and other aquatic plants, have been contributing toward the enrichment of diet with the subsistence of inhabitants from times immemorial (Williams, 2020).

According to MacNeish (1967), in the case of the ancient inhabitants of the Tehuacan Valley, Mexico, there were temporary changes in the composition of the diet between 9000 and 3000 years before the present. Since the settlement of the region, human beings have mainly fed on hunting animals (megafauna), an activity that represents the antecedent of the predominant subsistence pattern in human groups during the thousands of years that preceded this period. The extinction of megafauna was followed by continuous hunting, but perhaps with less and less success; however, the collection of wild plants increased in importance until the year 5000 BP where it began its decrease along with the appearance and availability of plants associated with agricultural processes, although it never ceased to be important (Casas et al., 2016b).

Some of the nonagricultural food resources that are still used, but undoubtedly was the basis of the diet of the ancient Americans are the following:

1. **Microalgae:** These are being consumed for thousands of years (Wells et al., 2017). Oldest known algal use as food is from Chile, dating back to 14,000 BP. However, none have expanded as a major crop. The reason may be social acceptance issues, being different

from traditional crops (Torres-Tiji et al., 2020). Nowadays, Spirulina has come to the forefront (Lafarga, 2019). In the 16th century, it was harvested from Lake Texcoco for use by Tenochtitlan (Mexico City now) and regarded as a food for the future as per the International Association of Applied Microbiology in 1967 (Costa et al., 2019). It has two species *Arthrospira platensis* and *Arthrospira maxima* as the most cultivated microalga worldwide — over 30% of microalgal biomass production is from *Spirulina* (Costa et al., 2019). It is rich in proteins which is around 60% on a dry weight basis (Rosa et al., 2015). If the conditions are not limited by nitrogen, values go up to 70% (Lafarga et al., 2020). This filamentous blue-green microalga is used as a nutraceutical food supplement because of its being rich in proteins, essential fatty acids, vitamins, polyphenols, and carotenoids (Pham et al., 2019). Its potential antioxidant activity too is investigated together with anti-inflammatory and hypolipidemic features. It shows great benefits against hypercholesterolemia, hyperglyceridemia, cardiovascular diseases, and inflammatory diseases (Wu et al., 2016). It contains many hydrophilic active ingredients like, phycocyanin and phycocyanobilin (Yang, et al., 2020).

2. **Native bees honey:** These are a large group of eusocial bees belonging to the family Hymenoptera and subfamily Meliponinae. They are stingless and are found in South and Central America, Africa, Southwest Asia, and Australia (Ávila et al., 2018). Their honey is used by the humans since ancient times (Vit et al., 2013). The breeding and raising of melipona bees have been a tradition among the people living in South Mexico and neighboring countries (the Mayan region) as they obtained honey for food and medicine. The beeswax has served as a sealant and an art tool (National Research and Council, 2007). *Melipona beecheii* is the most important species, widely evaluated by the Mesoamerican cultures like Maya since the pre-Columbian era (Yam-Puc et al., 2019). According to Mayan cosmogony, honey has been associated with fertility, the bees producing it are the guarantors of life (López-Maldonado, 2005). In Mayan culture, the stingless beekeeping was as important as the cultivation of maize (De Jong, 2001). They domesticated *M. beecheii* due to its nest size, the excellent flavor, therapeutic features, attractive golden appearance of honey, and docility of bees (Quezada-Euán et al., 2001). The propolis is produced by *M. beecheii*. It is a resinous apiarian product that has bitter flavor. It is basically a mixture of

wax and resin exudating from different plants. It is gathered by bees as an auxiliary material to protect their hives (Bracho Pérez et al., 2009). Nowadays it is used in the treatment of gastritis, inflammatory diseases, hemorrhoids, respiratory illnesses, and fatigue as well as the base of remedies and food products in traditional Mexican indigenous medicine (Yam-Puc et al., 2019).

"Honey is a very complex natural foodstuff; it contains exhibiting wide range of biological effects which act as natural antioxidants" (Ávila et al., 2018). Yam-Puc et al. (2019) have determined "13 pentacyclic triterpenes in the propolis from *M. beecheii* such as; α-amyrin, β-amyrin, lupenone, taraxerone, germanicol acetate, 24-methylencycloartan-3-one, and moretenol among others." In Mexico, the meliponiculture is an ancient tradition and highly beneficial for our health (Quezada-Euán et al., 2001).

3. **Cactaceae family:** Mexican territory is covered with lands with some degree of aridity in more than 50%, so, the evolution of flora is especially important because they have had to undergo various morphological, anatomical, and physiological modifications to overcome the lack of water in these environments. For people living in these environments, which is slightly more than 41 million people (Abd El-Ghani et al., 2017), producing their food through agriculture is not always possible, since the amounts of rainfall do not allow the development of conventional crops. For this reason, the use of wild species has represented a form of subsistence since prehispanic times. Among the species that offer products that are used by people settled in arid areas of Mexico are those belonging to the Cactaceae family, which is a botanical family of American origin. Cactaceae can adopt different forms of growth, including trees, shrubs, globose, creeping, and even climbing. The ancient Mexicans classified the cacti into two large groups: the *nochtlis* and the *comitls*. The former included all those species with articulated, discoid, and flattened stems (*Opuntia*, *Nopalea*, and *Epiphyllum* genera), while the latter included species with globose and some cylindrical stems (*Echinocactus*, *Ferocactus*, *Stenocereus*, *Cephalocereus*, *Lemaireocereus*, *Pachycereus* among others). "The cacti represent an important element in Mexico as seen in its coat of arms (Fig. 1.4). It is an eagle standing on a cactus prickly pear (nopal, current *Platyopuntia* genus) devouring a snake, regarded as a signal from the priests for the ancient Mexicans where they should build the capital of the Aztec Empire" (Abd El-Ghani et al., 2017).

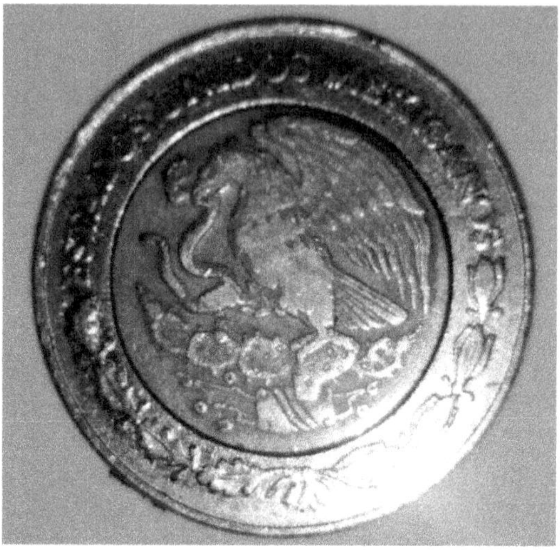

FIGURE 1.4 The Mexican coat of arms in a Mexican peso coin.
Source: Photo: Martín Huerta, self-elaboration.

Cactus prickly pear is a medicinal plant. Aztecs used its root with *Geranium* spp. (cranesbill) as a medicine to alleviate hernias and to soothe irritated livers. It has been used for more than 2500 years as basic food in ancient Mesoamerica, including Mexico. It spread from Mexico to other parts of South America and other continents. Many studies in rats as well as in humans have demonstrated many pharmacological properties, such as analgesic, anti-inflammatory, antiviral, hypoglycemic, and hypocholesterolemic effects of prickly pear pads or cladodes (Yarnell and Abascal, 2014), but most of the people in Mexico currently recognize the beneficial effect of nopal in the treatment of diabetes and weightloss.

Although there are many species of the genus *Platyopuntia*, there are few that are widely used as medicinal, that is the case of *Opuntia xoconostle*, a species with extremely acidic fruits that is used in the traditional cuisine of central Mexico, where they take advantage of the skin of the fruit to add it to the soup as one more vegetable (Fig. 1.5a). This is also used to prevent diabetes. Other species are consumed as sweet fruits (*Opuntia ficus-indica*) (Fig. 1.5b) and other varieties of *Opuntia* are used as vegetables to make salads (Fig. 1.5c, d).

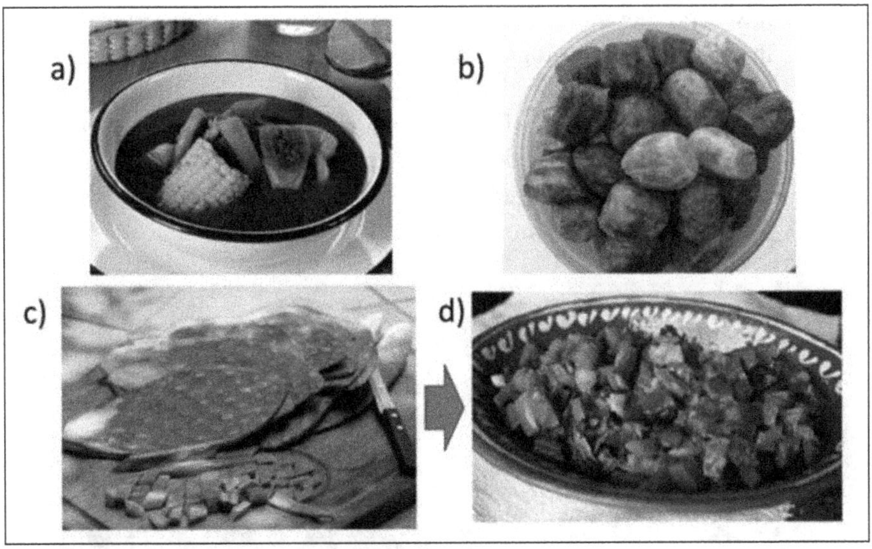

FIGURE 1.5 Different uses of prickly pear cactus.
Source: Photo: Martin Huerta.

Echinocactus platyacanthus a Mexican endemic distributed at several localities (Vargas-Luna et al., 2018) are nearly 2 m tall and 0.8 m in diameter. The thick and hard ribbed stems are light or dark green (Fig. 1.6), commonly known as "biznaga del dulce" in Mexico (Ramírez-Rodríguez et al., 2020). The same authors have reported its economical values as the stems and fruit are widely eaten by living beings. The useful part parenchyma of the stem is used as food, source of water, medicine, and commonly in the preparation of a traditional candy known as acitrón. In addition to being appreciated for its beauty, it has a relevant presence since prehispanic times because it was considered a protection amulet and was used to perform ceremonial rituals. With the arrival of the Spanish and the introduction of sugar cane to Mexico, the acitrón began to be elaborated. The root and pulp of *E. platyacanthus* are of medicinal value and are used in diabetes, period pain, headaches, chest pains, and inflammation due to impact. Very little data on *Echinocactus* species as well as its bioactive compounds is found in the literature (Ramírez-Rodríguez et al., 2020). There are many other species of cacti that produce fruits consumed by the rural population in different regions of Mexico;

however, they do not have a very wide use or consumption, because there is no technology that allows their commercialization to go beyond the places close to their natural distribution areas. They have a great value in their local use and just to mention some of them are the fruits of *Ferocactus* spp., *Escontria chiotilla*, *Myrtillocactus geometrizans*, *Hylocereus* spp., *Mammillaria* spp., *Stenocereus* spp., *Polaskia chichipe*, among others.

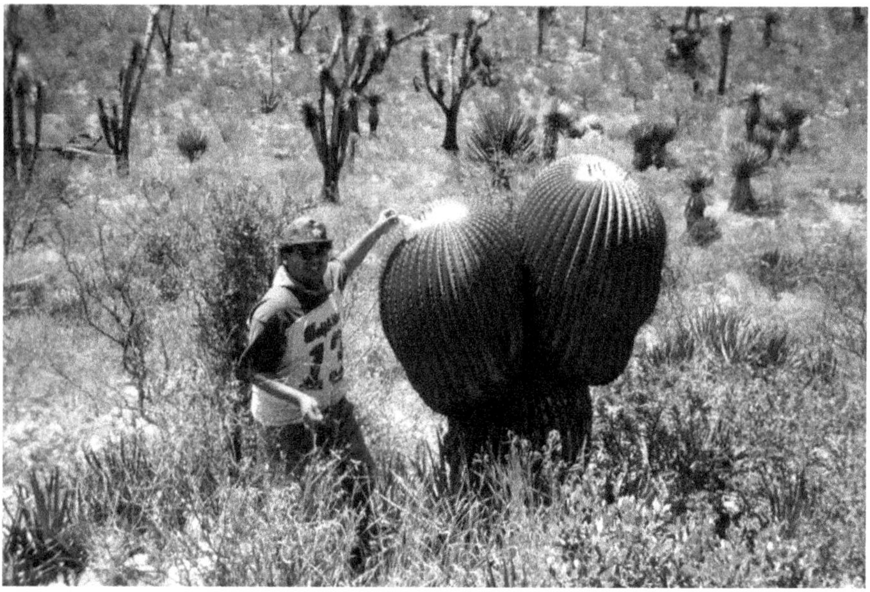

FIGURE 1.6 *Echinocactus platyacanthus* at San Luis Potosi, Mexico.

Source: Photo: Martin Huerta.

4. Mexican edible flowers: Mexico is one of the megadiverse countries in the world where the total known plant species are around 25,000 (1/10 of all plant species known in the world), and the endemic species numbers also are high in the total flora (1/2) (Velasco Lozano and Nagao, 2006). Edible flowers in Mexico are represented by 25 plant families and 50 genera (Mulík and Ozuna, 2020). The complex cosmovision of the Mexicans gives several meanings to xóchitl "flower" in Nahuatl. It was used to symbolize elegant and eloquent words in the poetry (Mulík and Ozuna, 2020). Before the Spanish colonization, the flowers were important among the Mesoamerican ethnic groups (Cáceres and Cruz, 2019); deity has been consecrated

with these, which was called Xochipilli, meaning "the prince of flowers." Following the colonization, important changes in the living took place compared with the pre-Columbian Mexico. It affected the indigenous gastronomy as well as in the use of edible flowers use. A complete replacement of all indigenous customs by Spanish customs, a kind of combination or syncretism was generated in many areas, including cooking, which was called miscegenation, and affected the culture and gastronomy until today in Mexico (Buchmann, 2016). Edible flowers possibly replaced meat during spring celebrations following the mix up of indigenous culture with Catholic customs of the Spanish colonizers. The edible flower consumption probably was related with poverty and low social status of indigenous people. For centuries, the Mexican edible flower cultivation has been a part of the cultivations by indigenous groups, being a marginal component of their agriculture even today (Manzanero-Medina et al., 2020). In 2010, traditional Mexican cuisine was recognized as Intangible Cultural Heritage by UNESCO for being a comprehensive cultural model including farming, ritual practices, ancestral skills, and culinary techniques (Mulík and Ozuna, 2020). A small sample of edible flowers is included in this because it seems impossible to make a complete list of whole country. Mulík and Ozuna (2020) have discussed this topic at length. In Mexico, *Cucurbita* spp. blossoms are known as "flor de calabaza" and in Nahuatl, the Aztec language as ayoxochquilitl or ayoxóchitl. It is eaten in many forms, but the most popular way is as soup or as a filling some other dishes such as "chiles rellenos" or "quesadillas."

The flowers of *Yucca* spp. are known as Desert candle (English Needle palm) or "flor de yuca" or "flor de izote" in Mexico. Mulík and Ozuna (2020) reported that salty water is prepared and flowers without stems and pistils are boiled in it to avoid bitterness, then water is changed during the cooking process many times by some people. The tomatoes, lime juice, and salt are mixed with it to serve as a nutritive salad. The cooked flowers are also used as a side dish to thick stew.

According to Mulík and Ozuna (2020), the Aztec marigold (*Tagetes erecta*) also called African marigold is endemic to Mexico; flowers have many ornamental uses all over the globe currently. In Mexico, every year on the first 2 days of November, the dead festivities take place where flowers are used. In Spanish, it is called "flor del cempoal" and "cempasúchil," related to its Nahuatl name cempoalxóchitl, meaning the flower of 20 petals. It is found in orange, gold, and yellow colors and has citrus-like and minty flavor. The sweet fresh petals of marigold are successfully used in salads and soups (Mulík and Ozuna, 2020).

In the Mesoamerican diet, nearly 1395 edible species have been reported by Castillo et al. (2020). This wide range of native gastronomic diversities includes insects up to 33%, 23% sea products, and 15% fungi. Only 6% of the total is mammals and birds. Nearly 906 edible species have been recorded from some provinces. These include nearly 62% of the known species as against the provinces of Coahuila, Chihuahua, Zacatecas, Durango, and San Luis Potosí, including just 10% of the food diversity (Fig. 1.7). These data are estimations lower than the great richness of edible species that exist in the country because many databases are not well justified, and the authors preferred to use only those that were solidly supported (Cerritos, 2021 personal communication).

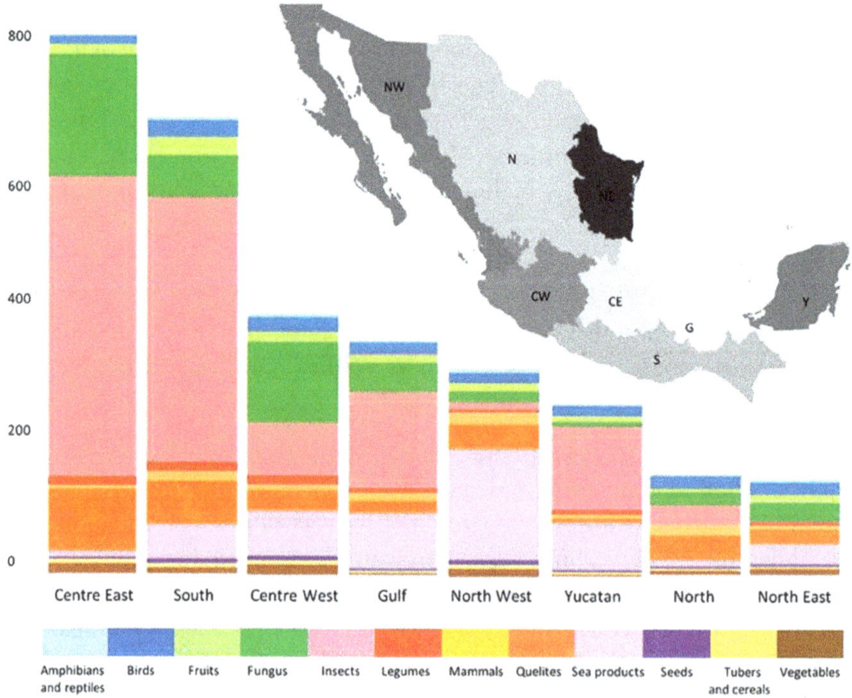

FIGURE 1.7 The number of edible species per category at Mexican ecoregions.

Source: Castillo et al. (2020) with permission.

For the case of northwestern North American indigenous people, Turner (2020) has reported that "carbohydrates have generally been in relatively short supply in the original diets, especially in the middle and northern regions. The inner bark, tree sap, greens, root vegetables, and berries are known for their sweet taste out of the 50 different plant foods from the region; some being and were appreciated as confections, others were used to sweeten foods as well as medicinal preparations. Among these are crystalline sugar from *Pseudotsuga menziesii* var. *glauca*); tree sap, pitch and/or inner bark from *Abies amabilis, Larix occidentalis, Pinus contorta, P. ponderosa, Acer macrophyllum, Alnus rubra, Betula papyrifera*, and *Populus balsamifera*; berries & fruits of *Amelanchier alnifolia, Fragaria chiloensis, F. vesca, F. virginiana, Gaultheria shallon, Gaultheria hispidula, Gaultheria ovatifolia*), *Maianthemum dilatatum, Maianthemum racemosum, Malus fusca, Prunus virginiana, Rubus ideaus, Rubus leucodermis, Rubus parviflorus, Rubus ursinus, Vaccinium membranceum, Vaccinium caespitosum*; greens from *Acer macrophyllum, Epilobium angustifolium, Opuntia fragilis, Fragaria vesca, F. virginiana*, shoots of *Rubus parviflorus* and *R. spectabilis*; Root vegetables (underground parts) *Allium acuminatum, A. cernuum, Asarum caudatum, Balsamorhiza sagittata, Camassia quamash, C. leichtlinii, Cirsium brevistylum, C. edule, C. undulatum* etc., *Erythronium grandiflorum, Lomatium dissectum, Osmorhiza berteroi* and *Osmorhiza* spp.; Flowers and nectar *Calochortus macrocarpus, Castilleja hispida, C. miniata, Comandra umbellata, Lonicera ciliosa, Menziesia ferruginea, Rosa nutkana, Rubus spectabilis* and *Trifolium pratense*). More detailed information on these is given in Turner (2020). The several original sweet foods are no longer widely consumed. These have been replaced by imported molasses, brown–white sugar, syrup, and honey, incorporated into Indigenous Peoples' food systems" with negative implications for health and well-being (Turner, 2020).

Traditional food systems in the world provide evidence about the relationship between diet and health, such as the importance of fiber in African diets, the antioxidants present in Asian diets, or omega-3 fatty acids in Mediterranean diets (Johns and Sthapit, 2004). Also, reliance on cereals, legumes, and fruits and vegetables of traditional food systems has lower energy and higher fiber content than the modern trend and might reduce the risk of disease (Johns and Eyzaguirre, 2006). Among the indigenous people, traditional eating habits originating from the cultural and biological richness are mostly getting lost. These people are changing their diets and turning toward the consumption of sugary soft drinks, instant soups, and highly processed foods (Castillo et al., 2020). In urban centers, of Mexico as well as in other countries, dietary patterns have changed dramatically in the last 4 decades, which has negatively impacted health, increasing their vulnerability to noncommunicable diseases (NCDs). "The dietary change is characterized by a decrease in the consumption of traditional foods, protectors of health, and the increase in the availability and consequently the consumption of highly processed foods with high energy density, high sodium content, saturated fats, sugars, colorings, preservatives, flavorings, and stabilizers; in turn, the consumption of products of animal origin has increased" (FAO, 2010). In Mexico, 29.8% of the total energy intake comes from the consumption of ultra-processed foods as per the nutrient use related to chronic NCDs (Marrón-Ponce et al., 2017). They have documented excessive intake of added sugar and saturated fat and lower consumption of dietary fiber (López-Olmedo et al., 2016), and high energy-density diets (Aburto et al., 2015) in the population. Mexico occupies first place in the sale of processed food among Latin American countries, and the fourth worldwide according to data from 2013 (FAO, 2019). Mexico has declared that the main challenges of taking processed food are the high rates of obesity. An estimated 57% of the Mexican population is overweight or obese (in 2016), with adults being the most affected with 73%. In urban areas, 35% of the children of school-going age are overweight or obese, and in rural areas it is 29%. Furthermore, 13.6% of Mexico's children under five suffer from chronic undernutrition, and in rural areas it is 21% (FAO, 2019). As per the highest number of diabetic population census, Mexico is number 5 in the world, with 12 million people between the ages of 20 and 79 years being diabetic. This number follows Brazil, USA, India, and China (Escalante-Araiza and Gutiérrez-Salmeán, 2020). This chaotic scene in which the high incidence of comorbidities is reflected explains why Mexico is the second place in the number of deaths from Coronavirus (SARS-CoV-2 or COVID-19) in Latin America, only after Peru (Fig. 1.8), and in the fourth place at the global level (Fig. 1.9). In Germany (Berlin), the role of visceral adiposity in the severity of COVID-19 has been discussed by Petersen et al. (2020). They have concluded that visceral adipose tissue and upper abdominal circumference specifically increase the likelihood of COVID-19 severity. This has been reinforced by Favre et al. (2021) who conducted their research in France (Paris and Nice). They mention that severe forms of COVID-19 in adults are associated with high visceral adiposity.

Moreno-Ulloa et al. (2018) carried out a study with an ethnic group from the northwest of Mexico called the Tarahumara, or Rarámuris (which in their language means foot runners). Their lifestyle include walking and running everyday in rural-dwellings as their physical capabilities allow running long distances that is nearly 100 miles/24 h with simple footwear "sandals" made by themselves with pieces of leather from some domestic animals is attracting global attention. The study refers to the metabolic syndrome among these people and the authors state that when Tarahumara Indians lifestyles change from rural to urban, the risk of prevalence of metabolic syndrome increases, being more in males than females.

A positive correlation has been reported between the sugar crop yields and obesity, overweight, and diabetes mortality rates in Mexico, Brazil, and Argentina following multiple correlation analysis (PCA) (Castillo et al., 2020). These are some among many other findings, which should be considered to initiate an important conversion in public policies related to health and nutrition in Mexico and other countries. The solution is that in culturally rich regions we must consume local diets together with reduction of organic waste or decrease in the consumption of unsustainable imported products (Tuomisto, 2019).

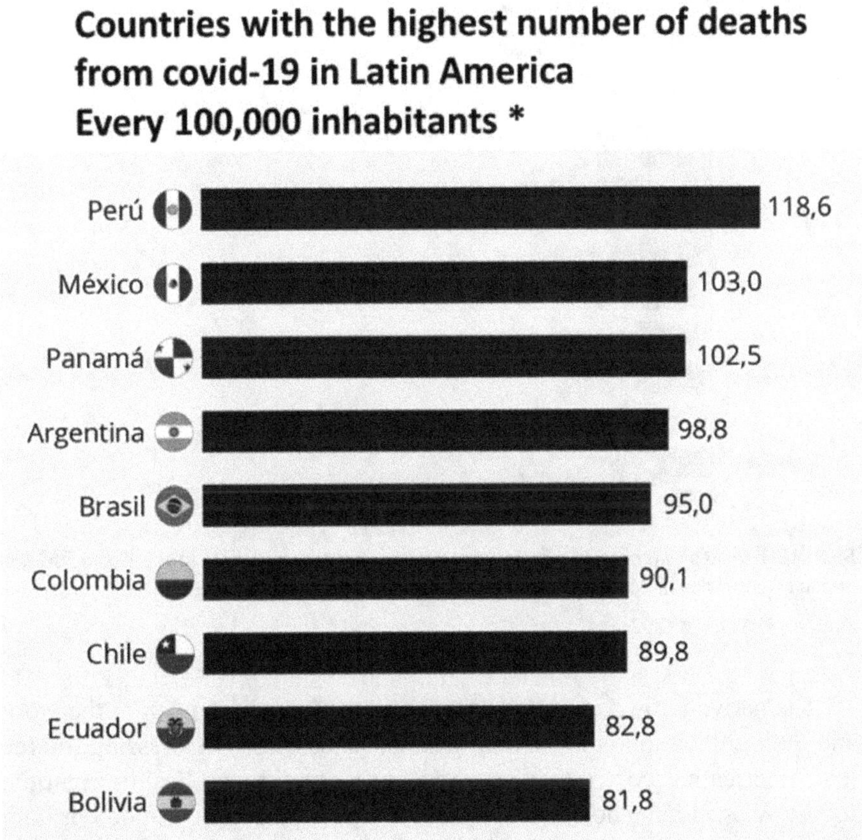

FIGURE 1.8 The most affected countries by SARS-CoV-2 (Coronavirus or COVID-19 pandemia) in Latin América.

Source: STATISTA (2021).

We find that nearly 15 crops are being consumed by humans in general during the last four decades (Harlan, 1975; Castillo et al., 2020). Almost 95% of the human nutrition is provided by only 30 plants (Myers, 1985; McNeely and Wachtel, 1988). The sugar cane, corn, wheat, rice, and potatoes are the top five crops; comprising major part of the human food (Vega et al., 2018). We must add other underutilized species to human diets, and production systems should be changed from intensive to extensive (Godfray et al., 2010; Ozturk et al., 2018; Castillo et al., 2020).

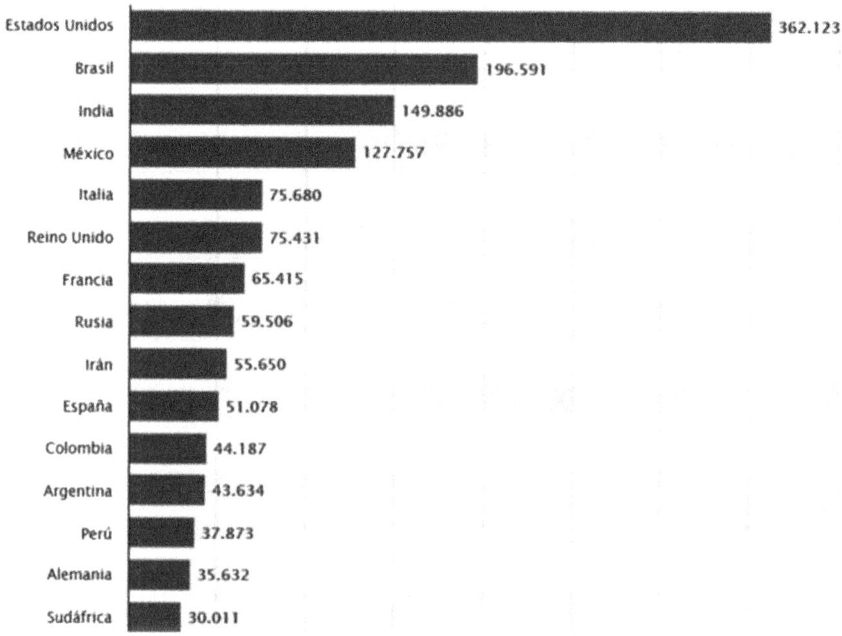

FIGURE 1.9 The number of people who died from the coronavirus in the first 15th more impacted countries in the world on January 5th, 2021.

Source: STATISTA (2021).

The native Latin American plant foods are spreading much in the world and their cultivation is more than in their lands of origin stressing the fact that America has contributed much to our globe through health-promoting foods. We still have no knowledge about many other native foods in Latin American countries. Some are hidden in the magnificent Andes mountain ranges together with Mexican forests, as well as in the rivers, lakes, and oceans surrounding the area (Masson-Salaue, 2019).

1.6 MEXICAN MEDICINAL KNOWLEDGE IN PREHISPANIC TIMES

Early Mexican indigenous people have left no written records of their knowledge (Casas et al., 2016a). The importance of plant resources in their life is traced by following archaeobotanical records (MacNeish, 1992). The pre-Columbian codices are accepted as the earliest records in Mexico which are scarce and were mostly burned. The wall impressions and other records belong to those of Olmeca and perfected by the Maya, Mixtec, and continued by Nahua people. All these serve as written records (Gutiérrez-Solana, 1992; Sahagún, 2006). Following the destruction ordered by the Catholic church, relatively few codices exist. During the conquest, many steles decorating the Mesoamerican temples have been destroyed or looted, therefore very little information has been left following all these catastrophes; not much has been left of the great botanical knowledge from regional Mexican cultures (Casas et al., 2016a). Only ethnographic documents from pre-Columbian Mexico are Spanish-translated version of friar Fray Bernardino de Sahagún from Náhuatl (the Aztec language) known as the Florentino Codex (Sahagún, 2006). These provide information from 15th and 16th centuries on the ways of living of Mexican indigenous people all cover the period just before the Spanish conquerors entered the area. There are some other chronicles of the conquest which write about the botanical gardens and zoos in Mexico Tenochtitlan and other cities (Sahagún, 2006; Díaz del Castillo, 2004). There were no living collections of plants and animals in that period in Europe. Other data comes from the work translated into Latin by Juan Badiano from De la Cruz and Badiano Codex, written by the Náhuatl physician Martín de la Cruz (De la Cruz, 1964). *Libellus de medicinalibus indorum herbis* is the original title of De la Cruz-Badiano Codex that discusses about 230 plants used as remedies as well as minerals and animals. The natural history of the New Spain (Historia natural de la Nueva España) written by Francisco Hernández de Toledo is another important document of this period. In 1571–1576, King Phillip's protophysician "Hernández de Toledo" has participated in an expedition and he compiled a monumental work. This title mentions about the medicinal uses and other facts practiced by indigenous people. It mentions about over 3000 plants together with 500 animals with references. Náhuatl medicine and information on the natural and cultural history of Mexico is the most important compendium by Francisco Hernández work (Hernández, 1959). In the 17th century, the original manuscript and much of the unique information it contained were lost because of the fire in the library of Escorial castle (Casas et al., 2016a).

The Spanish expedition led by Cristopher Columbus to America on October 12, 1492, saw the beginning of the conquest of America, whose first campaign was the one that the Spanish started in Cuba, by Velázquez; later, the two most important ones followed one is that of the Aztec Empire by Hernan Cortés and the other is that of the Inca Empire (by Francisco Pizarro). From there, began the "colonization of America," in which the Portuguese, English, Dutch, and French also intervened.

The new political and religious orders established by the Spanish from the 16th century destroyed much of the cultural and medical organization of the indigenous population of Mesoamerica and with it the information on the use of medicinal plants that had been accumulated for centuries was lost. Only the oral transmission of some practical aspects lasted after the complex theoretical body of indigenous medicine was fragmented. Historical research on the use of healing plants in prehispanic times is based, above all, on the study of the works that were written in Mexico toward the end of the 16th century and part of the 17th, the most important of which were disseminated in the 20th century. Other sources of documentation have different purposes and depth; some are part of the natural history that various European authors were interested in writing about the New World, who included a chapter on the American medicinal flora in their books. Still others, as a chronicle or stories, describe the customs of the conquered people, and when writing about the medicine of the aborigines, they incorporate concise data on medicinal herbalism. There are also medical books written by the Europeans settled in America, which include the description and use of medicinal plants of the indigenous people in the places where fate or curiosity led them to live (Lozoya, 1990).

In Mexico, there are 68 indigenous languages that are recognized to be spoken in different regions, for example, the Mayan language is spoken in the southern portion of the country (Yucatán, Quintana Roo, and Campeche), Otomí in the central portion (Querétaro, Hidalgo, Guanajuato, Mexico City, Tlaxcala, and the State of Mexico), but it is Nahua or Nahuatl that is most widely spread in Mexico, with 1,586,884 registered speakers until 2010. Nahuatl is spoken in 15 of the 31 states of the Mexican Republic and also has 30 variants with their respective self-denominations (INPI, 2020), this is the reason why the best-known records on traditional use of plants and animals are written in Nahuatl and denote a deep knowledge of plants, animals and their properties. The original Mexicans developed a nomenclature system to classify their plants, which was almost always formed by a single word composed of several phonemes united in a single word. The most frequent was the use of two phonemes forming a classification system like the current binomial classification system that uses genus and species of a plant developed very later by Western science. As is often the case in Nahuatl, the terms appear united in a single word where the ending *patli* (medicine) was the sound that was used in general to name the plant resources that the Mexica used in the treatment of diseases. In this way, plants of various genera were classified as medicinal, adding to their name the ending *patli*. For example, *tolpatli* is a medicinal plant of the *tollin* group, that is, the "tules," or reeds and it would mean "medicinal tule," *cuecuetzpatli* (*cuecuetzo*: which causes itching and would be called "medicine for itching"), it was the name given to another plant for its properties of irritating to the skin. The ending *patli* would correspond exactly to the Latin term *officinalis* (medicinal) of the scientific nomenclature that is currently used.

The De la Cruz-Badiano Codex "*Libellus de Medicinalibus Indorum herbis*" or "Little Book on indigenous medicinal herbs," from 1552 is the first catalog of Nahuatl indigenous medicine; it contains a mixture of pictographic–glyphic and alphabetic elements from prehispanic and colonial Mexico. There is currently a 1964 reprint made by the Instituto Mexicano del Seguro Social (the official institution responsible for health at the national level in Mexico). This is a compilation of remedies used by indigenous Mexicans with the help of plants. The son of the first governor of New Spain "Francisco de Mendoza" has commissioned the preparation to the Nahua doctor Martín de la Cruz. He collaborated with the College of Santa Cruz Tlatelolco during those days. Xochimilca Juan Badiano from the indigenous group translated the manuscript from Nahuatl into Latin, which was sent by Francisco de Mendoza to Spain in 1552 as a gift to King Felipe II after the completion of document. In 1902, it was incorporated into the collection of the Vatican Library. Following the restoration of diplomatic relations with Vatican, Pope John Paul II returned it to Mexico in 1991 and is currently in the National Library of Anthropology (Fig. 1.10). It is believed that the work was intended to communicate the wealth of medicinal remedies of the indigenous people in such a way that a European expert could understand it. From that place, a confluence of ideas was fostered in which indigenous knowledge should be translated and guided by the standards of the health and disease system of Galenic-Hippocratic Medicine recognized and practiced in the old world. In addition to the Martín de la Cruz and Juan Badiano, at least two *tlahcuilohqueh* (singular, *tlacuilo*; painter or illustrator) from Tlatelolco participated in the elaboration of the manuscript (Pardo-Tomás, 2013).

On each page, the remedy or prescription for a disease is presented, accompanied by the illustration/representation placed in the upper half of the sheet belonging to one or more plants used for the treatment. More detailed analyzes highlight the similarities and differences in the therapeutic use of water, salt, and organic substances described in *Libellus de Medicinalibus Indorum herbis*'s work concerning the European materia medica of the time (Hernández-Ramírez, 2020).

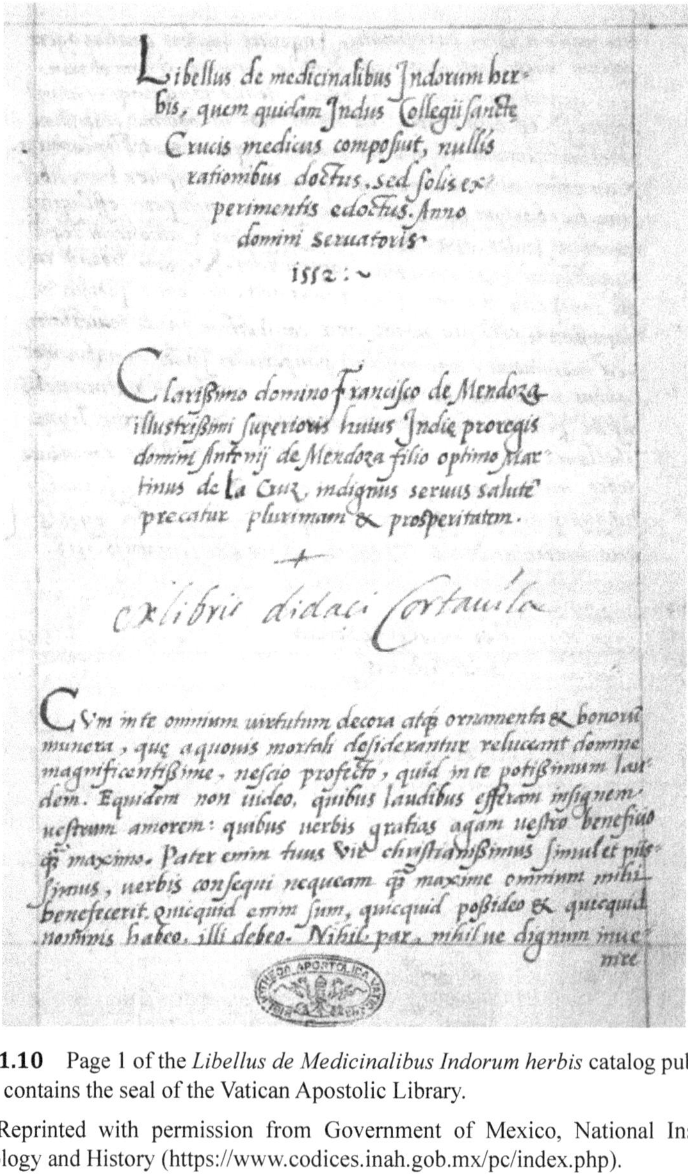

Libellus de medicinalibus Indorum herbis, quem quidam Indus Collegii sancte Crucis medicus composuit, nullis rationibus doctus, sed solis experimentis edoctus. Anno domini seruatoris 1552.

Clarissimo domino Francisco de Mendoza illustrissimi superioris huius Indie proregis domini Antonij de Mendoza filio optimo Martinus de la Cruz, indignus seruus salute precatur plurimam & prosperitatem.

ex libris didaci Cortavila

Cum in te omnium uirtutum decora atque ornamenta & bonorum munera, que a quouis mortali desiderantur, reluceant domine magnificentissime, nescio profecto, quid in te potissimum laudem. Equidem non uideo, quibus laudibus efferam insignem uestrum amorem: quibus uerbis gratias agam uestro beneficio quam maximo. Pater enim tuus Vir christianissimus simul et piissimus, uerbis consequi nequeam quam maxime omnium mihi benefecerit. Quicquid enim sum, quicquid possideo & quicquid nominis habeo, illi debeo. Nihil par, nihil ne dignum inuenire

FIGURE 1.10 Page 1 of the *Libellus de Medicinalibus Indorum herbis* catalog published in 1552 and contains the seal of the Vatican Apostolic Library.

Source: Reprinted with permission from Government of Mexico, National Institute of Anthropology and History (https://www.codices.inah.gob.mx/pc/index.php).

The therapeutic uses of various parts of body of about 80 animals are mentioned in the "*Libellus de Medicinalibus Indorum herbis*"; these include feathers, hair, nails, and horns; soft organs such as brain, liver, heart, blood, and other fluids formed inside the animal or located in the bone tissue of the animal (Aranda et al., 2003). The use of 251 medicinal plants and the iconographic contribution associated with the presence of 185 plant images is also highlighted, which are represented in detail, independently, and with a sense of dimension through shading (Valverde, 1984). The representation of plants includes details of their flowers, leaves, stems, and roots that resemble the criteria used in Europe to represent the herbs of the time (Valverde, 1984; Llach, 2011).

The first catalog related to the local flora and fauna too is *Libellus de Medicinalibus Indorum herbis*, with the traditional medical and pharmaceutical sciences of the time. In other words, it highlights species of therapeutic value that were recognized by the indigenous groups of Mexico, at the same time, it shows the confluence of two worlds: one in dominance and the other in resistance.

The disadvantage of the Nahua system is that they often used the same name to identify several plants that are botanically not always related. However, it must be recognized that indigenous botany reached a high degree of systematization in ancient times. The Mexica doctors (called *titici*) developed the classification of plants following criteria different from those that the current biologists require and use, but in some cases, the selection of vegetables made by the ancient Mexicans was so precise that centuries later, botanical science could include them in its modern classification and many of the plants in the same way that the indigenous culture had done. Such is the case of tomatoes (*tomatl*), for example, whose inclusion in the modern classification has been complete, or magueys (*metl*), which were also recognized as a well-differentiated specific group. The Nahuas named the agaves or magueys with surprising precision: *mexcalmetl* (*A. americana*), *centemetl* (*Agave potatorum*), *teometl* (*Agave atrovirens*), etc. (Lozoya, 1990).

The Mexica (the original group of the Aztec culture) divided the plants in different ways, among them, emphasizing the form of growth, thus, we can find that they referred to woody plants (*quahuitl*), shrubs (*quaquauhtzin*), and herbs (*xihuitl*), but there were also other ways to group them, for example, edible vegetables (*quilitl*), ornamental or sought for their flowers (*xochitl*) and the already mentioned medicinal ones (*patli*). More examples of the high degree of knowledge and development that Mexica botany had can be seen in Table 1.1.

TABLE 1.1 An Example of a Botanical Group Used in the Mexican Society Which Shows the Degree of Knowledge of the Pre-Hispanic Culture About Plants.

Group or Nahuatl family: ***tzapotl***, Meaning: **Sweet fruit**. Spanish name: **zapote**			
Nahuatl name	**Meaning**	**Properties or uses**	**current knowledge**
cochitzapotl	The sapote that produces sleep	It was used to make people sleep	*Casimiroa edulis* (Rutaceae) in addition to being sedative, today it is known that its fruits, seeds, and leaves contain substances that lower blood pressure
tliltzapotl	The black sapote	It was considered a laxative	*Diospyros ebenaster* (Ebenaceae) is an edible fruit, but if consumed in large quantities it can work as a powerful laxative
tezontzapotl	The sapote like tezontle stone	it was used to dye hair	Mammea americana (Caryophyllaceae) is an edible fruit, now it is also used for baldness
coztictzapotl	The yellow sapote	This name is referred to the color of the fruit, but traditional medicine has included the treatment of scalp infections, diarrhea, and eye and digestive problems	*Pouteria campechiana* (Sapotaceae) "canistel." The fruit is used in milkshakes, ice creams, or for making jellies, ice cream, jams, juices, various sweets, and pastries; the seed can be finely boiled roasted and mixed with cocoa to make a dark chocolate and in southern Mexico, the powdered seed is mixed with corn toasted, or cornmeal, sugar and cinnamon and prepared as a nutritious drink called "pozol"
xicotzapotl	The bumblebee sapote	It was used for chewing gum elaboration to freshen the breath	*Manilkara zapota* (Sapotaceae) It is used to make poultices against inflammation of the liver. Nowadays it continues the chewing gum elaboration.

1.7 A CASE STUDY IN AN ARID REGION OF MEXICO

1.7.1 WILD FLORA AND FAUNA USES AT EL HUIZACHE, SAN LUIS POTOSÍ, MEXICO

Hunting and gathering of wild species of flora and fauna have been an important subsistence form for inhabitants from semiarid lands of central Mexico since prehispanic times. In these habitats, the mean annual precipitation ranges between 400 and 600 mm, and the temperature ranging from 18 to 22°C (Huerta-Martínez et al., 2020). Water scarcity limits the development of traditional agriculture. The survival of these people has been possible because they have generated a broad knowledge of natural resources they possess and their uses, what is called in modern times as "traditional science." El Huizache region is one of the 155 priority regions for conservation in Mexico. It has a significant number of endemic species and is considered a center of origin and diversification of cacti. The area is characterized by four vegetation types, which are influenced by factors of the landscape (depth of the soil, geological substrate, slope of the slopes, exposure, and stony), of the soil (potassium, pH, calcium, and matter organic), and climatic factors, especially the temperature regime in the cold season of the year (Huerta-Martínez et al., 2020).

The use of flora in El Huizache is diverse, however, only nine categories of use are considered here: food, medicinal, drink, fiber, construction, living fences, forage, ornamental, and various. The cactus family contains the highest number of species with use (17), 10 of them are in some risk category (NOM-ECOL-059-2010), then there is the Agavaceae family (7), the families with the lowest number of species used were Anacardiaceae, Cucurbitaceae, Fouquieriaceae, Krameriaceae, and Loasaceae (1) (Table 1.2). Many species are used as food, either part of the plant or the whole plant, fruits, roots, leaves, or seeds. The flowers of *Yucca carnerosana* and *Y. filifera* are cooked like vegetables. The flower buds of *Hamatocactus crassihamatus*, *Ferocactus pilosus* are eaten as snacks. The fruits of *Echinocereus cinerascens*, *Lemaireocereus* sp., several species of *Mammillaria,* and *M. geometrizans*, are eaten fresh. *E. platyacanthus* is used for the elaboration of biznaga candy, *Lippia graveolens* is used as a condiment in meals, and the young individuals of *Hamatocactus* are used as a source of water. Young cladodes of various species of *Opuntia* are eaten as vegetables. The leaves and young shoots of *Buddleia scordioides* cooked are used as a supplement of children's diet (Table 1.2).

TABLE 1.2 Plant Species, Conservation Status According to the NOM-ECOL-059-2010 and Uses in El Huizache, San Luis Potosí, México.

Family	Scientific name	Status	Uses*
Agavaceae	*Agave asperrima* Jacobi		FP
	Agave lecheguilla Torr.		FP, O
	Agave scabra Salm-Dyck		F, Me, BE, C
	Agave striata Zucc.		FP, C, Or
	Dasylirion acrotriche (Sch.)Zucc.		BE, FP, Or, C, O
	Yucca carnerosana Trel.		F, FP, C, LF, O
	Y. filifera Chab.		F, FP, C, LF, O
Anacardiaceae	*Schinus molle* L.		Me
Bromeliaceae	*Hechtia glomerata* Zucc.		Fo
Cactaceae	*Ariocarpus trigonus* K. Schum.	*Threatened*	Me, Or
	Astrophytum myriostigma Lem.	*Threatened*	Or
	Echinocereus cinerascens (DC) Lemaire,		F, Me,
	Echinocactus platyacanthus Link & Otto	*Under special protection*	F, Fo, Or
	Echinocereus pectinatus (Scheid.) Engel.		Or
	Ferocactus pilosus (Galeotti ex Salm-Dyck) Werderm.	*Threatened*	F, Or
	Hamatocactus crassihamatus (Weber) Buxbaum	*Threatened*	F, Or
	Lemaireocereus sp.		F, LF
	Lophophora williamsii (Lemaire) Coulter	*Under special protection*	Me
	Mammillaria candida. Scheid.	*Threatened*	F, Or
	Mammillaria spp.		F, Or
	Myrtillocactus geometrizans (Bravo) Backeb.		F
	Neolloydia conoidea Britt. & Rose		Or
	Opuntia imbricata DC		LF, O

TABLE 1.2 *(Continued)*

Family	Scientific name	Status	Uses*
	Opuntia leptocaulis DC		Me, LF
	Stenocereus stellatus Riccob.		LF,
	Thelocactus hexaedrophorus (Lem.) Britt. & Rose	*Threatened*	Or
Compositae	*Artemisia confertifolia* DC,		Me
	Baccharis salicifolia Pers.		O
	Chrysactinia mexicana Gray,		Me, F
Cucurbitaceae	*Cucurbita foetidissima* H.B.K.		O
Euphorbiaceae	*Euphorbia antisyphilitica* Miranda		O
	Jatropha dioica Sessé ex. Cerv.		Me
Fouquieriaceae	*Fouquieria splendens* Engelm.		LF, Or
Krameriaceae	*Krameria lanceolata* Torr.,		Me
Labiatae	*Lippia graveolens* Kunth.		F
	Poliomintha longiflora Gray		Me
Leguminosae	*Acacia farnesiana* (L.) Willd.		O
	Dalea bicolor Humb. & Bonpl. in Willd.		Fo
	Mimosa biuncifera Benth.		O
	Prosopis spp.		C, Fo, O
Loasaceae	*Mentzelia hispida* Willd.		Me
Loganiaceae	*Buddleia scordioides* HBK		F
Zygophyllaceae	*Larrea tridentata* (DC) Coville		Me, LF, O

Note:* **F=Foods; **Me**=Medicinal; **BE**=Beverage; **FP**=Fiber; **C**=Construction; **LF**=Living fences; **Fo**=Forage; **Or**= Ornamental; **O**=Others.

1.7.1.1 MEDICINAL

Table 1.3 shows the species more commonly used as medicinal, the portions utilized, the uses, and the illness cured. They are *Agave salmiana ssp. crassispina*, *Ariocarpus trigonus*, *Artemisia confertifolia*, *Chrysactinia mexicana*, *Echinocereus cinerascens*, *Jatropha dioica*, *Krameria lanceolata*, *Larrea tridentata*, *Lophophora williamsii*, *Schinus molle*, *Mentzelia hispida*, *Opuntia leptocaulis*, *Poliomintha longiflora*.

1.7.1.2 BEVERAGE

One of the most utilized plant species in the elaboration of beverage is *Agave salmiana ssp. crassispina*, this species produces a beverage from its sap called "aguamiel" (when is consumed in fresh) or "pulque" (when is fermented). *Dasylirion* spp. is used the elaboration of the beverage called "sotol" in the same way as the elaboration of "mescal," which was elaborated with *Agave scabra* Salm-Dyck.

1.7.1.3 FIBER

The production of fiber from plants is a well-documented activity in the region; some of the species used for this purpose are *Agave lecheguilla*, *A. striata*, *A. asperrima*, *Yucca filifera*, *Y. carnerosana*, and *Dasylirion* spp. This use is frequent, but nowadays it is not at the industrial scale due to the substitution of natural fibers for synthetic ones.

1.7.1.4 CONSTRUCTION

The stems of many plant species, mainly shrubs or trees are used for construction, some of them are *Prosopis* spp., *Yucca filifera*, *Y. carnerosana*, the flowering stalks of *Agave salmiana* ssp. *crassispina*, *A. striata*, *Dasylirion acrotrichum* are used as beams.

1.7.1.5 LIVING FENCES

The main species used as hedges in the region are *Fouquieria splendens*, *Stenocereus stellatus*, *Yucca carnerosana*, *Y. filifera*, *Opuntia leptocaulis*, *Opuntia imbricata* and sometimes, *Larrea tridentata*.

1.7.1.6 FORAGE

Climate and soil are the two main limiting factors in the region. The production of forage is scarce and for this reason, the inhabitants feed the domestic livestock with wild plant species such as leaves of *Agave salmiana* ssp. *crassispina*, *Agave scabra* ssp. *potosinensis*, *Hechtia glomerata*, *Dalea bicolor*, and stems with singeing spines of *Opuntia* spp., *E. platyacanthus*, and *Prosopis* spp.

TABLE 1.3 Main Medicinal Plants Used at El Huizache, San Luis Potosi, Mexico.

Species	Part of the plant used	Disease used for
Agave salmiana ssp. crassispina Trel.	Leaves (a thin layer)	Stop bleeding
Ariocarpus trigonus	The juice of the plant	Muscular pain
Artemisia confertifolia DC	Leaves in infusion	Kidney pain
Chrysactinia mexicana Gray	Leaves in brew	Stomach pain
Echinocereus cinerascens (DC) Lemaire	Stem boiled	Fracture strengthen
Jatropha dioica Sessé ex. Cerv.	Root stem boiled	Gum Strengthening Hair, Baldness prevention
Krameria lanceolata Torr.	Root boiled	Blood thickness
Larrea tridentata (DC) Coville	Thin branches and leaves in an infusion	Stomach pain and rheumatism
Lophophora williamsii (Lemaire) Coulter	Stem in alcohol	Bone joints pain
Schinus molle L.	Leaves in infusion	Nausea
Mentzelia hispida Willd.	Root, branches, and leaves	Stomach infections
Opuntia leptocaulis DC	Fruits, roasted	Toothache
Poliomintha longiflora Gray	Leaves and young branches in infusion	Cough

1.7.1.7 ORNAMENTALS

The sale of plants as ornamentals is one of the ways the inhabitants of these regions have for getting some income. The Cactaceae family is the best represented, although some species have some conservation status. The species belonging to this family are collected, especially the big ones, since they are more attractive. Within this group are certain species of *Yucca*, several species of cactus, *Dasylirion* spp. and *Fouquieria splendens*; the prices of some species in United States dollars (USD) ranges from $0.07 to 0.15 for small cactus; $1.0–3.50 for *Fouquieria splendens* individuals; 2.0–3.50 USD for *Dasylirion* specimens; $1.0–1.50 USD for *Agave lecheguilla* individuals; *Euphorbia antisyphilitica* USD 1.00, Cholla cactus USD 1.00 and *Selaginella* sp. USD 45.00 per thousand.

In the study area, the most preferred species are *Astrophytum myriostigma, Thelocactus hexaedrophorus, E. platyacanthus, Echinocereus pectinatus, Neolloydia conoidea, Ferocactus pilosus*, and *Mammillaria candida*. The individuals of *Ferocactus pilosus*, and *E. platyacanthus* are selected between 8 and 20 cm in diameter. According to the inhabitants of the region, not long ago, all the hills around the town Charco Blanco had a very shiny red tonality, caused by the predominance of *Ferocactus pilosus* (Fig. 1.11). Nowadays, this species is not as abundant as before, and the hills do not have the same appearance. Three more species (not cacti) frequently preferred for this use are *Agave striata* Zucc., *Fouquieria splendens*, and *Dasylirion acrotrichum*.

1.7.1.8 OTHER USES

There is an important number of species that are considered because some of them have only one or two uses, nevertheless, important among them are: *Euphorbia antisyphilitica* Miranda is used to obtain wax; the branches of many species as *Prosopis* spp., *Acacia farnesiana* (L.) Willd., *Mimosa biuncifera* Benth. and *Larrea tridentata* and the stems of *Yucca carnerosana, Y. filifera*, and *Dasylirion acrotrichum* are used as fuel, the branches of *Baccharis salicifolia* are used to elaborate brooms and roofs construction. *Agave lecheguilla* and *Cucurbita foetidissima* are used as a soap substitute (Table 1.2).

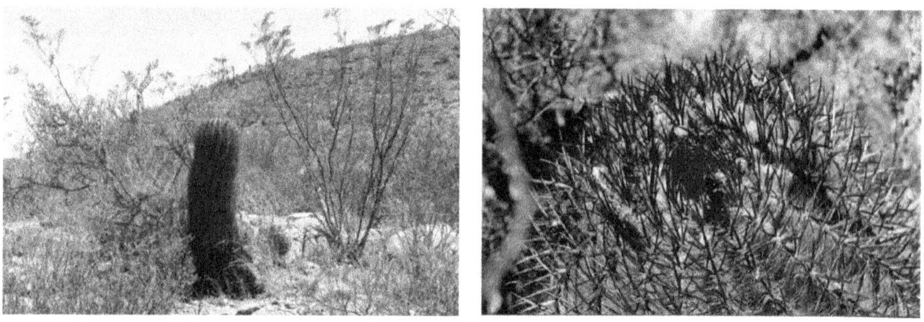

FIGURE 1.11 *Ferocactus pilosus* at El Huizache, San Luis Potosi, Mexico. Look at its red thorns.

Source: Photo: Martin Huerta.

1.7.2 FAUNA

Three main uses of fauna species were detected at El Huizache: food, medicinal, and pets (Table 1.4). The number of species considered in this chapter is not exhaustive, since some of them are difficult to obtain reliable information; however, it is a good sample of the species richness. The species in this section correspond to the information obtained from interviews with local people from Charco Cercado, Charco Blanco, and Guadalcanal towns.

1.7.2.1 FOOD

This use is probably the most important for the inhabitants of the study area because the species included representing a great part of the food resources, and their consumption is the result of their cultural inheritance. The consumed birds are represented by *Callipepla squamata* Vigors, 1830, *Colinus virginianus* Linnaeus, 1758, *Columbina inca* Lesson, 1847, *C. passerina Linnaeus* 1758, *Sturnella magna* Linnaeus, 1758, *S. neglecta* Audubon, 1844, and *Zenaida macroura* Linnaeus, 1758. Some of the most frequent mammals are *Lepus californicus* Gray 1837, *L. callotis* Wagler 1830, *Neotoma albigula* Hartley 1894, *Sylvilagus audubonii* Baird 1858, *S. floridanus* J. A. Allen 1890, *Odocoileus virginianus* Zimmerman 1780, and *Pecari tajacu* Linnaeus 1758. The reptiles are represented mainly by *Crotalus scutulatus* Cope 1883.

1.7.2.2 MEDICINAL

The richness of species used in medicine is not only important as food, but they are also the result of cultural inheritance. The inhabitants catch these species only when are needed, but in some cases, we found that in some stands located beside the highway, they are offered to the public, particularly species belonging to the genus *Crotalus*. The species most frequently used are *C. atrox* Baird & Girard 1853, *C. lepidus* Cope 1883, *C. molossus* Baird & Girard 1853, and *C. scutulatus*. Sometimes the inhabitants use the dry flesh, ground flesh, and the oil obtained from them as the cure for blood and bone diseases like leukemia, anemia, and arthritis (Fig. 1.12). *Phrynosoma modestum* Girard 1852 is another of the reptiles with medicinal use. The mammals registered were *Didelphis virginiana* Kerr 1792, *Dasypus novemcinctus* Linnaeus 1758, and *Taxidea taxus* Schreber 1778. The people named *Geococcyx californianus* Lesson, 1829 within the birds, but I never saw it at the cages (Table 1.4).

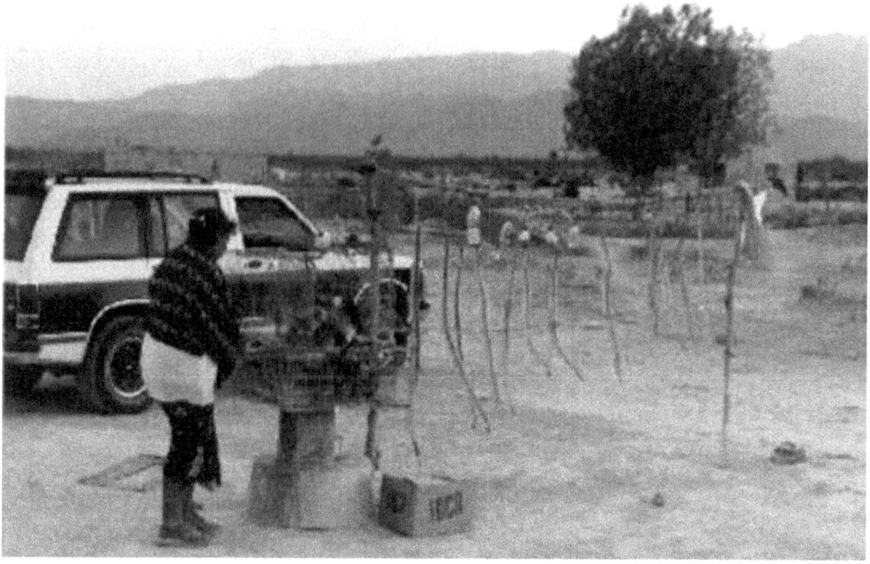

FIGURE 1.12 *Crotalus* spp. individuals sold in the stands beside the highway San Luis Potosi-Matehuala.

Source: Photo: Martin Huerta.

1.7.2.3 PETS

This group of species is very large, and many kinds of animals are captured for this purpose. Birds are the most used and include caged birds and noncaged birds. The first group is composed of small species that decorate the houses with their singing or eye-catching plumages. The main species are: *Aphelocoma ultramarina* Bonaparte, 1825, *Bombycilla cedrorum* Vieillot, 1808, *Cardinalis cardinalis* Linnaeus, 1758, *C. sinuatus* Bonaparte, 1838, *Carduelis psaltria* Say, 1823, *Carpodacus mexicanus* Müller, 1776, *Guiraca caerulea* Linnaeus, 1758, *Icterus galbula* Linnaeus, 1758, *Melanerpes auriphrons* Wagler, 1829, *Mimus polyglottos* Linnaeus, 1758, *Phainopepla nitens* Swainson, 1837, *Pheucticus melanocephalus* Swainson, 1827, *Pipilo fuscus* Swainson, 1827, *Piranga rubra* Linnaeus, 1758, *Ptilogonys cinereus* Swainson, 1824, *Serinus canaria,* Linnaeus, 1758, *Toxostoma corvirostre* Swainson, 1827, *Turdus migratorius* Linnaeus, 1766, *Tyrannus vociferans* Swainson, 1826, and *Zenaida asiatica* Linnaeus, 1758. The second group is represented by raptors like *Bubo virginianus* Gmelin, 1788, *Buteo jamaicensis* Gmelin, 1788, *Glaucidium gnoma* Wagler, 1832 (Fig. 1.13a, b, c respectively), *Falco mexicanus* Schlegel, 1851, *F. sparverius* Linnaeus,

1758, *Otus trichopsis* Wagler, 1832, *Parabuteo incinctus* Temminck, 1824 and *Polyborus plancus* Miller, 1777, in many cases are captured the young individuals together with the parents (Fig. 1.14).

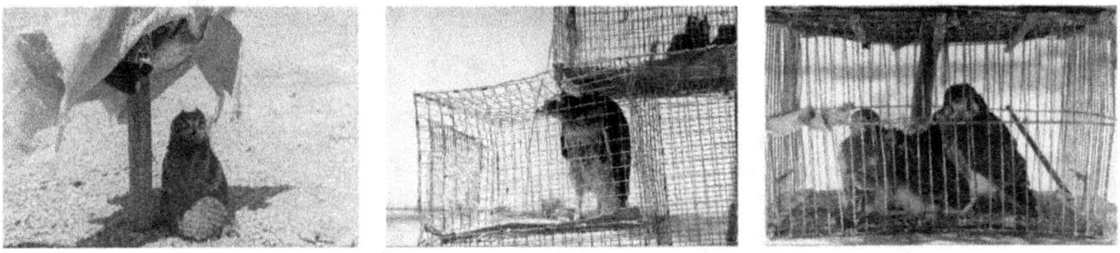

(a) (b) (c)

FIGURE 1.13 Some raptors caught and sold as pets (**a**) *Bubo virginianus*, (**b**) *Buteo jamaicensis*, (**c**) *Glaucidium gnoma.*

Source: Photo: Martin Huerta.

The mammals used as pets are *Bassariscus astutus* Lichtenstein 1830, *Mustela frenata* Lichtenstein 1831, young individuals of *Canis latrans* Say, 1823, *Procyon lotor* Linnaeus, 1758, *Lynx rufus* Schreber, 1777, *Taxidea taxus* Schreber, 1778, and *Spermophilus spilosoma* Bennett, 1833, *Urocyon cinereoargenteus* Schreber, 1775 (Fig. 1.15).

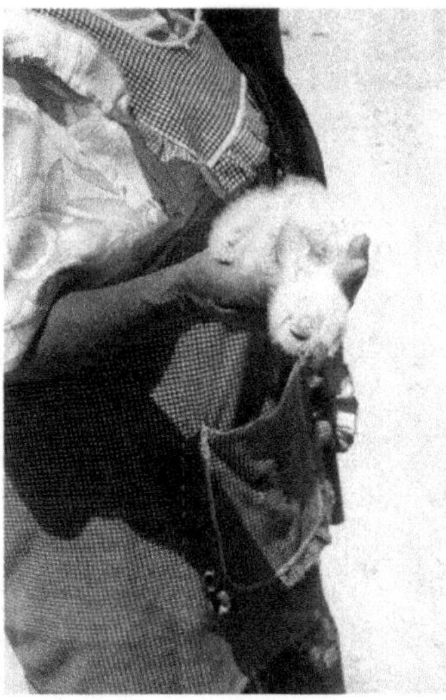

FIGURE 1.14 *Buteo jamaicensis'* brood caught for selling as pets.

Source: Photo: Martin Huerta.

1.7.2.4 OTHER USES

We found that the taxidermy is a frequent activity, particularly of *Canis latrans*, *Urocyon cinereoargenteus*, and *Lynx rufus*, between mammals, and seven species belonging to the genus *Crotalus* between the reptiles (Table 1.4).

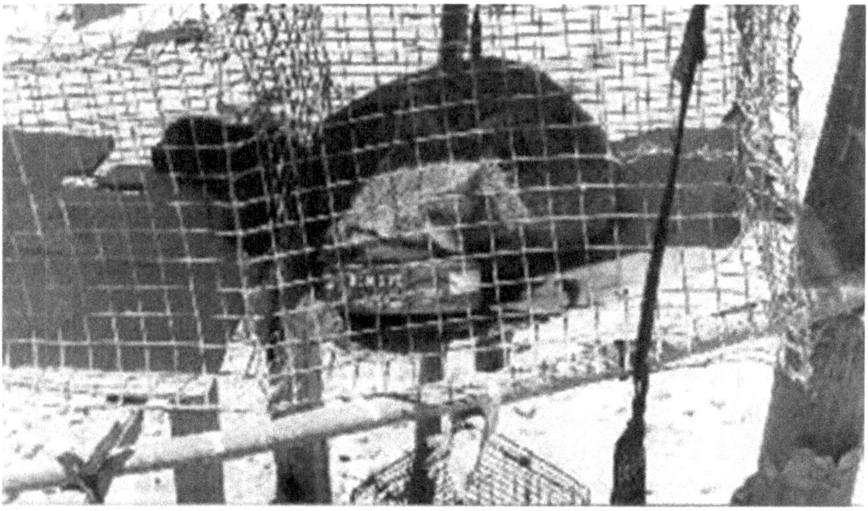

FIGURE 1.15 *Urocyon cinereoargenteus* sold as pet besides the highway San Luis Potosi-Matehuala.

Source: Photo: Martin Huerta.

The fauna uses at El Huizache Corridor are diverse and the region is considered as the biggest center for animals' trade in the country; Mellink et al. (1986), reported the use of 78 species, belonging to 42 families, mainly birds, and mammals.

The use of the biotic resources for self-consumption in this region is sustainable because the inhabitants only get the amounts of resource that they need at the moment, but there are 43 fauna species caught for sale that are used irrationally. In this case, the inhabitants go to the field and capture large quantities, a practice which may lead to reduce the populations' numbers. An example is the case of the collection of wild individuals of *Astrophytum myriostigma* and other cacti species, surely affecting the populations' recruitment.

TABLE 1.4 Fauna with use registered in El Huizache Corridor.

Family	Scientific name	Status	Uses*
REPTILES			
Crotalidae	*Crotalus atrox Baird & Girard, 1853*	Under special protection	F, M, O
	C. lepidus Cope, 1883	Under special protection	F, M, O
	C. molossus Bair & Girard, 1853	Under special protection	F, M, O
	C. scutulatus Cope, 1883	Under special protection	F, M, O
Iguanidae	*Phrynosoma modestum* Girard, 1852		M
Accipitridae	*Buteo jamaicensis* Gmelin, 1788	Under special protection	P
	*Parabuteo unicinctus*Temminck, 1824	Threatened	P
Bombycillidae	*Bombycilla cedrorum* Vieillot, 1808		P
Columbidae	*Columbina inca* Lesson, 1847		F
	C. passerina Linnaeus, 1758		F
	Zenaida asiática Linnaeus, 1758		P
Corvidae	*Aphelocoma ultramarina* Bonaparte, 1825		P
Cuculidae	*Geoccocyx californianus* Lesson, 1829		M
Emberizidae	*Icterus galbula* Linnaeus, 1758		P
	Pipilo fuscus Swainson, 1827		P
Falconidae	*Falco mexicanus* Schlegel, 1851	Threatened	P
	F. sparverius Linnaeus, 1758		P
	Polyborus plancus Miller, 1777		P
Fringillidae	*Cardinalis* Linnaeus, 1758		P
	Cardinalis sinuatus Bonaparte, 1838		P

TABLE 1.4 (*Continued*)

Family	Scientific name	Status	Uses*
	Carduelis psaltria Say, 1823		P
	Carpodacus mexicanus Müller, 1776		P
	Guiraca caerulea Linnaeus, 1758		P
	Pheucticus melanocephalus Swainson,1827		P
	Serinus canaria Linnaeus, 1758		P
Icteridae	*Sturnella magna* Linnaeus, 1758		F
	Sturnella neglecta Audubon, 1844		F
Mimidae	*Mimus polyglottos* Linnaeus, 1758		P
Muscicapidae	*Tordus migratorius* Linnaeus, 1766		P
Phasianidae	*Callipepla squamata* Vigors, 1830		F
	Colinus virginianus Linnaeus, 1758		F
Picidae	*Melanerpes aurifrons* Wagler, 1829		P
Ptilogonatidae	*Phainopepla nitens* Swainson, 1837		P
	Ptilogonys cinereus Swainson, 1824		P
Strigidae	*Bubo virginianus* Gmelin, 1788	Threatened	P
	Glaucidium gnoma Wagler, 1832	Rare	P
	Otus trichopsis Wagler, 1832		P
Thraupidae	*Piranga rubra* Linnaeus, 1758		P
Tyrannidae	*Tyrannus vociferans* Swainson, 1826		P
Didelphidae	*Didelphis virginiana* Kerr,1792		M
Dasypodidae	*Dasypus novemcinctus* Linnaeus, 1758		F, M

TABLE 1.4 (*Continued*)

Family	Scientific name	Status	Uses*
Sciuridae	*Spermophilus spilosoma* Bennett, 1833		P
Muridae	*Neotoma albigula* Hartley, 1894		F
Cervidae	*Odocoileus virginianus* Zimmermann, 1780		F
Tayasuidae	*Pecari tajacu* Linnaeus, 1758		F
Canidae	*Canis latrans* Say, 1823		P, O
	Urocyon cinereoargenteus Schreber, 1775		P, O
Procyonidae	*Bassariscus astutus* Lichtenstein, 1830		P
	Procyon lotor Linnaeus, 1758		P
Mustelidae	*Mustela frenata* Lichtenstein, 1831		P
	Taxidea taxus Schreber, 1778	Threatened	M
Felidae	*Lynx rufus* Schreber, 1777		P, O
Leporidae	*Lepus californicus* Gray, 1837		F
	L. callotis Wagler, 1830		F
	Sylvilagus audubonii Baird, 1858		F
	S. floridanus J. A. Allen, 1890		F

Note: **F**= Food; **M**= Medicinal; **P**= Pets.

1.8 CONCLUSION

American continent represents one of the most biodiverse continents in the world and it is recognized for its importance in the origin of agriculture and domestication of many species. Some of them now represent the base of the human diet. In America, there are ancient cultures that still use the natural resources in the same manner that the pre-Columbian cultures did. There is enormous knowledge of plants and animals, their medicinal and nutritional properties, and so on; however, with the arrival of the Spaniards to the continent, much of that knowledge was lost and only a few pictographic records were rescued, so knowledge has been transmitted orally from generation to generation with the imminent risk of being lost by modernity.

The system of classification of medicinal plants of the Aztecs constitutes a legacy that has been rescued, thanks to the Codex De la Cruz-Badiano. It contemplates precise information on plants, their uses, and forms of employment. On the other hand, the food production systems through agriculture, in many native peoples, maintain the tradition and use of creole races and with it the conservation of genetic material of their wild relatives. Many species that are currently used in rural areas of Mexico are not even cultivated, that is, wild individuals are used, and their use is local, but they represent an important part of the diet in the process of development of the towns.

Diet changes have revealed the poor quality of food under the modern food production systems, generating health problems and malnutrition, which is why a return to the incorporation of the components of the ancestral diet is urgently required.

KEYWORDS

- **Americas biodiversity**
- **prehispanic knowledge**
- **medicinal plants**
- **domestication**
- **traditional use**

REFERENCES

Abd El-Ghani, M. M.; Huerta-Martínez, F. M.; Hongyan, L.; Qureshi, R. *Plant Responses to Hyperarid Desert Environments*; Springer, 2017; pp 473–501.

Aburto, T. C.; Cantoral, A.; Hernández-Barrera, L.; Carriquiry, A. L.; Rivera, J. A. Usual Dietary Energy Density Distribution Is Positively Associated with Excess Body Weight in Mexican Children. *J. Nutr.* **2015,** *145* (7), 1524–1530.

Altieri, M. A.; Funes-Monzote, F. R.; Petersen, P. Agroecologically Efficient Agricultural Systems for Smallholder Farmers: Contributions to Food Sovereignty. *Agron. Sustain. Dev.* **2011,** *32*, 1–13.

Aranda, A.; Viesca, C.; Sánchez, G.; Sánchez, G.; de Viesca, M. R.; Sanfilippo, J. La materia médica en el Libellus de Medicinalibus Indorum Herbis. *Revista de la Facultad de Medicina* **2003,** *46*, 12–17.

Ávila, S.; Beux, M. R.; Ribani, R. H.; Rui C.; Zambiazi, R. C. Stingless Bee Honey: Quality Parameters, Bioactive Compounds, Health-Promotion Properties, and Modification Detection Strategies. *Trends Food Sci. Technol.* **2018,** *81*, 37–50.

Blancas, J.; Casas, A.; Rangel-Landa, S.; Moreno-Calles, A.; Torres, I.; Pérez-Negrón, E.; Solís, L.; Delgado-Lemus, A.; Parra, F.; Arellanes, Y.; Caballero, J.; Cortés, L.; Lira, R.; Dávila, P. Plant Management in the Tehuacán-Cuicatlán Valley, Mexico. *Econ. Bot.* **2010,** *64* (4), 287–302.

Bracho Pérez, J. C.; Rodríguez, B.; Llanes, F. Triterpenos pentacíclicos enpropóleo. *Rev. Soc. Quim. Perú* **2009,** *75*, 439–452.

Buchmann, S. *The Reason for Flowers: Their History, Culture, Biology, and How They Change Our Lives*; Simon and Schuster: New York, 2016.

Bye, R.; Linares, E. Los quelites, plantas comestibles de Mexico: una reflexión sobre intercambio cultural. *Biodiversitas* **2000,** *31*, 11–14.

Cáceres, A.; Cruz, S. M. Edible Seeds, Leaves and Flowers as Maya Superfoods: Function and Composition. *Int. J. Phytocosmetics Nat. Ingred.* **2019,** *6* (1), 2.

Casas, A.; Blancas, J.; Lira, R. Mexican Ethnobotany: Interactions of People and Plants in Mesoamerica. In *Mexican Ethnobotany: Interactions of People and Plants in Mesoamerica*; Lira, R., Casas, A., Blancas, J., Eds.; Springer Science+Business Media: New York, 2016a; pp 1–19.

Casas, A.; Caballero, J. Domesticación de plantas y origen de la agricultura en Mesoamérica. *Ciencias* **1995,** *40*, 36–45.

Casas, A.; Otero-Arnaiz, A.; Pérez-Negrón, E.; Valiente-Banuet, A. In Situ Management and Domestication of Plants in Mesoamerica. *Ann. Bot.* **2007,** *100*, 1101–1115.

Casas, A.; Torres-Guevara, J.; Parra, F. *Domesticación en el Continente Americano*. Vol. 1, Manejo de biodiversidad y evolución dirigida por las culturas del Nuevo Mundo. Universidad Nacional Autónoma de México., Cuidad de México. Universidad Nacional Agraria La Molina (UNALM) del Perú. Lima, República del Perú, 2016b; 504 p.

Castillo, A. M.; Alavez, V.; Castro-Porras, L.; Martínez, Y.; Cerritos, R. Analysis of the Current Agricultural Production System, Environmental, and Health Indicators: Necessary the Rediscovering of the Pre-hispanic Mesoamerican Diet? *Front. Sustain. Food Syst.* **2020,** *4*, 1–12.

Correa-Ascencio, M.; Robertson, I. G.; Cabrera-Cortés, O.; Cabrera-Castro, R.; Evershed, R. P. Pulque Production from Fermented Agave Sap as a Dietary Supplement in Prehispanic Mesoamerica. *Proc. Natl. Acad. Sci.* **2014,** *111* (39), 14223–14228.

Costa, J. A. V.; Freitas, B. C. B.; Rosa, G. M.; Moraes, L.; Morais, M. G.; Mitchell, B. G. Operational and Economic Aspects of *Spirulina*-Based Biorefinery. *Bioresour. Technol.* **2019,** *292*, 121946.

De Jong, H. La meliponicultura en la cosmovisión Maya. In: *II Seminario Mexicano sobre abejas sin aguijón*, Quezada-Euán, J. J. G., Medina, L., Moo-Valle, J. H., Eds.; Mérida, Yucatán: México, 2001; pp 10–18.

De la Cruz M. *Libellus de medicinalibus indorum herbis*. Manuscrito azteca de 1552. Según traducción latina de Juan Badiano. Instituto Mexicano del Seguro Social: Mexico, DF, 1964.

Delgado Salinas, A.; Bonet, A.; Gepts, P. The wild relative of *Phaseolus vulgaris* in Middle America. In *Genetic Resources of Phaseolus Beans*; Gepts, P., Ed.; Kluwer: Dordrecht, The Netherlands, 1988; pp 163–184.

Díaz del Castillo B. *Historia verdadera de la conquista de la Nueva España*; Editorial Porrúa: México, 2004.

Doebley, J. The Genetics of Maize Evolution. *Annu. Rev. Genet.* **2004,** *38*, 37–59.

Escalante A.; Giles-Gómez, M.; Hernández, G.; Córdova-Aguilar, M. S.; López-Munguía, A.; Gosset, G.; Bolívar, F. Analysis of Bacterial Community During the Fermentation of Pulque, a Traditional Mexican Alcoholic Beverage, Using a Polyphasic Approach. *Int. J. Food Microbiol.* **2008,** *124*, 126–134.

Escalante-Araiza, F.; Gutiérrez-Salmeán, G. Traditional Mexican Foods as Functional Agents in the Treatment of Cardiometabolic Risk Factors. *Crit. Rev. Food Sci. Nutr.* **2020,** 1–12.

FAO. Sustainable Diets and Biodiversity. Directions and Solutions for Policy, Research, and Action, 2010. http://www.fao.org/3/a-i3004e.pdf (accessed Sept 12, 2020).

FAO. El sistema alimentario en México—Oportunidades para el campo mexicano en la Agenda 2030 de Desarrollo Sostenible, 2019.

FAO Contributions to Rural Households. Use and Potential of Wild Plants in Farm Households, 1999. http://www.fao.org/3/w8801e04.htm (accessed Dec 18, 2020).

Favre, G.; Legueult, K.; Pradier, C.; Raffaelli, C.; Ichai, C.; Iannelli, A.; Redheuil, A.; Lucidarme, O.; Esnault, V. Visceral Fat Is Associated to the Severity of COVID-19. *Metabol. Clin. Exp.* **2021,** *115*, 154440.

Flannery, K., Ed. *Guilá Naquitz*; Academic Press: New York, 1986.

Godfray, H. C.; Beddington, J. R.; Crute, I. R.; Haddad, L.; Lawrence, D., Muir, J. F., et al. Food Security: The Challenge of Feeding 9 Billion People. *Science* **2010,** *327*, 812–818.

Gutiérrez-Solana E. *Códices de México*. Historia e interpretación de los grandes libros pintados prehispánicos. Mexico: Panorama Editorial, 1992.

Harlan, J. R. *Crops and Man*; American Society of Agronomy-Crop Science Society: Madison, WI, 1975.

Harlan, J. *Crops and Man*; American Society of Agronomy Inc.: Madison, WI, 2005.

Harris, D. R. Domesticatory Relationships of People, Plants, and Animals. In *Redefining Nature: Ecology, Culture, and Domestication*; Ellen, R., Fukui, K.; Eds.; Berg: Oxford, 1996; pp 437–463.

Hawkes, J. G. *The Diversity of Crop Plants*; Harvard University Press: Cambridge, 1983.

Hernández, F. *Historia natural de Nueva España*. Dos volúmenes. Universidad Nacional Autónoma de México: México, DF, 1959.

Hernández-Ramírez, A. M. *Libellus de Medicinalibus Indorum Herbis*: Códice Cruz-Badiano. *Cuadernos de Biodiversidad* **2020,** *58*, 1–8.

Huerta-Martínez, F. M.; Neri-Luna, C.; Muñoz-Urias, A.; Castruita-Dominguez, J. P.; Sahagún-Sánchez, F. J. Assessing the Relative Importance of Climate and Soil for Vegetation Patterns in a Semiarid Land of Central Mexico. *Egypt. J. Bot.* **2020,** *60* (3), 825–835.

ISC (International Science Council). Annual Report, 2019. https://council.science/publications/ (accessed Dec 20, 2020).

INPI Atlas de los Pueblos Indígenas de México. Gobierno de México, 2020. http://atlas.inpi.gob.mx/ (accessed Dec 20, 2020).

Johns, T.; Eyzaguirre, P. Linking Biodiversity, Diet, and Health in Policy and Practice. *Proc. Nutr. Soc.* **2006,** *65* (2), 182–189.

Johns, T.; Sthapit, B. R. Biocultural Diversity in the Sustainability of Developing-Country Food Systems. *Food Nutr. Bull.* **2004,** *25* (2), 143–155.

Joly, C. A. Biodiversity at Risk in the Americas. *Biota Neotropica* **2018,** *18* (3), e20180301.

Kinder, D. H.; Adams, K. R.; Wilson, H. J. *Solanum jamesii*: Evidence for Cultivation of Wild Potato Tubers by Ancestral Puebloan Groups. *J. Ethnobiol.* **2017,** *37* (2), 218–240.

Kwak, M.; Kami, J. A.; Gepts, P. The Putative Mesoamerican Domestication Center of *Phaseolus vulgaris* Is Located in the Lerma–Santiago Basin of Mexico. *Crop Sci.* **2009,** *49*, 554–563.

Lafarga, T. Effect of Microalgal Biomass Incorporation into Foods: Nutritional and Sensorial Attributes of the End Products. *Algal Res.* **2019,** *41*, 101566.

Lafarga, T.; Fernández-Sevilla, J. M.; González-López, C.; Acién-Fernández, F. G. *Spirulina* for the Food and Functional Food Industries. *Food Res. Int.* **2020,** *137*, 109356.

Llach, M. J. A. Nombrar y representar: escritura y naturaleza en el Códice de la Cruz-Badiano, 1552. *Fronteras de la Historia* **2011,** *16*, 13–41.

López-Maldonado, J. E. Ethnohistory of the Stingless Bees *Melipona beecheii* (Hymenoptera: Meliponinae) in the Mayan Civilization, Decipherment of the Beekeeping Almanacs Part I in the Madrid Codex and the Study of Their Behavioral Traits and Division of Labor; Ph.D. Dissertation, University of California, Davis, 2005.

López-Olmedo, N.; Carriquiry, A. L.; Rodríguez-Ramírez, S.; Ramírez-Silva, I.; Espinosa-Montero, J.; Hernández-Barrera, L., Campirano, F.; Martínez-Tapia, B.; Rivera, J. A. Usual Intake of Added Sugars and Saturated Fats Is High While Dietary Fiber Is Low in the Mexican Population. *J. Nutr*. **2016,** *146* (Suppl), 1856S–1865S.

Lozoya, X. *Los señores de las plantas*; Medicina y herbolaria en Mesoamérica. Consejo Nacional para la Cultura y las Artes. Editorial Pangea: México, DF, 1990; 58 p

MacNeish, R. S. A Summary of Subsistence. In *The Prehistory of the Tehuacán Valley: Environment and Subsistence*; Byers, D. S.; Ed.; Vol. 1, University of Texas Press: Austin, TX, 1967; pp 290–309.

MacNeish, R S. *The Origins of Agriculture and Settles Life*; University of Oklahoma Press: Chicago, 1992.

Manzanero-Medina, G. I.; Vásquez-Dávila, M. A.; Lustre-Sánchez, H.; Pérez-Herrera, A. Ethnobotany of Food Plants (Quelites) Sold in Two Traditional Markets of Oaxaca, Mexico. *South Afr. J. Bot*. **2020,** *130*, 215–223.

Marrón-Ponce, J. A.; Sánchez-Pimienta, T.; Louzada, M. L., Batis, C. Energy Contribution of NOVA Food Groups and Sociodemographic Determinants of Ultra-Processed Foods Consumption in Mexican Population. *Public Health Nutr*. **2017,** *21* (1), 87–93.

Masson-Salaue, L. 12th IFDC 2017 Special Issue—Foods from Latin America and Their Nutritional Contribution: A Global Perspective. *J. Food Compos. Analys.* **2019,** *82*, 1–15.

Matsuoka, Y.; Vigouroux, Y.; Goodman, M. M.; Sanchez, G. J.; Buckler, E.; Doebley, J. A Single Domestication for Maize Shown by Multilocus Microsatellite Genotyping. *Proc. Natl. Acad. Sci. USA* **2002,** *99*, 6080–6084.

McNeely, J. A.; Wachtel, P. S. *Soul of the Tiger: Searching for Nature's Answers in Southeast Asia*; Doubleday: New York, 1988.

Mellink, E.; Aguirre, R. J. R.; García-Moya, E. *Utilización de la Fauna Silvestre en el Altiplano Potosino-Zacatecano*; Colegio de Postgraduados. Chapingo: México, 1986.

Mexicanist. Domestication of Plants and Origin of Agriculture in Mesoamerica, 2021. https://www.mexicanist.com/l/domestication-of-plants-and-origin-of-agriculture-in-mesoamerica/# (accessed Feb 18, 2021).

Moreno-Ulloa, J.; Moreno-Ulloa, A.; Martínez-Tapia, M.; Duque-Rodríguez, J. Comparison of the Prevalence of Metabolic Syndrome and Risk Factors in Urban and Rural Mexican Tarahumara-Foot Runners. *Diab. Res. Clin. Pract.* **2018,** *143*, 79–87.

Mulík, S.; Ozuna, C. Mexican Edible Flowers: Cultural Background, Traditional Culinary Uses, and Potential Health Benefits. *Int. J. Gastronomy Food Sci.* **2020,** *21*, 100235.

National Research Council, Status of Pollinators in North America. The National Academies Press: Washington, DC, 2007. http://dx.doi.org/10.17226/11761.

Myers, N. *Gaia: An Atlas of Plant Management*; Doubleday: New York, 1985.

Nyberg, M.; Olsson, V.; Wendin, K. "Would You Like to Eat an Insect?" Children's Perceptions of and Thoughts About Eating Insects. *Int. J. Consum. Stud.* **2020,** 1–11.

Ozturk, M.; Hakeem, K. R.; Ashraf, M., Ahmad, M. S. A. *Global Perspectives on Underutilized Crops*; Springer Science+Business Media, 2018.

Paoletti, M. G. *Ecological Implications of Minilivestock. Potential of Insects, Rodents Frogs, and Snails*; NH, Science Publishers, Inc.: Enfield, 2005.

Pardo-Tomás, J. Conversions Medicine: Communication and Circulation of Knowledge in the Franciscan Convent and Collage of Tlatelolco. *Quaderni Storici* **2013,** *48*, 28–42.

Petersen, A.; Bressema, K.; Albrecht, J.; Thieß, H-M.; Vahldiek, J.; Hamma, B.; Makowski; M. R.; Niehues, A.; Niehuesa, S. M.; Adams, L. C. The Role of Visceral Adiposity in the Severity of COVID-19: Highlights from a Unicenter Cross-Sectional Pilot Study in Germany. *Metabol. Clin. Experimental* **2020,** *110*, 154317.

Pham, T. X.; Lee, Y.; Bae, M.; Hu, S.; Kang, H.; Kim, M. B.; Park, Y. K.; Lee, J. Y. *Spirulina* supplementation in a Mouse Model of Diet-Induced Liver Fibrosis Reduced the Pro-Inflammatory Response of Splenocytes. *Br. J. Nutr.* **2019,** *121*, 748–755.

Piperno, D.; Flannery, K. The Earliest Archaeological Maize (*Zea mays* L.) from Highland Mexico: New Accelerator Mass Spectrometry Dates and Their Implications. *Proc. Natl. Acad. Sci. USA* **2001,** *98*, 2101–2103.

Pyšek, P.; Dawson, W.; Essl, F.; Kreft, H.; Pergl, J.; Seebens, H.; van Kleunen, M.; Weigelt, P.; Winter, M. Contrasting Patterns of Naturalized Plant Richness in the Americas: Numbers Are Higher in the North But Expected to Rise Sharply in the South. *Global Ecol. Biogeogr.* **2019,** *28* (6), 779–783.

Quezada-Euán, J. G., May-Itzá, W., González-Acereto, J. A. Meliponiculture in Mexico: Problems and Perspective for Development. *Bee World* **2001,** *82*, 160–167.

Ramírez-Rodríguez, Y.; Martínez-Huélamoc, M.; Pedraza-Chaverrie, J.; Ramírez, V.; Martínez-Tagüeña, N.; Trujillo, J. Ethnobotanical, Nutritional and Medicinal Properties of Mexican Drylands Cactaceae Fruits: Recent Findings and Research Opportunities. *Food Chem.* **2020,** *312*, 126073.

Rodríguez, L. C.; Mendez, M. A.; Niemeyer, H. M. Direction of Dispersion of Cochineal (*Dactylopius coccus* Costa) within the Americas. *Antiquity* **2001,** *75*, 73–77.

Rosa, G. M. D.; Moraes, L.; Cardias, B. B.; Costa, J. A. V. Chemical Absorption and CO_2 Biofixation via the Cultivation of *Spirulina* in Semicontinuous Mode with Nutrient Recycling. *Bioresour. Technol.* **2015,** *192*, 321–327.

Sahagún, B. *Historia general de las cosas de la Nueva España*; Editorial Porrúa: México, 2006.

Smith, B. D. The Initial Domestication of *Cucurbita pepo* in the Americas 10,000 Years Ago. *Science* **1997,** *276* (5314), 932–934.

Smith, B. D. Documenting Plant Domestication: The Consilience of Biological and Archaeological Approaches. *Proc. Natl. Acad. Sci. USA* **2001,** *98*, 1324–1326.

Smith, B. D. Seed Size Increase as a Marker of Domestication in Squash (*Cucurbita pepo*). In *Documenting Domestication: The Intersection of Genetics and Archaeology*; Zeder, M. A. et al.; Eds.; University of California Press: Oakland, 2006; pp 25–31.

Smith, B. D. The Cultural Context of Domestication in Eastern North America. *Curr. Anthropol.* **2011,** *52* (S4), S471–S484.

Smith, B. D.; Yarnell, R. A. Initial Formation of an Indigenous Crop Complex in Eastern North America at 3,800 B.P. *Proc. Natl. Acad. Sci. USA* **2009,** *106*, 6561–6566.

Spengler III, R. N. Anthropogenic Seed Dispersal: Rethinking the Origins of Plant Domestication. *Trends Plant Sci.* **2020,** *25* (4), 340–348.

STATISTA. 2021. https://es.statista.com/estadisticas/1095779/numero-de-muertes-causadas-por-el-coronavirus-de-wuhan-por-pais/ (accessed Jan 20, 2021).

The Millennium Assessment. *Ecosystems and Human Well-Being*; Island Press, 2005.

Torres-Tiji, Y.; Fieldsa, F. J.; Mayfield, S. P. Microalgae as a Future Food Source. *Biotechnol. Adv.* **2020,** *41*, 107536.

Tuomisto, H. L. The Complexity of Sustainable Diets. *Nat. Ecol. Evol.* **2019,** *3*, 720–721.

Turner, N. J. "That Was Our Candy!" Sweet Foods in Indigenous Peoples' Traditional Diets in Northwestern North America. *J. Ethnobiol.* **2020,** *40* (3), 305–328.

Ulloa-Ulloa, C.; Acevedo-Rodríguez, P.; Beck, S.; Belgrano, M. J.; Bernal, R.; Berry, P. E.; Brako, L.; Celis, M.; Davidse, G., Forzza, R. C.; Gradstein, R.; Hokche, O.; León, B.; León-Yánez, S.; Magill, R. E.; Neill, D. A.; Nee, M.; Raven, P. H.; Stimmel, H.; Strong, M. T.; Villaseñor, J. L.; Zarucchi, J. L.; Zuloaga, F. O.; Jørgensen, P. M. An Integrated Assessment of the Vascular Plant Species of the Americas. *Science* **2017,** *358*, 1614–1617.

UNESCO. UNESCO—Traditional Mexican Cuisine—Ancestral, Ongoing Community Culture, the Michoacán paradigm [WWW Document], 2010. https://ich.unesco.org/en/lists (accessed Feb 22, 2020).

Valverde, J. The Aztec Herbal of 1552. Martín de la Cruz' "Libellus de Medicinalibus Indorum Herbis"; Context of the Sources on Nahualt Materia Medica. *Veroffentlichungen der Internationalen Gesellschaft fur Geschichte der Pharmazie* **1984,** *53*, 9–30.

Van Kleunen, M.; Pyšek , P.; Dawson, W.; Essl, F.; Kreft, H.; Pergl, J.; Weigelt, P.; Stein, A.; Dullinger, S.; König, Ch.; Lenzner, B.; Maurel, N.; Moser, D.; Seebens , H.; Kartesz, J.; Nishino, M.; Aleksanyan, A.; Ansong, M.; Antonova, L. A.; Barcelona, J. F.; Breckle, S. W.; Brundu, G.; Cabezas, F. J.; Cárdenas, D.; Cárdenas-Toro, J.; Castaño, N.; Chacón, E.; Chatelain, C.; Conn, B.; Dechoum, M. de S: Dufour-Dror, J. M.; Ebel, A. L.; Figueiredo, E.; Fragman-Sapir, O.; Fuentes, N.; Groom, Q. J.; Henderson, L.; Jogan , I. N.; Krestov, P.; Kupriyanov, A.; Masciadri, S.; Meerman, J.; Morozova, O.; Nickrent, D.; Nowak, A.; Patzelt, A.; Pelser, P. B.; Shu, W. S.; Thomas, J.; Uludag, A.; Velayos, M.; Verkhosina, A.; Villaseñor, J. L.; Weber, E.; Wieringa, J. J.; Yazlık, A.; Zeddam, A.; Zykova, E.; Winter, M. The Global Naturalized Alien Flora (GloNAF) Database. *Ecology* **2019,** *100* (1), e02542.

Van Vuuren, D. P.; Sala, O. E.; Pereira, H. M. The Future of Vascular Plant Diversity Under Four Global Scenarios. *Ecol. Soc.* **2006,** *11* (2), 25.

Vargas-Luna, M. D.; Hernandez-Ledesma, P.; Majure, L. C.; Puente-Martinez, R.; Macias, H. M. H.; Luna, R. T. B. Splitting Echinocactus: Morphological and Molecular Evidence Support the Recognition of Homalocephala as a Distinct Genus in the Cacteae. *Phytokeys* **2018,** *111*, 31–59.

Vavilov, N. I. *Origin and Geography of Cultivated Plants*; Cambridge University Press: Cambridge, 1992.

Vega, N.; Ponce, R.; Matínez, Y.; Carrasco, O.; Cerritos, R. Implications of the Western Diet for Agricultural Production, Health, and Climate Change. *Front. Sustain. Food Syst.* **2018,** *2*, 1–5.

Velasco Lozano, A. M. L., Nagao, D. Mitología y simbolismo de las flores. *Arqueol. Mex.* **2006,** *13*, 28–35.

Vit, P.; Pedro, S. R. M.; Roubik, D. *Pot-Honey a Legacy of Stingless Bees*, 1st ed., Springer-Verlag: New York, 2013.

Wells, M. L.; Potin, P.; Craigie, J. S.; Raven, J. A.; Merchant, S. S.; Helliwell, K. E.; Smith, A. G.; Camire, M. E.; Brawley, S. H. Algae as Nutritional and Functional Food Sources: Revisiting Our Understanding. *J. Appl. Phycol.* **2017,** *29*, 949–982.

Williams, E. The "Land of Fish": Reconstructing the Ancient Aquatic Lifeway in Michoacán, Western Mexico. *Ancient Mesoamerica* **2020,** 1–36.

Wu, Q.; Liu, L.; Miron, A.; Klímová, B.; Wan, D.; Kuˇca, K. The Antioxidant, Immunomodulatory, and Anti-Inflammatory Activities of *Spirulina*: An Overview. *Arch. Toxicol.* **2016,** *90*, 1817–1840.

Yam-Puc, A.; Santana-Hernández, A. A.; Yah-Nahuat, P. N.; Ramón-Sierra, J. M.; Cáceres-Farfán, M. R.; Borges-Argáez, R. L.; Ortiz-Vázquez, E. Pentacyclic Triterpenes and Other Constituents in Propolis Extract from *Melipona beecheii* Collected in Yucatan, México. *Revista Brasileira de Farmacognosia* **2019,** *29*, 358–363.

Yang, Y.; Du, L.; Hosokawa, M.; Miyashita, K. *Spirulina* Lipids Alleviate Oxidative Stress and Inflammation in Mice Fed a High-Fat and High-Sucrose Diet. *Mar. Drugs* **2020,** *18*, 148.

Yarnell, E.; Abascal, K. Herbs for Diabetes: Update-Part 1. *Alternative and Complementary Therapies* **2014,** *20*, 6328–333.

Zohary, D.; Hopf, M. *Domestication of Plants in the Old World*, 2nd ed.; Oxford University Press: Oxford, 1993.

CHAPTER 2

Traditional Medicinal Plants as Bioresources in Health Security

PRIYA SUNDARRAJAN[1] and LEKHA BHAGTANEY[2]

[1]Department of Life Science and Biochemsitry, St. Xavier's College (Autonomous), Mumbai, India

[2]Intern, Caius Laboratory for Interdisciplinary Research, St. Xavier's College (Autonomous), Mumbai, India

ABSTRACT

Humans have depended on nature for their existence since time immemorial. The use of biological resources for health care has been nurtured by the Indigenous people of every land. People of every culture have always tried and tested indigenous plants for thousands of years, identifying that almost all of nature is meant for food, clothing, shelter, and well-being and adapting based on available resources. Plants that exert beneficial pharmacological effects on human body are called medicinal plants and they possess therapeutic properties mainly due to their natural ability to synthesize secondary metabolites like alkaloids, tannins, and flavonoids, which are the sources of important drugs such as atropine, codeine, digoxin, morphine, quinine, and vincristine. The knowledge of medicinal plants and their use provide a vital combination of livestock and human health care in various parts of the world. This use of indigenous medicinal plants for health care has been developed over time in different cultures, based on the available natural resources in an area. Many of the traditional medicine are practiced in a nonformal way

Ethnic Knowledge and Perspectives of Medicinal Plants, Volume 1: Curative Properties and Treatment Strategies. Munir Ozturk, Kandikere R. Sridhar, Maryam Sarwat, Volkan Altay, & Francisco Martín Huerta-Martínez (Eds.)

by the local people as well as through recognized systematic medicinal systems like Ayurveda in India and similarly in other countries like China, Africa, and Egypt. According to many of these systems, the medicinal plants not only provide health security, but also involve an array of practices and resources that relate to mind-body-nature balance and nutritional well-being of the individuals. It has also been observed by researchers that in many of these practices, similar medicinal plants have been used for the treatment of same illness. Hence, it is necessary to increase awareness regarding the importance of medicinal plants and their benefits not only for curing diseases and ailments but also for supplementing nutrition. The chapter plans to shed light on the medicinal plants and Indigenous knowledge that have allowed for the human species in Indian subcontinent to thrive on natures' eco-system's services.

2.1 INTRODUCTION

Humans are majorly dependent on natural resources to satisfy their basic needs—food, clothing, and shelter. There are rising concerns over how long we will be able to enjoy these resources. These concerns are increasing our appreciation toward these essential reserves of nature, however, the clock is ticking. Natural resources are needed to support the growing population which is predicted to increase in the next 30 years by 2 billion people (Growing at a Slower Pace, June 17, 2019). Apart from the increase in population, the lives of older and frailer, younger (possibly lesser nourished) populations and populations suffering from increasing lifestyle disorders and other diseases, need to be secured. In addition to this, the economic discrepancy between the rich and the poor keeps growing which raises concern over the affordability of healthcare systems to the necessitous.

In principle, food and health security systems could help reduce the burden of adverse consequences related to health and curb the health risks related to food (Wahlqvist et al., 2019). The concept of health security of developing countries being assisted by traditional medicine systems has been recognized by the World Health Organization (WHO) (Rajeswara Rao and Rajput, 2010). The biggest challenges faced by the humankind in the year 2050 are going to be related to food where some people will experience starvation and undergo malnutrition, others will experience obesity as a result of excess of calories. Formulation of healthier diets and increasing the production of food is the need of the hour.

However, the solution to these problems does not lie in merely expanding the land for agriculture as the expense of such an activity will be borne by the surrounding ecosystem and the biodiversity which is already declining. Additionally, there is also a need for adaptation by the society to environmental changes driven by climate change that can threaten the production of food and livelihood of the people (Ulian et al., 2020). Food security can be directly affected by changing climates as it would result in reduction in availability of water, the weather getting warmer and arid soils. This in turn would raise food prices and decrease food availability. Therefore, understanding the technological and dietary potential of crops not commonly grown, as well as their tolerance to environmental stresses, is very valuable (Dias-Martins et al., 2018).

The survival of a number of medicinal plants is threatened due to climate change, global warming, over harvesting, and loss of habitat. Furthermore, livestock consume (by calorific value) about 36% of arable crops like sorghum, maize, and wheat, necessitating one-third of the total arable farming area currently in use. This is a complicated situation because it is necessary to secure the long-term development of healthy and nutritious food while still preserving biodiversity in order to provide other products and ecological services that are both directly and indirectly important to human well-being (Ulian et al., 2020). Cultivation is coming up as a financially viable choice for preserving the global resources of medicinal plants and their biodiversity (Rajeswara Rao and Rajput, 2010).

2.2 TRADITIONAL MEDICINAL PLANTS: CONVENTIONAL USES

Herbal preparations that utilize plant constituents as active components are described as Herbal Medicines. These preparations usually use parts of plants like flowers, bark, fruits, leaves, roots, berries, seeds, and sometimes even the entire plant (Pan et al., 2014). The administration of these preparations is usually in the form of syrups where honey or syrup are used along with plant extract, boiled plant extracts or decoctions, alcoholic extracts or tinctures, and infusions like herbal teas. For external application, essential oils, balms, and cataplasms are used (Ramalingum and Mahomoodally, 2014). Before the arrival of aspirin that was derived from *Spiraea ulmaria*, in order to maintain energy or treat diseases, humans relied on crude ingredients of plant. Egyptian papyri show that *S. ulmaria* was prescribed for swelling and fever whereas the Greek Hippocrates suggested it for fever and pain. Excavational studies suggest that the use of medicinal plants goes back to 8000 years in China and 6000 years in Iraq. Sumerians of southern Mesopotamia, who existed 5000 years ago, maintained written accounts of use of herbal medicines and reported firmly-established medicinal uses for plants like thyme, caraway, and laurel (Pan et al., 2014).

According to the WHO Global Report on Traditional and Complementary Medicine (World Health Organization, 2019), over 90% of member states in the regions—Western Pacific, South-East Asia, and Eastern Mediterranean, use traditional medicine systems (World Health Organization, 2019). Traditional medicine is highly prevalent in developing countries where a significant proportion of the population is dependent on it for therapy (IARC, 2002). For instance, the ratio of traditional practitioners to the population is 1:500 and that of the medical doctors to the population is 1:40,000 in sub-Saharan Africa (Karunamoorthi et al., 2013). The reason for this prevalence lies in its historical use and its connection to culture, even though Western medicine coexists in these nations (IARC, 2002). The reliance on traditional medicine systems will only rise in the coming times as it is culturally valid and likely to retain its affordability in comparison to the modern health care system which has its own limitations along with being expensive. The factors that influence the patient to pick traditional medicine system over modern medicine have been given in Figure 2.1 (Karunamoorthi et al., 2013).

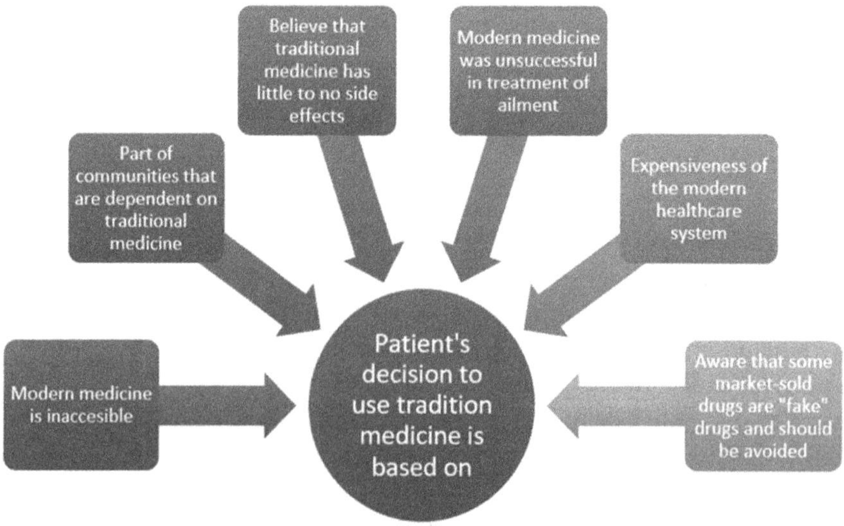

FIGURE 2.1 Factors influencing the decision of a patient to opt for traditional medicine for treatment (Karunamoorthi et al., 2013).

All over the world, there is extensive and successful usage of medicinal plants. The continent with proper established documentation of medicinal plants is Asia. Consequently, the majority of internationally recognized medicinal plants originate in this area, especially in China and India. Herbal medicine is becoming increasingly popular in North America and Europe, particularly in context of increasing lifestyle disorders and remedying the imbalances brought about because of it. Since ancient times, plants utilized in structured traditional medicine systems such as Traditional Chinese Medicine, Kampo, Unani, and Ayurveda have prospered as medical systems. In addition to being well-established structured systems, these systems have multicomponent mixtures at the core of their medium of therapy (Karunamoorthi et al., 2013).

In today's times, in comparison to chemical products that are harmful to both humans and nature, products made from medicinal plants represent safety. However, even though natural products have been treasured for their numerous qualities including aromatic, flavoring, and medicinal, the demands of the contemporary times have been met by synthetic products. Thus, the current requirement is substituting the chemicals with compounds derived from plants (Karunamoorthi et al., 2013).

2.3 TRADITIONAL MEDICINAL SYSTEMS IN THE WORLD

Traditional medicine as defined by WHO is "The sum total of the knowledge, skill, and practices based on the theories, beliefs, and experiences indigenous to different cultures, whether explicable or not, used in the maintenance of health as well as in the prevention, diagnosis, improvement or treatment of physical and mental illness." The policymakers and general practitioners all over the world are trying to overcome hurdles in reference to the regulations, preservation, availability, quality, effectiveness, and safety of traditional medicinal systems. However, the use of these systems is only increasing in various parts of the world. The matters regarding the practices and practitioners are also gaining more attention along with the products of these systems. WHO's responsibility in promoting traditional medicine is outlined in Figure 2.2 (World Health Organization, 2013).

Some of the well-recognized traditional medicinal systems include Ayurveda, Unani, Chinese Medicine, Siddha, and Kampo among many others. Despite having major application differences, the core philosophy behind all these systems is the natural affinity between the universe or the macrocosm and an individual or the microcosm. In theory, there are some common resemblances among traditional medicinal systems such as the significance of a practitioner's knowledge, focus on prevention, individualized care, multicausal way of diagnosis, systemic expertise in health and disease, understanding the operational aspects of health and diseases and so on (Payyappallimana, 2010).

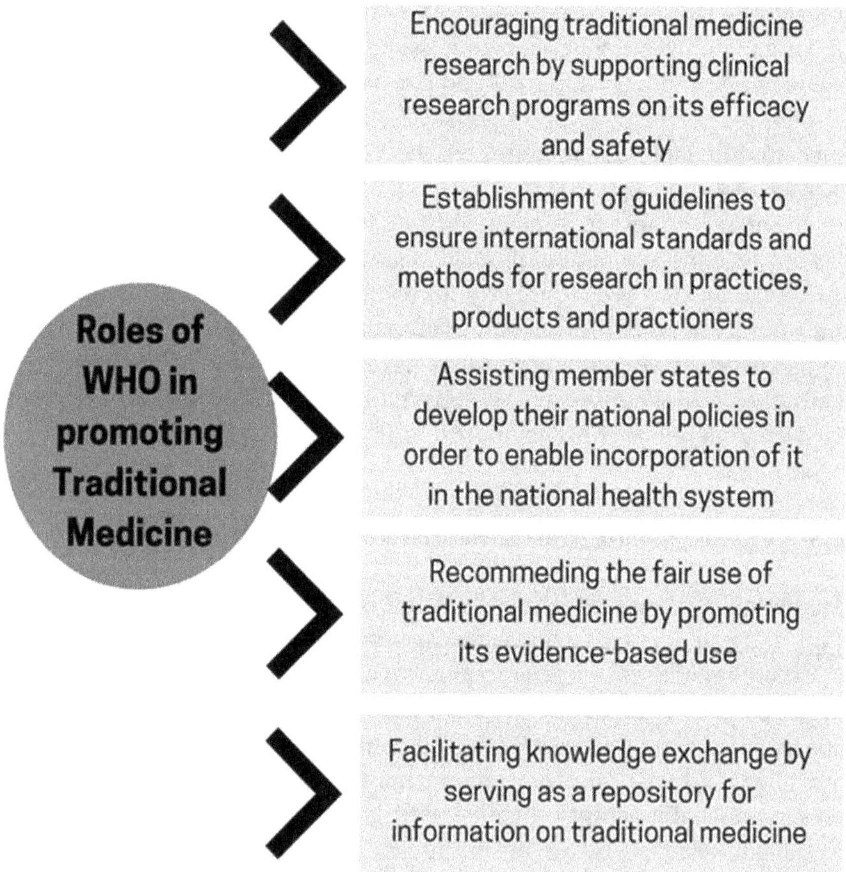

FIGURE 2.2 Roles of WHO in promoting traditional medicine systems (World Health Organization, 2013).

The famous traditional systems have come to be well-established and ordered medicinal systems. Despite there being persistence of a few flaws, these medicinal systems hold a valuable archive of knowledge collated by humans. A great deal of knowledge has been accumulated and progress has been made over countless generations in terms of the optimal time to acquire different herbs, medicinal material identification, herb selection, and preparation techniques. However, there is an urgent need for regulation of dose and suitable processing for the reduction in toxicity of the drug and enhancement of drug efficacy. Due to clinical experiments, a significant amount of data has been collected and thus, modern medicine is being developed with the help of traditional medicine. In case any type of traditional medicine is successfully implemented, it can unexpectedly aid in the development of novel drugs, leading to a number of advantages, including substantial cost savings (Yuan et al., 2016). Some of the most popular traditional medicine systems have been mentioned in the following paragraphs.

The Indian traditional system of medicine known as Ayurveda utilizes natural elements to eliminate the disease's root cause thereby restoring equilibrium in the body. The philosophy of Ayurveda emphasizes living a balanced lifestyle to prevent disorder and excessive pain. Various herbs are combined in a specific quotient in many Ayurvedic therapies to reduce toxicity and produce an optimal therapeutic effect. There are over 400,000 registered practitioners of Ayurveda. An official body has been established by the Government of India to oversee the practice, quality, and efforts directed toward education in Ayurveda. Ayurvedic medicine's biologically active components and their efficacy in treatment are becoming more widely known.

Traditional Chinese medicine has become an integral part of the Chinese healthcare system and has started to gain acceptance an alternative or complementary system of medicine in the Western world. The extremely essential factor of this traditional system, the Chinese herbal medicine, has reportedly 1.5 billion users around the world. Traditional Chinese medicine uses a combination of different herbs in accordance with a set of stringent guidelines to prescriptions or formulas (*fang ji*), as referred to by the Chinese. A traditional formula is typically made up of four components—the "monarch," "minister," "assistant," and "servant," each of which contains one to many drugs and serves a different purpose in the formula. These drugs should ideally form an organic group to achieve the desired beneficial effect while minimizing side effects.

The traditional system of medicine in Japan is called Kampo. The traditional Chinese medicine was launched in Japan in the fifth or sixth century. Further, it was substantially modified and adapted by the practitioners in Japan as a result of their unique circumstances and eventually evolved into Kampo. According to recent reports, some Japanese doctors use Kampo prescriptions in their everyday practices, often as the favored mode of treatment. Certain physicians in Japan use Kampo medicines in conjunction with chemotherapy or radiotherapy to treat patients suffering from cancer. This demonstrates how well modern medicine and traditional medicine can work together. While the use of Kampo in combination with modern medicine becomes more common, there is an increasing awareness of the imminent necessity to research the interactions between both of these modes of therapy (Yuan et al., 2016).

One of the most historic and multifaceted medicine systems is that of the African Traditional Medicine, despite of poor maintenance of records. The African Traditional Medicine is regarded as a wholesome system that involves the body which is healed through traditional practices and the mind which is healed by the people's faith in religion. There are reports indicating that the African countries are increasingly familiarizing the populations with the traditional medicine system. Regulatory frameworks and national policies on traditional medicine are being improved along with building their institutional capacity. Progress was also observed in the advancement of traditional medicine in ministries of health by implementation of national programmes and introduction of board of experts. People from all walks of life, different ages, occupations, education levels, and religions constitute the market of African Traditional Medicine. This suggests that the use of traditional medicine is not restricted to particular sections of the society but is prevalent across African populations (Mothibe and Sibanda, 2019).

Many Western medical professionals believe that traditional systems of medicine are unreliable however they have a large number of users all around the world. By combining advanced techniques of modern medicine and traditional medicine's practical ethnomedicinal and ethnobotanical perspectives, it is possible to produce substantial advantages in the development of novel drugs and reformed medicines (Yuan et al., 2016).

2.4 PLANT-BASED FOOD AS THERAPY: A HISTORY

In recent years, there has been a lot of discussion on established concepts in nutrition and the use of pharmaceuticals. The idea of having a diet providing nutrients in enough quantities to fulfill organic needs of an individual also known as "adequate nutrition" is slowly being replaced by the term "optimal nutrition." This term focuses on having a diet that prevents the possibility of infliction of disease, enhance general well-being, and encourage good health. By performing intensive research on the various ways food can provide protection to the human body, health specialists found that there is presence of substances known as phytochemicals in abundance in food. On the basis of this, there came about a concept of "functional food" which is also described by various terms like "medicinal food," "vitafoods," "medifoods," or "pharmafoods." The parts of food plants that can provide therapeutic effects on consumption as described by a traditional, ethnomedical, or biomedical system are called medicinal food plants. In addition to supplying the body with essential nutrients and satisfying hunger, medicinal food has the capability of providing good mental and physical health by reducing the occurrence of diseases related to nutrition. This is possible due to the presence of bioactive compounds in the plants. The intake and type, however, should be in the normal amounts, as expected in a diet.

Early 1980s saw the establishment of functional foods as a separate class of food called the Foods for Specific Health Use in Japan. Functional Food Science in Europe, a European project, defined functional food as "A food can be regarded as functional if it is satisfactorily demonstrated to affect beneficially one or more target functions in the body, beyond adequate nutritional effects, thus either improving the general physical conditions or/and decreasing the risk of the generation of diseases (Ramalingum and Mahomoodally, 2014)." One of the first instances of a functional food being released into the market that claimed specific health benefit was of Unilever. Unilever created polyunsaturated fatty acid-rich spreads in the late 1960s with the aim of lowering blood cholesterol levels. This example demonstrates how functional foods can help meet unique customer needs while also contributing to improved public health (Weststrate et al., 2002).

The use of plants as health supplements dates back to 3300 BC with records on Egyptian hieroglyphics, which described more than 700 such plants and herbs. The Ebers Papyrus also describe many herbs that are used till this day such as *Aloe vera* L. History has seen a strong link between pharmacology and food for the treatment of a variety of disorders and promotion of good health. "Let food be your medicine and medicine be your food," as expressed by Hippocrates in 500 BC. Spices, for instance, are many a times considered as enhancers of taste or flavors but in the olden times spices were used in cooking as they had significant impact on the metabolism of an individual. *Curcuma longa*, more commonly known as turmeric, has been a part of Indian cooking since historic times. Turmeric shows the presence of a bioactive compound curcumin which is known to display many health-promoting properties such as anticarcinogenic, anti-inflammatory, and antioxidant properties. Its mechanism of action includes its influence on the functioning of angiogenesis and cell–cell adhesion, modulation of the immune system, glutathione S-transferases and cyclooxygenases enzyme inhibition, and inhibition of various cell signaling pathways. The allicin containing *Allium sativum* or garlic has displayed many positive effects on health such as enhanced circulation, lowering hypertension, and improve levels of HDL while reducing LDL levels. It can be consumed both cooked and raw. The herb *Mentha piperita* or peppermint has been used for a long time for its properties helpful in solving any digestive troubles such as problem in evacuation of bowel can be resolved because it is a smooth muscle relaxant and some other troubles like abdominal distension and bloating. The herbs of the Lamiaceae family—sage (*Salvia officinalis*) and thyme (*Thymus vulgaris*) were used to treat tonsilitis, laryngitis, bronchitis, cough, troubles related to spasmodic gastrointestinal tract, and also used as an anthelminthic in Egypt during the ancient times.

The bioactive compounds in plants were then used as blueprints for developing novel drugs with the advancements in pharmacological research. An example of this is the development of aspirin in 1897 which was a derivative of salicylic acid. After this discovery came a rapid progress in the field of pharmacology where chemical drugs were used for the treatment of many of the diseases (Ramalingum and Mahomoodally, 2014).

2.5 FOODS WITH THERAPEUTIC POTENTIAL

Since the beginning of the practice of agriculture, over thousands of species of plants have been cultivated. However, the society today, hinges on around 200 of these species thereby greatly narrowing the genetic diversity range of the crops. Almost half of the global calorie intake is supported by the crops—maize, rice, and wheat, putting the security of our food supply at extreme risk. Intensification of agriculture resulted in a reduction in the diversity of diets as well as food culture. Additionally, traditional crops, which provided essential micronutrients like zinc, vitamin A, and iron to poor communities, were lost. All things being said, recently, there has been increasing awareness about sustainable development, sustenance of the locals, biodiversity, and its impact on the security of food and nutrition. Due to this, there has been a wide promotion of researching more efficient means of production for mainstream crops and the advantages of using underutilized conventional crops.

There is immense potential in the underutilized traditional crops yet to be realized in terms if sustainable food production and food security. These crops can often adapt to the changing climatic conditions and are of great importance to the locals. Conditioning these crops to normal agriculture would be of help considering the challenge we are facing with respect to sustainable food production. Many a times these underutilized crops serve more than one purpose and are part of production of medicines, fibers, and timbres. Some of these were major crops, but have since been supplanted by new commercial varieties, for instance, lesser in popularity pulses like lablab have been replaced by millets. A valuable amount of traditional information on these varieties of plants such as about usage and cultivation are rapidly becoming extinct. Fungi and crops that contribute to food security like cereals and domesticated legumes can have varying chemical, antioxidant, and nutritional content and therefore access to these become important as they have might have a direct impact on human health. This impact could be positive or negative, for instance, the impact on the microbiome of the human intestine (Ulian et al., 2020).

Sago Palm: One of the characteristic underutilized traditional food crops known as sago palm (*Metroxylon sagu* Rottb.) is widely found in regions of the Pacific and Asia and very little research has been performed on this plant. It can grow in areas such as peat swamps and wetlands where economically important food crops are hard to cultivate. It can produce high amounts of starch (150–300 kg of dry starch per plant) and is therefore an important plant with respect to food security as it can provide as a staple food without competing for arable land. Noodles and breads can be made comfortably without change in taste or quality when sago starch is mixed in wheat flour (60%). Accordingly, the volume of edible starch that is present in the markets can be enhanced with addition of sago starch. However, the wetlands and swamps where sago palms are growing are being converted into lands for growth of commercial crops like rubber trees and oil palm, thereby resulting in a significant reduction of the sago palm population. The growth of such crops desperately require recognition, policy formation, and funds by national governments (Regional Expert Consultation, 2017).

Grass Pea: A plant called grass pea or *Lathyrus sativus* L. is of great significance economically in many of the developing countries like Ethiopia, Nepal, Pakistan, Bangladesh, and India. One or two weeks prior to the harvest of rice, its seeds are usually scattered into standing crops of rice. This way the remaining moisture following the rice harvest is exploited by the grass pea seeds. Due to its nutritional value, it is used for a variety of purposes such as fodder, feed as well as food. In addition to being a highly drought-resistant crop, it is also resistant to excess water and flood conditions. Grass pea also has the ability to grow on diverse soils ranging from heavy clays to poor soil. Therefore, grass pea shows great potential in terms of food security as well as for sustainable food production. A major drawback of this plant, however, is that it produces a neurotoxin β-N-oxalyl-L-α,β-diaminopropionic acid

(ODAP) due to which consumption of this crop for extended periods leads to lathyrism, a neurological disorder that affects domestic animals and humans. A number of factors influence the accumulation of ODAP into *Lathyrus* such as abiotic stresses, nutrients, and growth stage of plant. This has resulted in very less research on this plant. Due to this lack of research, there is limited biotechnological investment and there is little understanding of the complex genome. Extensive plans allowing for detection of genotypes with lower ODAP content as well as combining increased yield with low ODAP content and efficient seed detoxification techniques are urgently needed. Genomic tools that are breeder-friendly are becoming more widely available, therefore allowing breeding protocols to be more efficient. The use of next-generation sequencing has provided a way to tap into the wealth of genomic resources available for this underappreciated crop (Dixit et al., 2016).

Pulse Crops: Other crops that would help to prevent possible protein malnutrition in the future are pulses. Pulse crops can be profitable as they are excellent sources of protein, resistant to change in climate, and sustainable. A variety of pulses can account for 33% of dietary requirements as they comprise of high levels of albumins and globulins. However, problems like presence of antinutritional factors, allergenicity, or digestibility still need to be addressed if they are to be workable alternative sources of proteins. Using pulses as a source of protein requires a significant amount of effort such as selection of the best species or implementation of optimized processing and production. Pulse proteins' mechanical flexibility, which allows them to produce soft gel particles comparable to whey proteins or fibril-like structures to imitate meat, is an added benefit. However, in order to gain consumer acceptance, it may be necessary to decrease or remove unwanted flavors. Studies have also found ways to significantly lessen the content of antinutritional factor by treatments with specific enzymes, modulation of the vegetative cycle, heat treatment, or physical processes (Bessada et al., 2019).

Cowpea: Cowpea is high in protein and contains a wide range of nutrients. It also contains high levels of nutraceuticals like polyphenols, polyunsaturated fatty acids, antioxidants, and dietary fibers. The widely consumed and grown cowpea is an essential legume for millions around the world in regards to health and nutrition. Cowpea is a staple food in the region of the Americas, Africa, southern Europe, Oceania and tropical, semiarid and arid regions of Asia. Additional points of benefits are that cowpea is resistant to environmental stresses, stability in production, and high relative productivity. Through usage of suitable genotypes and enhancements in production systems, cowpea productivity and commercial feasibility can be increased in all major areas, reducing reliance on foreign inputs. Cowpea helps in improving the nitrogen and phosphate fertility of the soil, which will favor the succeeding cereal crops. Aside from nitrogen fixation, the crop's involvement in the system of rotation crop promotes the quantities of organic matter produced and increases carbon fixation. The accumulation of organic matter improves the fertility of the soil and physical attributes like production system sustainability, soil conservation, infiltration rate, and nutrient retention. Certain studies were able to acquire high-yielding potential genotypes of cowpea with early maturity and plant morphology that was conducive to mechanized harvesting owing to the investments in research and broad genetic variation. These genotypes are more resistant to pests and pathogens, as well as unfavorable environmental conditions (such as dryness and temperature variation). Cowpeas have piqued the interest of large farmers in the last decade, having ceased to be a subsistence crop cultivated primarily by family farmers. Cowpea production increased at a faster rate than all other pulses in the first decade of the 21st century (Carneiro da Silva et al., 2019).

Pearl Millet: *Pennisetum glaucum* (L.) R. Br. or pearl millet is a crop popularly grown in regions of Asia and Africa. In other parts of the world like Brazil, this crop serves as a feed and cover crop rather than food for human consumption. It is well-known for producing nutritional cereal grains that can withstand drought as well as heat. These grains also have higher levels of amino acids compared to traditionally grown crops like rye and wheat, maize-like lipid levels, increased content of dietary fiber as compared to rice and gluten-free. Furthermore, in comparison to corn, pearl millet is more affordable, and resistant to aflatoxin contamination. Possessing a low glycaemic index, makes pearl millet a substitute food for weight management and lowers the risk of developing chronic illnesses like diabetes. As a result, there should be greater emphasis on genetic improvement for launching novel cultivars with increased grain yields as well as evaluation of the benefits and potential use of pearl millet in the diet, since this cereal is important for food safety as well as a viable option for consumers looking for sustainable, nutritious, and low-cost food items (Dias-Martins et al., 2018).

These constitute a few of the potential food crops among many others that are being currently researched.

2.5.1 UP-AND-COMING TECHNOLOGIES FOR DISCOVERY AND IMPROVEMENT OF FOOD CROPS

With increasing urban population, there has been a rise in curiosity about urban farming although this type of farming has restrictions in many cities.

There are a number of new farming methods that have minimal impact on the environment and can be used in regulated indoor conditions, even in cities. Among these techniques, aeroponic where roots dangling in the air are sprayed with water that is nutrient rich, aquaponic where fish waste and water are used and hydroponic where solutions that are nutrient-rich are used to grow plants, hold most potential. Hydroponic greenhouses, for instance, on the roofs of houses in Chicago and New York now provide fresh vegetables for farmer's stores with shorter routes of transportation and storage times.

Rising demand for food that is healthy as well as sustainable, has the food industry keep an eye out for any novel technologies or food items. Also of significance is novel food, which is traditional food prepared for new markets. Aquatic plant cultivation (like seaweed) is a rapidly expanding traditional industry, where algaculture for consumption is now being exercised in around 50 countries. New food products that have reduced impact on the environment are being created as a result of evolving technologies and innovations. For instance, protein alternatives like mycoproteins are being derived from fungal biomass. Cellular agriculture is a growing industry that uses plant and animal cells to produce food in vitro such as gelatine, eggs, milk, and meat. Despite their potential, more research on the benefits and drawbacks of newly emerging food products as well as their involvement in nutritional and sustainable food systems, is required (Lindgren et al., 2018).

Ethnobotany is a science that studies the interactions between humans and plants. It is centered at the intersection of natural and social sciences. Bioprospecting for new botanically derived drugs and new food crops has traditionally relied on ethnobotanical data. For identification and detection of bioactive compounds from medicinal plants bioprospecting, which is ethnobotanically-led is becoming more effective than random assays. For example, oseltamivir was derived from *Illicium verum* Hook.f., amid the epidemic of bird flu, on the basis of ethnobotanical information from Chinese traditional medicine. Developing novel molecular tools have given rise to new perspectives. DNA sequencing allows for phylogenetic reconstruction with clustering of hot nodes of prospective plant species known traditionally for medicinal value. The use of identical or closely linked species of plants in varied cultures suggests that the knowledge was gained independently by distinct and noninteracting groups of humans. This is attributable to the reality that certain plants have similar morphological traits as a result of their close placement in terms of phylogeny, a concept called "evolutionary convergence." It was also proposed by certain research groups to label plants in one phylogenetic node, having resemblance in uses, with the expression "ethnobotanical convergence." Plants that have evolved in the same lineage have far more uses medicinally as compared to species that have evolved separately and the variation in medicinal use is linked to the species' evolutionary history. The use of spices as seasoning for two foods from distinct cultural and geographical regions act as a good example of ethnobotanical convergence. *Origanum vulgare* L. is used to season pizza in Western cultures, while another species of the same genus, *Origanum syriacum* L., is used to season a similar dish in the Near East called manousheh. Along with the approach of phylogeny, "omic" techniques producing large data sets and their analyses with the help of bioinformatics are valuable in detection of plants with established ethnobotanical uses, the plant taxa with most potential in culinary or medicinal use (Garnatje et al., 2017).

General metabolite profiles, both quantitative and qualitative in nature, are presented by metabolomics studies. When these profiles are derived from plants susceptible to a variety of environments, the information produced helps in evaluating the temporal and spatial distribution of phytochemicals in study and the impact of geographical and plant developmental cues. The impact of complex mixtures, like those commonly utilized in Chinese traditional medicine, can also be better understood with the help of metabolomics. The major challenge in research of natural products is understanding complex mixtures and designating the bioactive compounds. Untargeted metabolite profiling along with fractionation based on bioassays enhances bioactive compound identification. Detection of loci of significant metabolic quantitative trait through metabolomics can improve breeding techniques of medicinal plants. Thoroughly researched medicinal products and culinary ingredients may be developed through this approach of metabolomics. Combination of the two approaches—metabolomics and functional characterizations of products of genes based on genomic studies, enhance the speed of discovery of significant bioactive compounds and their novel biosynthetic pathways. This way the production and discovery of culinary and medicinal products is also improved. An example of this combination of ethnobotanical approach with "omic" technique is the FAD2 phytochemicals discovery, which took place in a bioengineered, nonplant host system. The discovery occurred after the metabolomes and transcriptomes of unusual fatty acid accumulating developing seeds were compared (Garnatje et al., 2017).

2.6 SUSTAINABLE USE OF TRADITIONAL MEDICINAL PLANTS

There is an increase in threat to extinction and erosion of medicinal plants in the wild and the general biodiversity in plants due to a rise in the pressure on forest ecosystems and unpredictable weather patterns. Urgent strategies that assist sustainable supplies catering to a rise in world demand in products derived from medicinal plants are required for the protection of these medicinal plants (Rajeswara Rao and Rajput, 2010). There has been considerable amount of study on utilization of medicinal plants in a sustainable manner. A number of suggestions regarding conservation have been gathered, along with adoption of structures for species monitoring as well as inventorying in combination with practices of conservation that involve both approaches of in situ and ex situ (Figure 2.3). These involve biodiversity management while maintaining its potential of satisfying the needs of the populations that come after us (Chen et al., 2016).

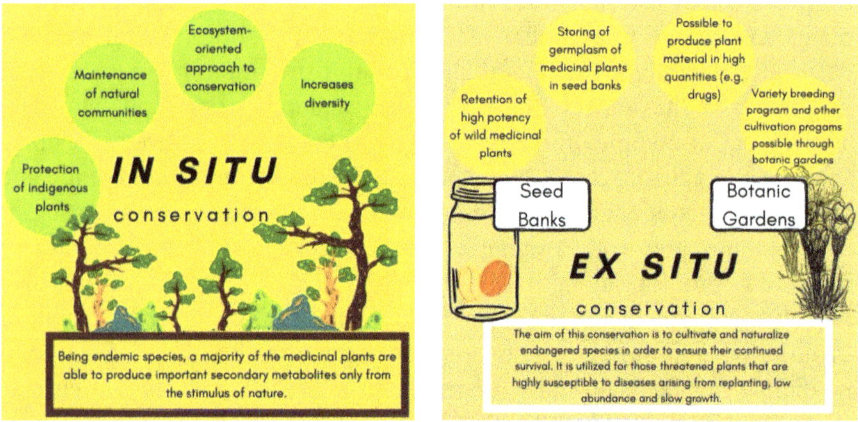
Maintenance of natural communities
Ecosystem-oriented approach to conservation
Increases diversity
Protection of indigenous plants
IN SITU
conservation
Being endemic species, a majority of the medicinal plants are able to produce important secondary metabolites only from the stimulus of nature.
Retention of high potency of wild medicinal plants
Storing of germplasm of medicinal plants in seed banks
Possible to produce plant material in high quantities (e.g. drugs)
Variety breeding program and other cultivation progams possible through botanic gardens
Seed Banks
Botanic Gardens
EX SITU
conservation
The aim of this conservation is to cultivate and naturalize endangered species in order to ensure their continued survival. It is utilized for those threatened plants that are highly susceptible to diseases arising from replanting, low abundance and slow growth.

(A) (B)

FIGURE 2.3 (A) In situ conservation and its advantages. (B) Ex situ conservation and its advantages (Chen et al., 2016).

The fact that medicinal plants have supplies that are extremely limited in nature, a viable conservation strategy might be utilization of wild resources in a sustainable manner. Over 50,000 species of plants are used in medicines and other products related to health, accounting for more than one-tenth of all species of plants. Yet, there is no uniformity in their worldwide distribution. The countries with the highest usage of medicinal plants are China with around 11,000 plant species and India with around 7500 plant species succeeded by 19 other nations with medicinal plant percentages varying from 7 to 44% in Malaysia and India, respectively. Particular families of plants have a greater percentage of endangered species than others, not just in terms of the number of medicinal plants they have. It is necessary to understand the biological properties and geographic distribution of medicinal plants in order to direct efforts related to conservation such as determining whether conservation of species should be carried out in a nursery or in nature.

The practice of domestic cultivation is a widely accepted one even though medicinal plant resources harvested from the wild are considered to be higher in efficacy. The production of medicinal plants encounters troubles such as erroneous identification of botanical origin, presence of active components in low amounts, contamination by pesticides, and presence of toxic components. Through the utilization of new techniques in cultivation, overcoming these troubles becomes easy. The advantages of controlled conditions of growth are—the production stability is ensured and production of bioactive components is enhanced. By practicing cultivation techniques, there is recovery of the wild resources of medicinal plants as there will be a decrease in the harvest of these plants and the cost is also reduced to a more affordable level (Chen et al., 2016).

There are arguments in support of and against the inclination toward cultivated or wild plants. This is mainly due to the outlook of communities who prefer wild plants as opposed to scientific facts and data. Wild plants differ in the secondary metabolites' concentration compared to cultivated plants. But these concentrations can be regulated under cultivation. Most companies merchandising in herbs are partial toward material from cultivated plants as their certification as organic or biodynamic is possible. International trade has been increasingly insisting on wild collections being certified. It is almost impossible to bring all species under cultivation immediately. Impetus should be given to cultivation at a smaller scale. This would mean an involvement of local communities also regulated harvests with regards to availability of populations thus encouraging natural proliferation (Rajeswara Rao and Rajput, 2010).

Certain medicinal plants are slow in growth and have a limited prevalence, therefore, overexploitation of their resources or overharvesting leads to exhaustion of resources and sometimes even extinction of species. This is why it is important to develop plans for good harvesting practices and use medicinal plants in a sustainable manner. Collection of flowers or buds and leaves of medicinal plants is a far less damaging than harvesting an entire plant or roots. A favorable alternative to drugs that are produced from root or whole plants, is utilizing the leaves as treatment. The discovery that roots and leaf stems of ginseng have equivalent pharmacological activities, for instance, makes the utilization of leaf stems more advantageous in terms of sustainability (Chen et al., 2016).

Nonscientific and unsustainable methods are used more often than not to source most of the biomass of medicinal plants from forests. CITES (Convention on International Trade in Endangered Species of Wild Flora and Fauna) guidelines are repeatedly ignored and exports and collections end up damaging local communities. Adverse effects of this are observed in the way of: reduced livelihood opportunities for locals, decline in government revenue, and biodiversity loss. This also goes against the essence of Convention on Biological Diversity objectives. The plethora of existing acts and laws fall short in curbing the menace. The administration of nations that undertake exports should emplace viable strategies for the protection of the biodiversity of medicinal plants as well as the interest of the locals. They should further ensure that the collections abide with the guidelines put in place by Guidelines of the Conservation of Medicinal Plants, WHO/IUCN/WWF (World Wide Fund for Nature), WHO Guidelines for Good Agricultural and Collection Practices for Medicinal Plants, International Standard for Sustainable Wild Collection of Medicinal Plants.

Due to globalization, markets have opened up benefitting transnational companies in countries that export medicinal plants. Indigenous knowledge needs protecting from biopiracy thus giving rise to threats and issues surrounding intellectual property rights. There is a clear increase in the worldwide demand for products derived through medicinal plants thus paving way for numerous opportunities to wisely utilize this resource via technology value addition, exports, and creation of employment in developing countries. Newer business can be established and technologies and innovations can advance if countries start to share resources, expertise, and ideas with each other. Some of the indicators of the direction of the medicinal plants field are nanotechnology, bioinformatics, inflammation technology, and biotechnology (metabolomics, proteomics, genomics). These are playing a vital role in fashioning the trends in future research.

The focus of the administrations needs to be directed toward creating an inventory of the resources of medicinal plants and native traditional knowledge thus aiding in cultivation as well as conservation of medicinal plants along with creation of wealth via this resource. Failures in regulated mechanisms deprive nations that are rich in biodiversity as well as the locals that strived to preserve it, their fair share in enterprise profits. There will be a continuous rise in harvesting natural population and depletion of species of medicinal plants unless necessary measures are initiated to remedy these concerns by cultivating these resources for a sustainable supply. R&D toward medicinal plants requires strengthening in developing economies to deal with the rivalry from multinational companies. The export of crude dried drugs should be discouraged while the export of value-added commodities should be encouraged. With a worldwide emphasis on natural elements in consumer goods, there seems to be a bright future for the medicinal plants field (Rajeswara Rao and Rajput, 2010).

2.7 HEALTH SECURITY: CHALLENGES AND ISSUES

A crucial element of human security is health security. For the promotion of food security and minimization of chemical and microbiological risks, for a number of populations, sanitation is provided and hygiene is ingrained. In a few places, occupational safety and controls for environmental contamination co-exist. But such protection is subject to the access to and existence of evidence-based, affordable and equitable management measures, diagnostic and preventive health.

Where there is an absence of health systems supporting populations, for a lot of people, fear of poverty because of catastrophic diseases or even slight injuries is real. There is a disparity with regards to the sector of global health where there are huge advances in success in some areas of the world while the others face a high scarcity. As reminded by the WHO, one-third of the world's population in underdeveloped and transition nations still lack access to important advanced health care. Due to improper financing by government administrations, even though there is a rise in financing by private sectors, access to human resources, and material for health care is limited.

Humanity in these regions is perennially plagued with the weight of communicable diseases such as tuberculosis, malaria, HIV, diarrheal diseases, and pneumonia along with chronic diseases like ischemic heart diseases, diabetes, etc. High child and maternal mortality and re-emerging diseases (lifestyle, chronic, and infectious) are the usual constraints to positive impacts of factors such as social (urbanization and fast changes in demographics), institutional (increase in health costs and privatization, centralized and vertical programmes having little regard to the local conditions, poor utilization of community health care, brain drain of medical practitioners), and biophysical (related epidemics and environmental changes). Conversely, health challenges faced by developed economies are ageing population, low fertility, lifestyle-related and chronic ailments, and growing fiscal burdens due to an increase in health care expenditure.

The urban-centered, advanced-technology-based, curative medicine has found a place across nations along with the global model for healthcare. In such systems, health planners have been confronted with many challenges of optimally combining promotive and preventive health with therapeutic medicine. Because of these continuing complex challenges, fundamentals of universal access basis contextual needs along with stress on primitive and preventive health via self-reliant, participatory, intersectoral alliance in various health plans remains an unaccomplished ideal. This reinforces the need of relying on independent models of healthcare distribution.

It is very clichéd to comment that regions rich in biodiversity in the southern parts are the ones that suffer most from partisanship in accessibility, availability, and inexpensive healthcare. With an increase in alienation of populations from natural environments because of numerous factors, a collateral depletion of cultural set-ups including health resources and applications base occurs giving rise to a situation in which even though relevant knowledge persists, the practice is quite poor.

Such depletion of practices is more accentuated by education systems that fail to understand the importance of such inherent methods or practices, thus distancing youngsters from exploring these areas. The implication of this is that it is not often for the absence of potency that traditional knowledge is rejected but it is due to inadequate socio-political structures. There is a well thought out social implication of this traditional knowledge being inexpensive, safe, and accessible health option for guaranteeing health security to scores of rural families. Therefore, traditional knowledge medicines are important to support due to the failures of mainstream medicine in delivery primary healthcare.

In the same way, traditional health professionals in a community health situation are understood as bridging a gap in mainstream healthcare access. It is necessary to understand that in a lot of societies traditional medicine does play a vital complementary role parallel to the mainstream modern healthcare system and this fact needs to be better acknowledged and appreciated. This requires a multidimensional approach where numerous resources need convergence, including the ones in relation with local healthcare traditions.

As the last 20 years have shown us, there is an increased relevance in bringing biodiversity conservation objectives in line with the public health approach. At present, traditional knowledge health practices are being boosted either by states, which majorly focus on healthcare delivery; by organization of civil society whose focus is on health and conservation; or private sectors via marketing and production of supplements, healthcare services, and medicines. Coordinated policy focus on various junctions providing health resources, various governance measures, and practices remains insufficient. Even though there exist several reports independently highlighting concerns related to the use of traditional medicines or biological resources (for instance, IUCN and WHO reports); studies comprehensively addressing issues related to sustainable use, conservation, and biological resources related equity; along with concerns related to impartial access to efficacious nutrition and healthcare, and biocultural resources and human resources required there under to accomplish development objectives at the governance of local level are very few. Most studies concentrate on health linkages and biodiversity of resources in relation to modern pharmaceuticals and only some focus from the perspective of community health (Biodiversity, 2013).

The idea of global health security supports the current regulations for global response and preparedness to the emergence of infectious diseases. The agenda of Global Health Security that is a collaboration among governments had been launched in the year 2014, and it aimed at the safety of the interconnected world from threats of infectious diseases. The governments participating in the agenda of Global Health Security focus on building up their nations' capacities for prevention, detection, and response. In the public health-related emergencies context, political and financial support has been received for the Agenda from almost 50 countries and international organizations.

Global health security leans toward emphasizing containment of diseases in the interest of protection of national security as against prevention of upcoming local outbreaks. Containment of diseases is a common practice in the action of controlling emergence of infectious diseases. Perspective of national security more often than not results in neo-colonial, unilateral, short-term solutions fashioned to protect the national borders. For instance, several nations and their airline industries-imposed travel curtailments during the outbreak of the Ebola virus in 2013–2016 in West Africa, contradictory to the recommendations of the WHO.

Respect toward human values and rights such as solidarity and equity should underlie every agenda of national security. These values are aligned with motives of a lot of people providing healthcare services in emergencies of public health. The agenda of health security should concentrate on building resilience to infectious disease outbreaks that may arise in the future, and necessitate a systematic long-term approach basis surveillance as well as strengthening of the national health systems. Shielding the populations from the threats of infectious disease requires that governments shoulder the responsibilities of serving the ones in need on priority, wherever they may live (Flahault et al., 2016).

2.8 CONCLUSION

Populations around the world are increasingly accepting the traditional knowledge of medicines to satisfy their healthcare needs. Although ongoing public support is retaining as well as encouraging the growth of traditional systems in both developed and developing nations, there is a disconnect in preference of the people and the efforts made nations and institutions for integration. It is obvious that any healthcare model relying on a single system of medicine would struggle to meet potential demands in terms of healthcare in the foreseeable future. It is critical not to glamourize traditional medicinal systems but rather to critically consider issues of quality, efficacy, and safety as well as rational usage and access through effective policy interventions and incorporate them into the conventional healthcare sector without jeopardizing their key characteristics and diversity.

The contribution of neglected crops in regions where they were adopted are too numerous. These crops were able to survive for many years despite the everchanging climate and provided for the necessitous rural populations. This is reason enough for the promotion of these crops as contributors in nutrition and food security. Allocation of resources, research and development initiatives, policy support, and strong advocacy will be needed.

The question on how we can make the discovery of new plants more orderly is answered by the use of ethnobotanical data along with molecular tools such as DNA sequencing. Even though the combination of "omics" and metabolomics have demonstrated to be of great value, metabolite identification at a large scale still remains a challenge. That being said, with further development in this field, we can look forward to improved tools of discovery.

Advances in medicinal plant tissue culture have emerged as a powerful tool for the large-scale and highly efficient processing of valuable bioactive components, and advances in genetic engineering have made large-scale natural product biosynthesis feasible, thereby boosting conservation and sustainable use of medicinal plants. It is a strong belief that the idea of global health security should be broadened to include sustainability and solidarity. This is how we can ensure the development of a long-term strategy as well as overcome the constraints relating to the current responses toward emergencies of global health.

KEYWORDS

- **health security**
- **human health**
- **medicinal plants**
- **nutritional value**
- **traditional knowledge**

REFERENCES

Bessada, S. M. F.; Barreira, J. C. M.; Oliveira, M. B. P. P. Pulses and Food Security: Dietary Protein, Digestibility, Bioactive and Functional Properties. *Trends Food Sci. Technol.* **2019,** *93*, 53–68.

Biodiversity, Traditional Knowledge and Community Health: Strengthening Linkages, 2013. Iuncbd.org. http://www.iuncbd.org/biodiversity-and-health/biodiversity-traditional-knowledge-and-community-health-strengthening-linkages.

Carneiro da Silva, A.; da Costa Santos, D.; Lopes Teixeira Junior, D.; Bento da Silva, P.; Cavalcante dos Santos, R.; Siviero, A. Cowpea: A Strategic Legume Species for Food Security and Health. In *Legume Seed Nutraceutical Research*. IntechOpen, 2019.

Chen, S.-L.; Yu, H.; Luo, H.-M.; Wu, Q.; Li, C.-F.; Steinmetz, A. Conservation and Sustainable Use of Medicinal Plants: Problems, Progress, and Prospects. *Chin. Med.* **2016,** *11* (1), 37.

Dias-Martins, A. M.; Pessanha, K. L. F.; Pacheco, S.; Rodrigues, J. A. S.; Carvalho, C. W. P. Potential Use of Pearl Millet (*Pennisetum glaucum* (L.) R. Br.) in Brazil: Food Security, Processing, Health Benefits and Nutritional Products. *Food Res. Int. (Ottawa, Ont.)* **2018,** *109*, 175–186.

Dixit, G. P.; Parihar, A. K.; Bohra, A.; Singh, N. P. Achievements and Prospects of Grass Pea (*Lathyrus sativus* L.) Improvement for Sustainable Food Production. *Crop J.* **2016,** *4* (5), 407–416.

Flahault, A.; Wernli, D.; Zylberman, P.; Tanner, M. From Global Health Security to Global Health Solidarity, Security and Sustainability. *Bull. World Health Org.* **2016,** *94* (12), 863.

Garnatje, T.; Peñuelas, J.; Vallès, J. Ethnobotany, Phylogeny, and "Omics" for Human Health and Food Security. *Trends Plant Sci.* **2017,** *22* (3), 187–191.

Growing at a Slower Pace, World Population Is Expected to Reach 9.7 Billion in 2050 and Could Peak at Nearly 11 Billion Around 2100, June 17, 2019. https://www.un.org/development/desa/en/news/population/world-population-prospects-2019.html

IARC Working Group on the Evaluation of Carcinogenic Risks to Humans. Some Traditional Herbal Medicines, Some Mycotoxins, Naphthalene and Styrene. *IARC Monogr. Eval. Carcinogenic Risks Humans* **2002,** *82*, 43–68.

Karunamoorthi, K.; Jegajeevanram, K.; Vijayalakshmi, J.; Mengistie, E. Traditional Medicinal Plants: A Source of Phytotherapeutic Modality in Resource-Constrained Health Care Settings. *J. Evid.-Based Complement. Altern. Med.* **2013,** *18* (1), 67–74.

Lindgren, E.; Harris, F.; Dangour, A. D.; Gasparatos, A.; Hiramatsu, M.; Javadi, F. et al. Sustainable Food Systems-a Health Perspective. *Sustain. Sci.* **2018,** *13* (6), 1505–1517.

Mothibe, M. E.; Sibanda, M. African Traditional Medicine: South African Perspective. *Trad. Complem. Med.* IntechOpen, 2019.

Pan, S.-Y.; Litscher, G.; Gao, S.-H.; Zhou, S.-F.; Yu, Z.-L.; Chen, H.-Q. et al. Historical Perspective of Traditional Indigenous Medical Practices: The Current Renaissance and Conservation of Herbal Resources. *Evid.-Based Complemen. Altern. Med.: ECAM* **2014,** *2014*, 525340.

Payyappallimana, U. Role of Traditional Medicine in Primary Health Care: An Overview of Perspectives and Challenges. *Yokohama J. Soc. Sci.* **2010,** *14* (6), 57–77.

Rajeswara Rao, B. R.; Rajput, D. K. Global Scenario of Medicinal Plants. Researchgate.net, 2010. https://www.researchgate.net/publication/274341699_GLOBAL_SCENARIO_OF_MEDICINAL_PLANTS

Ramalingum, N.; Mahomoodally, M. F. The Therapeutic Potential of Medicinal Foods. *Adv. Pharmacol. Sci.* **2014,** *2014*, 354264.

Regional Expert Consultation on Underutilized Crops for Food and Nutritional Security in Asia and the Pacific, 13–15 November 2017, Bangkok, Thailand, 2017. Apaari.org. https://www.apaari.org/web/regional-expert-consultation-uuc.

Ulian, T.; Diazgranados, M.; Pironon, S.; Padulosi, S.; Liu, U.; Davies, L. et al. Unlocking Plant Resources to Support Food Security and Promote Sustainable Agriculture. *Plants, People, Planet* **2020,** *2* (5), 421–445.

Wahlqvist, M. L.; Keatinge, J. D. H.; Butler, C. D.; Friel, S.; McKay, J.; Easdown, W. et al. A Food in Health Security (FIHS) Platform in the Asia-Pacific Region: The Way Forward. *Asia Pac. J. Clin. Nutr.* **2019,** *18* (4), 688–702.

Weststrate, J. A.; van Poppel, G.; Verschuren, P. M. Functional Foods, Trends and Future. *Br. J. Nutr.* **2002,** *88* (S2), S233–S235.

World Health Organization. WHO Global Report on Traditional and Complementary Medicine. World Health Organization, 2019. https://apps.who.int/iris/handle/10665/312342.

World Health Organization. WHO Traditional Medicine Strategy: 2014–2023. World Health Organization, 2013. https://apps.who.int/iris/handle/10665/92455.

Yuan, H.; Ma, Q.; Ye, L.; Piao, G. The traditional medicine and Modern Medicine from Natural Products. *Mol. (Basel, Switzerland)* **2016,** *21* (5), 559.

PART II
Ethnomedicinal Flora

CHAPTER 3

Traditional Herbal Treatments in Karabakh-Azerbaijan

SAYYARA J. IBADULLAYEVA[1], AYTEKIN A. ASGEROVA[2], ASMAR E. HUSEYNOVA[3], AFIG T. MAMMADOV[4], and IRADA M. HUSEYNOVA[5]

[1]*Institute of Botany, Azerbaijan National Academy of Sciences, Baku, Azerbaijan*

[2]*Azerbaijan State Agrarian University, Ganja, Azerbaijan*

[3]*Baku State University, Baku AZ, Azerbaijan*

[4]*Genetic Resources Institute, Azerbaijan National Academy of Sciences, Baku, Azerbaijan*

[5]*Institute of Molecular Biology & Biotechnologies, Azerbaijan National Academy of Sciences, Azerbaijan*

ABSTRACT

This chapter is devoted to the ethnic use of wild medicinal plants in the flora of the Karabakh region in Azerbaijan. The species reported from the center are 1316 and from the southern parts 1250 species. The area belongs to the botanical–geographical regions of the Lesser Caucasus. The current study is based on surveys of local communities because the territories were under the occupation of Armenia for during the last three decades. Previous published

Ethnic Knowledge and Perspectives of Medicinal Plants, Volume 1: Curative Properties and Treatment Strategies. Munir Ozturk, Kandikere R. Sridhar, Maryam Sarwat, Volkan Altay, & Francisco Martín Huerta-Martínez (Eds.)

data has revealed that more than 2500 plants are distributed in Karabagh. Out of these ethnobotanical features, nearly 101 species have been recorded in the scientific literature, being widely used in folk medicine. The data presented reveals that some of the plants are characteristic for a specific area, and their distribution areal is limited to Karabagh, for example, *Sanguisorba officinalis* and *Salvia karabachenses*. Nearly 61 species of perennial grasses are found to predominate in the area, followed by 13 species of trees and shrubs and 8 tree species. These are used differently when compared to the other regions. Some of the species are not found in the wild in the Karabagh region, they are cultivatd and used as medicinal plants like, *Tanacetum vulgare, Rosmarinus officinalis, Pimpinella anisum, Papaver somniferum,* and *Mentha piperita.*

3.1 INTRODUCTION

Long-term and detailed botanical-systematic, geobotanical studies, as well as the data published in the classical sources show that 70% of the species from Karabakh are found in other parts of Azerbaijan as well. It is a small part of the Caucasus (Grossheim, 1949; Conspectus of the Caucasus Flora, 2003–2006). According to the latest data, 4961 higher plant species belonging to 159 family and 1117 genera are distributed in Azerbaijan (Askerov, 2016), of which more than 1500 are medicinal (Damirov, 1970; Ibadullayeva and Alakbarov, 2013), up to 800 aromatic—spice plants (Ibadullayeva and Jafarli, 2007), about 200 wild vegetables (Gasimov et al., 2009) and other useful plants (Gasimov et al., 2006; Ibadullayeva et al., 2010, 2012; Ibadullayeva and Shahmuradova, 2015). More than 26.52% of the plants recorded from Azerbaijan (1316 species) are distributed in Garabakh as well (Flora of Azerbaijan, 1952–1961).

Karabakh is located in the central part of the Lesser Caucasus botanical–geographical region of Azerbaijan. The area has a rich flora and dense vegetation, including dense forests, mountain meadows, and other types of plant cover. There are different versions of the origin of the name Karabakh. The most accepted one is in the ancient Azerbaijani-Turkish language, the word “black” means “large,” and bakh means the “garden,” that is, Karabakh means “Large Black Garden.” The region is also distinguished by the richness of medicinal plants. According to ancient Greek scholars, in the antique period and the early Middle Ages, Karabakh was part of the Albanian state. Based on manuscripts, in the first century AD, Caucasian Albania exported medicinal plants in glass boxes to Rome. Apparently, since ancient times, Karabakh has served as a rich source of medicinally valuable plants in the world (Alekperli, 2001). The territory of Azerbaijan is one of the "hot-spots of biodiversity" in the world. Garabakh is one of the ancient and eternal territories of Azerbaijan. The importance of studying the cultural interactions of this region includes cultural richness, antiquity, and diversity of manifestations in its territories. A large part of the region's population has lived as refugees and settled in other areas for many years as a result of aggression by other nations. Our main goal is to enlighten the ethnic use of medicinal plants from Karabakh, following the return of this terretory to the Azerbaijan. In view of the latest developments, we have conducted an ethnobotanical analysis of this area. It was important to collect information on the experience of the people regarding plant use at present and in the past (Damirov et al., 1988; Ibadullayeva et al., 2013). Since the Stone Age, people living in groups around Karabakh have used plants both as medicine as well as food. We are presenting the data here about the medicinal plants.

Out of over 300,000 flowering plants in the world, more than 60% have been and are used as medicine and food (Ozturk et al., 2021a, b). In recent years, people are collecting medicinal plants not only from the wild but are also growing these in the controlled greenhouses, as an integral part of human civilization currently (Ozturk and Hakeem, 2018, 2019a, b; Ozturk et al., 2017a, b, c, 2018a, b, c, 2020, 2021a, b).

There is great need to pool up and renew the information about plants constantly which should be communicated to the people (Ozturk et al., 2018a, b, c). In Karabakh, the protection of plants is an emotional task and "occupies the main agenda" as an issue of Azerbaijan after the liberation of occupied territory. The war in the area during last three decades, overgrowth of invasive plants, and excessive collection of some plants has led to a decline in plant sources in the area, together with noncompliance with post-harvest regulations as well as lack of control mechanisms, have increased a great pressure on its biodiversity. Ethnobotanical studies in the region can help in the production of new medicines for the treatment of diseases. The both ethnobotany and ethnopharmacology are widely used to search for new compounds (Oksana et al., 2021; Ibadullayeva, 2020).

There is great wisdom in the saying of Hippocrates (460–370 BC) which mentions that "let the food be your medicine, and medicine your food." The traditionally used herbal medicines occur naturally and are used to treat the diseases depending on the local or regional healing customs used. These are prepared from the selective plants without industrial processing. Traditional herbal medicines growning in Karabakh also play an important role in the strategy of prevention and the treatment of acute respiratory syndrome, and the antiviral diseases. Many new preparations from these plants are currently being developed. The research on traditional herbal remedies is expected to play a crucial role in global health cure system. Significant research investments in traditional herbal medicines are being made by China, India, Nigeria, the United States (US), and the WHO (Ghulam et al., 2018). With increasing attention and public funding on the study of traditional herbal medicines, more detailed analysis of regions and ethnic applications are needed. For years, the classical world pharmacopeias have described a large number of herbal medicines used to treat various diseases (Pleskanovskaya et al., 2019; Hamzah et al., 2020; Khan et al., 2020; Masoodi et al., 2020; Ozturk et al., 2020, 2021a, b). These are today considered alternative medicine. Scientific evidence and clinical validation of herbal medicines require a rigorous approach that includes chemical standardization, biological analysis, animal models, and clinical trials (Ibadullayeva et al., 2017; Ozturk et al., 2020, 2021a, b). In industrialized countries, methodologies take into account the complexity of chemicals and how they can be used for treating human diseases (Ozturk and Hakeem, 2018, 2019a, b). Even during surgery (before and after surgery), treatment with herbal medicines is continued and more satisfactory results are obtained from such applications. All this has created a need for ethnobotanical research in different regions of the Lesser Caucasus botanical–geographical region of Azerbaijan, and such studies were conducted by us (Ibadullayeva and Shahmuradova, 2015; Ibadullayeva and Abbasova, 2018; Ozturk et al., 2018a, b, c).

The plants traditionally used in the territory of Karabakh were analyzed by Petrov (1940) about 80 years ago. His work has its own characteristics, both in terms of theme and approach to the topic. The book contains extremely important materials not only for ethnobotanists but also for phytopharmacists. During the present evaluations we found that some plants (trees and perennial grasses) do not play an important role in the economic activity of the population. However, in olden days, plants were used not only for domestic purpose but also occupied the ideology and culture of the public in the area. Authors have noted that the materials collected from Karabakh did not fully cover the plants used by the population. They studied wild food plants and determined whether they were used as medicine. The occupation of 20% of the lands of Azerbaijan over the past 30 years has prevented any research in the region. The occupation forces did not write a single sentence about the plant diversity and ethnobotany of the area.

Taking all this into account, after independence of Karabakh, our first task was to pool up the ethnobotanical data on traditional medicinal plants used in

Karabakh. We feel ethnobotany is a hybrid science therefore it is necessary to draw conclusions from historical, political, archeological, economic, and scientific facts.

3.2 HISTORY OF FOLK MEDICINE IN KARABAKH

Ancient Azerbaijani manuscripts have revealed that more than 700 medicinal plants were used by the inhabitants of Karabakh in the Middle Ages. The territory is famous for its rich vegetation, amazing greenry, dense forests, mountain meadows, vast fields, and the wide range of landscapes rich in medicinal plants. Among these, the "Khari-bulbul" (*Ophris caucasica*) is a symbol of the city of Shusha, the historical center of Karabakh. Information about the development of medicine in Caucasian Albania can be found in the work of local historian Moisey Kalankatuylu "History of the Albanian country." He noted that "in order to achieve perfection, it is necessary to deal with sciences such as mathematics, agronomy, and medicine" (Figure 3.1).

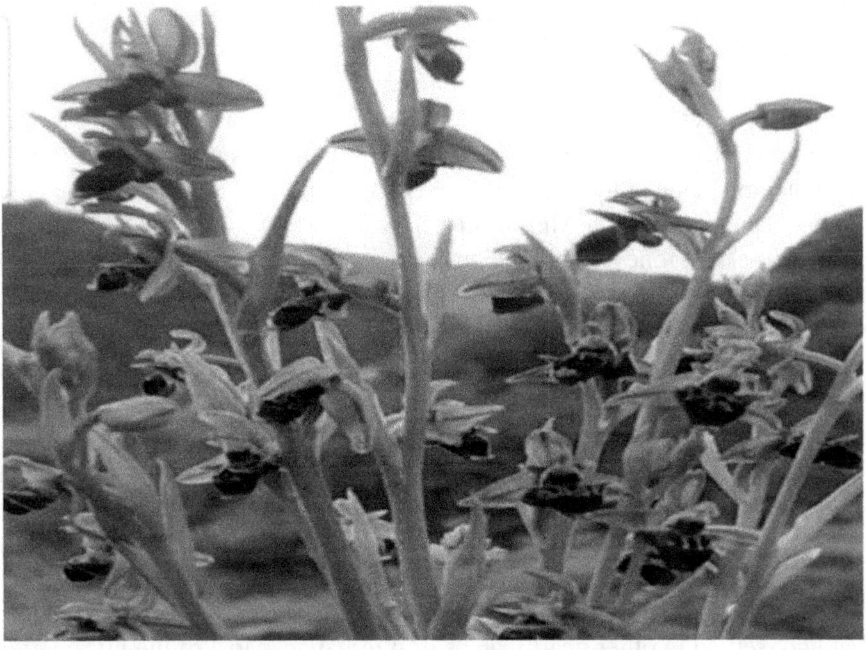

FIGURE 3.1 "Khari-bulbul" (*Ophris caucasica* Woronow ex Grossh).

During the Christian era in Caucasian Albania in the first century AD, Syrian and Greek medicine found way to the area. This happened through Albanian church schools in Karabakh, where students got acquainted with the work of ancient doctors like Hippocrates and Galen. Nestorian physicians came to this area from the Byzantine Empire, Syria, Greece, and Iran. All these played an important role in the development of medicine in Karabakh in the 4th–5th centuries. They established the famous Jundishapur (Gondishapur) Medical Academy in Iran and staff from this place repeatedly visited Karabakh, providing medical services to the local population. Alongside the professional medicinal treatments, common remedies widespread in Karabakh were treated by the national medicine men. In the Middle Ages, medicinal plants were widely used in witchcraft and surgery by Turkish people. National surgeons, specialists who treated fractures, were popularly called "sinikhchi," and otolaryngologists were called "chopchu." One of the most famous doctors of Azerbaijan in the 16th century was Yusif Karabakhi, who was called a "genius teacher." He was born in Karabakh, spent most of his life and work in Central Asia, and taught at a madrasa in Samarkand. Turkish people created a historical treasure with national ethnobiological features by using plants extensively in medicine, food, clothing, dyeing, and other household activities. The Azerbaijan scientists and physicians described 724 species of plants and 150 species of animals, 115 medicinal minerals, and more than 800 medicines with complex components in their works long back (Alekperli, 2001). Abu Ali ibn Sina (980–1037) moved from Hamadan to Azerbaijan in about 1001–1010. He studied the features of national medicine in the cities of Karabakh, Ganja, and Khoy, and noted this in his manuscripts (Abu Ali Ibn Sina, 1982).

Karabakh is one of the ancient settlements of the Turkish (Albanian) people, but in the 19th century Armenians from Iran, as well as the inhabitants from Udin ethnos from the Gabala region of Azerbaijan moved to this area and formed a community of different ethnic groups, all accepted the Gregorian religion. The newcomers had partially acquired traditional knowledge and skills from the local population, including the use of plants. In the 1990s, Karabakh was occupied by other nations, the surrounding areas were devastated during the three decades of occupation. The local inhabitants were looted, pastures, meadows, natural resources, and forests where medicinal plants grew were repeatedly burnt during 30 years. Azerbaijanis living in Karabakh and surrounding areas were expelled from their homes and got settled in other nearby areas of Azerbaijan. Most of the information on the use of useful plants has been lost in this way.

One of the ancient centers of herbal treatment is the Gabala-Ismayilli zone. The city was located in the territory of Caucasian Albania in ancient and medieval times. Excavations have uncovered the remains of a medical pharmaceutical laboratory, as well as a large number of medicines and perfumes stored in clay and glass containers; a distillation device for extracting oil from medicinal plants has also been found. The Udin tribes moved to Karabakh from Gabala surroundings and spread their ethnic knowledge in the area. During excavations near Karabakh, containers for storing medicines were also found in the city of Beylagan.

In the 12th century, Karabakh was already a part of the Atabey Eldeniz state of Azerbaijan, with Tabriz as its capital. During this period, there were medical schools, pharmacies, and hospitals in Beylagan and Barda, and well-known specialists in medicine conducted experiments there. Karabakh doctors attended medical schools in large cities of Azerbaijan, such as Tabriz, Ganja, and Shamakhi. In Shamakhi, they took lessons from Kafiyaddin Omar (12th century), the uncle of the famous poet Khagani Shirvani and the founder of the "Melhem" Medical Academy. In the 16th century, Yusif Karabakhi, one of the most famous doctors of Azerbaijan, was already known throughout Asia. The search for and discovery of new remedies for diseases and similar issues have long been influenced by Sufi ideas and views. In the Middle Ages, despite all external influences in Karabakh and nearby territories, the search for new remedies, as well as more affordable forms and methods of application, continued. The names and rules of use of many medicinal plants are available shown in the works of Nizami Ganjavi in the 12th century, and four centuries later in the works of Mohammad Fuzuli. The therapeutic value of mummy (in organ damage), saffron (in cold and fever), pumpkin (against worms and diarrhea), mint (in gastrointestinal diseases) have been described in Nizami Ganjavi's famous "Khamsa." The great Azerbaijani poet and thinker of the 16th century M. Fuzuli gave extensive medicinal information in his works "Sahhat and Maraz," "Sohbatul Asmar." For example, "Sohbatul Asmar" discusses the medicinal value, benefits, and harms of fruits. Well-known scientists and artists from Karabakh also mentioned the useful plants used in the area and provided information on their use.

Karabakh borders Iran. It has its own peculiarities in folk medicine. Two directions in the development of medicine and pharmacology have been noted. First, besides local medicines, preparations imported from neighboring countries and other developed countries were widely used in the cities, suburbs, and border areas. In the cities, this work was carried out by special people, professionals in this field, doctors, and physicians who knew different languages. Based on the achievements of medicine, they used Arabic books on pharmacology and pharmacy ("Garabaddini")—pharmacopeias. The Attars were mainly engaged in the purchase and sale of medicines and were less involved in treatment. They were the owners of pharmacies called "Eastern pharmacies" and were popularly known as "nuskhaband"s (nuskha-prescription, band-letter). In addition to selling and using ready-made medicines, "nuskhaband"s were also involved in the production of prescription drugs. Solutions of some cultivated plants (Pepper—*Piper capsicum*, Saffron—*Crocus sativa*, Cumin—*Cuminum cyminum*, Dill—*Anethum graveolens*, Pomegranate—*Punica granatum*, etc.) are examples of medicines used during those periods. The preparation of opium from the heads of tulips (*Papaver somniferum*) was also known. Information about all this is found in the poems of Natavan, the daughter of Karabakh Khan.

The second direction of folk medicine was developed far from the cities—in the remote mountainous provinces. One of such territories was the Karabakh region. Karabakh had its unique flora and vegetation, and the local Albanian-Turkish population was well acquainted with and used medicinal plants. Later, the Armenian tribes settled in Karabakh, used the plants for the same purpose. It should also be noted that the population of Karabakh was composed entirely of Azerbaijanis until the early 19th century. After the invasion of Azerbaijan by the Russian Empire, Armenians from neighboring countries were relocated from time to time, thereby displacing the local population. In Armenian-language sources, the region is called "Arsakh," but it is interesting that the root of this word originates from the ancient Turks. The original form of the word was "Arsak," which was also associated with the existence of Turkic-speaking Sak tribes in that area.

The first inscriptions on the ancient monuments discovered in the territory of Karabakh indicate that the plants were used for medicinal purposes. Azerbaijani Turks have created a historical treasure with national ethnobiological features in medicine, food, clothing, dyeing, and household activities.

Throughout the history, Azerbaijan has been in contact with the culture, science, and medicine of other nations and countries, especially the occupying powers. This, in turn, certainly had an impact on the development of medicine. For example, during the rule of the Arab caliphate, the culture, science, and medicine of the Arabs spread throughout the territory of the caliphate, including Karabakh in Azerbaijan. One of the significant events in the field of medicine and pharmacology at that time was the establishment of first treatment and prevention centers, albeit in a primitive form. These included hospitals (darush-shefa), pharmacies (ajzachikhana), and medical educational institutions (medical madrasas). The discovered historical data and manuscripts of those periods are characterized by the emergence of the first pharmaceutical centers in Karabakh. These centers of medicine were headed by Attars. The Attars were mainly engaged in the collection, drying, and processing of medicinal plants, as well as the sale of medicines in their primitively organized small shops. According to the manuscripts of Attars and doctors from that time, herbs, flowers, roots, seeds, fruits, fruit barks, rhizomes, and leaves of various plants were widely used in the folk medicine of the area in various medicinal forms (infusions, preparations, aromatic waters, solutions, etc.).

The spread of Azerbaijani science and historical treasures in the world, which has ancient roots, is a powerful blow to the myth that our neighbors are the most ancient people in the Caucasus. It should also be noted that each field of science and research has its own origin, history, and path of development. Historical origin and development have ethnic bases in all spheres of life. Certain features are tested over the centuries and passed down from generation to generation to create a national-ethnic style. The analysis of the national ethnobiological aspects of Azerbaijan confirm the deep intellectual power of our people since ancient times.

3.3 KARABAKH FLORA—PRESENT

Azerbaijan is floristically divided into 20 botanical–geographical regions: around the Caspian Sea. The flora is represented by 1200 species; distributed in Absheron (1000), Gobustan (1200), Kur-Araz lowland (1215), Kur plain (1205), Bozdagh range (1190), Lankaran—Mughan (1500), mountainous part of Lankaran (1107), Diabar-Zuvand (1107), Lankaran lowland (1205), Nakhchivan plains (1175), mountainous part of Nakhchivan (2700), Samur-Davachi lowland (1145), Greater Caucasus—Guba Mountain Range (1700), East of the Greater Caucasus (1205), West of the Greater Caucasus (1105), North of the Lesser Caucasus (1203), Central of the Lesser Caucasus (1316), South of the Lesser Caucasus (1250), and Alazan-Ayrichay Valley (1100). No information has been obtained for many years on the state of forests, steppes, meadows, and wetlands of two of the three botanical geographical regions (central and southern parts of the Lesser Caucasus), including Karabakh. Only from the research carried out till the 1990s, the collected literature data and satellite images have provided necessary information on these territories. Based on this information, 400 species of trees and shrubs are spread in Karabakh, 70 of these are native and some are endemics: *Taxus baccata*, *Quercus boissieri* (=*Q. araxina*), *Pterocarya fraxinifoli*, *Pinus eldarica*, *Buxus microphylla*, *B. sempervirens*, *Pyrus eldarica*, *P. salicifolia*, *Vitis sylvestris*, *P. granatum*, *Platanus orientalis*, etc. (Figure 3.2). The mountainous areas of the Lesser Caucasus consist of six ranges. The flora of half of these territories (Karabakh, Zangazur, and Daralayaz ranges) was under occupation for many years. The forest fund of Karabakh was 247,352 ha, of which 13,197.5 ha consisted of valuable forest trees. Before the occupation, 152 natural monuments and five geological objects were registered from the area. During the occupation, 986 ha of the state forest fund, 560 ha of tugai forests (riverine forests), and 710 ha of kolkhoz forests consisting of valuable tree species were destroyed and nothing remains today. Six oriental plane (*P. orientalis*) trees (150–250 ages old) in Aghdam city, 8 in the villages of Shelli, Seyidli, Sarihajili, Aliaghali villages (200–250 years old), and 71 in the vicinity of Boyahmedli village (400 years old) which had been protected as a natural monument and certified have been destroyed.

Valuable beech, linden, hornbeam, and oak trees have been cut down and burned. These areas include 26,000 ha of forest in Lachin, Kalbajar, and Aghdara districts, and forests were destroyed. The only natural Platanus forest in Europe was in the western part of the Lesser Caucasus in the Zangilan region, but during the long occupation, a wood processing plant was built there, and Platanus trees were cut from 117 ha.

The areal range of some plants is limited to Karabakh. Because the area has not been completely cleared of mines and few other security problems, it was not possible to conduct monitoring in the area, to obtain full information about the current state of the plants belonging only to Karabakh. The centers of basic diversity, distribution of the hereditary diversity, the intensity of species formation need to be determined using plant systematics approach. We do not have full information about the current plant diversity, their population indicators, habitats, and the latest state of phytocenology in the region which remained under occupation for almost 30 years. In some of its territories, wild plants have been completely destroyed by the invaders and narcotic plants grown on these sites. The anthropogenic impact on the nature of Karabakh has led to a reduction or complete extinction of several valuable plants. In the broad-leaved forests of the Lesser Caucasus, the Goygol National Park has been established to preserve the genepool of *Quercus iberica*, *G. macranthera*, especially *P. eldarica*, one of the world's rare

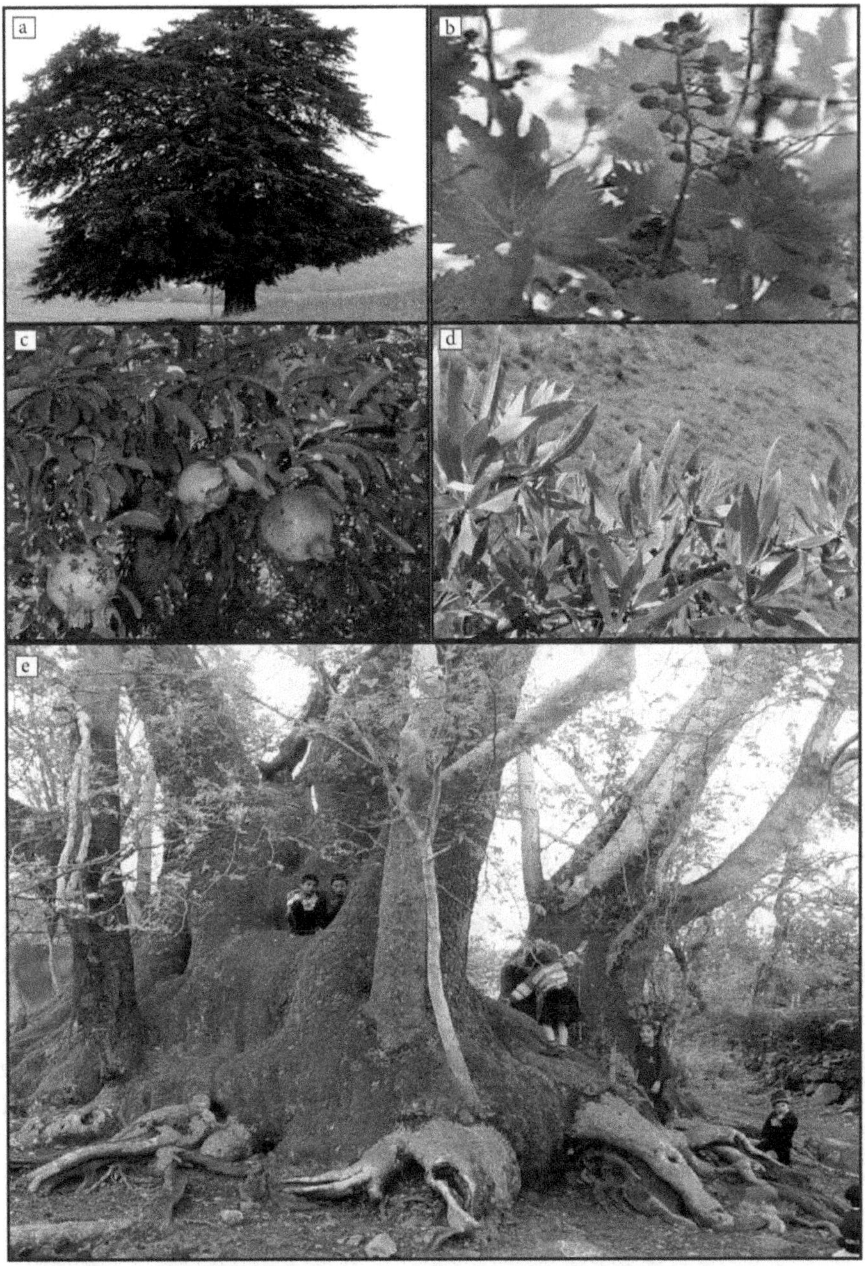

FIGURE 3.2 Some represantive examples of trees and shrubs of Karabagh.

(*Note*: **a**: *Taxus baccata;* **b**: *Vitis sylvestris*; **c**: *P. granatum*; **d**: *Pyrus eldarica*; **e**: *P. orientalis* (870 years old tree)).

"pearls." This park, where most Karabakh plants were collected, is located 20 km from the Kalbajar region.

The first proposal in this connection will be to create a new national park after studying the biodiversity of the area.Vegetation of Karabakh includes semideserts and semisteppes in vertical zoning (up to 400 m above sea level) followed by steppe vegetation (400–800 m), mesophilic forests (1000–2000 m), high mountain vegetation (2000–2500 m), alpine-subalpine vegetation (2200–3000 m), rocky vegetation (Murovdagh area over 3000 m), and wetland vegetation around the rivers and lake deltas. Sugovushan and other wetlands of Karabakh and plants of these territories with their unique features must be investigated at length.

Typical landscapes of Karabakh are highly notable for their scenic views, endemics, relict and endangered species, trees, gardens and parks, waterfalls, caves, lakes, wells, and other places. More than 2000 plants are included in the list of natural monuments. They include oriental plane, pine, chestnut, pear, beech, oak, mulberry, linden, buxus, etc. Most of the 140 rare and endangered plants included in the first edition of the Red Book of Azerbaijan ("Red Book" of the Azerbaijan SSR, 1989) were found in Karabakh. The current state of "nature pearls" such as *Ophrys caucasica*—mountain orchid (khari-bulbul), Shusha astragalus, yew (garachohre), Karabakh tulip, Maryam pea, Shusha sainfoin, Azat tree (*Zelkova*), *Shtrenbergiya* is still less known globally.

The second edition of the "Red Book" of the Republic of Azerbaijan was published in 2013. However, it was impossible to obtain any new information about the plants distributed in the occupied territories of Karabakh, including Fizuli, Agdam, Jabrayil, Zangilan, Gubadli, Kalbajar, Shusha, etc. reserves (Garagol and Basitchay reserves). All these were occupied and the state reserves (Gubadli, Arazboyu, Dashalti, and Lachin) were negatively affected by such anthropogenic impacts. The Basitchay State Nature Reserve is located in the Basitchay valley of the Zangilan region, an area of 100 ha covered with plane tree forests. Theser shold be re-evaluated. Garagol State Nature Reserve covers the highlands of the Lachin region. More than 100 plants were protected there before the occupation. The most memorable of the reserves is the Hajishamli forest in Lachin, where red oak was protected. Another protected area had been created in Gubadli and Lachin and named as Gubadli State Nature Reserve. This reserve was covered with Golden oak, walnut, hornbeam, maple, hawthorn, juniper, and other valuable tree species. Currently no information was available on the latest status of the Dashalti State Nature Sanctuary in the Shusha and Khojaly territories and the Arazboyu State Nature Sanctuary in the Zangilan region bordering Iran.

These reserves and sanctuaries should become new topics for scientific research. Reserves and sanctuaries created in the territory of Karabakh should gain the status of Karabakh National Park. As a result of research to be conducted in the liberated territories, new information on rare and endangered species should be included in the third edition of the Red Book of the Republic of Azerbaijan and their protection ensured.

3.4 KARABAKH MEDICINAL PLANTS

The researchers are gathering information about the human use of plants in the past and create the basis for the opening of new industrial enterprises. A significant part of the collected material based on verbal information is quickly forgotten; as such, books on this issue should be published in the national language. The beginning of the integration of science into the economy is deeply connected with ethnobotany.

In addition to fresh herbs, dried herbs, horse milk, and sour milk have been widely used in the area. Among plants considered a remedy by local communities, sagebrush was used in increasing appetite, tutsan in infectious diseases of the internal organs, violet and rose in the treatment of headache. Studies are going on related to the general ethnobotanical methods and surveys in the settlements of IDPs and refugees from most regions of the Karabakh region, based on the experience of the people on the use of different plant species (Guber, 2001; Martin, 2001). No field research has been conducted in some areas so far; however, in a short period, a lot of material has been collected about the methods and application ways of different species, some very important plants have not as yet played a significant role in the economic set up of the population, as refugees have already settled in large cities. Continuation of the research in other districts and regions inhabited by IDPs has facilitated the completion of the work carried out in Karabakh. Figure 3.3 provides information on the results of the interviews, indicating the age limit. The most valuable information in the interviews was obtained mainly from the older generation (Figure 3.3).

For the last 25 years, IDPs have been engaged in new forms of farming, the use of wild flora, and information about some plants has been completely lost. The folkloric information collected by ethnographers and archeologists in connection with material and cultural monuments really allows us to describe the history of Karabakh better way. Much of the past has probably been erased from the memory of the younger generation. For this reason, the best way is to investigate the materials collected so far after people return to their ancestral lands. We believe that the establishment of a regional ethnographic museum in Karabakh will unite ethnographers from all regions. The materials collected will help ethnographers of the region to gather new information for the restoration of the existing landscape and related forms. The detailed study of modern technological methods—the archaeological approach in the medicinal evaluations will open new and unexpected horizons for future economic uplift.

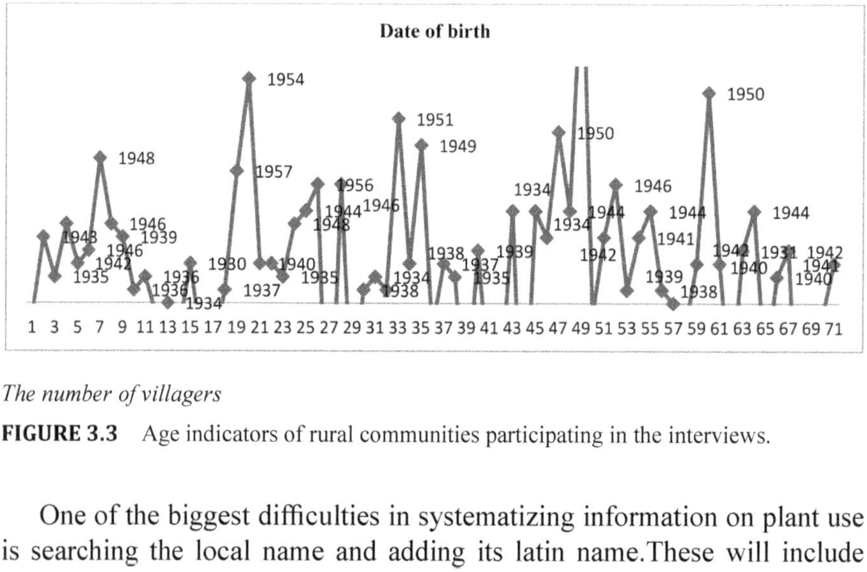

The number of villagers

FIGURE 3.3 Age indicators of rural communities participating in the interviews.

One of the biggest difficulties in systematizing information on plant use is searching the local name and adding its latin name.These will include botanical names given during linguistic expeditions. The most important factor to consider is the presence of collective names, which are specific to different plant species for any particular economic feature, in the national nomenclature. For example, in Karabakh, "pytrakh" refers to all plant species with small thorny fruits that easily cling to human clothes or livestock. The representatives are; Stickseeds—*Lappula* genus *L. barbata, L. patula, L. squarrosa* (Boraginaceae), Sticklewort—*Agrimonia eupatoria* (Rosaceae), *Torilis arvensis* (Apiaceae) and *Circaea lutetiana* (Onagraceae).

Genista dracunculoides (Fabaceae) has broom-shaped twigs corresponding to the word "broom" in the Azerbaijani language and dried flowers are included in the broom flower group, *Xeranthemum cylindraceum* (Asteraceae), short stature with rod-shaped branches is Bushy jasmine—*Jasminum fruticans* (*Oleaceae*). In Karabakh, *Genista dracunculoides*, *Reseda luteola* (Resedaceae) in the Kura-Araz lowland, *Datisca cannabina* (Datiscaceae) in the Greater Caucasus, botanical geographical regions are known as *Genista*.

Although these plants belong to different families, they possess some similar technological features (for obtaining yellow paint) and are therefore grouped under by the same name. In Karabakh, Pigweed or amaranth—*Amaranthus retroflexus* (Amaranthaceae) and goosefoot or wild spinach—*Chenopodium album* (Chenopodiaceae) are also called pigweed. These are two separate plants under a common name, which are used in the spring for the same purpose as spinach.

Sometimes the semantic relationship of names in the regions remain controversial. In Karabakh, the mountainous form of *Festuca ovina* (Poaceae) of the genus *Festuca* (Fescue) and Oregano, containing purple spike flowers—*Origanum vulgare* (Lamiaceae) with purple spike flowers are pronounced the same way locally. *O. vulgare*, along with the branches of *Cornus mas* are used to obtain black dye for wool. *O. vulgare* ("Garaginikh" in the Azerbaijani language) has long been used in folk dyeing technology. *O. vulgare* and *Festuca ovina* ("Garaot" in the Azerbaijani language) species are united under the local toponym "garaot" ("*gara*" is black and "*ot*" is grass) due to the black color originating from the anthocyanin. However, our research has proven that *O. vulgare* is a high-quality essential oil plant. The aromatic essential oil obtained from this plant can be used in pharmaceutical industry, soap making, and cosmetics.

Botanists have combined some mints under a common Latin name—*Mentha longifolia* (Long-leaved mint). Due to different tastes of mint varieties used in food, local people name these differently: yarpiz, nane, dags. It should also be noted that *Mentha* species are the most commonly used medicinal plants (for stomach pain, headache, and toothache). Although three wild species of the *Rumex* genus are used for the same purpose, they have different local names: *Rumex acetosa, R. crispus, R. pulcher*—avalik. It should be noted that *avalik* (fiddle dock) is the most powerful remedy for diarrhea. The porridge made from avalik and yogurt can quickly stop diarrhea.

In the general ethnic translation, the species called "raspberry (morug)" or "blackberry (böyürtkən)" (both differ in color), belong to the genus *Rubus*. The words in front of the common name reflect the diversity of the *Rubus* genus according to the color of the fruits of the plant: grayish blackberry—*R. caesius*, Caucasian raspberry—*R. caucasicus*-bloody blackberry—*R. sanguineus*. Occupants have changed their names during occupation and named these as "mosh." This nomenclature is unstable even within a region. It is possible to name some species according to this "binary type" in the vernacular, and in determining the ethnic name. The plant species that are systematically distant from each other are sometimes united. For example, thorn in the Azerbaijani language sounds like "tikan"; "Boyurtkan"—all *Rubus* species (Rosaceae), "Garatikan"—*Paliurus spina-christi* (Rhamnaceae), "Saritikan" *Centaurea solstitialis* (Asteraceae) belong to different families, but are called by the common toponym "tikan" in Azerbaijani language; "boyur" is flank, "gara" is black, "sari" is yellow. However, the fruits of the blackberry are used as a diaphoretic and antipyretic, and leaves are used as an astringent in diarrhea and bleeding.

The species with little economic value have taken their folk names from species that are similar to them but have high economic value. *Hypomaratrum* (in Azerbaijani—Atboyanasi)—*Hippomarathrum crispum* belongs to the *Apiaceae* family. *Peucedanum ruthenicum* (in Azerbaijani—daghchetiri) and *Prangos ferulacea* (in Azerbaijani—chashir) are in the same family and have economic value. They are called by one name "chashir," as these species are very similar and taste bitter. It should be noted that "chashir"—*Prangos ferulacea* is one of the plants used in the treatment of tumors worldwide. "Daghchetiri"—*P. ruthenicum* seeds and roots are also used against tumors. *Iris sulfurea*—"kash-chirish" belongs to the *Iris* genus, it has no economic value and is very different from the real resinous "chirish"—*Eremurus spectabilis* MB of high economic value, with young edible leaves and dense roots. It is quite risky to say exactly which botanical species belongs to the referred local name, without any investigation. The real reason why we have difficulty in understanding the role of plants in the lives of the local population in the past is that it is impossibile to break away from modern advancements. It is also interesting, looking at the plant through the eyes of a person living in a completely different economic environment. It will be risky to use plants in Karabakh unless new field research is conducted and plants from local communities are studied at length.

Interestingly, people use some plants only for religious purposes buit some of these are medicinally valuable. One of the most important features of the ancient culture of the Karabakh territory is the unity of mystical and mythological ideas of folk medicine associated with medicinal plants. An example of this is the dog rose plant (*Rosa canina*). According to the mythology, it is forbidden to collect the fruit of the plant after sunset. The fruit collection of *Juniperus, Peganum*, and *Ferula* species must be performed using special sacred words, which, according to the legends, have a positive effect on the patient's psyche. This way religious beliefs connected to the collection timing of plants help to preserve such examples in nature. Although the advantages of traditional medicinal plants in Karabakh are indisputable, their application requires therapies in Eastern tradition integrated with global applications which should encompass natural philosophy, theology, empirically based clinical practice, and spiritual and moral principles. Ethnic Karabakh people, like other Eastern people have used the same plants for the treatment of the same diseases. The survey performed has allowed collecting information on the use of medicinal plants in Karabakh. The leaves with and without stalks, dried in shady and airy places are used as raw materials, which are reported to be collected during the flowering period. Simple or complex fresh leaves that are fully developed should be collected and dried with a stalk over a specified period. Flower groups or individual flowers are usually collected during the flowering period of the plant. In dry raw materials, the type of flower group, the flower, the presence or absence of hairs, size, color, smell, and taste are determined. Fresh flowers should be collected and dried during the flowering period and dried in an airy place. The above-ground parts should be dried well. The above-ground parts of grasses are mainly collected during the flowering period. Therefore, the raw material contains also flowers and unripe fruits. There are different methods of collecting herbs. Only the above-ground part of some grasses (shoots) is gathered, whereas other grasses are gathered entirely, together with the root. The hairs of all parts of the dry raw material, the length of the stem, the size, smell, and taste of the leaves and flowers are studied. Herbs must be collected and dried in accordance with certain norms, or used in the form of whole grass in combination with above-ground parts, sometimes leaves, stems, flowers, and fruits are evaluated. The stems of the mature or young shrubs are collected and dried, whereas the bark of trees and shrubs must be collected and dried according to the established standards, without serious damage to the plant.

Fruit refers to true and false fruits, berries, complex fruits, as well as their separate parts. These should usually be harvested at full maturity or shortly before ripening. When analyzing fruits, attention needs to be paid to their shape, size, color, smell, and taste. The fruits consist of pericarp, seed, or stone; it can be dry (dried fruits) and juicy, whereas fresh fruits or parts of them must be dried during the ripening period. The whole seed or its individual kernels are used during ripening. These consist of a shell, endosperm, and embryo. For raw material identification, its shape, size, color, and surface of the shell are studied. The color and smell are determined when it is crushed or scratched. To separate very small seeds, they are sifted. Seeds or their parts (kernels) are collected and dried during the ripening phase.

Roots of some plants are used as a medicinal raw material (*Bryona alba*, *Inula helenium*, *Daucus carota*, etc.) (Ozturk and Mert, 1983; Ozturk et al., 1983a). In this case, the roots are collected during the fruit ripening period.

Rhizomes and roots must be collected, peeled, and dried according to certain norms. Rhizomes and bulbs should be harvested within a specified time, the remains of dry leaves should be peeled and dried using airflow. Fresh or dried tubers must be collected within the established time period, peeled and dried, whole or cut. Rhizomes together with tubers—individual roots, whole, or chopped tubers are peeled and air dried. Rhizomes should be collected, cleaned from above-ground parts, and dried whole or chopped. Bulbs should be collected and peeled, cleaned from above-ground parts; dried pulpy leaves, their outer parts, and immature small leaves should be dried. Examples are onion and garlic. The buds as immature vegetative shoots are separated from the scales, collected and dried. Spores are valuable plant raw material and excipients such as salt, essential oil, etc. are obtained from them. Sclerosion is multicellular and adheres firmly to the vegetative body of the fungus. It is collected and used following known standards.

In folk medicine, special norms for the collection of medicinal plants have been formed. According to the representatives of the communities in the Karabakh region, the medicinal plant must first be clearly identified. During the initial processing, after the raw material has dried, the useless parts must be removed. Above-ground plant parts (leaves, flowers, shoots, fruits) should be collected in the morning when it is dewy (between 8 and 10 am) and underground organs in the evening after 5 pm (roots, rhizomes). Only well-developed healthy raw materials need to be collected. Plants damaged by insects or microorganisms should be removed. People need licenses for gathering (partial and limited) of rare and other protected species, local communities do not touch them.

Plants can be damaged by different types of anthropogenic impacts. It is not advisable to collect material from contaminated ditch edges, pond areas, dirty reservoirs (upto 100 m from the road) close to large industrial enterprises. Allergic reactions to some plants cause dermatitis, inflammation of the mucous membranes of the eyes, and diseases of the nose and throat. To comply with safety regulations, gathering poisonous plants should be avoided. The conditions of gathering medicinal plants depend on the active compounds in their content, as well as the formation and accumulation of maximum phytomass. The collection of each species depends on the calendar date. Moreover, there are general standards and methods for individual morphological groups formed on the basis of many years of experience. The swollen buds should be collected in early spring. The buds of the pine tree (*Pinus sylvestris*) should be cut in the form of a "crown" of more than 3 mm in length. Before drying, the scales on it should be removed. Unauthorized collection of plants in parks, forestry enterprises, and recreation areas close to residential territories is prohibited. It is advisable to collect the bark during the juice movement (in April–May) when the bark is easily separated. Circular cuts at a distance of 20–30 cm from each other should be made with a steel knife.

Moss, lichen, and other particles on the bark should be cleaned before drying. The leaves are usually collected during budding and flowering. However, it can also be done at other times. For example, the leaves of *Trifolium* species (14 species are found in Karabakh) should be collected after flowering, and the leaves of *Tussilago farfara* should be gathered in the first half of summer. The leaves of *Eucalyptus cinerea* should be collected in late autumn, winter or spring, whereas, the leaves of *Vaccinium arstostaphylos* should be gathered at the onset of flowering and in autumn when fruits ripen. Many plant leaves (*Nepeta* sp., *Salvia* sp.) can be harvested during the summer (*Datura stramonium*, *Atropa caucasica*), from flowering to the fruit ripening period. The leaves should be gathered without a stalk using a sharp knife, sickle, or by hand. Plants should be pruned clean in the stalks or cut off the above-ground parts. The leaves should be collected after plucking (*Urtica dioica*) and left for drying (*M. piperita*, *Myrtus communis*) (Ozturk and Vardar, 1973; Vardar and Ozturk, 1973; Ozturk et al., 1983b, 2004, 2011). It is not allowed to gather all the leaves completely during the collection of wild perennials. Flowers (individual or whole flowers) should be collected at the beginning or end of budding. They are gathered usually by hand (*Anthemis austriaca—A. zangelana*, *Calendula persica* and *C. officinalis*), or using a sharp knife, scissors, a sickle (*Crataegus pentagyna*, *Tilia cordata*) or a special mower (*Tanacetum kotschyi*). *Helichrysum plicatum* and *Anthemis austriaca* should be gathered when the height of plant reaches 1, and 3 cm, respectively. Immediately after harvesting, the unwanted parts must be torn off (initial processing). Buds (*Artemisia* species) should be collected before flowering. Some species of grasses should be collected at the beginning of flowering (*Artemisia abthintium*, *Convallaria majalis*), others at the flowering stage (*Primula algida*), and some at the end of flowering, fruiting, and fruit ripening (shrubs). After removing the stems of plants with a knife, scissors, a sickle, "clean" shoots should be cut with a mower. When gathered, the above-ground parts of some plants should be at the level of 5–10 cm above the soil surface (*Convallaria majalis, Primula algida*). Some plants should be cut in the lower parts of the root (*Ephedra procera*, *Hypericum perforatum*, *Chelidonium majus*, *Equisetum arvense*, *Berberis vulgaris*), some should be gathered together with the apex flowers (*Artemisia absthintium*—length 25 cm, stem thickness 3 mm, *Achillea millefolium*—length 15 cm, stem thickness 3 mm, *Equisetum arvense*—length 40 cm, stem thickness 5 mm) or with side branches, and sometimes annual plants should be collected along with the roots. For this purpose, fully developed shoots should be cut in an area of 1 m^2, before drying, wood, contaminated parts, thick stem parts (initial processing) should be removed, and threshed (*Thymus* sp., *Anthemis* sp.). It is usually recommended to collect juicy soft fruits during technical ripening, at 60–70% maturity (*Ricinus communis*, *Phaseolus*, *Linum alexeenkoanum* (=*L. orientale*), *Sinapis arvensis*). Above-ground parts of the plants with dried fruits and seeds should usually be pruned after drying (*Carum carvi*, *Foeniculum vulgare*, *Linum alexeenkoanum*). Juicy fruits should be collected by hand as much as possible so as not to damage the integrity of the membranes. Sometimes fruits need to be processed because they are contaminated with various pests. Species of the *Hippophae rhamnoides*, *Crataegus* and *Rosa* genera, should be subjected to the initial processing after fruit gathering. The damaged, unripe and insect-contaminated fruits should be removed. Underground organs (roots, rhizomes, tubers, and bulbs) should usually be collected in autumn or spring before the vegetative activity begins. For example, species of the *Alchemilla* genus should be gathered during the flowering period, whereas the root and tubers of *Bryonia alba* should be collected with a hook-shaped tool during flowering and fruiting periods, the rotten parts should be separated from the basal leaves, roots, and rhizoids. These parts should be collected in a wicker basket after washing in cold water. The raw material consists of mucus, saponins, which contain highly soluble substances. Some raw materials *(Liquorice, Acorus, Althaea*) do not have fungus (Ozturk et al., 2017a). The best containers for drying and transporting raw materials are baskets, wooden boxes, and cloth bags. Transport of leaves, grass, and flowers in plastic bags is not safe. The collected raw material should be spread on a cloth or tarpaulin in the shade for 2–3 h.

3.5 DRYING OF THE RAW MATERIALS OF MEDICINAL PLANTS

A vast majority of the raw materials of medicinal plant are used in medicine in a dried form. Only certain species (aloe, saffron, kalanchoe) are allowed to be used after initial processing. Ensuring the safety of biologically active substances during drying, the simplest and the most effective way to protect medicinal raw materials is a must. Medicinal plants lose 70–90% of moisture during harvesting and 10–15 (20)% after drying. First, living cells accumulate biologically active substances as a result of biochemical processes. Moisture, disruption of food metabolism, and natural dehydration led to a decrease in the content of biologically active substances in raw materials. Enzymes get denatured during temperature drying. If the temperature is maintained, the lysis process begins. However, in some cases, the drying process of raw materials is necessary to increase the content of active substances. To maintain certain groups of biologically active substances during the optimal drying regime, drying should be performed using special methods based on experimental data. It should be carried out gradually under the cover (in attic, etc.) at normal temperature. Sometimes the reagent increases the course of procedure or accelerates the subsequent dehydration process. There are various methods currently used to dry medicinal plants.

Without artificial heating: (a) outdoor air-shade, under the canopy, and wind dryers; (b) special drying in the sun–air drying.

With artificial heating: (a) leaves, grass, and flowers are dried following shade-air method. In simple cases, the raw material is dried under the canopy or around special drying points. (b) The drying chamber with air dryers is equipped with shelves located inside the canvas or metal grid.

Quality raw materials are obtained by drying with air dryers very slowly in the open air. The hot arid climate mainly causes almost no damage to the rhizomes, roots, and other underground organs under the influence of solar radiation.

During sun drying, the amount of alkaloids and tannins in the raw material decreases to some extent (*Scopolia, Senecio*). Therefore, plants containing pigments should be dried only in the shade. In a hot dry climate, raw materials from different morphological groups are collected and dried under any condition. Such drying is called convective and thermoradiation drying. Convective drying is a continuous process performed in the drying cabinet. The drying cabinet is designed as a stationary and portable type. Stationary dryers are usually used for medicinal plants in large areas. Their drying chamber consists of a boiler, a metal grid, and an insulated drying chamber. Dryers are heated with water, steam, or flue gases. Simple dryers are mainly designed for medicinal plants.

Individual collectors also use heat drying ovens and hot plates.

Radiation drying is performed by infrared rays and significantly reduces dehydration processes. This method is used in the laboratory.

Experiments have shown that microwave drying of herbs is more efficient. General norms for drying should be followed. When drying medicinal plants, raw materials should be spread in a thin layer in all cases (except for the method of obtaining essential oils). The temperature regime for the extraction of substances from barberry root, leonurus, crataegus fruit, ginseng root, and lily-of-the-valley should be 60–90°C, and during drying, the temperature limit follows the general norms. It is recommended to dry the rhizomes and roots of Syrian juniper, flowers of mountainous Arnica at a temperature of 50°C, to isolate the essential oils and lactone belonging to sesquiterpenes. Podophyll should be dried at 40°C and the eleutherococcus at 70°C. In the experimental study, during drying, the loss in the mass of various plant parts is as follows: 65–70%—buds; 70–80%—flowers; 55–90%—leaves; 65–90%—shoots; 60–80%—roots and rhizomes; 50–70%—bark; 30–60%—fruit and 20–40%—seeds.

3.6 PLANTS AND PHYTOTHERAPY

The plant species in nature synthesize a large number of biologically active compounds, and these have been used by healers and doctors for centuries (Ozturk and Hakeem, 2018, 2019a, b). Healers were engaged not only in the preparation of medicinal products from plants, animals, and mineral substances but also in their application. Studying wild medicinal plants by healers has created possibilities of using these and their physiologically active substances—resins, nectars, essential oils, etc. It has also been determined in which phase these substances were and in which organ of the plant they were more. Knowing the accumulation patterns of physiologically active substances in plants allows choosing the methods of their drying, storage, and use. The source of raw materials includes dried or freshly harvested medicinal plants or their parts; a mixture of oils, resins, fats, snake venom, honey, and animal waste, etc (Altay and Karahan, 2012, 2017; Altay et al., 2015a; Younessi-Hamzekhanlu et al., 2020; Ozturk et al., 2021a, b). Healers have studied the combined effects of these substances and herbs. Based on historical facts, it can be said that for centuries, the healers cultivated the plants, which were used to serve in the healing. Some plant-derived substances are not used directly for therapeutic purposes. Some herbs are especially important in improving the overall tone of the body and stimulating metabolism. Many medicinal plants are used not only in medicine but also in other sectors of the economy—perfumery, cosmetics, and food industry (Altay and Çelik, 2011; Altay et al., 2015a, b; Karahan et al., 2015; Kafi et al., 2018; Letchamo et al., 2018; Mercimek et al., 2019; Taşpınar et al., 2019; Altay and Ozturk, 2020; Ozturk et al., 2019, 2020b, 2021c).

The work of analysts and organizers familiar with the characteristics of medicinal plants and products has been done by healers and positive results were obtained. One of the main goals of healers was the search for natural biologically active substances, including those of plant, animal, and mineral origin, as well as development of therapeutic agents based on these. The healing practices passed from generation to generation and hundreds of healers grew up in the territory of Karabakh. As a result of the occupation of Karabakh in the 1990s, the population became victims as refugees and the healers disappeared. During the survey, information was obtained on the use of the same plants in the treatment of many diseases, and this was reported by different rural communities. The frequency of use of these plants by rural communities in the treatment of the diseases is presented in Table 3.1. Habits have been taken into account in the information on the plant parts used in the treatment of the diseases.

Use value (UV) of the plants was calculated using the quantitative method showing the relative importance of species in the area by the formula: UVi ¼ XUi = Ni, where UV is the cost of using one species; U is the number of citations per species; and N is the number of informants (Phillips and Gentry, 1993).

As seen in Table 3.1, different people show the therapeutic effect of the same plant on different diseases. These treatments are carried out by infusions (extracts), oral drugs, rubbing (smearing), applying to the skin, and sometimes by spraying dry plant powder on open wounds.

3.7 BIOLOGICALLY ACTIVE SUBSTANCES IN THE MEDICINAL PLANTS

Medicinal substances include natural compounds derived from plants, animals, fungal, mineral, or synthetic derivatives, and compounds with pharmacological activity (Hamzah et al., 2020; Khan et al., 2020; Ozturk et al., 2020). The plant parts and their physiologically active substances—resins, nectars, essential oils, etc., are evaluated, together with the fact in which organ of the plant and in which phase of development the active compounds accumulate. This information allows the choosing of the methods of drying, storage, and use of plants. Plant products, animal and fungal derivatives—exogenous and endogenous plant secretions, etc., are used in medicine. For example, in plants—resin, gummi, essential oil, in animals—snake venom, bee products (honey and wax), etc.

3.8 ETHNOBOTANY, PHARMACOLOGY, MOLECULAR BIOLOGY

Almost three decades of occupation of Karabakh have caused serious damage to forests. New systems formed due to deforestation reflect complex

TABLE 3.1 Results of Surveys on the Treatment of Diseases with Herbs in the Territory of Karabakh- Azerbaijan.

Cardiovascular	Degenerative	Digestion	Other diseases	Pain	Reproductive	Lung diseases	Venereal diseases
Blood viscosity (pollution) $5^{a}9^{b}$	Breast cancer $11^{a}3^{b}40^{c}$	Constipation $3^{a}11^{b}$	Internal parasites $3^{a}11^{b}$	Abdominal pains $3^{a}11^{b}$	Immune deficiency in humans $5^{a}2^{b}1^{c}$	Acute respiratory infections $2^{a}12^{b}$	Herpes $15^{a}2^{b}$
Heart problems $3^{a}11^{b}3^{c}$	Childhood cancer $6^{a}8^{b}24^{c}$	Diarrhea $1^{a}13^{b}5^{c}$	Mental illness $4^{a}10^{b}$	Headache 4^{a} 10^{b}	Difficult pregnancy $8^{a}6^{b}$	Asthma $5^{a}9^{b}15^{c}$	Ulcers $3^{a}11^{b}$
High blood pressure 4^{a} 10^{b} 14^{c}	Diabetes $10^{a}4^{b}7c$	Gallbladder disease $2^{a}12^{b}$	–	Toothache 2^{a} 12^{b}	Infertility $9^{a}5^{b}$	Cough $1^{a}13^{b}$	Trophic wounds $2^{a}12^{b}$
Numbness and swelling of the muscles 2^{a} 12^{b}	Internal tumors $7^{a}7^{b}$	Hiccup $2^{a}12^{b}$	–	Stomach ache 6^{b}	Prostate $1^{a}13^{b}$	Tuberculosis $7^{a}1^{b}9^{c}$	–
–	Liver problems $3^{a}11^{b}$	Intestinal disorders $4^{a}10^{b}$	–	Menstrual pains 1^{a}	Ovary $1^{a}13^{b}$	–	–
–	–	Sputum $3^{a}11^{b}$	–	–	Syphilis $1^{a}2^{b}4^{c}$	–	–
–	–	Hemorrhoids $3^{a}11^{b}$	–	–		–	–
–	–	Stomach pains $8^{a}6^{b}$	–	–	Uterine disorders $2^{a}12^{b}$	–	–
–	–	Vomiting $1^{a}13^{b}$	–	–	–	–	–
–	–	–	11^{d}	9^{d}	7^{d}	12^{d}	20^{d}

Note: The figures show the number of villages. (a) frequently mentioned in interviews; (b) sometimes mentioned; (c) fatal diseases (following WHO); (d) infectious diseases. Numbers define the people interviewed.

feedbacks between biotic and abiotic, as well as cultural features (Kellogg et al., 2016). Medicinal plants of different families have been observed all over the world and their distribution is not random (Huy et al., 2018). The similar medicinal properties of plants belonging to the same family with close evolutionary connections are largely due to the fact that they contain the same secondary components. Such features have been discovered by the community in nearby phytogeographical areas based on traditional intuition. Integration of ethnobotanical, phytochemical, and molecular data has improved the prospects for the use of medicinal plants in Azerbaijan like other countries (Karimov et al., 2010; Mustafayeva et al., 2015). The use of closely related plants in different cultures (nations) in a similar way shows that people living differently have general knowledge about the use of the beneficial plants (Ozturk et al., 2014, 2016, 2017a, b, c, 2018a, b, c, d, e, f, g, h; Imanberdieva et al., 2018a, b). Some plants have similar morphological features due to their close phylogenetic location and people know this (Nimet, 2009; Ozturk et al., 2021a, b).

Ethnobotanical research has revealed that plant resources play a key role in the development of new drugs for the treatment of diseases (Altay and Karahan, 2012; Altay et al., 2015a, b; Karahan et al., 2015; Younessi-Hamzekhanlu et al., 2020). Plants and humans are in constant dynamic contact, and as a result, people are developing strategies and methods to use plants. Thus, plants create secondary metabolites to protect themselves from overuse, and people are looking for ways to use these metabolites to their advantage, for example, the role of essential oils has not been fully evaluated although these have been used by the local population in aromatherapy since years (Ibadullayeva and Jafarli, 2007; Ozturk et al., 2020). The recorded medicinal uses and analysis of ethnobotanical data together with identifying phylogenetic and genetic links between plants is a convenient tool for the discovery of new drugs. In particular, new perspectives are gained in the development of molecular tools in the DNA sequence, and this process allows for the phylogenetic reconstruction and grouping of potentially beneficial plants (Robertson and Richards, 2015; Maestri, 2017). The species of genus *Altheae* distributed in the territory of Karabakh are used in the same way in phylogenetically distant areas. This type of ethnobotanical data shows that people from different cultures and remote areas have discovered plants belonging to the same areal type for the treatment of similar diseases. An application of two different species belonging to various geographical areas for the same purpose is another example of ethnobotanical compatibility. In Western cultures, *Satureja* species are used in dishes, while in the

East, *Mentha* species belonging to the same genus are used (Ozturk et al., 2004). Both plants are phylogenetically very close, have a similar chemical composition, and are used similarly. The methods of molecular biology too are used to identify plants or genes of plants suitable for pharmaceutical evaluations (Keatinge et al., 2011). With the passage of time research done gets older as new species emerge, or species migrate from neighboring countries. Therefore, it is important to periodically study these and explore their new, as well as useful features. During our ethnobotanical survey a new species for the Caucasus, *Helociadium nadiflorum* (L.) W.D.J.Koch was recorded. Its phylogeny was confirmed through the determination of nucleotide sequence of the ribosomal DNA (nrDNA) in the internal transcribed spacer (ITS) region (Pimenov et al., 2018). This study on sequence analysis of the nuclear ribosomal DNA internal transcribed spacer (nrDNA-ITS) based on the morphological characteristics helped in the determination and confirmation of this species. Using the SYM + G substitution model (19950 trees), a consensus tree of the species was compiled following Bayes method. The predominant phytocenoses (abundance, height, phenophase, and stratification) were identified, characteristic vegetation of the distribution area described and nomenclature summary together with an areal map was compiled. Similar studies are being conducted on *Artemisia* species. They are widely used in veterinary medicine following ethnic methods.

3.9 MEDICINAL PLANTS FOUND IN KARABAKH AND THEIR USES

Earlier a large group of plants were used for the preparation of medicines and consumed as food in Karabakh. This was more common among people who traditionally collected wild plants and knew their health benefits. Today it is mentioned that wild plants generally have higher useful values, fiber and polyphenol content, and antioxidant capacity than the corresponding cultivated species. The people from local communities know many wild plants which are effective in preventing chronic health problems like cardiovascular diseases and diabetes. Much of this knowledge has been passed down orally from generation to generation and has led to the development of traditional treatment systems at global level (Savo et al., 2015; Qureshi et al., 2016; Huy et al., 2018; Ozturk and Hakeem 2018, 2019a, b, 2020). People trust in phytomedicines due to the long-term tradition of herbal treatments and this type of application in the use of health-promoting herbs is increasing globally.

This chapter presents information about common diseases which are easily treated with simple herbal medicines. Nearly 102 plant taxa are used in Karabakh and herbal medicines have been easily prepared and used in primary health care. During the survey, information was obtained from different rural communities on the use of plants in the treatment of diseases (Appendix 3.1). The table summarizes the bioecological features, description of the disease for which each plant is applied, form, and composition of the traditional preparation, latin name and family of the plant, part of the plant used, basic chemical components, quality standards, methods of preparation, therapeutic properties, indications, dosage and mode of application, safety precautions, and important references. This is an attempt to promote the rational, safe, and appropriate use of herbal medicines. This data can be used by health planners, national health authorities, and others involved in the development of the health sector.

People are aware of the therapeutic effect of the same plant on different diseases. These treatments are usually given orally as an infusion (extract) no more than 1–2 times a day, applied to the skin as a poultice, and sometimes by spraying dry plant powder on open wounds. As can be seen from Appendix 3.1, 101 types of folk medicines are used in the treatment of various diseases in Karabakh. Many of these have been confirmed in scientifically and included in the State Pharmacopoeia. Regarding the life forms of these species, it seems that most of them are perennial grasses (61 species), followed by trees and shrubs (13 species). In addition, eight species of trees are widely used in the region (Figure 3.4).

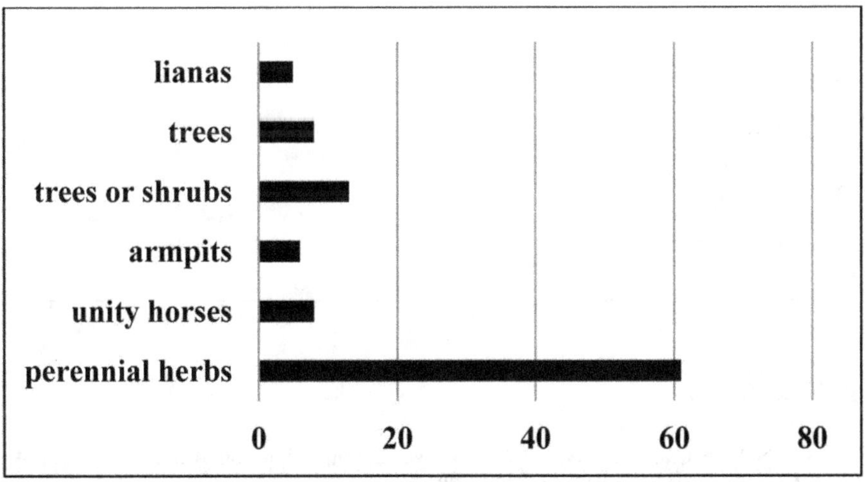

FIGURE 3.4 Life forms of plants used in folk medicine.

The areal of the *S. officinalis* and *S. karabachenses* species is limited to Karabakh but there are reports of the use of these plants in other regions of Azerbaijan.

Some plants are not found in the wild but are cultivated by locals and used as medicine. The examples are; *Tanacetum vulgare, Rosmarinus officinalis, P. anisum, P. somniferum, M. piperita, Matricaria matricarioides, Iris germanica, Kalanchoe pinnata, Ficus carica, Ephedra aurantica, Cucurbita maxima, Coriandrum sativum, Calendula officinalis, Bidens tripartita, Allium sativum,* and *Aesculus hippocastanum.*

H. plicatum and *S. karabachenses* are known as the endemics of Caucasus, these are distributed in Karabakh.

3.10 CONCLUSIONS

In conclusion, we can say that the information gathered and presented here was pooled up to substantiate the importance and relevance of ethnobotanical work in Karabakh-Azerbaijan. We have tried to briefly review the information collected from the area; to identify some issues in the context of ethnobotanical research for the future development and identify the ways to be followed to solve the existing problem and finally emphasize the possible areas of the practical application of ethnobotanical knowledge.

KEYWORDS

- **Azerbaijan**
- **ethnic use**
- **Karabagh**
- **traditional herbal plants**

REFERENCES

Abu Ali Ibn Sina. *Canon of Medical Sciences*, Vol. 2, translation from Arabic by Zavadovsky, Yu. N.; Mirzayeva, S.; Tashkent, FAN, 1982.

Alekperli F. U. *A Thousand and One Secrets of the East*, Vol. I.; Tural Publishing House: Baku, 2001.

Altay, V.; Çelik, O. Antakya semt pazarlarındaki bazı doğal bitkilerin etnobotanik yönden araştırılması. *Biyoloji Bilimleri Araştırma Dergisi* **2011,** *4* (2), 137–139.

Altay, V.; Karahan, F. Tayfur Sökmen Kampüsü (Antakya-Hatay) ve çevresinde bulunan bitkiler üzerine etnobotanik bir araştırma. *Karadeniz Fen Bilimleri Dergisi* **2012,** *2* (7), 13–28.

Altay, V.; Karahan, F. Anadolu geleneksel tıbbında güneş çarpması ve güneş yanığı tedavisinde kullanılan tıbbi bitkiler. *Erzincan Univ. J. Sci. Technol.* **2017,** *10* (1), 124–137.

Altay, V.; Ozturk, M. The Genera *Salsola* and *Suaeda* (Amaranthaceae) and Their Value as Fodder. In *Handbook of Halophytes*; Grigore, M.-N., Ed.; Springer Nature: Switzerland AG, 2020. https://doi.org/10.1007/978–3-030–17854–3_97–1.

Altay, V.; Keskin, M.; Karahan, F. An Assessment of the Plant Biodiversity of Mustafa Kemal University Tayfur Sokmen Campus (Hatay-Turkey) for the View of Human Health. *Int. J. Sci. Technol. Res.* **2015a,** *1* (2), 83–103.

Altay, V.; Karahan, F.; Sarcan, Y. B.; Ilçım, A. An Ethnobotanical Research on Wild Plants Sold in Kırıkhan District (Hatay/Turkey) Herbalists and Local Markets. *Biol. Diversity Conserv.* **2015b,** *8* (2), 81–91.

Askerov A. M. *Flora of Azerbaijan*; Elm: Baku, 2016.

Conspectus of the Caucasus Flora. Vols. 1 and 2. Publishing House, St. Petersburg University, 2003–2006.

Damirov I. A. *On the History of the Use of Medicinal Plants in Azerbaijan*; Baku, 1970.

Damirov I. A.; Prilipko, L. I.; Shukurov, D. Z., et al., *Medicinal Plants of Azerbaijan*; Baku, 1988.

Flora of Azerbaijan. Vols. 1–8; Publishing House of the Academy of Sciences of Azerbaijan SSR: Baku, 1952–1961.

Gasimov, G. Z.; Guliyev, V. B.; Ibadullayeva, S. J. Wild Food Plants in the Nakhchivan Autonomous Republic of Azerbaijan Based on Ethnobotanical Research Materials. *J. Plant Resour., St. Petersburg* **2009,** *45* (2), 109–115.

Gasimov, M. A.; Gasimov, T. A.; Gadirova, G. S. *Medicinal Plants of the XXI Century*; Elm: Baku, 2006.

Ghulam, Y.; Mushtaq, A.; Daniel, P.; Muhammad, Z.; Shazia, S.; Sehrosh, Mir. Ethnobotany of Medicinal Plants for Livelihood and Community Health in Deserts of Sindh-Pakistan. In *Herbs and Human Health, vol. 1—Ethnobotany and Physiology*; Ozturk, M.; Hakeem, K. R., Eds.; Springer: Berlin/Heidelberg, Germany, 2018; pp 767–793.

Grossheim A. A. *Determinant of the Caucasus Plants*; State Publishing House Sov. nauka, 1949.

Guber R. *La Etnografia*. Metodo, campo y reflexividad; Norma, Bogota, 2001.

Hamzah, T. N. T.; Ozturk, M.; Altay, V.; Hakeem, K. H. Insights into the Bioactivite Compounds of Endophytic Fungi in Mangroves. In *Biodiversity and Biomedicine—Our Future*; Ozturk, M.; Egamberdieva, D.; Pesci, M., Eds.; Chapter 15, Elseiver, Academic Press, 2020; pp 277–292.

Huy, H. V.; Hung, H. V.; Buckney, R. T., De Filippis, L. F. Molecular Biodiversity Convergence with Biogeography and Ethnobotany of Rare and Endangered Medicinal Plants from Northern Vietnam. In *Herbs and Human Health, Vol. 1—Ethnobotany and Physiology*; Ozturk, M.; Hakeem, K. R., Eds.; Springer: Berlin/Heidelberg, Germany, 2018; pp 1–52.

Ibadullayeva, S. J. Ethnobotany of Local Used Medicinal Plants in Azerbaijan Republic. *J. Med. Biol.* **2020,** *2* (2), 72–81.

Ibadullayeva S. J., Alakbarov, R. *Medicinal Plants (Ethnobotany and Phytotherapy)*; Baku: Elm, 2013.

Ibadullayeva, S. J.; Mamedova, S. E.; Sultanova, Z. R.; Movsumova, N. V.; Jafarli, I. A. Medicinal Plants of Azerbaijan Flora Used in the Treatment of Certain Diseases. *Int. J. Pharm. Pharmacol.* **2010,** *4* (5), 545–548.

Ibadullayeva, S. J.; Shahmuradova, M. *Ethnobotanical Researches in Azerbaijan (Goygol region)*; Tahsil: Baku, 2015.

Ibadullayeva, S. J.; Abbasova, V. N. Ethnopharmacological Importance of Medicinal Plants Spread in Tovuz-Gazakh Territory. *ANAS News, Biol. Med. Sci.* **2018,** *2*, 47.

Ibadullayeva, S. J.; Gahramanova, N. J.; Shahmuradova, M. J. Use of Wild Plants at Dermatosis (Skin Diseases): Ethnobotany. *J. Appl. Pharma. Sci.* **2012,** *2* (8), 64–67.

Ibadullayeva, S. J., Jafarli, I. A. *Essential Oils and Aromatherapy*; Elm: Baku, 2007.

Ibadullayeva, S. J.; Shahmuradova, M. J.; Mustafayev, A. B. Protection of Some Rare and Critically Threatened Medicinal Plants in the Azerbaijan Flora. *J. Biol. Life Sci.* **2013,** *4* (1),145–152.

Ibadullayeva, S. J.; Mohammad, Z.; Jafarli, I.; Asbghian, N. Folk Medicine (Ethnobotany in Azerbaijan Region). IIR, Tehran, 2017.

Imanberdieva, N.; Severoğlu, Z.; Kurmanbekova, G. et al., Plant Diversity of Ala-Archa Nature Park in Kyrgyzstan with Emphasis on Its Economic Potential. In *Vegetation of Central Asia and Environs*; Egamberdieva, D.; Öztürk, M., Eds.; Chapter 16, Springer Nature: Switzerland AG, 2018a; pp 365–381.

Imanberdieva, N.; Imankul, B.; Severoğlu, Z. et al., Potential Impacts of Climate Change on Plant Diversity of Sary-Chelek Biosphere Reserve in Kyrgyzstan. In *Vegetation of Central Asia and Environs*; Egamberdieva, D.; Öztürk, M., Eds.; Chapter 16; Springer Nature: Switzerland AG, 2018b; pp 349–364.

Kafi, M.; Kamili, A. N.; Husaini, A. M. et al., An expensive spice—Saffron (*Crocus sativus* L.)—Case study from Kashmir, Iran and Turkey. In *Global Perspectives on Underutilized Crops*; Ozturk. M. et al., Eds.; Chapter 4; Springer International Publishing AG, part of Springer Nature, 2018; pp 109–149.

Karahan, F.; Altay, V.; Keskin, M. An Ethnobotanical Study on Woody Plants Benefits from Handicrafts in Antakya District (Hatay-Turkey). *Int. J. Sci. Technol. Res.* **2015,** *1* (1), 1–18.

Karimov, Y. B.; Suleymanov, T. A.; Isayev, J. I.; Khalilov, J. S. *Pharmacognosy: Tutorial, Baku*: "Herba Flora," 2010.

Keatinge, J. D.; Yang, R.-Y.; Hughes, J. D.; Easdown, W. J.; Holmer, R. The Importance of Vegetables in Ensuring Both Food and Nutritional Security in Attainment of the Millennium Development Goals. *Food Sci.* **2011,** *3*, 491–501.

Kellogg, J. J.; Todd, D. A.; Egan, J. M.; Raja, H. A.; Oberlies, N. H.; Kvalheim, O. M.; Cech, N. B. Biochemometrics for Natural Products Search: Comparison of Data Analysis Approaches and Application to Identification of Bioactive Compounds. *J. Nat. Prod.* **2016,** *79*, 376–386.

Khan, F.; Szmigielski, R.; Gul, A. et al., Advancements in Plant Transgenomics Approach for the Biopharmaceutics and Vaccines Production. In *Biodiversity and Biomedicine—Our Future*; Ozturk, M.; Egamberdieva, D.; Pesci, M., Eds.; Chapter 18; Elseiver, Academic Press, 2020; pp 317–333.

Letchamo, W.; Ozturk, M.; Altay, V. et al., A Alternative Potential Natural Genetic Resource: Seabuckthorn [*Elaeagnus rhamnoides* (syn.: *Hippophae rhamnoides*)]. In *Global Perspectives on Underutilized Crops*; Ozturk, M. et al., Eds.; Chapter 2; Springer International Publishing AG, part of Springer Nature, 2018; pp 25–82.

Maestri, R. Using Phylogenetic Clade Composition to Understand Biogeographical Variation in Functional Traits. *Front Biogeogr.* **2017,** *9* (3), e34435.

Martin, G. J. *Etnobotany*. Manual de Methods. Nordan—Comunidad. Montevideo, Uruguay, 2001.

Masoodi, K. Z.; Amin, I.; Mansoor, S. et al., Botanicals from the Himalayas with Anticancer Potential—An Emphasis on Kashmir Himalayas. In *Biodiversity and Biomedicine—Our Future*; Ozturk, M.; Egamberdieva, D.; Pešić, M., Eds.; Chapter 11; Academic Press, 2020; pp 189–234.

Mercimek, H. V.; Altay, V.; Ozturk, M.; Akçiçek, E.; Gucel. S. An Overutilised Industrial Crop Tobacco—*Nicotiana tabacum* L. Case Study from Turkey. In *Crop Production Technologies for Sustainable Use and Conservation*; Ozturk, M. et al., Eds.; Apple Academic Press, Chapter 15, 2019; pp 365–394.

Mustafayeva, I. R.; Ibadullayeva, S. J.; Alakbarov, R. A.; Ismayilov, A. H.; Qasimov, H. Z.; Qasimova, S. S. *Pharmacognosis with the Basis of Botany*; Science-Education: Baku, Azerbaijan, 2015.

Nimet, Ö. *Fitoterapi (Bitkilerle tedavi) ve Aromaterapi (Uçucu yağlarla tedavi)*. İstanbul, 2009.

Oksana, S.; Marian, B.; Shokoofeh, H.; Milan, S.; Jan, K.; Laura, L.-T.; Ulkar, I.; Ibadullayeva, S. J.; Marco, L. COVID-19 Prophylaxis Efforts Based On Natural Antiviral Plant Extracts and Their Compounds. *Molecules* **2021,** *26*, 727.

Ozturk, M.; Vardar, Y. Distribution and plasticity of *Myrtus communis* L. *Phyton (Austria)* **1973,** *15*, 145–150.

Ozturk, M.; Mert, H.H. Water Relations and Germination of Seeds of *Inula graveolens* (L.) Desf. *Biotronics* **1983,** *12*, 11–17.

Ozturk, M.; Hakeem, K. R. *Plant and Human Health—Vol. 1—Ethnobotay and Physiology*; Springer Science + Business Media: NY, 2018.

Ozturk, M.; Hakeem, K. R. *Plant and Human Health—Vol. 2—Phytochemistry and Molecular Aspects*; Springer Science + Business Media: NY, 2019a.

Ozturk, M.; Hakeem, K. R. *Plant and Human Health—Vol. 3—Phytochemistry and Therapeutic Uses*; Springer Science + Business Media: NY, 2019b.

Ozturk, M.; Secmen, O.; Segawa, M. Ecological Aspects of Seed Germination in *Myrtus communis* L. *Mem. Fac. Integ. Arts-Sci. Hiroshima* **1983b,** *8*, 63–68.

Ozturk, M.; Secmen, O.; Gork, G.; Kondo, K. Productivity and Biotic Relations of *Inula graveolens* (L.) Desf. *Mem. Fac. Integ. Arts-Sci. Hiroshima* **1983a,** *8*, 77–84.

Ozturk, M.; Gork, C.; Gork, G. Ethnoecology of Wild Mints in Turkey. 2nd Intern. Cong. on Traditional Medicine and Materia Medica, 4–7 October, Iran, 2004.

Ozturk, M.; Gucel, S.; Celik, A.; Altundag, E.; Mert, T.; Akcicek, E.; Celik, S. *Myrtus communis* in Phytotheraphy in the Mediterranean In *Genetic Resources, Chromosome Engineering & Crop Improvement:Medicinal Plants*; Singh, R., Ed.; Chapter 28, Vol. 6; CRC Press: Boca Raton, USA, 2011; pp 923–934.

Ozturk, M.; Altay, V.; Gucel, S.; Guvensen, A. Halophytes in the East Mediterranean-Their Medicinal and Other Economical Values. In *Sabkha Ecosystems: Volume IV: Cash Crop Halophyte and Biodiversity Conservation Tasks for Vegetation Science*, Vol. 47; Springer Netherlands, 2014; pp 247–272.

Ozturk, M.; Altay, V.; Altundağ, E.; Gucel, S. Halophytic Plant Diversity of Unique Habitats in Turkey: Salt Mine Caves of Çankırı and Iğdır. In *Halophytes for Food Security in Dry Lands*; Khan, M. A.; Ozturk, M.; Gul, B.; Ahmed, M. Z., Eds.; Chapter 18; Elsevier, 2016. http://dx.doi.org/10.1016/B978–0-12–801854–5.00018–2

Ozturk, M.; Altay, V.; Hakeem, K. R.; Akçiçek, E. *Liquorice from Botany to Phytochemistry*; SpringerBriefs in Plant Science, 2017a. https://doi.org/10.1007/978–3-319–74240–3

Ozturk, M.; Altay, V.; Gonenç, T. M. Herbal from High Mountains in the East Mediterranean. In *Drug Discovery from Herbs-Approaches and Applications*; Bhojraj, S. et al., Eds.; NAM S & T Centre, DAYA Publishing House: New Delhi, India, Chapter 24, 2017b; pp 327–367.

Ozturk, M.; Altay, V.; Gucel, S.; Altundağ, E. Plant Diversity of the Drylands in Southeast Anatolia-Turkey: Role in Human Health and Food Security. In *Plant Biodiversity: Monitoring, Assessment and Conservation*; Ansari, A. A.; Gill, S. S., Eds.; Chapter 5, CABI UK, 2017c; pp 83–124.

Ozturk, M.; Hakeem, K. R.; Ashraf, M.; Ahmad, M. S. A. *Global Perspectives on Underutilized Crops*; Springer Science+Business Media, 2018a.

Ozturk, M.; Altundağ, E.; Ibadullayeva, S. J.; Altay, V.; Aslanıpour, B. A Comparative Analysis of Medicinal and Aromatic Plants Used in the Traditional Medicine of Iğdır (Turkey), Nakhchivan (Azerbaijan), and Tabriz (Iran). *Pak. J. Bot.* **2018b,** *50* (1), 337–343.

Ozturk, M.; Altay, V.; Altundağ, E.; Ibadullayeva, S. J.; Aslanipour, B.; Gönenç, T. M. Herbals in Iğdır (Turkey), Nakhchivan (Azerbaijan), and Tabriz (Iran). In *Plant and Human Health*; Ozturk, M.; Hakeem, K.R., Eds.; Vol. 1; Springer: Cham, Chapter 6, 2018c; pp 197–266.

Ozturk, M.; Altay, V.; Latiff, A. et al., A Comparative Analysis of the Medicinal Pteridophytes in Turkey, Pakistan, and Malaysia. In *Plant and Human Health*; Ozturk, M.; Hakeem, K.R., Eds., Vol. 1; Springer: Cham, Chapter 9; Springer International Publishing AG, 2018d; pp 349–390.

Ozturk, M.; Altay, V.; Latiff, A. et al., A Comparative Analysis of the Medicinal Plants Used for Diabetes Mellitus in the Traditional Medicine in Turkey, Pakistan, and Malaysia. In *Plant and Human Health*; Ozturk, M.; Hakeem, K.R., Eds.; Vol. 1; Springer: Cham, Chapter 11, Springer International Publishing AG, 2018e; pp 409–461.

Ozturk, M.; Altay, V.; Latiff, A. et al., Potential Medicinal Plants Used in the Hypertension in Turkey, Pakistan, and Malaysia. In *Plant and Human Health*; Ozturk, M.; Hakeem, K.R., Eds., Vol. 1; Springer: Cham, Chapter 16, Springer International Publishing AG, 2018f; pp 595–618.

Ozturk, M.; Gökler, I.; Altay, V. Medicinal Bryophytes Distributed in Turkey. In *Plant and Human Health*; Ozturk, M.; Hakeem, K.R., Eds., Vol. 1; Springer: Cham, Chapter 8, Springer International Publishing AG, 2018g, pp 323–348.

Ozturk, M.; Altay, V.; Orçen, N. et al., A Little Known and a Little Consumed Natural Resource: *Salicornia*. In *Global Perspectives on Underutilized Crops*; Ozturk, M. et al., Eds., Chapter 3, Springer International Publishing AG, 2018h; pp 83–108.

Ozturk, M.; Altay, V.; Guvensen, A. Sustainable Use of Halophytic Taxa as Food and Fodder—An İmportant Genetic Resource in Southwest Asia. In *Ecophysiology, Abiotic Stress Responses and Utilization of Halophytes*; Hasanuzzaman, M.; Nahar, K.; Öztürk, M., Eds.; Springer: Singapore, Chapter 11, 2019; pp 235–257.

Ozturk, M.; Egamberdieva, D.; Milica, P. *Biodiversity and Biomedicine-Our Future*; Academic Press, Elsevier Inc., 2020.

Ozturk, M.; Altay, V.; Guvensen, A. *Portulaca oleracea*: A Vegetable from Saline Habitats. In *Handbook of Halophytes*; Springer Nature: Switzerland AG, 2020b; pp 1–14.

Ozturk, M.; Altay, V.; Efe, R. *Biodiversity, Conservation and Sustainability in Asia: Volume I: Prospects and Challenges in West Asia and Caucasus*; Springer Nature: Switzerland AG, 2021a. DOI: 10.1007/978–3-030–59928–7

Ozturk, M.; Khan, S. M.; Altay, V.; Efe, R.; Egamberdieva, D.; Khassanov, F. *Biodiversity, Conservation and Sustainability in Asia: Volume II: Prospects and Challenges in South and Middle Asia*; Springer Nature Switzerland AG, 2021b. DOI: 10.1007/978–3-030–73943–0

Ozturk, M.; Altay, V.; Gönenç, T.M.; Unal, B.T.; Efe, R.; Akçiçek, E.; Bukhari, A. An Overview of Olive Cultivation in Turkey: Botanical Features, Eco-Physiology and Phytochemical Aspects. *Agronomy* **2021c,** *11*, 295.

Petrov, V. A. *Ethnobotany of Nagorno-Karabakh*; Baku, 1940.

Phillips, O.; Gentry, A. H. The Useful Plants of Tambopata Peru: I. Statistical Hypotheses Tests with a New Quantitative Technique. *Econ. Bot.* **1993,** *47*, 15–32.

Pimenov, M. G.; Nabiyeva, F. Kh.; Degtyareva, G. V.; Samigullin, T. Kh.; Ibadullayeva, S. J.; Ibragimov, A. Sh., Zulfugarova, P. V. *Helasciadium nodiflorum*—New Genus and Species of Umbelliferae for the Flora of Azerbaijan and the Entire Caucasus. *Bot. J., St. Petersburg* **2018,** *103* (4), 517–528.

Pleskanovskaya, S. A.; Mamedova, M. A.; Ashıralıyeva, M. A. et al., *Glycyrrhiza glabra* (Liquorice) in Turkmenistan—Medicinal and Biological Aspects. In *Plant and Human Health,—Pharmacology and Therapeutic Uses*; Ozturk, M.; Hakeem, K. R., Eds.; Vol. 3, Chapter 2, Springer Nature: Switzerland 2019; pp 23–35.

Qureshi, R.; Ghazanfar, S. A.; Obied, H.; Vasileva, V.; Tariq, M. A. Ethnobotany: A Living Science for Alleviating Human Suffering. *Evid. Based Complement. Alternat. Med.* **2016,** *2016*, 9641692.

"Red Book" of the Azerbaijan SSR. *Rare and Endangered Species of Animals and Plants*; Ishiq: Baku, 1989.

"Red Book" of the Republic of Azerbaijan. Rare and Endangered Plant and Mushroom Species; Edition II: Baku, 2013.

Robertson, M.; Richards, C. Opportunities and Challenges of Next Generation Sequencing Applications in Ecological Epigenetics. *Mol. Ecol.* **2015,** *24*, 3799–3801.

Savo, V.; Caneva, J. R. G.; McClatchey, W. C. Plant Selection for Ethnobotanical Uses on the Amalfi Coast (Southern Italy). *J. Ethnobiol. Ethnomed.* **2015,** *11*, 58.

Taşpınar, K.; Ozturk, M.; Altay, V.; Polat, H. Sugar beet—An overutilised ancient crop. In: *Crop Production Technologies for Sustainable Use and Conservation*; Ozturk, M. et al., Eds.; Apple Academic Press, Chapter 14, 2019; pp 321–363.

Vardar, Y.; Ozturk, M. Some Ecological Aspects of *Myrtus communis* L. *Bot. Jahrb. Syst.* **1973,** *93*, 562–567.

Younessi-Hamzekhanlu, M.; Ozturk, M.; Altay, V. et al., Ethnopharmacological Study of Medicinal Plants from Khoy City of West Azerbaijan-Iran. *Indian J. Trad. Knowl.* **2020,** *19* (2), 251–267.

APPENDIX 3.1 Bioecological and pharmacological features of the main medicinal plants used in the treatment of various diseases in the territory of Karabakh.

Botanical name (taxa-family)	Months of use	Part used	Use in the diseases
Achillea millefolium L. (Asteraceae)	6–10	Leaves and flowers	Leaves and flowers are quality raw materials. The plant contains general strengthening, anti-inflammatory, antispasmodic, astringent, and weak local anesthetics. Used in the treatment of uterine, lung, gastrointestinal, nasal bleeding, burns, trophic ulcers, chronic boils, and skin diseases. The plant and flowers have been successfully used in gastric and duodenal ulcers, enterocolitis, nephritis, non-specific colitis, spastic pain in the stomach and intestines. It activates and normalizes metabolism, included in the mixtures used in hypertension, atherosclerosis, and obesity. When consumed, platelets in the blood increase. In particular, the use in thrombosis is not allowed. It increases blood clotting. Due to its antiallergic properties, it is successfully used in diathesis, eczema, erysipelas, and bronchial asthma; is indispensable in bleeding, especially in the lungs, intestines, nose, uterus, and kidneys; very useful in neuroses (spastic parametropathy), inflammation of the mammary glands, menstrual disorders, convulsions, and vomiting. It is included in the mixtures used for general strengthening, in asthenic condition, neurosis, and hysteria. Two teaspoons of herb should be infused in 250 mL of hot water for 15 min (in a thermos) (daily dose). It is advisable to consume 2–3 cups a day. For external use, 3 tablespoons of the plant should be infused in 1.5–2 cups of hot water. In diseases of the bile, stomach, and intestines, it is necessary to take 30 g of yarrow, 50 g of chamomile, and 50 g of mint as infusion. For taking a bath, 50–75 g of the plant are infused in 1 L of hot water for 20 min and filtered. This amount is enough for one bath. The plant is widely used in the preparation of fat and meat products (sausages). As an extract, the yield is 17% in 70% alcohol, moisture 13%, total ash 15%, essential oil 0.1%, blackened particles 2%, 4 cm body parts 5%, particles of flowers, stems, and others with a diameter of 0.5 mm 3%, organic matter 0.5%, mineral substances not more than 1%. It is prescribed as a bath and antiseptic for oral administration, also useful as a diaphoretic in lung diseases. It contains bitter substances in leaves and flowers thus used in appetizing, choleretic, anti-hemorrhoidal, and emollient ingredients. The plant is well-known in folk medicine

APPENDIX 3.1 *(Continued)*

Botanical name (taxa-family)	Months of use	Part used	Use in the diseases
			as a hemostatic and wound healing drug. It has been used successfully in liver diseases, gout, rheumatism, lymph node tuberculosis, as well as in deworming, leg pains, purulent wounds, anemia, and pulmonary tuberculosis, and menstruation disorders. In ancient times, Achilles, Patroclus, Giron, Telephus, and Dioscorides called this plant a "miracle plant."
A. hippocastanum L. (Hippocastanaceae)	5–10	Leaves and tissues	The extract made from the seeds is used as a tonic in venous thrombosis. It reduces capillary permeability, improves microcirculation, and eliminates inflammatory processes. The extract of the seeds reduces blood clotting. Drugs derived from seeds are used in varicose veins, acute and chronic thrombophlebitis, trophic ulcers of the shin veins, disorders of peripheral arteries (atherosclerosis of peripheral arteries, arthritis, thromboembolism of small vessels), inflammation of hemorrhagic nodules. Aescin in the leaves is used in acute and chronic diseases of the veins (phlebitis, thrombophlebitis) and rectal fissures and hemorrhoids.
Alnus incana (L.) Moench (Betulaceae)	9–3 Only in winter	Fruit	An astringent, anti-inflammatory, hemostatic, and disinfectant drug. The infusion made from the fruit is an astringent and quality medicine for acute and chronic colitis and enterocolitis.
A. sativum L. (Alliaceae)	5–7	Roots and leaves	It is a mucus-secreting, antiseptic, antitussive, and tonic for the immune system, enhances the secretion of enzymes in the gastrointestinal tract by increasing appetite, has a strong effect on food digestion. Ethereal substances in its content have a bactericidal effect and are disinfectant. The extract is also used in intestinal atony, as part of complex therapy in colds of the upper respiratory tract (bronchitis, tracheitis). The powder and oil are mainly used to increase the resistance of the organism to arterial hypertension, atherosclerosis, hyperlipidemia, and colds.
Althaea officinalis L. (Malvaceae)	4–5; 9–10	Roots, leaves, and flowers	Mainly used in inflammatory diseases of the upper respiratory tract, as a cough suppressant and emollient. The root is widely used in gastric and duodenal ulcers, gastritis, colitis, and diarrhea. In Eastern medicine, it is used in kidney and urinary

APPENDIX 3.1 *(Continued)*

Botanical name (taxa-family)	Months of use	Part used	Use in the diseases
			tract stones, cystitis, tumors of the urinary tract, chronic prostatitis, joint pain. 2–3 tablespoons of the root are infused in 0.5 L of hot water for 10–12 h in a thermos. Half a cup of the infusion should be consumed 20–40 min before meals, 3 times a day. Powder, solution, and syrup made from the roots have anti-inflammatory and antitussive properties.
Ammi visnaga (L.) Lam. (Apiaceae)	6–7	Fruit	It is a spasmolytic and vasomotor drug; relieves smooth muscle spasms, spasms of the urinary tract, intestines, bronchial and coronary arteries. The plant has a spasmolytic effect, reduces vascular tone, dilates the coronary arteries of the heart, intestine, urinary and biliary tract, and bronchi. It is used in inflammatory and stone diseases of the kidneys and urinary tract.
Anabasis aphylla L. (Chenopodiaceae)	7–8	Stem	It has a peculiar faint odor and indeterminate taste. All parts of the plant are poisonous. It is a cough suppressant. The seeds are respiratory analeptic. In large doses it has an analeptic and reflective tonic effect on the respiratory center.
Anethum graveolens L. (Apiaceae)	6–8	Seeds and Shoots	Has fragrant fruit and raw materials, used as a diaphoretic and antispasmodic with very good effect on gastrointestinal and urological problems. As a diaphoretic, it should be used after adding 1000 g water to 1g dill. The fruit has a mild diuretic effect. The mixture with fennel raw material is very valuable as a high-quality anti-flatulent and diaphoretic drug. The leaves are applied during hypochromic anemia and used as a diuretic in hypertension.
Artemisia absinthium L. (Asteraceae)	7–9	Inflorescence and leaves	Used in the treatment of diseases of the gastrointestinal—respiratory tract, inflammation of the kidneys and bladder, pulmonary tuberculosis, purulent wounds, ulcers, fissures. Used to increase appetite. The plant (whole and divided) and flowers are used in infusions and mixtures as a quality appetizer, strengthener of the gastrointestinal tract. Useful as a raw material for brewing and cooking. The bitter substance (absinthe) and other substances in sagebrush stimulate the function of the gastrointestinal tract, especially the pancreas. It increases the activity of the central

APPENDIX 3.1 *(Continued)*

Botanical name (taxa-family)	Months of use	Part used	Use in the diseases
			nervous and hematopoietic system, guarantees a complete cure for asthenia, fatigue, anemia, and epilepsy. Due to its antipyretic and antitussive properties, it is used in the prevention and treatment of malaria, influenza, and acute respiratory diseases accompanied by fever. Successfully used especially in gastric diseases accompanied by hypersecretion, also included in mixtures for the treatment of various liver and biliary tract diseases. It is rich in diuretics and anti-inflammatory substances, infusion is used as an external drug, compresses and soaks, and as an enema against ascarids and pinworms. 1 teaspoon of the plant infused in 250 mL of hot water, and cooled for 10 min and consumed 3 times a day, 1.5 h before or after meals (daily dose). The course of treatment is 2–3 weeks.
Arctium lappa L. (Asteraceae)	9–10	In the first year of life, the roots are collected in autumn	It has a peculiar faint odor; floury, starchy taste. Infused and cooked root is an indispensable tool as a diuretic, choleretic, diaphoretic, in diseases such as rheumatism, gout, cholecystitis, cholangitis; also used in furunculosis, eczema, skin rashes, trophic wounds, burns and externally for washing and soaking.Used as soaking in eczema, furunculosis, rashes, trophic wounds, and burns. Infusion of the root is used in combination with olive or peach oil to strengthen the hair. The leaves are used as a compress for joint pain.
Asparagus officinalis L. (Asparagaceae)	5–7	Roots	Used for scurvy, rheumatism, otitis, angina, late-healing wounds, as an expectorant, and in anorexia.
Astragalus dasyanthus Pall. (Fabaceae)	6–7	Plant parts during mass flowering	Hypotensive and sedative, rich in biologically active substances with pharmacological effects. Contains high amounts of α-tocopherol (vitamin E) and selenium, the plant increases muscle function and normalizes the blood clotting system. Infusion of the plant is used in hypertension, chronic cardiovascular insufficiency, coronary artery spasm, acute and chronic nephritis.
Berberis vulgaris L. (Berberaceae)	5–9	Leaves, roots, fruit	Green leaves are anti-inflammatory, choleretic, antispasmodic, and hemostatic. The roots of the common barberry, a wild perennial shrub, are considered a quality raw material and medicine. The infusion increases bile secretion, due to the antispasmodic effect, dilates the bile duct and creates a choleretic effect. The fruit lowers the blood sugar.

APPENDIX 3.1 *(Continued)*

Botanical name (taxa-family)	Months of use	Part used	Use in the diseases
Betula pendula Roth = *B. verrucosa* Ehrh. (Betulaceae)	1–3	Buds and leaves	The buds are disinfectant and diuretic, when cooked they are useful for kidney disease, heart edema, and as a cholagogue.
B. tripartita L. (Asteraceae)	7–10	Flowers, leaves	An astringent with a peculiar smell and bitter taste, top flowers and leaves are used, an antiseptic, diuretic, choleretic, and anti-inflammatory. The extract destroys gram-positive bacteria and pathogenic fungi as antimicrobial, has weak sedative, choleretic, diaphoretic, diuretic, wound healing, antiallergic and hypotensive properties. Used in the treatment of anorexia, liver, biliary tract, rickets, gout, burns, intractable wounds, ulcers of various etiologies, and infectious diseases. A good blood purifier and antiallergic drug in folk medicine. Used in skin diseases, eczema, diathesis, and erysipelas in children and adolescents is highly effective. External application of the plants in the practice of pediatrics is very useful, effective in the treatment of diathesis, rickets, and eczema. The leaves are put on the snake-bitten area of the skin. The mixture containing Bidens—10 g, Greek walnut—5 g, *Viola tricolor*—20 g, cockleburs roots—15 g, *Urtica* flowers—10 g, black currant leaves—10 g, and strawberry leaves is used in blood purification, skin diseases, and rickets. 20 g of this mixture are boiled in 1 L of water over low heat for 10 min. During the day, adults can take 30 g per h, and children—1 tablespoon. In chronic kidney diseases, 30 g of bearberry and 15 g of birch cones should be added to this composition.
Bistorta major Gray (= *Polygonum bistorta* L.) *Bistorta carnea* (C.Koch) Kom. (=*P.carneum* C. Koch) (Polygonaceae)	5–8	Rhizomes and thin roots	A medicinal plant having astringent properties and strengthening the organism. It manifests astringent, anti-inflammatory, and hemostatic properties. Cooked rhizomes are used in chronic diseases of the intestine, diarrhea, and diseases of the nasopharynx, oropharynx, and hypopharynx. Rhizomes are astringent, anti-inflammatory and hemostatic. Used in acute and chronic intestinal diseases, especially diarrhea, in dental practice in stomatitis, gingivitis, chronic tonsillitis, and other diseases of the mouth and throat.

APPENDIX 3.1 *(Continued)*

Botanical name (taxa-family)	Months of use	Part used	Use in the diseases
Brassica juncea (L.) Czern. *Brassica nigra* L. (Brassicaceae)	6–7	Seeds	A local irritant, distractor, and analgesic, as well as an appetizer. The seeds have active substances. Sinigrin glucoside breaks down sugar into potassium bisulfate, allyl oil, and water. This oil has a specific odor and is flammable, so it warms the area of the skin by reddening it. A mustard leaf 8 × 12.5 cm in size is a local sedative and distractor.
Bryonia aspera Steven ex Lede. (Cucurbitaceae)	5–9	Roots and Rhizomes	Used in diseases of the gastrointestinal tract and duodenum, bronchitis, to treat colds, coughs, worms, as well as in psychological disorders.
Bryonia alba L. (Cucurbitaceae)	5–9	Roots and Rhizomes	The roots are used for medicinal purposes. Two amorphous toxic glucosides—brionine and brionidine, tannins, starch, resin, polysaccharides, etc. are found in the root and other parts. The plant extract increases the cardiac muscle tone and raises blood pressure. The alcoholic extract of the plant has a mild laxative effect. Due to its toxicity, this plant is used in rheumatoid arthritis by rubbing it externally. According to folk medicine, the boiled roots, are used in the treatment of stiff joints and are an effective tool in the treatment of epilepsy.
C. officinalis L. (Asteraceae)	6	Flowers	Used in folk medicine as an anti-tumor drug, also used in diseases of the mouth and throat, injuries and trophic ulcers, gynecological diseases, erosions, trichomonas colpitis, in ophthalmic practice because of its anti-inflammatory properties.
Capsella bursa—pastoris (L.) Medik. (Brassicaceae)	5–6	Above-ground parts	It has hypotensive, antipyretic, astringent, and diuretic properties. Juice made from fresh herbs is strong antihemorrhagic. The infusion is mainly used in the diseases of gastrointestinal tract, diarrhea, bile and kidney stones, gout, and rheumatism with metabolic disorders. Also used as a good hemostatic agent in uterine, gastric, and renal hemorrhage. 2 teaspoons of herbs are infused in 2 cups of hot water for 10 min and consumed 2 cups a day (daily dose). In the case of heart and circulatory disorders, the mixture should be prepared with 10.0 g of Capsella, 10.0 g of hawthorn, 5 g of valerian, 5 g of Melissa, 2 teaspoons of the mixture infused in 250 mL of water for 10 h,

APPENDIX 3.1 *(Continued)*

Botanical name (taxa-family)	Months of use	Part used	Use in the diseases
			and consumed hot. The same dose is taken in combination with horsetail in lung, rheumatism, liver, gout, nasopharyngeal, and throat infections. The liquid and aqueous extracts are used in uterine atony and uterine bleeding. Fresh leaves are used in the treatment of diabetes.
Carum carvi L. (Apiaceae)	7–8	Leaves and fruit	The leaves and fruit are high-quality diaphoretics, successfully used in the treatment of flatulence and included in gastric mixtures, has appetizing, antispasmodic (intestinal muscles, uterus, urinary tract) activity, increases bronchial mucus, enhances lactation in women. 2–3 teaspoons of the plant infused in 200 mL of boiling water (in a thermos) is consumed daily. Effective in coughs of inflammatory origin in the bronchi, gastritis, enterocolitis, intestinal pains in children, flatulence, chronic atonic constipation as diaphoretic, and emollient. Enhances lactation in breastfeeding women. One tablespoon of fruit should be mixed with 1 cup of sour cream and boiled for 3 min. One tablespoon of the obtained mixture should be consumed 3 times a day.
Centaurium umbellatum Gilib. (Asteraceae)	6–10	Roots and Rhizomes	Used as a remedy for rheumatism, diabetes, lung diseases, whooping cough, kidney pain, inflammation of the bladder, epilepsy, as a diuretics improving liver function.
Centaurea cyanus L. (Asteraceae)	5–9	Flowers, roots, and rhizomes	Flowers of the plant are used in the treatment of diseases of the urinary tract, especially glomerulonephritis (does not irritate the renal parenchyma), and prepare the diuretic tea. It contains bitter glucosides, which have a choleretic and antispasmodic effect in liver diseases. In medical practices, the infusion and extract are used as a diuretic in nephritis, cystitis, urethritis, as a cholagogue in the liver, and duodenal ulcers, as an antitussive in diphtheria, neurological and gastric diseases, diarrhea in children, and uterine bleeding; as a diuretic in edema caused by liver and heart diseases. 1 tablespoon of flowers infused in 0.5 L of boiled water (daily dose) should be consumed 2–3 times a day for 30 min before meals. In medical practices, the flowers of the plant are used as a diuretic in inflammation of the urinary tract. Roots and rhizomes (whole, cut) are used as an antitussive medicine. In the cooked form, it is also included in laxative

APPENDIX 3.1 *(Continued)*

Botanical name (taxa-family)	Months of use	Part used	Use in the diseases
			mixtures. As a diuretic in edema due to heart and kidney diseases, as a diuretic in urinary tract diseases (pyelonephritis, cystitis, urethritis), as a diuretic in prostate diseases, as an anti-inflammatory and antispasmodic drug, in metabolic disorders (kidney and gallbladder) as a diuretic and for the regulation of salt metabolism, also prescribed for cholecystitis, cholangitis, biliary dyskinesia, and hepatitis. In folk medicine, the flowers or leaves are mixed with other plants and successfully used in eye practice, uterine bleeding, chronic skin diseases—in the treatment of furunculosis, eczema, trophic wounds. Fresh leaves are used in malaria, edema, conjunctivitis, skin injuries. In Bulgarian medicine, the infusion is used as a tonic for the stomach and appetizing medicine.
Chelidonium majus L. (Papaveraceae)	5–9	Stems and leaves during flowering, fruit	A high-quality and useful raw material. The stem is poisonous, with an odor and an undefined taste. An external anti-inflammatory, antiseptic, antispasmodic, choleretic drug, has mainly antispasmodic, choleretic, and anti-inflammatory (bactericidal) properties. As a drug, it has fungicidal and bacteriostatic effects in cancer, metastases. The juice is obtained from fresh plants. The extract is used in laryngeal and intestinal papillomatosis, lupus erythematosus, 2.5% aqueous infusion in diseases of the liver and biliary tract. Due to its strong toxic properties, overuse can cause nausea, vomiting, and respiratory paralysis.
Cichorium intybus L. (Asteraceae)	7–10	Capitulum	Used in intestinal spasms and inflammation, flatulence, diarrhea, convulsions, as a diuretics, in furuncles, purulent wounds, rheumatism, bronchial asthma, eczema, gastritis, enteritis.
C. sativum L. (Apiaceae)	5–6	Above-ground part	The infusion and aqueous extracts of the plant are quality medicines. Used in the content of mixtures for gastrointestinal, bile diseases, and hemorrhoids.
Convallaria majalis L. (Convallariaceae)	5–7	Leaves, flowers, seeds	Plant is applied since the Middle Ages, used in the treatment of cardiac type neurocirculatory dystonia, hysteria, mild toxic goiter. One tablespoon of the plant infused in 200 mL of boiling water (in a thermos) should be consumed (daily dose).

APPENDIX 3.1 *(Continued)*

Botanical name (taxa-family)	Months of use	Part used	Use in the diseases
			1–2 tablespoons should be taken 3–4 times a day before meals. As a raw material, flowers, leaves, and stems contain corglycone, which is used in cardiovascular diseases and has a strong effect. In folk medicine it is used in the treatment of many diseases: heart, as a diuretic in edema of various etiologies, neurosis, epilepsy, fever, eye diseases, and as an external lotion. As it is a poisonous plant, it should be prescribed by doctors.
Crataegus transcaucasicus Pojark. (Rosaceae)		Flowers and fruit	A cardiotonic drug. The ripe juicy fruit is used as a quality medicinal plant raw material. Stimulates the heart muscle, reduces sensitivity and has an antiarrhythmic effect, dilates peripheral blood vessels, lowers blood pressure by dilating heart and brain blood vessels, hypocholesterolemic effect lowers blood cholesterol, especially lecithin. Used in folk medicine for various purposes. Infusion of flowers and fruit is used as a cardiotonic agent in heart failure, heart palpitations, angioneurosis, early stages of hypertension, insomnia, hyperthyroidism accompanied by tachycardia, especially in menopausal circulatory failure and atherosclerosis.
C. maxima Duch. (Cucurbitaceae)	7–8	Seeds and fruit	The healing properties of the seeds have long been known in folk medicine. It has been studied in detail both experimentally and clinically, used in the preparation of diuretic, anti-ulcer, reparative, anti-inflammatory drugs. Most successfully used in the treatment of tapeworms (pork tapeworm, dwarfs, long tapeworms) and pinworms. The oil of the seeds is used as a hepatotropic and choleretic drug in hepatitis, fatty dystrophy of the liver, dyskinesia of the biliary tract, gastritis, gastric and duodenal ulcers; as a qualitative antidizuritiv agent in prostate adenoma; oil from the seeds has a very good effect on cervical erosion, dermatitis, eczema, and burns. Diuretics, choleretics, and mild laxatives are made from the pulp of the fruit. It improves intestinal function, thus used in constipation, excretion of chlorides from the body, increasing diuresis.
Datisca cannabina L. (Datiscaceae)	Throughout the year	Leaves, stems, stalks, and inflorescences	Has a faint odor and a bitter taste, has mainly choleretic and anti-inflammatory, anti-ulcer and antispasmodic effects. Affects the large intestine smooth muscles and bile ducts. The toxic effect is small. It is prescribed as a cholagogue in cholecystitis, as a spasmolytic in hypoacidity, gastritis, and gastric and duodenal ulcers.

APPENDIX 3.1 *(Continued)*

Botanical name (taxa-family)	Months of use	Part used	Use in the diseases
Dryopteris filix-mas (L.) Schott (Drypteridaceae)	4–5; 9–10	Leaves, roots, and rhizomes	As an anthelmintic drug, used in kidney and urinary tract diseases. Filixanum in its content is used to treat tapeworms. The extract obtained from rhizomes is successfully applied as an anthelmintic, sometimes overdose can cause shortness of breath, vomiting, diarrhea, headaches, cardiovascular distress, and difficulty breathing.
Echinops ritro L. (= *E. ruthenicus* Bieb.) (Asteraceae)	9–10	Flowers and ripe fruit	An analeptic and immune tonic medicinal plant, increases the reflex activity of the spinal cord, tones skeletal muscles, less toxic, has wide therapeutic effects. Used in injuries of the central and peripheral branches of the central nervous system—paresis of the facial nerve, vascular dystonia in asthenic conditions, and hypotension and atrophy of the optic nerve.
Equisetum arvense L. (Equisetaceae)	5–7	Vegetative stems and branches	Has anti-inflammatory, disinfectant, diuretic, hemostatic, cardiotonic, tonic, wound healing, and astringent properties. It normalizes water-salt metabolism, lowers cholesterol, and removes toxic slags from the body (especially in lead poisoning). Used in the treatment of hypertension, atherosclerosis, gout, and wounds that are difficult to heal, rheumatism, eye, gallbladder, and kidney diseases, tumors of the stomach and intestines, internal and external bleedings, edema of the lower extremities. External application is prescribed for chronic hard-to-heal ulcers of the skin and dandruff (seborrhea). Included in diuretic teas, used in many cases of edema (pleurisy, heart, kidney, tuberculosis, chronic lead poisoning) and gout. An herbal mixture is the best anti-asthma and anti-cancer remedy. 1–2 tablespoons of the plant infused in 2 cups of boiling water (thermos) (daily dose) should be consumed. The infused and cooked plant is considered a good remedy for inflammation of the bladder and urinary tract in heart disease. It is prescribed for skin rashes, obesity, microhematuria, hemorrhage, especially in tuberculosis etiology, and pulmonary heart failure. 2 teaspoons of the mixture containing horsetail 10 g, *Plantago lanceolata* 10 g, anise 5 g, elderberry flowers 5 g, and thyme 5 g should be infused in 250 mL of water for 15 min and consumed 2–3 cups every day. Solution for external use: 4–5 tablespoons of the plant is brewed in 2 cups of hot water.

APPENDIX 3.1 *(Continued)*

Botanical name (taxa-family)	Months of use	Part used	Use in the diseases
Ephedra aurantica Takht.et Pachom. (Ephedraceae)	4–10 (except the 6. month)	Above-ground organs	Stimulates the respiratory system, increases blood pressure, improves the nutrition and volume of the heart, increases the tone of peripheral blood vessels, reduces the tone of the bronchial smooth muscles. Improves liver blood circulation. It creates mydriasis and lowers the intraocular pressure by dilating the pupils. Normalizes blood pressure, used in asthma attacks in infectious diseases, spring fever, urticaria, and other allergic diseases, in rheumatism, malaria, asthma, hypertension, gastrointestinal diseases, and ascites. Ephedrine obtained from the plant stimulates and calms the cardiovascular system, used in bronchial asthma due to the reduction of smooth muscle tone in the bronchi, whooping cough, asthmatic bronchitis, allergic diseases (spring fever, urticaria, vasomotor rhinitis, serum sickness), lowering blood pressure, infections, intoxications, acute trauma, and inflammation.1 teaspoon of the plant dissolved in 250 mL of water for 10 min and consumed 3 times a day and 1 cup 2 times a week.
Ficus carica L. (Moraceae)	5–8	Leaves and fruit	The leaves are used as a photosensitizing drug in the treatment of vitiligo (leukoderma), alopecia, wounds, and boils. The fruit is used as an emollient and laxative.
Filipendula ulmaria (L.) Maxim. (Rosaceae)	6–7	Flowers	The flowers are used to prepare anti-inflammatory, hemostatic, diuretic, anti-hemorrhoid, wound, and anti-burn medicines. Cooked (1:20 and 1:50) and brewed (1:50 and 1: 100) flowers are evaluated. Used as an anti-inflammatory, astringent, to facilitate healing of wounds, in baths for wounds, as bandages to dry wounds; for gargling, to treat eczema, trophic wounds, itchy dermatoses, and rashes; very effective as an enema in hemorrhoids.
Frangula alnus Mill. (Rhamnaceae)	5–9	Roots	Like the *Senna plant*, it also contains weak laxatives, affects 8–12 h after consumption; used in constipation, spastic colitis, hemorrhoids, rectal fissures, pregnancy constipation; has anti-inflammatory and diaphoretic properties. One tablespoon of roots should be brewed in 1 cup of hot water for 10–15 min over low heat. It is possible to consume 1/2 cup 2 times a day in the mornings and evenings.
Foeniculum vulgare Mill. (Apiaceae)		Ripe fruit and a central umbel	The solution made from the fruit is used as an antitussive, intestinal emollient in flatulence, and a cholagogue.

APPENDIX 3.1 *(Continued)*

Botanical name (taxa-family)	**Months of use**	**Part used**	**Use in the diseases**
Fumaria officinalis L. (Papaveraceae)	6–7	Seeds	Used against pancreatitis, cholecystitis, chronic hepatitis, chronic gastritis, enterocolitis, as an anthelmintic, to increase urinary and sweat excretion, in eczema, and as an antitussive.
Glycyrrhiza glabra L. (Fabaceae)	Year round	Roots and stems	In folk medicine used for colds accompanied by cough, 0.5 teaspoons of *Glycyrrhiza* roots mixed with 1 teaspoon of honey should be consumed 3 times a day. In gastric ulcers and various biliary diseases, the root should be chewed 5–7 times a day. The dry and concentrated extract made from the roots is a cough elixir; *Glycyrrhiza* syrup is an antitussive.
Kalanchoe pinnata (Lam.) Pers. (Grassulaceae)	4–9	Stems and leaves	Anti-inflammatory drug, stimulates tissue regeneration; juice from the plant is anti-inflammatory and activates the exudation phase. Used in wounds, burns, frostbite, when antibacterial agents are required, in the purification of pus, epithelialization. Under the influence of the juice, the body produces anti-enzyme substances, used as an antivirus in poliomyelitis and enteroviruses. The juice made from fresh stems is used as a local anti-inflammatory, tissue cleaner. Also prescribed for the treatment of purulent necrotic processes, trophic wounds, bedsores, perforated wounds, skin transplants, and burns; to put tampons in purulent wounds, abscesses, paronychia, furunculosis, used in erysipelas, eye diseases, dystrophy of the eye, burns, trauma, and keratitis.
Helichrysum plicatum DC. (Asteraceae)	6–8	Inflorescence and leaves	Used in diseases of the gastrointestinal tract, liver, diarrhea, headaches, joint pains, jaundice, itching, worms; more effective in liver diseases, especially in acute hepatitis of various etiologies; widely used in indigestion, poor appetite, deficiency of gastrointestinal enzymes, atherosclerosis, fat metabolism disorders, obesity, diabetes, coronary heart disease as a hypolipidemic drug, for the removal of cholesterol and related compounds from the body; successfully used in the complex therapy of giardiasis.

APPENDIX 3.1 *(Continued)*

Botanical name (taxa-family)	Months of use	Part used	Use in the diseases
H. rhamnoides L. (Elaegnaceae)	6–9	Leaves, fruit, and seeds	The oil, fruit juice, and extracted products are widely used in the formation of epithelial cells and as a painkiller. The oil obtained from the pulp of the fruit is very valuable in the treatment of skin wounds, trauma, eczema, lupus. In colds and fevers, it is advisable to consume 1 tablespoon of fruit juice and puree 3 times a day. The oil is anti-inflammatory, analgesic, used for wound healing, participates in the regeneration of epithelial tissues. The oil has been used successfully in the prevention and treatment of cancer (stomach cancer) by radiation. Used in gastric and duodenal ulcers, erosions, and colpitis of the cervix in obstetric practice; leaves are used in cases of scurvy, hypo-, and avitaminosis, skin burns, frostbite, rashes, and injuries.
Hedysarum caucasicum Bieb. (Fabaceae)	7–8	Leafy stem	An astringent with a faint odor and an antiviral drug. The ointment destroys the herpes virus. The above-ground part is an indispensable medicine for strengthening the body of the elderly in respiratory diseases and chronic diseases in spring and autumn.
Hypericum perforatum L. (Hyperiacaceae)	7–8	Stems, flowers, and leaves during flowering	Recently, the antidepressant effect of this plant has been discovered. An astringent, antiseptic, anti-inflammatory, and antidepressant drug; above-ground part (stems, flowers, and leaves) widely used. It strengthens the body, shows hemostatic properties. Used as a stimulant and antispasmodic in myocarditis and endocarditis, asthenic cases, neurosis, neurasthenia, headache, weakness, as an anti-inflammatory and analgesic agent; in diseases of the gastrointestinal tract (gastritis, gastric and duodenal ulcers, enterocolitis, diarrhea, hemorrhoids, ulcerative colitis), liver, duodenum (cholecystitis, cholelithiasis, jaundice, chronic hepatitis). Infused and cooked plants are prescribed for intestinal colitis, skin burns, gingivitis and stomatitis. The mixture containing this plant is used in combination with antibiotics in the treatment of gram-positive microorganisms and staphylococci; also used in abscesses, phlegmon, and infiltrative processes. It has also been shown to relieve high psychoemotional sensitivity and stress, shows photosensitizing properties. Its mixture with biologically active substances (alcohol, carotenoids, tocopherols) has an inflammatory effect.

APPENDIX 3.1 *(Continued)*

Botanical name (taxa-family)	Months of use	Part used	Use in the diseases
			The infusion is a quality antispasmodic, astringent, disinfectant, and anti-inflammatory drug; used in gastritis, acute and chronic enteritis and colitis, biliary dyskinesia, cholecystitis, gallstone disease, hepatitis, and flatulence. Infusion in the rinsing form is used in tonsillitis, angina, gingivitis, and stomatitis. The solution is prepared by brewing 1 tablespoon of herbs in 1.5 cups of boiled water (in a thermos) and consumed 1/3 cup 3 times a day 20–40 min before meals. For external use, 2–3 tablespoons of the plant parts are infused in 2 cups of boiling water and taken as a solution. 2 teaspoons of the plant parts are brewed in 250 mL of boiled water and taken 2–3 cups a day. It should be taken for several weeks in a row. To prepare the alcohol solution it should be stored in 70–96% ethyl alcohol in a ratio of 1:10 for 10 days. 30–50 drops of solution are solved in 1/3 cup of water and used for rinsing.
			In folk medicine, it is used in joint diseases of the metabolism, infectious and rheumatic etiology, wounds, ulcers, and various traumas, acute infectious diseases: tuberculosis, fever, and benign derivatives. In mastopathy—mastitis, it is useful for the treatment of inflammatory diseases of the female genital organs. Due to the photosensitizing properties of the plant, it is used in the treatment of the *vitiligo* disease, treatment of mouth and throat diseases, burns, and injuries. Also used in the cases of unpleasant sensations in the liver, bitterness in the mouth, constipation, loss of appetite. Not recommended for those who are prone to hypertension because it raises blood pressure. The plant should be brewed in 250 mL of water for 5 min. A cup of the infusion should be consumed 2–3 times a day (in case of cough, its mixture with honey is used). It is not recommended to drink for more than 24 h. Used in folk medicine for neurosis, palpitations, and weakness.
Humulus lupulus L. (Cannabaceae)	7–8	Inflorescence (female flowers), fruit	A sedative, somnolent, appetizing, and analgesic. The ripen swollen fruit of ordinary hop is quality raw material. The flowers (whole and divided) are used as a quality sedative and general body-strengthening drug.

APPENDIX 3.1 *(Continued)*

Botanical name (taxa-family)	Months of use	Part used	Use in the diseases
Inula helenium L. (Asteraceae)	7–10	Lower leaves and young tips, roots	Used in bronchitis, pneumonia, bronchial asthma, tuberculosis, and diphtheria due to its antitussive and inflammatory properties. It is prescribed for gastritis, colitis, diseases of the liver and bile ducts, urinary tract due to its high anti-inflammatory properties. Also evalauted in diarrhea, chronic enterocolitis, constipation, anorexia. Rhizomes and roots are useful in bronchitis, tracheitis, pulmonary tuberculosis, asthma. A quality antitussive and disinfectant herb. Used in gastric diseases—gastritis, ulcers, nervous diseases, radiculitis, endemic ur, and duodenal ulcers, 1 tablespoon infusion taken 2–3 times a day. Very effective in heart diseases, hypertension, toothache, shortness of breath and weight loss, colitis, liver, bile, urinary tract diseases, and edema. Highly effective anthelmintic (especially against ascarids); especially effective against worms at concentrations of 1:100 and 1:1000. Cooked rhizomes and roots (crushing, briquettes) are used in diseases of the respiratory system, especially in mixtures such as cough suppressants. A preparation called Alanton, used at a dose of 0.12 g, 3 times a day for 6–8 weeks after meals, has a very good effect on diseases of the stomach and duodenum. Two teaspoons of the plant parts added to 1 cup of boiled water are kept in a thermos. 1/3 cup 3 times a day should be taken 20–40 min before meals. For infusion, 1 tablespoon of the root should be brewed in 2 cups of water over low heat for 10–15 min. It is advisable to take 1–2 tablespoons every hour. Acute kidney disease and pregnancy are contraindicated. In skin diseases (leishmaniasis, eczema, skin rashes) the roots are filtered and the ointment is applied to the skin while hot. Inula is considered valuable in Tibetan medicine. In Bulgarian medicine, the infusion of the roots is used as a remedy for palpitation, headaches, epilepsy, and diphtheria. The composition of the ancient recipe (ointment) for skin diseases is as follows: 180 g of the Inula root is boiled in 360 g of water and mixed with 120 g of pork fat and butter. It is used in rheumatism in combination with the root of cockleburs.

APPENDIX 3.1 *(Continued)*

Botanical name (taxa-family)	Months of use	Part used	Use in the diseases
			* 2 tablespoons of the Inula roots are brewed in 1 cup of water for 30 min, cooled for 10 min, 0.5 cup of the infusion is taken 2–3 times a day 1 h before meals. * 2 teaspoons of the crushed Inula roots are kept in cold boiled water for 8 h, 0.5 cup is consumed 4 times a day 30 min before meals. * 20 g of the Inula roots are kept in 100 g of 70% alcohol for 8–10 days. 20 drops are consumed 3 times a day 20 min before meals. In gynecological diseases, 1 teaspoon of the crushed Inula roots are added to 1 cup of hot water, kept over low heat for 10–15 min, set aside for 4 h, and filtered. In premature painful menstruation, one tablespoon is taken, 3–4 times a day.
Iris germanica L. (Iridaceae)	5–6	Above-ground parts	Used in avitaminosis, gastrointestinal diseases, bloating, flatulence, anemia, jaundice, bleeding. The plant has also an appetizing effect.
Juniperus oblonga Bieb. (Cupressaceae)	8–10	Fruit	The fruit has a tonic, general strengthening, phytoncide, anti-inflammatory, antitussive, emollient, and strong diuretic effect; used in asthenia, anemia, furunculosis, joint diseases, chronic skin diseases, gallstones, and kidney stones, and gout. It is very effective in the treatment of liver and bile diseases. The fruit also used in the treatment of kidney and urinary tract diseases (chronic nephritis, pyelonephritis, cystitis, nephrolithiasis, acute and chronic urethritis). It is prescribed as a high-quality diuretic in the treatment of edema of various etiologies. In various joint diseases, a solution of fruit and twigs (200–300 g of raw material in 1 L of water) are used in the form of a bath, the twigs are used also for disinfection in various infectious diseases. As it has essential oil, it irritates the digestive system, increases peristalsis, dilutes sputum, and increases diuresis.
Leonurus quinquelobatus Gilib. (=*L. cardiaca* L.) (Lamiaceae)	6–7	Stems, flowers, and leaves during flowering	As a sedative, lowers blood pressure and slows the heart pulpitation rate; improves carbohydrate and fat metabolism, normalizes protein metabolism. The extract is used in neurosis, hypertension, coronary heart disease, thyrotoxicosis, insomnia, and vegetative-vascular dystonia; also in gastrointestinal neurosis, flatulence, and spastic colitis.

APPENDIX 3.1 *(Continued)*

Botanical name (taxa-family)	Months of use	Part used	Use in the diseases
Matricaria matricarioides (Less.) Porter (Asteraceae)	6–7	Capitulum	Has a sedative effect on the nervous system; anti-inflammatory, antiseptic, hemostatic, analgesic, anti-bloating, diaphoretic, choleretic, astringent, emollient, astringent, and antiallergic properties; used in the diseases of the respiratory system as a weak antitussive, in the gastrointestinal tract—gastritis, ulcers, enterocolitis, non-specific ulcerative colitis, cholecystitis, hepatitis, intestinal dyskinesia, and flatulence. Included in many mixtures in the diseases of kidneys, urinary tract, and diathesis; prescribed for angina, stomatitis, and periodontitis, eczema, furunculosis, and burns. 2–3 tablespoons of flowers are infused in 2 cups of hot water (in a thermos) and consumed 3 times a day. When applied externally, 4–6 tablespoons of flowers should be brewed in 2 cups of hot water. The flowers are anti-inflammatory, antispasmodic, antiallergic, and diaphoretic. It is taken orally as a solution and in the composition of mixtures; has a weak antiseptic and astringent effect.
Melissa officinalis L. (Lamiaceae)	5–7	The plant is collected along with the stem and leaves at the top when budding and flowering begins	The crushed leaves are sedative and antispasmodic. Applied to facial rashes, has a sedative, antispasmodic and antibacterial effectİ; relieves shortness of breath, heart pain, reduces the number of breaths, tones and strengthens the nervous system. The high therapeutic effect is due to the essential oil it contains; plant regulates the secretion of gastric juice, reduces spasms, eliminates flatulence, dyskinesia, enzyme deficiencies, and improves metabolism. The infusion is used successfully in neuroses, fatigue, vegetative-vascular dystonia; also in intestinal dyskinesia and intestinal pains, cholecystitis, cholangitis, kidney stones, urinary tract diseases, angina, and menopausal syndromes. When used externally, it has good antibacterial, antiviral effects on the skin against furunculosis, herpes, stomatitis, and periodontitis. The juice of the young leaves cut before flowering is used in cooking.
Melilotus officinalis (L.) Pall. (Fabaceae)	7–9	Top flowers (30 cm), leaves	It is fragrant and bitter. It is an anticoagulant herb for the treatment of convulsions; is sedative, venotonic, and angioprotective drug; a local emollient. Inflammatory processes in the skin are treated with poultice and compress; used in folk medicine as an antitussive, emollient, diaphoretic, analgesic; prescribed for diseases of the respiratory system and hypersensitivity of the organism.

APPENDIX 3.1 *(Continued)*

Botanical name (taxa-family)	Months of use	Part used	Use in the diseases
M. piperita L. (Lamiaceae)	7–8	Leaves and flowers	Has antispasmodic, analgesic, antiseptic, choleretic, and astringent properties; used in the treatment of hypertension, angina, rheumatism, toothache, and atherosclerosis because it stimulates the cardiovascular system and relieves pain (especially headaches); recommended for the treatment of diseases of the upper respiratory tract—bronchial asthma and bronchiectasis; has a good effect on the biliary tract and intestinal dyskinesia; increases digestion and appetite. It is used in gastritis, ulcers, colitis, enterocolitis, flatulence, shortness of breath, vomiting, and diarrhea; included in herbal teas for gallstones, hepatitis, and cholecystitis; constant use strengthens the organism. As a sedative, the plant has a positive effect on hysteria, fatigue, migraines, as well as a diuretic effect. Due to the menthol content of the leaves, it is used in angina, stomach, and intestinal pains. Used externally in baths and recommended in neuralgia, toothache, bronchitis, and bronchiectasis due to its antiseptic, analgesic, and inflammatory properties; leaves are used to increase appetite, against shortness of breath, and vomiting.
Nigella sativa L. (Ranunculaceae)	5–6	Petals	Used for whooping cough, eczema, lichen, bronchitis, bronchial asthma, gastrointestinal diseases, pleurisy, as anti-convulsive, emollient, and anti-inflammatory. Mentioned to be effective in all health problems except death.
Ononis arvensis L. (Fabaceae)		Above-ground part	Infusion of the plant is used as hemostatic in hemorrhoids and during inflammatory processes; used in rectal fissures, post-dysentery, and proctological constipation, in the form of infusions and extracts; prescribed for the high tone of the rectum, hemorrhagic veins, painful defecation. Successfully used in thrombophlebitis, in varicose enlarged phlebothrombosis.
Origanum vulgare L. (Lamiaceae)	7–8	Flowering period, above-ground part	A fragrant, sweet and bitter, slightly astringent plant, used as quality cough medicine and a drug that increases intestinal peristalsis. It is prescribed as an infusion for oral administration, bath, and as an antiseptic; also useful as a diaphoretic in lung diseases, strengthens the central nervous system: used in neurosis, fatigue, hysteria, epilepsy, hypertension, atherosclerosis, in neurotic complaints related to menopause; increases

APPENDIX 3.1 *(Continued)*

Botanical name (taxa-family)	Months of use	Part used	Use in the diseases
			the secretion of the bronchial gland, has a spasmolytic, antitussive effect, causes strong sweating; used in the treatment of bronchitis, pneumonia, bronchiectasis, bronchial asthma, and diphtheria. Also evalauted in anorexia, gastritis, gastrointestinal spasms, gastric and duodenal ulcers, atonic constipation, as a cholagogue and anti-inflammatory; used in rheumatism when joints are swollen, in gout, amenorrhea, eczema, skin rashes and various injuries. To prepare the solution, 2 tablespoons of the plant should be infused in 2 cups of boiled water (in a thermos). It should be taken 3 times a day 20–40 min before meals.
Padus avium Mill. (Rosaceae)	10	Leaves, flowers, bark, and fruit, rhizomes, and roots	An astringent, anti-inflammatory, hemostatic, antimicrobial drug that contains tannins; reduces capillary permeability due to anthocyanin and vitamin P. Tannins and anthocyanins have an anti-inflammatory and a phytoncide effect. Cooked and liquid extracts of roots and rhizomes are prescribed as a quality medicine having astringent and hemostatic properties in chronic intestinal diseases, diarrhea, colitis, enterocolitis, stomatitis, gingivitis, and cervical erosion.
P. somniferum L. (Papaveraceae)	7–9	Fruit and capsule	A herbaceous plant, ripe capsules are used to prepare opium, has a unique smell, a painkiller and analeptic. The crushed capsules and seeds (raw material) of poppy, are a quality hypnotic and analgesic.
Phaseolus vulgaris L. (Fabaceae)	8–9	Fruit	The fruit is a hypoglycemic, diuretic, and hypotensive drug; is used in mild and moderate diabetes.The infusion is prescribed in the early stages of kidney disease, rheumatism, hypertension, and disorders of salt metabolism.
Peganum harmala L. (Peganaceae)	4–5	Above-ground parts	Stems, leaves, buds, and flowers are considered raw materials, having a specific odor and indefinite taste. Quinazoline-containing indole alkaloids are present in all organs of the plant. Local communities use its seeds as a painkiller. To relieve pain 1–2 seeds are kept at the base of the tooth. Increases skeletal muscle tone and intestinal motor function; used in various diseases of the peripheral nervous system and brain disorders. For religious reasons it is burned to prevent the evil eye, the smoke improves mood and relieves the pain.

APPENDIX 3.1 *(Continued)*

Botanical name (taxa-family)	Months of use	Part used	Use in the diseases
Persicaria hydropiper (L.) Spach (Polygonaceae)	6–7	Above-ground parts and roots during flowering	A drug with hemostatic as well as analgesic properties; used in modern medicine for hemorrhoids, chronic endometritis, uterine fibroids, and heavy menstrual bleeding. In medical practice, the infusion and aqueous extract of the plant are used as a hemostatic drug in disorders of uterine menopause and dysmenorrhea, and hemorrhagic bleeding; prescribed as a painkiller together with *Claviceps purpurea*. The infusion is prepared in a ratio of 12:200 and a tablespoon of the drug should be consumed 3 times a day. In folk medicine, it is used as an astringent, analgesic, hemostatic agent; also used in the treatment of kidney stones, edema, gastric ulcers, eczema, asthma, and thyroid diseases.
Picea abies (L.) Karst. (Pinaceae)	7–8	Cones	Used for rinsing the mouth and inhalation during inflammation of the upper respiratory tract.
P. anisum L. (Apiaceae)	10	Seeds and above-ground parts	An antitussive medicine; fruit and above-ground parts are considered to be medicinal raw materials. Anetol in the plant oil affects the mucous membranes of the respiratory tract; increases the secretion and causes the evacuation of sputum by activating the ciliated epithelial cells in the respiratory tract; also has antiseptic properties by affecting the muscles in the bronchi and intestines, it relieves spasms, has an anti-inflammatory, diuretic effect, and increases the milk supply of lactating women. It is prescribed as an antitussive in inflammation of the upper respiratory tract, diphtheria. Pharmacologically, the essential oil has an absorbing and antispasmodic effect. This oil has a bactericidal effect, accelerating the removal of sputum from the bronchi, affecting its dilution; very effective in the diseases of trachea, laryngitis, bronchitis, diphtheria, chronic bronchopneumonia, and tonsillitis; successfully used in gastritis, flatulence, atonic constipation, and other diseases of the gastrointestinal tract. The fruit has a mild diuretic effect in cystitis, pyelonephritis, urethritis, as well as antiseptic and antispasmodic effect. In obstetrics and gynecology, the fruit as an adjuvant also stimulates menstruation and childbirth.

APPENDIX 3.1 *(Continued)*

Botanical name (taxa-family)	Months of use	Part used	Use in the diseases
Pinus sylvestris L. (Pinaceae)	2–3	Cones	The infusion of the buds is a quality medicine, used as an antitussive, disinfectant, and diuretic. Its extract is included in body-strengthening baths.
Plantago major L. (Plantaginaceae)		Leaves and seeds	The briquetted leaves are used as a quality anti-inflammatory and antitussive; juice made from fresh roots of the plant is considered indispensable for the treatment of anacid gastritis and chronic colitis. The plant has anti-inflammatory, bactericidal, wound healing, antitussive and hemostatic, diuretic, and hypotensive effects; more widely used in hypertension and atherosclerosis. The juice and infusion of the leaves are a good cough suppressant, therefore used successfully in acute and chronic respiratory diseases; also used in diseases of the gastrointestinal tract, gastritis, gastric and duodenal ulcers, acute and chronic enteritis, ulcerative colitis. It is very effective in the treatment of diarrhea, dysentery, and tuberculosis. For this purose 1–3 teaspoons (5–15 g) of the plant infused in 2 cups of hot water should be consumed 3 times a day, 30 min before meals (daily dose). 1 g of the plant powder can be taken 3–4 times a day, 30–40 min before meals. In the case of lung and stomach cancer, it is necessary to crush the fresh leaves of the plant, add powdered sugar until saturated, and keep it in a warm place for 2 weeks. One tablespoon of the preparation should be consumed 3–4 times a day, 20 min before meals. It is recommended for the treatment of malignant tumors, diseases of the stomach, intestines, liver, kidneys, diabetes, infertility, chronic ulcers, eye, and lung diseases, bleeding. Infusion of plantain is an analgesic in pulmonary tuberculosis, accompanied by fever and cough, and is indispensable in the removal of toxins from the body in various insect and snake bites. Leaves and seeds are used in chronic diarrhea.
Plantago squalida Salisb.=*Plantago psyllium* L. (Plantaginaceae)	6–7	Leaves	The plant is collected during the flowering period. Seed collection done during fruiting. Freshly harvested plant is used as a medicinal raw material for making juice. Cultivated forms and mature seeds are used as quality medicine. Fresh leaves are used to make juice, which is used in the treatment of gastritis and chronic colitis.

APPENDIX 3.1 *(Continued)*

Botanical name (taxa-family)	Months of use	Part used	Use in the diseases
Primula veris L. (Primulaceae)	5–6	Leaves	Has a specific smell and a bittersweet taste; leaves contain large quantity of vitamins (especially ascorbic acid) used against scurvy. The rhizomes and roots are used in infectious inflammatory diseases of the respiratory tract, difficult expectoration, and coughing fits.
Polygonum aviculare L. (Polygonaceae)	6–7	Flowers	Has a diuretic, anti-inflammatory, astringent, tonic, hemostatic, and choleretic effect. It is prescribed for enterocolitis accompanied by diarrhea; used especially in diseases of the kidneys and urinary tract, nephritis, pyelonephritis, cystitis, gastritis, diseases of the liver, gallbladder, gynecological diseases of inflammatory etiology, infertility, gout, tuberculosis, malaria, diphtheria, rickets, and diathesis. Also used in many hemorrhages (gastrointestinal, kidney, lung, and uterine) and lung diseases accompanied by cough. 2–3 tablespoons of the plant parts are heated in 2 cups of cold boiled water until boiling (daily dose). In spring and autumn, for prophylactic purposes, 1 cup can be consumed 2–3 times a day, each time. The course of treatment is several weeks. It is recommended to take 3 cups a day during diarrhea. Also used in rheumatism, gout, urinary tract, and kidney diseases, urinary retention, and hemorrhoids. Externally used on skin rashes. The infusion of the plant is used in the removal of kidney calculi and inflammatory processes. The mixture prepared is used and the juice of the plant is prescribed for malignant tumors. In folk medicine, it normalizes metabolism, is included in the ingredients used in diseases of the kidneys and gallbladder. Fresh juice made from the plant is mainly used in the treatment of burns.
Populus nigra L. (Salicaceae)	5–8	Buds, side stems, and leaves	The plant stem is a diuretic, analgesic, sedative, and antiseptic. The water-alcohol extract is an antiseptic and anti-inflammatory drug. Infusion of the leaves is used in burns, wounds, dermatitis, cystitis, intestinal atony, as a diuretic in edemas, in cystitis, intestinal atony, and hemorrhoids. The buds are applied against rheumatism.

APPENDIX 3.1 *(Continued)*

Botanical name (taxa-family)	Months of use	Part used	Use in the diseases
Potentilla erecta (L.) Raeuschel (Rosaceae)	4–5, 9–10	Rhizomes are collected during flowering, especially in spring and autumn	It has a faint odor, is fragrant, and has a strong astringent effect; accepted as a quality herbal medicine for diarrhea and nasopharyngeal diseases—gingivitis, stomatitis, enteritis, enterocolitis, dyspepsia, dysentery, bleeding ulcerative colitis, diseases of the esophagus, larynx, digestive, respiratory and other organs. Used in angina, chronic tonsillitis, hemorrhoids, burns, eczema, neurodermatitis, skin and mucous membrane damage, and excessive sweating of the feet.
P. granatum L. (Punicaceae)	5–11	Fruit and peel, rhizomes	Increases appetite, improves digestion, has an anti-bloating effect, increases the tone of the central nervous system, has a choleretic effect; is a psychostimulant and astringent. Pomegranate fruit is widely used in dysentery and intestinal disorders due to its astringent properties. The juice is used in the treatment of anemia. The roots, stems, and bark are used to treat tapeworms. It is considered an effective remedy for anemia.
Quercus robur L. (Fagaceae)	3–4	Root and stem bark	Roots are astringent. Its broth has astringent and anti-inflammatory properties, recovers denatured proteins. Antimicrobial, antiprotozoal properties are due to the presence of gallic acid and catechins. The bark of the wild and cultivated Oak plant is harvested as a raw material in early spring and used as a quality medicine. Due to its astringent properties, it is an indispensable medicinal plant in gingivitis, stomatitis, diseases of mouth, throat, esophagus, larynx, and the digestive and respiratory organs.
Rhamnus cathartica L. (Rhamnaceae)	8–9	Flowers	A wild shrub, the ripe fruit is used as a quality laxative. Increases the peristalsis of the large intestines, bowel movement occurs 10–14 h after a meal. The solution, infusion, and fresh fruit are used in spastic and atonic constipation, hemorrhoids, rectal prolapse. Has a diuretic effect. When used as a mild decoction and dry medicine, the effect is visible after 8–10 h in atonic and spastic constipation. Very useful in hemorrhoids and anal fissures. In this case, 1 tablespoon of fruit (15–20 pieces) is boiled in 1 cup of water for 10–15 min and half a cup is taken in the evenings. To prepare the solution, 1 tablespoon of the plant is brewed in 1 cup of boiled water for 2 h. 0.5 cup of the solution should be consumed at night. In folk medicine, it is used for edema, gout, skin rashes. The fruit is known in medicine as an anti-tumor agent.

APPENDIX 3.1 *(Continued)*

Botanical name (taxa-family)	Months of use	Part used	Use in the diseases
Rubus idaeus L. (Rosaceae)	6–8	Fruit, flowers	In folk medicine fresh fruit is used in alcohol poisoning, hypermenorrhea, hemorrhoids and skin rashes. Dissolving 1 tablespoon of roots in 2 cups of water is very effective in the treatment of bronchitis. Infusion of the leaves is very effective in gargling in diseases of the mouth and throat, redness and rashes on the skin, conjunctivitis. The fruit is used as a diaphoretic and antipyretic, and the leaves as an astringent in diarrhea and bleeding. Infused and cooked leaves as an emollient in coughs and angina, infusion of the leaves used in hemorrhoids and gynecological diseases. An ointment made from fresh raspberry leaves is used for the treatment of acne and rashes on the skin. Infusion of flowers is used in acne, erysipelas, and conjunctivitis. Raspberry flowers, fruit, and leaves are used as antisclerotic, anti-inflammatory, antipyretic remedies and as vitamin-rich substances in hypertension and atherosclerosis. Used in the confectionery industry to produce juices, kvass, syrups, tinctures. Pies and jams are made from both fresh and dried fruits.
Rhus coriaria L. (Anacardiaceae)	4–5, 8	Leaves, fruit	Leaves collected before flowering and green fruit after flowering. It is an astringent and tanning medicine, used as an anti-inflammatory as well as antiseptic. The plant has cholagogue properties. Sumac leaves are used as a quality medicine. The leaves are a source of raw materials for tannin production.
Rosa canina L. (Rosaceae)	9–10	Roots and fruit	Infusion of the root removes all stones and salts from the body, weakens, and destroys plasmodium malaria. Two tablespoons of finely chopped root infused in 200 g of hot water for 15 min is taken every other day, 1 cup 3 times a day. The fruit and seeds are a valuable remedy for tapeworms, urinary stones, rheumatism, gout, and as a diuretic.
R. officinalis L. (Lamiaceae)	4–10	Above-ground parts	The infusion of rosemary leaves is used as a tonic, anti-inflammatory, in fatigue, cardiac neurosis, biliary excretion, neuritis and colds, severe injuries, boils and gynecological practice, and menstrual disorders. Fresh leaves and stems are used for inhalation in colds, and the ointment is used for rubbing painful areas in rheumatism and radiculitis.

APPENDIX 3.1 *(Continued)*

Botanical name (taxa-family)	Months of use	Part used	Use in the diseases
Rubia tinctorum L. (Rubiaceae)	2–4, 8	Roots	It has a specific faint odor, sweet taste, is slightly bitter and astringent. Rose madder helps to gradually break down uric acid concretions. Ruberitric acid facilitates this process making fragile the salts of phosphorus, calcium, and magnesium in the urine. It has a bactericidal effect, destroys the coccal flora, reduces muscle tone but increases the tone of the transverse muscles, helps to remove stones, sand, and concretions from the kidneys and urinary tract. In kidney disease, it is used to dissolve, remove small concretions, especially salts of phosphorus, calcium, and magnesium, and relieve spasms.
Rumex confertus Willd. (Polygonaceae)	8–9	Roots	Has a faint odor, a peculiar bitter taste. Anthracene derivatives increase intestinal peristalsis. Contains astringents, anti-inflammatory and resinous substances also have a laxative effect. Due to its astringent properties, the roots are used in small doses in gastrointestinal diseases such as colitis, enterocolitis, and in high doses as a laxative. Used in veterinary practice in intestinal and skin diseases. Solutions and cooked forms are used.
Sambucus nigra L. (Sambucaceae)	5–6	Flowers	It is diaphoretic; flowers have a diaphoretic (sambunigrin), antipyretic, diuretic, antitussive, carbohydrate-regulating, blood-sugar-lowering, general, and local anti-inflammatory as well as a weak disinfectant and astringent effect. Infusion of flowers is prescribed for colds, flu, and bronchitis. It is used in liver disorders, kidney diseases as a quality diuretic.
S. karabachenses Pobed. (Lamiaceae)	6–7	Above-ground parts	In folk medicine, sage is used externally as an anti-inflammatory and disinfectant mostly in skin diseases; also used in angina, influenza, stomatitis, gingivitis, and in the form of enemas. For oral administration, 1–2 tablespoons of the plant parts are infused in 2 cups of hot water for 10 min (in a thermos) (daily dose). Also externally applied. In our opinion, sage has a very good effect on inflammatory diseases of the mouth and throat in the form of external application of compresses and bandages. Two teaspoons from each, sage and matricaria are brewed in 250 mL water for 15 min and used as a

APPENDIX 3.1 *(Continued)*

Botanical name (taxa-family)	Months of use	Part used	Use in the diseases
			diaphoretic. According to the local people, it is taken orally in the diseases of liver and kidneys, gastritis, ulcers, enterocolitis, diarrhea, and bronchitis. It normalizes the sex glands; very effective in infertility and climacteric conditions. The infusion strengthens the nervous system and reduces sweat secretion; can be used to improve lactation. Its mixture with honey strengthens the organism of physically weak children.
Sanguisorba officinalis L. (Rosaceae)	8–9	Rhizomes and roots	An odorless and astringent, anti-inflammatory, hemostatic, and tonic drug; prescribed in lamblia, trichomoniasis, dysentery, typhoid, and paratyphoid. Cooked and extracted forms of rhizomes and roots of the plant show astringent, antiseptic, and hemostatic properties; prescribed in chronic diseases of the gastrointestinal tract, enterocolitis, diarrhea and dysentery, pulmonary diseases, hemorrhage, and uterine bleeding.
Senecio rombifolius (Adams) Sch.Bpi. (Asteraceae)	6–9		The raw material is the roots and shoots of biennial plants; collected during budding, flowering, and fruit formation; a spasmolytic and sedative drug. S. *platyphylloides*, a wild perennial herb, is a quality analgesic during flowering. Its flowers and fruit are also used as pain relievers.
Silybum marianum (L.) Gaertn. (Asteraceae)	8–9	Fruit	An odorless plant, slightly bitter in taste; used in toxic liver damage, acute and chronic hepatitis, liver cirrhosis, lipid metabolism disorders, and hepatic dystrophy.
Sorbus persica Hedl. (Rosaceae)	8–9	Fruit	Juice and cooked form of fresh fruit are used in gastrointestinal dysentery, scurvy, avitaminosis, diabetes, hemorrhoids, and the liquid extract is used as an emollient and hemostatic drug. The infusion has a diaphoretic and appetizing effect.
T. vulgare L. (Asteraceae)	6–9	Capitulum, roots	A choleretic and antihelminthic drug. The flowers have antihelminthic (ascarids and pinworms), antibacterial, choleretic, antispasmodic, and astringent properties. Used to increase appetite, hypersecretion, increase liver function in hepatitis, increase the bactericidal and bacteriostatic effect in the fight against insecticides.
			One tablespoon of the plant is infused in 0.5 L of hot water (in a thermos) (daily dose). 5% solution (70–105 mL) is taken 2–3 times a day in gastric and duodenal ulcers. 5 g of flowers are brewed in 1 L of boiled water and taken 1–2 times a day. In rheumatism,

APPENDIX 3.1 *(Continued)*

Botanical name (taxa-family)	Months of use	Part used	Use in the diseases
			50 g of flowers should be kept in 1 L of wine for 8 days. It is necessary to consume 30–40 g each time in the afternoons and evenings. 8 g- sagebrush, matricaria, and *Tanacetum* are brewed in 250 mL of boiled water and used as enemas against worms.
			In America, the liqueur is made with Tanacetum and walnuts and used in canning meat. In medical practice, the infusion of the flower is widely used as a choleretic drug in ascariasis, enterobiasis, liver diseases, chronic cholecystitis, hepatitis, biliary dyskinesia, as an anthelmintic, and against lamblia.
			Widely used in folk medicine in diseases of nervous system, epilepsy, migraine, acute infectious respiratory diseases, pulmonary tuberculosis, bile duct diseases, hepacholecystitis, and cholangitis. Raises blood pressure. This plant has a good anthelmintic effect; used mainly against ascarids and pinworms. It has insecticidal properties and helps to repel various insects. It is used as a cholagogue in hepatitis, cholecystitis, and as an antispasmodic. Also used in neurosis, epilepsy, inflammation of the respiratory tract, tuberculosis, headache, biliary diseases. Due to toxicity, use during pregnancy is contraindicated. A anthelmintic and insecticidal drug.
			The essential oil of the plant is considered the best worm repellent. It is an effective drug in the expulsion of pinworms and ascarid helminths. Used in English medicine to prevent migraines. Tanacetum increases the secretion in hepatitis, reduces the amount of mucus and bile, normalizes the tone of the gastrointestinal muscles. The infusion reduces the amplitude and rate of the heart, increases blood pressure and bile secretion. Essential oil is extremely toxic, has worm repellent and antimicrobial properties. It is an antiseptic, antispasmodic. and anthelmintic in Bulgarian medicine. Low doses are used in gastrointestinal diseases.
Taraxacum officinale Wigg. (Asteraceae)	5–8	Bark and fruit	Used in gastrointestinal and kidney diseases, worms, angina, gingivitis, fever, diabetes, cough, thirst, rheumatism, and for strengthening the body. An appetizing and choleretic stimulant. The root of this wild perennial herb is a quality raw material.

APPENDIX 3.1 *(Continued)*

Botanical name (taxa-family)	Months of use	Part used	Use in the diseases
			Qualitative bitter substances in the roots (whole and divided) are medicines that have an appetizing, digestive, and choleretic effect. Used in a cooked form, tablets, and mixtures.
Tilia cordata Mill. (Tilliaceae)		Flowers and receptacle	Evaluated in the treatment of neurosis, inflammatory diseases of the upper respiratory tract, angina, and influenza. Used as a diuretic, analgesic, and anti-inflammatory agent in the treatment of pyelonephritis, cystitis, rheumatism, gout, gastrointestinal spasms, kidney and gallbladder pains, inflammatory diseases of the female genital organs. Also evaluated as an external remedy for hair loss, inflammatory diseases of the mouth and tonsils, mastitis, ulcers, burns, hemorrhoids, joint pain, and also for taking aromatic baths.
Thymus kotschyanus Boiss.et Hohen. (Asteraceae)	5–6	Flowers, leaves, and stems	Contains bitter substances, has an appetizing effect and used in the treatment of gastrointestinal, liver, and pancreas diseases. The infusion, extract, and a cooked form are used successfully in inflammation of the upper respiratory tract, tuberculosis, diphtheria, and bronchial asthma. An aromatic bath prepared from this plant is used in the diseases of joints, muscles, and peripheral nervous system. Infusions and extracts are used in acute and chronic respiratory diseases, bronchial asthma, and tuberculosis. As a bactericidal medicine, it is an anticonvulsant, strengthening, analgesic, wound healing, and anti-worm. It is a very productive plant. In folk medicine, it is used in bronchial asthma, ulcers, anorexia, flatulence, and diarrhea. A bath including this plant is recommended for rheumatism, angina, nervous, and skin diseases. In children suffering from rheumatism: 2 g of plant extract, 1 g of rosemary, 1 g of lavender, baking soda 350 g are used in the form of baths. Also used as a disinfectant for gastritis, flatulence, convulsions, and against worms. To obtain a concentrated infusion, 5 g of the plant is brewed in 250 mL water. The daily dose is 500 g. The following mixture is very effective in cases of upset stomach and coughing fits.

APPENDIX 3.1 *(Continued)*

Botanical name (taxa-family)	Months of use	Part used	Use in the diseases
			It has strong anti-inflammatory (contains thymol), anti-convulsive, sedative, antitussive, analgesic, wound healing, and deworming effects. Used in hypertension, atherosclerosis, neuralgia, radiculitis, thyrotoxicosis (goiter), neurosis, and hysteria; also as a worm repellent and diaphoretic, in neuralgia and gastrointestinal pain. In Azerbaijani medicine, the infusion and solution of the leaves are used as an anti-inflammatory agent in heart diseases, constipation, liver diseases, as well as in hypertension and atherosclerosis.
Tussilago farfara L. (Asteraceae)	3–6	Inflorescence	Used in various diseases of kidneys, bile ducts, in ascariasis, as a restorer of the blood, and in some skin diseases. Contains anti-inflammatory, antitussive, astringent, diuretic, and diaphoretic substances. The plant is used in the treatment of acute and chronic diseases of the upper respiratory tract: bronchitis, pleurisy, pneumonia, diphtheria, bronchial asthma, bronchiectasis, and influenza. Due to its high-quality antitussive and choleretic properties, it is effective in the treatment of tuberculosis, inflammatory diseases of the gastrointestinal tract, liver and bile diseases, malaria, eczema, kidney diseases, and cystitis. It is prescribed externally for burns, furunculosis, thrombophlebitis, angina, and stomatitis. Also recommended to infuse 3 tablespoons of flowers or leaves in 2 cups of hot water (in a thermos) (daily dose). Should be consumed 3 times a day, 20–40 min before meals. This infusion can also be applied externally. It is used in folk medicine as an anti-burn agent.
Urtica dioica L. (Urticaceae)	6–7	Leaves	Evaluated in asthenia, anemia, arterial hypotension, neurosis, hysteria, bronchitis, pneumonia, bronchial asthma, tuberculosis, diphtheria, anorexia, diarrhea, constipation, gastritis, enterocolitis, epilepsy, and atherosclerosis. Used in the treatment of nephritis, pyelonephritis, and cystitis as a diuretic and anti-inflammatory drug in diseases of the liver, kidneys, and bile ducts. As a diuretic and tonic, it has a positive effect on I-II degree cardiovascular diseases; has a hemostatic effect by increasing the tone of the uterus, used in menopausal bleeding, uterine fibroids, bleeding after labor and abortion, inflammatory processes. 3 tablespoons of the plant should be infused in 2 cups of hot water (thermos) and taken 3 times a day 20–30 min before meals (daily dose).

APPENDIX 3.1 *(Continued)*

Botanical name (taxa-family)	Months of use	Part used	Use in the diseases
			For external use, the dose is twice a day in high concentrations.
			Used in gout, rheumatism, diathesis, eczema, hypogalactia (low milk secretion), diabetes, hemorrhoids, malaria, and obesity. The infusion normalizes the process of skin regeneration in burns, wounds, and injuries. The juice of the young plant helps to dissolve bile and kidney stones. Nettle roots are a very good remedy for stones "stuck" in the bile and kidneys. Nettle seeds are considered to be the best for this purpose. It is considered indispensable for external application in burns (weak moisturizer), wound healing, eczema, itchy skin, rheumatism of the joints.
Vaccinium myrtillus L. (Monotropaceae)	6–8	Leaves and ripe fruit	The leaves are collected in spring and autumn, when the fruit is fully ripe. It is used in liver diseases, hypoacidity, gastritis, the articular form of rheumatism, nocturnal enuresis, scurvy, deworming, diarrhea. The infusion made from the fruit is prescribed for diarrhea because it is astringent, and the stem is prescribed as a quality anti-diabetic drug. It is also prescribed for urinary tract stones, pyelonephritis, cystitis, prostatitis, gonorrhea. For disinfection, demineralization, and stimulation of nitrogen metabolism. Together with *Arctostaphylos*, it is effective in kidney and gastrointestinal diseases. Also used successfully in edematous nephropathy of pregnant women, diabetes, pyelonephritis, and the postpartum period. Aerosol inhalation is used in chronic pneumonia, bronchiectasis, and bronchitis; as an astringent and anti-inflammatory drug in gastritis, enterocolitis, and diarrhea, as a gargle in angina, stomatitis, periodontitis, avitaminosis, chronic tonsillitis, gingivitis, mouth wounds, and ulcers.
Valeriana grossheimii Vorosch. (=*V. officinalis* L.) (Valerianaceae)		Rhizomes and roots; Above-ground parts	Mostly used in fatigue related to neurosis, nervous system disorders. Due to its hypotensive and antispasmodic properties, it is used in hypertension, cardioneurosis, and angina. Valerian is also used successfully in spastic colitis, chronic diarrhea, gastrointestinal neurosis; has a very good effect on hyperthyroidism, chorea, epilepsy, and early menopausal complaints; is very effective in anorexia, strengthening the body in diseases of the bile, stomach, and pancreas.

APPENDIX 3.1 *(Continued)*

Botanical name (taxa-family)	Months of use	Part used	Use in the diseases
			One tablespoon of roots are infused in 1 cup of boiled water in a thermos and taken 3–4 times a day, 1/3 cup each time.
Viburnum opulus L. (Viburnaceae)	5–9	Leaves, flowers, fruit, and roots	The fruit is used for antispasmodic purposes in gastrointestinal ulcers, polyps, and hyposecretion; fruit juice is mixed with sugar and 2–3 tablespoons of the preparation consumed with water 3–4 times a day. 3–4 tablespoons of dried fruit are brewed in 0.5 L of boiled water (thermos) (daily dose), the extract and the aqueous solution are diuretic, laxative, and disinfectant. Also used in diathesis and nosebleeds, the extract and cooked forms of the leaves are used as hemostatic in uterine bleeding; the fruit contains high-quality antipyretics, diaphoretics, vitamins, and weak laxatives. Used in rheumatoid arthritis, raises blood pressure by increasing the tone of the heart muscle, has a mild laxative effect.
Viola arvensis Murr. *Viola tricolor* L. (Violaceae)	5–6	Above-ground organs	Has a faint odor, unique sweet taste and contains mucus; an antitussive and diuretic drug. A solution and extract are prepared from the raw material, which is successfully used as a cough suppressant and diuretic; also used as cough medicine in inflammatory diseases of the lungs and upper respiratory tract, nasopharyngeal diseases, especially diphtheria; successfully used in the iseases of kidneys and urinary tract, as a diuretic and anti-inflammatory drug; as a laxative and "blood purifier" in diseases of the joints, skin, furunculosis, rash, diathesis, and eczema. It is applied externally as a bath in joint and skin diseases. Herbal infusion is used for diphtheria and bronchitis, as an antitussive and diuretic. Recently, a pharmacological study of the plant has revealed its anti-allergic activity. A high content of biologically active substances guarantee its successful use in the field of cosmetology. Thus, by applying the infusion, it is possible to treat oily seborrhea, scratches, and purulent wounds on the face and hair.
			1–2 tablespoons of the plant parts are infused in 500 mL of hot water (in a thermos) (daily dose). 1 tablespoon of the solution (10.0: 200.0) is taken 3 times a day.

CHAPTER 4

Ethnic Knowledge on Medicinal Flora and Application by the Tribals of Southwest India: A Review

SIDDARAMAIAH LOKESH[1], VENKATESHU SRINIVAS[2], BENDARAVAADI R. MANJUNATHA[1], MYSORE R. GANGADHAR[1], SHIVANNEGOWDA MAHADEVAKUMAR[3], and KANDIKERE R. SRIDHAR[4,5]

[1]*Department Studies in Anthropology, University of Mysore, Manasagangotri, Mysore, Karnataka, India*

[2]*Department Studies in History, University of Mysore, Manasagangotri, Mysore, Karnataka, India*

[3]*Department Studies in Botany, University of Mysore, Manasagangotri, Mysore, Karnataka, India*

[4]*Department of Biosciences, Mangalore University, Mangalagangotri, Mangalore, Karnataka, India*

[5]*Centre for Environmental Studies, Yenepoya (Deemed to be University), Mangalore, Karnataka, India*

ABSTRACT

Documentation of ethnobotanical and ethnomedicinal knowledge of tribes in India is valuable although it is challenging. The current review focused mainly on the ethnomedicinal knowledge of selected tribes residing in the regions of Western Ghats of southwest India (Karnataka, Kerala, and

Ethnic Knowledge and Perspectives of Medicinal Plants, Volume 1: Curative Properties and Treatment Strategies. Munir Ozturk, Kandikere R. Sridhar, Maryam Sarwat, Volkan Altay, & Francisco Martín Huerta-Martínez (Eds.)

Tamil Nadu states). Based on the literature and repeated visits to tribal communities, documentation of medicinal plant species was possible along with part of plant used and their value to cure specific diseases. Detailed account has been provided about the tribes of Karnataka residing in different regions (Bandipur, Biligiri Ranga Hills, Heggadadevana Kote, Hunsur, Male Mahadeshwara Hills, and Nagarahole). In addition to tribal knowledge in Karnataka, studies carried out on the Kani tribe of Kerala and Tamil Nadu have been highlighted. Kani tribes residing in Tamil Nadu has the highest choice of plant species for medication. Leaves of medicinal plant species are used extensively by the tribes of Karnataka, Kerala, and Tamil Nadu. This study facilitates a comparison of tribal knowledge on the medicinal plants used as first aid, to treat or to cure different human ailments. Understanding the tribal knowledge and impart it into the modern medicine is an exciting task. This study hopes to find solution to combat the emerging lifestyle diseases caused by the climatic change or destruction of forest ecosystems, which highlights the importance of forest conservation for future life sustenance. This documentation of use of medicinal plant diversity based on tribal folklore serve as a valuable baseline data toward conservation, further research, and possible commercialization.

4.1 INTRODUCTION

The Indian subcontinent is geographically located in a strategic location with tropical, subtropical, and temperate climatic conditions with a wide variety of forests ecosystems. Tribal population in India largely depends on the forest produce for their nutrition, medicine, shelter, and other essential livelihoods. The Indian subcontinent is rich tribals as many as 550 communities with about 50 million population residing in different pockets of the Western Ghats, Deccan Plateau, Himalayas, and other regions (Binu et al., 1992; Nair and Daniel, 1986; Rao and Razi, 1981; Ramesh and Pascal, 1997; Prasad and Kumar, 2013). The Western Ghats is one among the renowned hotspots biodiversity of the world supplies enormous amount of crude drug to the pharmaceutical industries. Endemic flora and their valuable phytochemical constituents drawn a lot of attention of researchers to document the plants which are used to treat or cure many dangerous diseases. Diverse medicinal floras are used in the Indian traditional medicinal systems (Ayurveda, Siddha, and the Unani). Contribution of ethnic knowledge on the floral biodiversity in health-promoting medicinal practices of tribes has been documented in different parts of the country. More than 8000 plant species have been used in ethnic as well as modern medicines in India. About 90–95% of the medicinal plants derived from the wild and up to 70% of such collections involve destructive or unscientific extraction. Tribals and their adjoining environment are intricately linked and they rely on natural forest resources to meet their primary health care. Ethnic knowledge of medicinal plants is very important for modern pharmaceutical industries, which provide basis and helps to identify novel therapeutics used in various health related applications.

Based to the World Health Organization (WHO), up to 65–80% global population in developing countries is depending on the flora for primary healthcare owing to poverty as well as lack of access to the modern medicine (Calixto, 2005). Medicinal plants occupied a key position in the world to treat and prevent many diseases for several years. Modern day discovery of new drug molecules is rooted to the ethnic medicinal plants. Many of the plants used by tribes have not been explored and exploited for the fullest extent for pharmacological applications. In the recent past, application of ethnobotanical knowledge has attained considerable momentum in the scientific communities (Heinrich, 2000). Awareness on medicinal plants has been geared up due to the escalating cost of drugs in keep up human health or wellness and bioprospects of new plant-derived products (Hoareau and DaSilva, 1999). Generally, all medicinal products are obtained from plants, either in simple form using specific parts or more complex form of consortium of extracts, combinations, decoctions consortium, and others. The prime benefits of use of plant-derived drugs are relatively safer compared to the synthetic substitutes offer unlimited therapeutic benefits with affordable cost (Iwu et al., 1999). Around 200 years ago, the pharmacopoeia was conquered by the herbal drugs derived from plant species and up to 25% of them were prescribed worldwide (Ernst, 2005). Among the 252 drugs earmarked as basic necessity by the WHO, up to 11% are solely derived from plants and a substantial number of synthetic drugs were derived from the precursors of plant origin (Rates, 2001). The knowhow and application of medicinal plants is one of the basic concerns in the development of pharmaceuticals and validation of new drugs (Posey and Plendrleith, 2002).

This chapter provides an insight into the medicinal plants documented for the last decade used by various tribes of Karnataka with special emphasis on the Kani tribes residing in Karnataka, Kerala, and Tamil Nadu.

4.2 ETHNOMEDICINAL FLORA

Plants have been considered as the basic resources for production of medicines in Ayurveda and other Indian systems of medicine, which serve as basic necessity to establish pharmaceutical industries. Forests in India, including most of the protected areas are known to have sizeable local communities deriving a variety of the ecosystem products. The Indian subcontinent has been considered as one of the richest plant medicinal sources in the world and possesses tremendous contemporary relevance owing to health security to millions of people. However, the growing pressure of population and urbanization has resulted in exploitation of the floristic resource of forests leading to deforestation and loss of valuable plant species. Trade studies indicate that there are up to 880 medicinal plant species in the Indian trade, among them 100 species are from cultivated sources, 14 are imported/exotic to India and the remaining are collected from wild from forests (De, 2016). It has been assessed that in United States, plant-derived drugs account to about 25%, whereas in the developing countries like India and China, the share is up to 80% (Joy et al., 1998). Therefore, the economic value of medicinal plants is highly significant to the countries like India than the rest of the countries. Up to two-thirds of the plant species are required in modern system of medicine, while the rural population rely on their own indigenous system of medicine.

The Western Ghats is one of the globally renowned biodiversity hotspots that provide substantial plant wealth useful in traditional as well as modern medicine. Phytogeographers call this region as the "Malabar Botanical Province," which exists as a narrow stretch starts from the hills of river Tapti in the north up to Kanyakumari in the south all along the west coast running through the states of Maharashtra, Goa, Karnataka, Kerala, and Tamil Nadu. It has approximately 1500 km in length and embraces a steep gradient of climatic conditions, which has supported a wide range of forests such as scrub jungles, evergreen forests, and semievergreen forests including shola forests. The expansion of the tropical rain forests in the southern part of Western Ghats with shola forests in the Kudremukh (Karnataka) and Nilgiris (Tamil Nadu) are the most fascinating landscapes of Western Ghats. There are as many as 5800 flowering plant species documented in Western Ghats, among them 56 genera (in 2100 species) have been identified as endemic. There are many unidentified and underexplored flora, fauna, and microbial wealth associated with Western Ghats (Rao, 2012).

4.3 ETHNOMEDICINAL FLORA OF KARNATAKA

In the recent past, several research papers dealt on the ethnomedicine of various districts, tribes, and local people (nontribals) of Karnataka. Although they are mainly concerned to document the medicinal plants used and their applications, they have not focused to explore the medicinal values like extraction and validation to prove their efficacy in the era of modern biology. In many such efforts, the ethnomedicinal practices followed by the tribals and local people in many districts like Bangalore, Belgaum, Bidar, Chikmagalur, Gadag, Kodagu, Mysore, Raichur and Tumkur have been documented (Yoganarasimhan et al., 1982; Pushpalata et al., 1990; Gopakumar et al., 1991; Kshirsagar and Singh, 2000a, b, 2001; Kattimani et al., 2001; Prashantkumar and Vidyasagar, 2006; Ramana et al., 2007; Upadhyay et al., 2010). Data collection of traditional medicinal performances has also been made from specific to regions such as Bhadravati, Bidar, Davangere, Gadag, Raichur, Sringeri, Sagar, Shivamogga, Subramanya, and coastal locations of Karnataka (Dwarakan and Diwakar, 1997; Gunaga et al., 2012; Harihar and Kotresha, 2012; Murthy, 2015; Bhandary and Chandrashekar, 2002; Parinitha et al., 2004; Shivanna and Rajakumar, 2010; Prakasha and Krishnappa, 2006; Rajakumar and Shivanna, 2010a,b; Poornima et al., 2012; Shiddamallayya et al., 2010a,b).

In the last decade, there is a growing concern on the ethnomedicinal plants and their usefulness in different traditional health practices. Data on the traditional practices toward specific disease conditions involves intermixed information by the tribal as well as non-tribal population of a specific region. The main efforts on such lines include dermal diseases, wounds, snakebite, oral health, bone fractures, gynecological problems, reproductive care, jaundice, and malaria (Shantamma and Sudarshana, 1986; Maruthi et al., 2000; Bhandary and Chandrashekar, 2001; Hegde et al., 2003; Hebbar et al., 2004a, b; Hegde et al., 2007; Vidyasagar and Prashantkumar, 2007; Prashantkumar and Vidyasagar, 2008; Bhat et al., 2012; Upadhya et al., 2012; Prakash and Unnikrishnan, 2013; Bhat et al., 2014). Recently, many reports were generated on the uses of ethnomedicinal plants by various tribes in India (Savithramma et al., 2007; Pattanaik et al., 2008; Kosalge and Fursule, 2009; Namsa et al., 2009; Upadhyay et al., 2010). However, the studies carried out pertain to specific tribe or tribes are meagre and many of them are not comprehensive.

Tribal people residing in various locations in Karnataka and other southern states of India are following their own unique practices through utilization of natural resources especially the medicinal plant to treat various ailments. These patterns differ significantly between tribes as well as the geographic locations. In Karnataka, ethnicity diversified large number of tribes residing in various parts of the state. Similarly, use and application of medicinal plant resources for the traditional health practices also diversified. These changes may be attributed to the varying cultures, geography, different ecological conditions, and variations in climatic factors including the vegetation. Interestingly, specific district in Karnataka has its own traditional health practices. The availability of plant resources and the association of tribals with forest ecosystems have strengthened the ethnic knowledge in these regions.

The tribal health and associated issues are closely linked with forest ecosystem and those are dependent on the various socioeconomic and political factors. In spite of Government and non-Governmental efforts toward the primary health care of these marginalized people, report on the health status of tribal communities is meagre. Studies are very limited to a few tribes (e.g., *Hakki-Pakki, Iruliga, Jenu-Kuruba, Koraga* and *Siddi).* With exception of a few reports, incidence of many communicable and noncommunicable diseases is prevalent in the tribal communities. Thus, it is highly challenging to the Government to formulate suitable strategies to combat the health-related complications of tribes.

4.3.1 TRIBES OF KARNATAKA

In Karnataka, a total of 56 tribes have been recognized (Roy ct al., 2015). The ethnomedicinal practices of some of the tribes have been documented include Gowlie (Dandeli), Jenu-Kuraba (Kodagu and Mysore), Khare-Vokkaliga (Uttara Kannada), Kunabi (North Karnataka), Siddi (Ankola, Haliyal, Sirsi, Uttara Kannada and Yellapura), Soliga (Biligiri Ranga Hills or BR Hills, Gundlupet, Heggadadevana Kote or HD Kote, Hunsur, Piriyapatna and Nanjangud), and others.

Gowlie: The Gowlie community is distributed in Maharashtra, Goa, and Karnataka. In Karnataka, the Gowlie tribe is known from Dandeli region of Uttara Kannada district. This tribe has its own roots from Yadava community and their major occupation is animal herding and trading milk. The ethnomedicinal knowledge of Gowlie tribe is poorly followed. So for there is only one report on ethnomedicinal documentation from Gowlie of Karnataka, which has documented 41 ethnomedicinal plants used to treat various diseases from traditional practitioners of the Gowlie residing in Uttara Kannada (Bhandary et al., 1996).

Jenu-Kuruba: Jenu-Kuruba is an important tribe in Nilgiris (Tamil Nadu) and they are concentrated in Karnataka (Kodagu and Mysore districts: HD Kote, Hunsur and Piriyapatna) (Hathur et al., 2013). Kshirsagar and Singh (2000b) recorded the ethnomedicinal plants used by Jenu-Kuruba of Mysore district and provided the scientific and local names of 25 medicinal plant species along with the geographic distribution in the district (family of plants, mode of preparation, applications, and the modes of administration). Nanjunda (2010) has documented uses of 20 traditional medicinal plant species to treat or cure 21 ailments from the Jenu-Kuruba tribe from Kodagu district. Srinivas et al. (2019) reported up to 67 plant species (62 genera in 37 families) used to treat various ailments. These documentations help to find out the practices of tribals and their intimate association with indigenous plants.

Khare-Vokkaliga: In the district Uttara Kannada, several ethnic tribes exist, among them Khare-Vokkaliga is one of the tribes. The ethnomedicinal plants used by Khare Vokkaliga was recorded by Achar et al. (2010) by documenting uses of 57 ethnomedicinal plant species to treat 39 diseases. Achar et al (2010) is the only study on the diversity and floristic wealth of Uttara Kannada used by Khare-Vokkaliga tribe.

Kunabi: The Kunabi (or Kunbi) tribes are residing in Northern Karnataka and Vidarbha region of Maharashtra. They are also centered in Gujarat, Goa, Kerala, and Madhya Pradesh. In Karnataka, these tribes are inhabiting in the semievergreen forests of the district Uttara Kannada. Harsha et al. (2002) documented the ethnomedicinal aspects of the tribe Kunabi. This includes 45 plant species used to treat 24 ailments (e.g., allergy, skin diseases, sores, inflammation, fever, cuts, wounds, and urinary tract infections).

Siddi: The ethnic tribe, Siddi in Karnataka, is the descended from the Southeast Africa. They are concentrated in Uttara Kannada (Ankola, Haliyal, Joida, Mundgod, Sirsi, and Yellapura), Belgaum (Khanapur), and Dharwar (Kalghatgi). Ethnomedicinal plants of Siddi tribe was documented by Bhandary et al. (1995) and reported 98 preparations employed to treat different diseases. Bhat et al. (2019) recorded the medicinal plant species used by the local population residing in Siddapur region of Uttara Kannada district where Siddi tribe exists.

Soliga: Hosagoudar and Henry (1993) documented the ethnobotanical plants used by the Soliga tribe. They reported usefulness of 57 plant species by the tribe for treating various ailments. A detailed account is available on the lifestyle, culture, rituals of Soliga tribe, and their traditional ethnomedicinal practices from Chamarajanagar district (Madegowda, 2009; Madegowda and Usha, 2015). It was understood that the Soliga tribe has maintained a constant and close rapport with the forests to meet most of their essential needs. Owing to their intimate association with the nature, the Soliga tribe has a holistic viewpoint on their ethnic knowledge.

Other Tribes: Rajasab and Isaq (2004) documented up to 51 ethnomedicinal plant species frequently used by Lambani tribe to treat various ailments. Prashantkumar and Vidyasagar (2006) recorded the ethnomedicinal applications of 30 medicinal plant species treating various ailments by many ethnic groups residing in Bidar district (e.g., Halakki, Kadu-Kuruba and Lambani). Bhagya and Sridhar (2009) documented the traditional use 25 legume species in health promotion among the ethnic fishermen community from 12 locations of west coast of Dakshina Kannada (e.g., Besta, Bovi, Gangamathasta, Mogaveera and Karvi). Ethnomedicinal plants from Chitradurga district was reported by Hiremath and Taranath (2010), which includes 15 plant species with 12 formulations as ethnic therapy for snakebites in the four tribes (Hakki-Pikki, Iruliga, Jenu-Kuruba and Lambani). During the data acquisition on the plant species used to treat herpes, 34 formulations derived from 57 species of plants by various tribes in Uttara Kannada district (e.g., Hallakki-Vokkaliga, Koraga and Malekudiya) (Bhandary and Chandrashekhar, 2011). A recent study revealed the use of 102 plant species to treat dermal diseases by the tribes in Uttara Kannada (e.g., Gowlie, Hallakki-Vokkaliga, Kunbi and Siddi) (Bhat et al., 2014).

4.3.2 HILLY REGIONS OF KARNATAKA

Chamarajanagar district is known for diversity of medicinal plants as well as tribal population. However, there are no substantial scientific literatures to justify the ethnic medicinal values of plants by these tribes. This district has been blessed with two major hills called Biligiri Ranga Hills (BR Hills) and Male Mahadeshwara Hills (MM Hills). A large number of tribals residing in these regions utilize the natural resources for their day-to-day requirements and they are highly knowledgeable on the medicinal plants. Gireesha and Raju (2013) recorded a total of 38 medicinal plants belonged to 26 families from the BR Hills used for various ailments. Sushma et al. (2019) also listed 130 plant species (in 60 families) used by the tribal communities from the BR hills. Diversity of medicinal plants from Chamarajanagar district along with their ethnomedicinal values are documented (Nandini and Shiddamallayya, 2013; Murugeswaran et al., 2015). Gireesha (2019) performed the ethnobotanical explorations during 2012–2016 in BR and MM Hills, where majority of tribal population is housed. In BR Hills, the locations surveyed include Bhothanni Podu, Kannera, and Bhangle Podu, while in the MM Hills Indiganetta, Kokware, Nagamale, and Thulasikere. In BR Hills, 50 medicinal plants were found (22 herbs, 44%; 15 trees, 30%; 11 shrubs, 22%; two climbers, 4%). A total of 97 medicinal plants have been documented in MM Hills (36 herbs, 37.1%); 34 trees, 35.1%; 19 shrubs, 19.6%; eight climbers, 4.2%). Similar study has been carried out based on the tribes in HD Kote by Srinivas et al. (2019). They documented 67 species of medicinal plants from Jenu-Kuruba, Betta-Kuraba, and Yerava tribes.

Table 4.1 lists 125 medicinal plants (in 105 genera and 53 families) used by the ethnic groups in Karnataka state (BR Hills, MM Hills, HD Kote, and Chamarajanagar). The family Fabaceae has been represented with nine plants followed by the families of Lamiaceae and Asclepiadaceae with eight species each (Figure 4.1a). Further, six species each of families, Amaranthaceae and Apocynaceae, while five species each of Euphorbiaceae and Sapotaceae are used by the tribals. Plants are used by the tribes in Karnataka to treat 61 ailments (Figure 4.1b). Among them, a number of species to treat fever stand first (25 species) followed by leprosy, dermal (19 species each), cough (18 species), piles (15 species), wounds (14 species), diarrhea (13 species), diuretic, and hemorrhage (11 species each). Up to nine plant parts are used for medication by different tribals in Karnataka (Figure 4.2a). Among them leaves stands first followed by root, bark, whole plant, fruits, flowers and stem. Latex and bulb/rhizome are also used for preparation of medicine by the tribals.

4.4 ETHNOMEDICINAL FLORA OF KERALA AND TAMIL NADU

4.4.1 KERALA AND TAMIL NADU

In the recent past, a large number of reports are available for documenting the ethnomedicinal plants from Kerala (Binu, 2012; Dilipkumar and Janardhana, 2012; Sudeesh, 2012), and Tamil Nadu (Aadhan and Anand, 2017; Alagesaboopathi, 2009; Arul-Manikandan, 2005; Ganesh et al., 1996; Sivakamasundari et al., 2015; Sivaperumal et al., 2010; Subbaiyan et al., 2014). Kani, Kaniya, Kaniyan, and Kaniyaar tribes are the indigenous tribes belong to the oldest ethnic community in Southern India. This community is traditionally nomadic and currently settled in the forests of Agasthyamalai Hills (Kerala) and Tirunelveli Hills (Tamil Nadu) of the Western Ghats (Anuradha 2000; Ayyanar and Ignacimuthu, 2005, 2011). They are also

TABLE 4.1 Distribution Parts Used and Medicinal Uses of Medicinal Plants Used by the Tribes in Karnataka State (BR Hills, Biligiri Ranga Hills; MM Hills, Malamahadeshwara Hills; HD Kote, Heggadadevana Kote).

Medicinal plant	Family	Distribution	Parts used	Medicinal use
Abrus precatorius L.	Fabaceae	MM Hills and HD Kote	Root, leaves, and seeds	Rheumatism and diuretic
Abutilon indicum L. Sweet	Malvaceae	BR Hills	Whole plant	Tuberculosis, ulcers, and blood bleeding
Acacia decurrens Willd.	Fabaceae	MM Hills and HD Kote	Bark	Dysentery
Acacia leucophloea (Roxb.) Willd.	Fabaceae	MM Hills	Bark, root, leaves, seeds, and gum	Bronchitis and rheumatic fever
Acacia nilotica (L.) Willd.	Fabaceae	BR Hills and MM Hills	Bark, root, leaves, seeds, and gum	Bronchitis and rheumatic fever
Achyranthes aspera L.	Amaranthaceae	BR Hills, MM Hills and HD Kote	Whole plant and root	Arthritis
Acorus calamus L.	Araceae	MM Hills	Rhizome and leaves	Epilepsy, mental illness, chronic diarrhea, and dysentery
Acronychia pedunculata (L.) Miq.	Rutaceae	BR Hills	Leaves and bark	Purgative, scabies, bone fractures, soars, and ulcers
Adenanthera pavonia L.	Papilionaceae	MM Hills and HD Kote	Seeds, wood, leaves, and root	Pulmonary infection, fever, skin disease, joint pain, and emetic
Adhothoda zeylanica Medicus.	Acanthaceae	BR Hills	Whole plant	Respiratory stimulant
Aegle marmelos (L.) Correa	Rutaceae	MM Hills	Root, bark, fruits, flowers, and resin	Stringent, digestive and stomachache, diarrhea, and dysentery
Aerva javanica (Burm. f.) Juss.	Amaranthaceae	BR Hills and MM Hills	Whole plant	Diuretic and purgative
Aerva lanata (L.) Juss.	Amaranthaceae	MM Hills and HD Kote	Whole plant	Skin irritation
Albizia lebbeck (L.) Willd.	Fabaceae	MM Hills	Bark, seeds, wood, and flowers	Skin disease, herpes infection, and poison bites

TABLE 4.1 (*Continued*)

Medicinal plant	Family	Distribution	Parts used	Medicinal use
Albizzia odorotissima (L.f.) Benth.	Fabaceae	MM Hills and HD Kote	Bark, seeds, wood, and flowers	Skin disease, herpes infection, and poison bites
Allamanda cathartica L.	Apocynaceae	MM Hills	Leaves and bark	Hydrogogue
Alstonia scholaris (L.) R.Br.	Apocynaceae	BR Hills, MM Hills and HD Kote	Bark	Wounds, sinus, and skin diseases
Alternanthera pungens Kunth.	Amaranthaceae	MM Hills and HD Kote	Whole plant	Diuretic and gonorrhea
Amaranthus spinosus L.	Amaranthaceae	MM Hills and HD Kote	Root, stem, and leaves	Urinary disorders and piles
Amaranthus tricolor L.	Amaranthaceae	MM Hills and HD Kote	Root, stem, and leaves	Urinary disorders and Piles
Annona reticulata L.	Annonaceae	MM Hills and HD Kote	Root	Anthelmintic and pitta
Annona squamosa L.	Annonaceae	MM Hills and HD Kote	Root, seeds, bark, and fruits	Anthelmintic and pitta
Anthocephalus chinensis (Lam.)	Rubiaceae	MM Hills and HD Kote	Bark, fruits, stem, leaves, and seeds	Febrifuge, burns, poisoning, wounds, gynecological problems, and cough
Argemone mexicana L.	Papavaraceae	MM Hills and HD Kote	Whole plant, seeds, and latex	Scabies, opthalmia, skin diseases, stomachache, and leprosy
*Argyreia cuneata (*Willd.) Ker.	Convolvulaceae	BR Hills, MM Hills and HD Kote	Leaves	Wounds, bleeding, carminative, and liver disorders
Artocarpus heterophyllus Lam.	Moraceae	BR Hills, MM Hills and HD Kote	Fruits, seeds, leaves, and latex	Wounds, liver disorders, indigestion, stomachache, and phlem
Asclepias curassavica L.	Asclepiadaceae	MM Hills and HD Kote	Whole plant, root, and latex	Semitic, piles, gonorrhea, anthelmintic, epilepsy, cough, and leprosy
Asparagus racemosus Willd.	Liliaceae	BR Hills	Whole plant	Infertility and loss of libido
Azadirachta indica A. Juss.	Meliaceae	BR Hills, MM Hills and HD Kote	Bark, leaves, flowers, and seeds	Skin disease, antiseptic, skin burns, ulcers, purgative, and toothache

TABLE 4.1 (*Continued*)

Medicinal plant	Family	Distribution	Parts used	Medicinal use
Basella rubra L.	Basellaceae	MM Hills and HD Kote	Whole plant	Blood cancer and burns
Basilicum polystachyon (L.) Moench.	Lamiaceae	BR Hills, MM Hills and HD Kote	Leaves	Sprains, sedative, epilepsy, and neurologic problems
Bauhinia variegata L.	Caesalpiniaceae	BR Hills, MM Hills and HD Kote	Root, bark, and flowers	Worm infestation, leprosy, wounds, cough, urinary disorder, and glandular swelling
Biophytum reinwardtii (Zucc.) Kiotzch.	Oxalidaceae	MM Hills and HD Kote	Root, bark, and flowers	Carminative, diarrhoea, laxative, anthelmintic, cough, bleeding, piles, and stomachache
Biophytum sensitivum (L.) DC.	Oxalidaceae	BR Hills	Leaves	Febrifuge and insomnia
Boerhavia diffusa L. nom. Cons.	Nyctaginaceae	BR Hills	Whole plant	Chest pain and to reduce heat
Borassus flabellifer L.	Arecaceae	MM Hills and HD Kote	Root, leaves, and seeds	Renal disorder, kidney stone, and nephritis
Brassica juncea (L.) Czern. and Coss.	Brassicaceae	MM Hills and HD Kote	Roots, leaves, inflorescence seeds, and ash	Bleeding, leprosy, constipation, stomachache, and cardiac disease
Breynia retusa (Dennst.) Aist.	Euphorbiaceae	MM Hills and HD Kote	Seeds oil	Headache, worm infestation, emetic, and leprosy
Breynia vitis-idaea (Burm. f.) Fisch.	Euphorbiaceae	MM Hills and HD Kote	Leaves and bark	To treat nervous disorders, oedema, and bleeding
Butea monosperma (Lam.) Taub.	Papilionaceae	BR Hills, MM Hills and HD Kote	Leaves	Hemorrhage
Caesalpinia pulcherrima (L.) Sw.	Caesalpiniaceae	MM Hills and HD Kote	Bark, flowers, seeds, and resin	Piles, tumors, and menstrual disorder

TABLE 4.1 (*Continued*)

Medicinal plant	Family	Distribution	Parts used	Medicinal use
Calamus thwaitesii Becc.	Arecaceae	MM Hills and HD Kote	Bark, leaves, and flowers	Purgative
Calotropis gigantea (L.) Dryand.	Asclepiadaceae	MM Hills and HD Kote	Leaves and bark	bleeding disorder, diarrhoea, fever, skin diseases, and ulcer
Calotropis procera (Aiton) W.T.Aiton	Asclepiadaceae	MM Hills and HD Kote	Root, bark, leaves, flowers, and latex	Nervous system disorder, leprosy, abdominal pain, worm infestation, cough, snake bite, and joint pain
Cannabis sativa L.	Cannabinaceae	BR Hills, MM Hills and HD Kote	Root, bark, leaves, flowers, and latex	Nervous system disorder, leprosy, abdominal pain, worm infestation, cough, snake bite, and joint pain
Canscora diffusa (Vahl) R.Br.	Gentianaceae	MM Hills and HD Kote	Leaves and resin	Piles, kapha, fever, and skin disease
Canthium parviflorum Lam.	Rubiaceae	MM Hills and HD Kote	Whole plant	Piles, abdominal disorder, sterility in female, and skin problems
Capparis spinosa L.	Capparidaceae	MM Hills and HD Kote	Fruits, seeds, and root	Anthelmintic and throat problems
Careya arborea Roxb.	Lecythidaceae	MM Hills and HD Kote	Bark	Diuretic, expectorant, rheumatism, and liver infections
Caryota urens L.	Arecaceae	MM Hills and HD Kote	Root and bark	Sinus, anthelmintic, poison bite, and ulcers
Cassia fistula L.	Caesalpiniaceae	BR Hills, MM Hills and HD Kote	Leaf bud, seeds, and toddy	Diarrhoea, migraine, and poison bites
Centella asiatica (L.) Urban	Apiaceae	BR Hills	Fruits and leaves	Wounds, diabetes, tumors, skin diseases, and herpes infection
Cissampelos pareira L.	Menispermaceae	BR Hills	Leaves and stem	Fever and diarrhoea
Cocos nucifera L.	Arecaceae	MM Hills and HD Kote	Whole plant, seeds, bark, leaves, and root	Heart complaints, kidney stones, asthma, arthritis, and stomachache

TABLE 4.1 (*Continued*)

Medicinal plant	Family	Distribution	Parts used	Medicinal use
Colocasia esculenta (L.) Schott	Araceae	MM Hills and HD Kote	Root, flowers, fruits, oil, shell, ash, and spadix	Urinary disorders, gastritis, hemorrhage, pitta, and fever
Commelina benghalensis L.	Commelinaceae	BR Hills, MM Hills and HD Kote	Corm and leaves	Piles, cough, and cold
Commelina paludosa BI	Commelinaceae	MM Hills	Whole plant	Hemorrhage, fever, laxative, and leprosy
Cordia obliqua Willd.	Boraginaceae	BR Hills, MM Hills and HD Kote	Whole plant and roots	Laxative
Coriandrum sativum L.	Apiaceae	MM Hills and HD Kote	Bark, leaves, fruits, and seeds	Expectorant, fever, worm infection, cough, skin disease, and dental disorders
Crotalaria albida Heyne	Papilionaceae	MM Hills	Whole plant, fruits, oil, leaves, and seeds	Diuretic, carminative, cough, fever, indigestion, and headache
Cryptolepis buchanani R. and S.	Asclepiadaceae	MM Hills	Root	Purgative
Curculigo orchioides Gaertn.	Hypoxidaceae	BR Hills	Root	Hemorrhage, wounds, leprosy, jaundice, and anemia
Curcuma longa L.	Zingiberaceae	BR Hills, MM Hills and HD Kote	Leaves	Piles and bronchitis
Cycas circinalis L.	Cycadaceae	MM Hills	Rhizome	Leprosy, skin diseases, jaundice, fever, and pox
Cyperus rotundus	Cyperaceae	BR Hills	Stem and leaves	Urinary disorder, bronchial asthma, fever, and hemorrhage
Dalbergia lanceolaria L.f.	Papilionaceae	MM Hills	Rhizome	Vomiting, indigestion, cough, and bronchitis

TABLE 4.1 (*Continued*)

Medicinal plant	Family	Distribution	Parts used	Medicinal use
Datura innoxia Mill	Solanaceae	MM Hills	Whole plant, seeds, and oil	Indigestion, rheumatism, oedema, and arthritis
Decalepis hamiltonii Wt. and Arn.	Asclepiadaceae	MM Hills	Leaves	Cerebral depressant and narcotic antispasmodic
Dioscorea alata L.	Dioscoreaceae	MM Hills	Roots, leaves, flowers, fruits, and whole plant	Appetizer, polyuria, hemorrhage, wounds, jaundice, and fever
Emblica officinalis Gaertn.	Phyllanthaceae	BR Hills, MM Hills and HD Kote	Tuber	Piles, anthelmintic, and leprosy
Euphorbia hirta L.	Euphorbiaceae	BR Hills	Fruits, bark, leaves, flowers, and seeds	Anemia, jaundice, diabetes, and asthma
Euphorbia tirucalli L.	Euphorbiaceae	MM Hills	Leaves and shoot	Dysentery
Ficus racemosa	Moraceae	BR Hills	Latex	Toothache, skin diseases, and leprosy
Gendarussa vulgaris Nees.	Acanthaceae	MM Hills	Bark, root, latex, and fruit	Burns, fatigue, urinary problems, and leprosy
Gymnema sylvestris R. Br.	Asclepiadaceae	MM Hills	Leaves	Emetic, hemorrhage, and rheumatism
Helicteres isora L.	Sterculiaceae	BR Hills	Leaves and root	Diabetes, cardiac stimulant, headache, poisoning, and bronchial asthma
Hemidesmus indicus (L.) R.Br. ex.Schult.	Apocynaceae	MM Hills	Leaves, root, fruits, stem, and bark	Wounds, polio, asthma, and diabetes
Hemidesmus indicus (L.) R.Br.	Asclepiadaceae	BR Hills	Root, flowers, leaves, and fruit	Skin disease, burns, and leucoderma
Hibiscus rosasinensis L.	Malvaceae	BR Hills	Whole plant	Wounds and laxative

TABLE 4.1 (*Continued*)

Medicinal plant	Family	Distribution	Parts used	Medicinal use
Holarrhena pubescens Wall. Ex. G.Don	Apocyanaceae	BR Hills	Bark and seeds	Hemorrhage and leprosy
Holoptelia integrifolia (Roxb.) Pianch.	Ulmaceae	MM Hills and HD Kote	Bark	Tuberculosis, piles, leprosy and vomiting
Ichnocarpus frutescence (L.) W.T. Aiton	Apocyanaceae	MM Hills and HD Kote	Root	Dyspepsia, skin problems, and kidney stone
Lantana camera L.	Verbenaceae	MM Hills	Leaves	Diaphoretic, carminative, rheumatism, and hemorrhage
Leonotis nepatifolia (L.) R.Br.	Lamiaceae	MM Hills and HD Kote	Flowers and leaves	Skin infection, scalds, rheumatism, nasal disorder, and worm infection
Leucas aspera (Willd.) Link.	Lamiaceae	MM Hills and HD Kote	Flowers and leaves	Skin problems, antipyretic, fever, eye disease, snakebite, and poisoning
Leucas cephalotes (Roth) Spreng.	Lamiaceae	BR Hills	Whole plant	Headache, jaundice, itching, and cold
Litsea stocksii Hook.f	Lauraceae	MM Hills	Leaves and seeds	bladder irritations, sprains, and itching
Lobelia leschenaultiana (Presl.) Skottsb.	Lobelliaceae	MM Hills	Leaves	Poison bites
Madhuca longifolia Koen.	Sapotaceae	MM Hills and HD Kote	Flowers, seeds, root, bark, stem, and oilcake	Rheumatism, laxative, piles, leprosy, and fever
Melia azadirach L.	Meliaceae	MM Hills	Leaves, gum, seeds, and root	Anthelmintic, diuretic, leprosy, blood disorder, fever, and worm infestation
Memecylon umbellatum Burm. f.	Melastomataceae	MM Hills	Leaves, root, and bark	Astringent, eye problems, and dysentery

TABLE 4.1 (*Continued*)

Medicinal plant	Family	Distribution	Parts used	Medicinal use
Mimosa pudica L.	Mimosaceae	MM Hills	Root, whole plant, and leaves	Diarrhoea, hemorrhage, and urinary calculi
Morinda pubescens Sm.	Rubiaceae	BR Hills, MM Hills and HD Kote	Root, leaves, fruits, and bark	Fever, ulcers, and digestive disorders
Murraya koinighii (L.) Spreng	Rutaceae	BR Hills, MM Hills and HD Kote	Leaves, root, and bark	Sickness and nausea
Nelumbo nucifera Gaertn.	Nelumbonaceae	MM Hills and HD Kote	Root, flowers, seeds, tuber, and anther	Hemorrhage, sterility, diarrhea, and pitta
Nothapodytes nimmoniana (J. Grah.) D.J.	Icacinaceae	BR Hills	Bark, root, and leaves	Fever, dog bite, and poison bite
Nymphaea pubescens Willd.	Nymphaeaceae	MM Hills	Rhizome, flowers, and seeds	Dysentery, cardiotonic, skin problems, burns, and diarrhoea
Ocimum americanum L.	Lamiaceae	BR Hills	Whole plant	Verminosis, toothache, cough, and fever
Ocimum tenuiflorum L.	Lamiaceae	BR Hills	Leaves	Cough
Oscimu adscendens Wild.	Lamiaceae	MM Hills	Leaves and seeds	Fever, mental disorder, cold, cough, and ulcers
Oscimum sanctum L.	Lamiaceae	MM Hills and HD Kote	Leaves and seeds	Fever, mental disorder, cold, cough, and ulcers
Oxalis corniculata L.	Oxalidaceae	BR Hills	Whole plant	Hemorrhoids and dysentery
Paspalum scrobiculatum L.	Poaceae	MM Hills	Stem and grain	Polyuria, sinus, and wounds
Passiflora foetida L.	Passifloraceae	MM Hills	Fruits and leaves	Emetic and asthma
Pennisetum americanum (L.) Leeke	Poaceae	MM Hills and HD Kote	Grains	Cold, cough, fever, and headache

TABLE 4.1 (*Continued*)

Medicinal plant	Family	Distribution	Parts used	Medicinal use
Phyllanthus acidus (L.) Skeels	Phyllanthaceae	MM Hills	Root and fruits, seeds	Stomachache, diuretic, diarrhea, and laxative
Phyllanthus niruri L.	Phyllanthaceae	MM Hills and HD Kote	Whole plant	Stomachache, diuretic, diarrhoea, laxative, jaundice, and urinogenital disorders
Piper longum L.	Piperaceae	BR Hills	Fruits, root, and stem	Cholera, diarrhea, and viral hepatitis
Plectranthus aimboinicus (Lour.) Spreng.	Lamiaceae	BR Hills	Whole plant	Cold, cough, fever, and headache
Pongamia pinnata (L.) Pierre.	Fabaceae	MM Hills and HD Kote	Bark, leaves, seeds, flowers, and root	Poisoning, piles, uterine disorder, wounds, stomachache, and poison bites
Pterocarpus marsupium Roxb.	Fabaceae	MM Hills and HD Kote	Heart wood, leaves, gum, stem, and bark	Leprosy, worms, wounds, poison bites, pitta, and leprosy
Rauwolfia serpentina (L.) Benth.	Apocyanaceae	BR Hills, MM Hills and HD Kote	Root	Poison bites, hypertension, mental disorders, and insomnia
Riccinus communis L.	Euphorbiaceae	MM Hills and HD Kote	Root, leaves, seeds, and oil	Abdominal pain, piles, chest pain, constipation, fever, and jaundice
Rubia cordifolia L.	Rubiaceae	BR Hills	Root, stem, fruits, and leaves	Rheumatism, bronchitis, and dysentery
Ruta chalepensis L.	Rutaceae	BR Hills	Leaves and flowers	Cough
Solanum indicum L.	Solanaceae	BR Hills	Root and berries	To treat bronchitis and asthma
Solanum nigrum L.	Solanaceae	BR Hills, MM Hills and HD Kote	Leaves, fruits, and whole plant	To treat cancerous sores, boils, and leucoderma
Solanum torvum Sw.	Solanaceae	MM Hills and HD Kote	Whole plant and root	Cough, sedative, diuretic, and digestive

TABLE 4.1 (*Continued*)

Medicinal plant	Family	Distribution	Parts used	Medicinal use
Strychnos nux-vomica L.	Loganiaceae	BR Hills	Bark, leaves, and seeds	To treat heart ailments, eye ache, migraine, and headache
Terminalia belerica (Gaertn.) Roxb.	Combretaceae	BR Hills	Fruit	To treat piles and diarrhoea
Terminalia chebula Retz.	Combretaceae	MM Hills and HD Kote	Fruits and bark	Laxative, stomachache, diuretic, cardiotonic, asthma, and jaundice
Tinospora cordifloia (Thunb.) Miers.	Menispermaceae	BR Hills, MM Hills and HD Kote	Leaves	Fever, anemia, jaundice, leprosy, worms, and fever
Tylophora indica (Burm. F.) Merrill.	Asclepiadaceae	BR Hills	Leaves	To treat respiratory issues and asthma
Vitex negundo L.	Verbenaceae	BR Hills, MM Hills, and HD Kote	Leaves, root, fruits, and bark	Rheumatism, antifungal, to treat cancer, and diuretic
Zingiber officinale Roscoe	Zingiberaceae	MM Hills and HD Kote	Rhizome	Cardiac disease, wounds, indigestion, diarrhea, and stomachache

Source: Gireesha and Raju, 2013; Srinivas et al., 2019; Gireesha, 2019).

settled in different regions of Karnataka after migration leading a settled life (Kollegala, Mysore, Mandya, Chamarajanagar and Hassan).

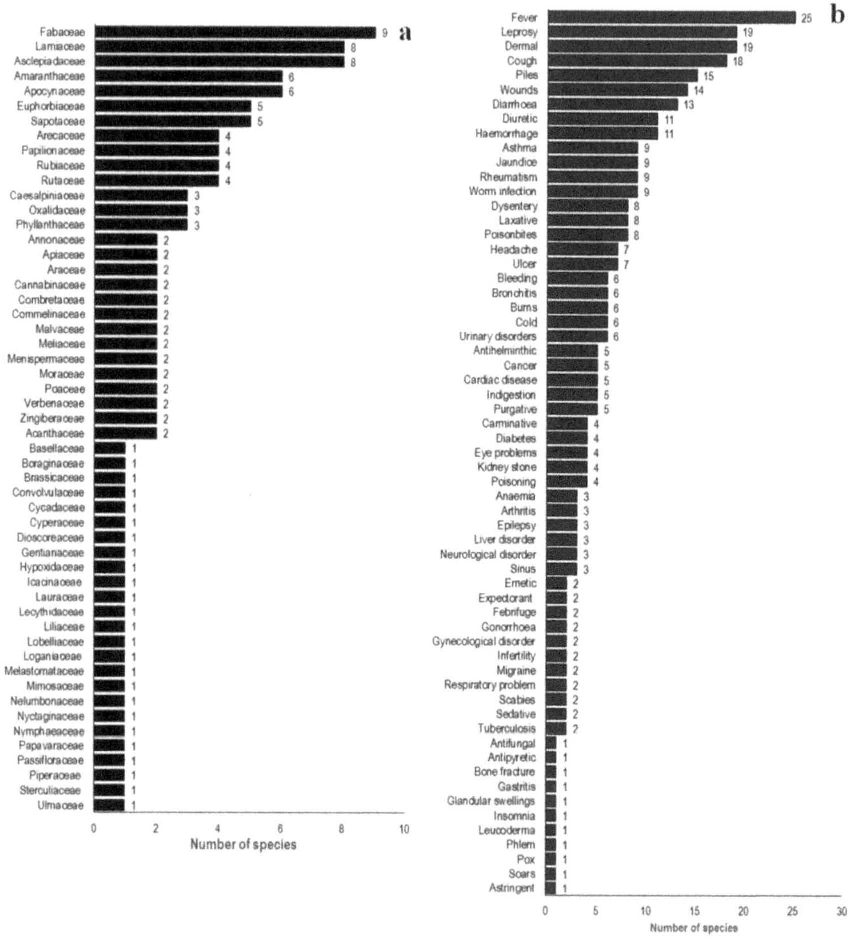

FIGURE 4.1 Family-wise distribution of medicinal plants used by the tribes of Karnataka state (a) and their uses to treat different diseases (b).

Kani tribe lives together in small communities called Muttu-Kani or headman and some are residing in the vicinity of towns. The main occupation of Kani is gathering of cane to supply it to the artisans nearby and also weave themselves (mats and baskets). They also collect the minor nontimber forest products (e.g., bee wax, honey, gums, medicinal plants and others) depending on the seasons. The Muttu-Kani are popular in curing severe diseases even among their population. Their knowledge of treatment of diseases originated from their ancestors. Although they are settled far away from their origin, they are still following the traditional practice of Ethnomedicine to their own and outside the community. Kani tribe traces their ethnic knowledge about medicinal plant species way back to the saint of Hindu called Agasthiyar Muni. The Kani tribe possesses substantial knowledge on medicinal plant resources, which are useful to serve as first aid other ailments (e.g., poisonous bites, cold, cough, headache, fever, and other problems).

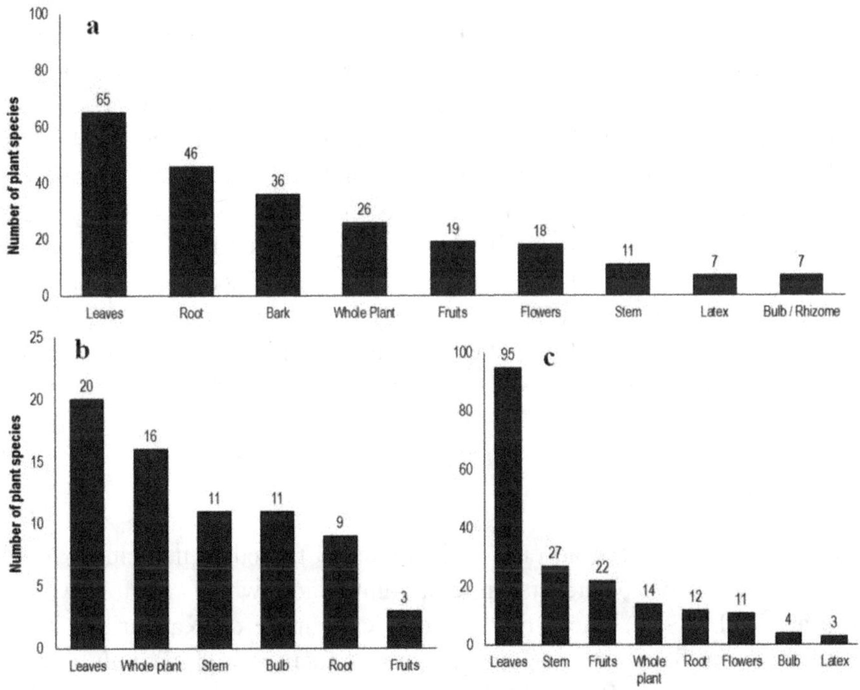

FIGURE 4.2 Plant parts used for medicine by the tribes in Karnataka state (a), plant parts used by the Kani tribes in Kerala (b), and Tamil Nadu (c) for medicinal purposes.

There are several ethnic practitioners in the Kani tribe and there are five major research contributions related to medicobotanical aspects. Since they have been largely recognized to reside in Tamil Nadu and Kerala, considerable information has been gathered by various researchers. Kani tribes residing from Kerala are also endowed with sufficient knowledge on medicinal plants and some researchers gathered information on ethnomedicinal plants. Vijayan et al. (2007) recorded the ethnomedicinal plants from Agasthya Vanam (part of Western Ghats known for floral diversity). Kani tribe residing in Kottoor Reserve forest were interviewed and recorded a total of 50 medicinal plant species used in the treatment of 39 diseases. Xavier et al. (2014) has documented 36 species of medicinal plant species used by the Kani tribes in Kerala.

4.4.2 KERALA

Detailed literature analysis yielded a total of 72 medicinal plant species (in 62 genera and 45 families) employed by the Kani tribe in Kerala (Table 4.2). Further, among the 72 plant species, the family Fabaceae represented a highest of seven plants followed by four plants of Asteraceae, while Aristolochiaceae, Convolvulaceae, Lamiaceae, and Verbenaceae are represented by three species each (Figure 4.3a). Plants used by the Kani tribes in Kerala to treat 47 ailments (Figure 4.3b). Among them, poison bits stand first (nine species) followed by jaundice (eight species), headache (seven species), blood purification, and fever (five species). Up to six plant parts are used by the Kani tribes of Kerala for medication purposes (Figure 4.2b). Among them leaves were the highest followed by the whole plant, stem, bulb, and root.

4.4.3 TAMIL NADU

Janaki Ammal and Prasad (1984) documented the ethnomedicinal knowledge of Kani tribe for the first time in Tamil Nadu, which was followed by Prasad et al. (1987). Medico-ethnobotanical survey on Kani tribes in the Mundanthurai Sanctuary of Tamil Nadu was focused by Ignacimuthu et al. (1998). Viswanathan et al. (2001) recorded the ethnomedicinal plants of Kani tribes from the Kalakad Mundanthurai Tiger forest reserve of Tamil Nadu. Ayyanar and Ignacimuthu (2005) conducted ethnomedicinal survey among the Kani tribes residing in Kouthalai region of Tirunelveli Hills of Tamil Nadu. They have documented ethnic uses of 54 plant species (in 26 families). Subitha et al. (2011) conducted an ethnobotanical survey and acquired data on the ethnomedicinal plant species used by the Kani tribe in the Pechiparai forest region of Kanyakumari district in Tamil Nadu (the southern part of the Western Ghats). Ayyanar and Ignacimuthu (2011) recorded up to 90 plant species (in 83 genera and 52 families) employed by traditional healers of

TABLE 4.2 Details of Ethnomedicinal Plant Species Used by the Kani Tribes Residing in Kerala State.

	Family	Parts used	Disease	Mode of administration
Abrus precatorius L.	Fabaceae	Root	Jaundice	Oral
Acacia pennata Willd.	Mimosaceae	Bark	Odontalgia	Decoction
A. calamus L.	Acoraceae	Stem	Jaundice	Oral
Adenia hondala (Gaertn.) de Wilde	Passifloraceae	Tubers	Promote lactation	Paste
Allium cepa L.	Amaryllidaceae	Bulb	Cut wounds	Topical
Anaphyllum wightii Schott.	Araceae	Whole	Snakebite	Paste
Andropogon muricatus Retz.	Poaceae	Root with rhizome	Fever, inflammation, and skin irritation	Oral, topical, and inhalation
Aristolochia indica L.	Aristolochiaceae	Roots	Headache	Paste
Aristolochia tagala Cham.	Aristolochiaceae	Leaves	Snake bite	topical
A. heterophyllus Lam.	Moraceae	Leaves	Centipede bite	topical
Artocarpus hirsutus Lam.	Moraceae	Flower, leaves, and stem bark	Arthritis, pitta, and sexual weakness	Topical and oral
Averrhoa bilimbi L.	Oxalidaceae	Leaves and flower	Scurvy and cholesterol	Oral
Begonia malabarica Lam.	Begoniaceae	Leaves	Timea-pedis	Paste
Biophytum sensitivum (L.) DC.	Oxalidaceae	Whole plant	Cancer	Oral
Caesalpinia bonduc (L.) Roxb.	Caesalpiniaceae	Roots	Piles	Juice
Calycopteris floribunda Lam.	Combretaceae	Leaves, fruit, and flower	Malarial fever, dysentery, and jaundice	Oral
Capscicum frutescens L.	Solanaceae	Fruits	Cholesterol, postnatal care	Oral
Centella asiatica (L.) Urb.	Apiaceae	Whole plant	Hair diseases	Topical
Chlorophytum laxum R. Br	Liliaceae	Bulb and tubers	Snake and insect bite	Paste

TABLE 4.2 *(Continued)*

	Family	Parts used	Disease	Mode of administration
Chromolaena odorata (L.) King and Robins.	Asteraceae	Leaves	Injuries	Paste
Clerodendrum nfortunatum L.	Lamiaceae	Leaves	Itching	Topical
Clerodendrum viscosum Vent.	Verbenaceae	Leaves	Injuries	Paste
Clitoria ternatea L.	Fabaceae	Leaves	Wounds	topical
Coscinium fenestratum (Gaertn.) Coleb.	Menispermaceae	Stem	Jaundice and diabetes	Oral
Costus speciosus (Koenig) J. E. Smith	Zingiberaceae	Stem	Ottalgia	Juice
Croton tiglium L.	Euphorbiaceae	Leaves	Pyoderma	Paste
Curculigo orchioides Gaertn.	Hypoxidaceae	Whole plant and tubers	Menstrual problems, asthma, and diabetes	Oral
Cyclea peltata (Lam.) Hook. f. and Thomas.	Menispermaceae	Aerial parts	Frothy stool	Paste
Dalbergia lanceolaria L. f.	Fabaceae	Bark	Jaundice	Oral
Dioscorea hispida Dennst.	Dioscoreaceae	Tubers	Pyrosis	Raw and chew
Elephantopus scaber L.	Asteraceae	Whole plant	Blood clotting	Oral
Emilia sonchifolia (L.) DC.	Asteraceae	Leaves	Eye injuries	Juice
Evolvulus alsinoides (L.) L.,	Convolvulaceae	Whole plant	Chest infection	Powder
Glycyrrhiza glabra L.	Fabaceae	Whole plant	Tuberculosis	Paste
Gossypium hirsutum L.	Malvaceae	Leaves	Poison infection	Oral, topical, and inhalation
Helicteres isora L.	Sterculiaceae	Flowers and leaves	Cold, fever, and cancer	Oral

TABLE 4.2 *(Continued)*

	Family	Parts used	Disease	Mode of administration
Hemidesmus indicus (L.) R. Br	Apocynaceae	Tubers and roots	Abdominal colic, cough, pyrosis, and blood purification	Oral
Holostemma ada-kodien Schult.	Asclepiadaceae	Tubers	Promote lactation	Paste
Humboldtia unijuga Bedd.	Caesalpiniaceae	Roots	Headache	Paste
Indigofera tinctoria L.,	Fabaceae	Leaves	Headache	Dermal
Ipomea pes-tigridis L	Convolvulaceae	Leaves	Spider bite	Paste
Ipomea quamoclit L.	Convolvulaceae	Leaves	Throat pain	Paste
Justicia adhatoda L.	Acanthaceae	Leaves	Pneumonia and pain	Topical and oral
Morinda reticulata Gamble.	Rubiaceae	Whole plant	Blood purification and jaundice	Oral
Moringa pterygosperma Gaertn.	Moringaceae	Stem bark	Burning injury	Topical
Myxopyrum smilacifolium (Wall.) Blume	Oleaceae	Stem	Migraine	Paste
Naravelia zeylanica (L.) DC.	Ranunculaceae	Stem	Rhinitis	Powder
Naregamia alata Wight and Arn.	Meliaceae	Whole	Headache and ottalgia	Paste
Ocimum tenuiflorum L.	Lamiaceae	Leaves and root	Cold and fever	Oral
Oryza meyeriana (Zoll and Mor. ex Steud.) Baill.	Poaceae	Seeds	Chickenpox	Paste
Pergularia daemia (Forrsk.) Chiov.	Asclepiadaceae	Whole plant	Blood clotting	Oral
Phyllanthus amarus Schum. and Thonn.	Euphorbiaceae	Whole plant	Jaundice	Oral
Phyllanthus urinaria L.	Phyllanthaceae	Whole plant	Chest infection	Paste

TABLE 4.2 *(Continued)*

	Family	Parts used	Disease	Mode of administration
Pisonia grandis R. Br.	Nyctaginaceae	Leaves	Elephantoid swellings and arthritis	Topical
Plectranthus ambonicus (Lour.) Spreng.	Lamiaceae	Whole plant	Headache and ottalgia	Paste
Plumbago zeylanica L.	Plumbaginaceae	Roots	Arthritis, cold, and fever	Oral, topical, and inhalation
Protasparagus racemosus (Willd.) Oberm.	Liliaceae	Tubers	Diarrhoea, fever and leucorrhoea	Juice
Pterospermum rubiginosum Heyne ex Wight and Arn.	Sterculiaceae	Bark	Bone fracture, injuries, laceration, and sprain	Paste and powder
Pyrrosia heterophylla (L.) M.G.Price	Polypodiaceae	Leaves and root	Jaundice	Oral
Scleria lithosperma (L.) Sw.	Cyperaceae	Tubers	Sebaceous cyst	Powder
Scoparia dulcis L.	Scrophulariaceae	Leaves, flowers, and fruits	Kidney stone	Oral
Senna alexandrina Gars. Ex Mill.	Fabaceae	Whole plant	Blood purification and bee bite	Oral, topical, and inhalation
Smilax zeylanica L.	Smilacaceae	Rhizome and leaves	Blood purification and piles	Oral and paste
Spatholobus parviflorus (Roxb. ex DC.) O. Ktze.	Fabaceae	Leaves	Conjunctivitis	Paste
Spermacoce articularia L. f.	Rubiaceae	Leaves	Injuries	Paste
Strychnos nux-vomica L.	Loganiaceae	Leaves and seeds	Snakebite and eye infection	Topical

TABLE 4.2 *(Continued)*

	Family	Parts used	Disease	Mode of administration
Thottea siliquosa (Lam.) Ding Hou	Aristolochiaceae	Tubers	Snakebite	Paste
Trichopus zeylanicus Gaertn.	Trichopodaceae	Whole plant	Obesity	Powder
Vernonia cinerea (L.) Less.	Asteraceae	Leaves	Conjunctivitis	Juice
Vitex negundo L.	Verbenaceae	Leaves	Dyspnoea and tuberculosis	Juice
Vitex trifolia L.	Verbenaceae	Whole plant	Wound and cancer	Oral, topical, and inhalation
Zingiber officinale Rose.	Zingiberaceae	Tubers	Stomachache	Oral

Source: Vijayan et al. (2007); Xavier et al. (2014).

Kani tribes residing in Tirunelveli Hills and they are useful to treat up to 65 different diseases.

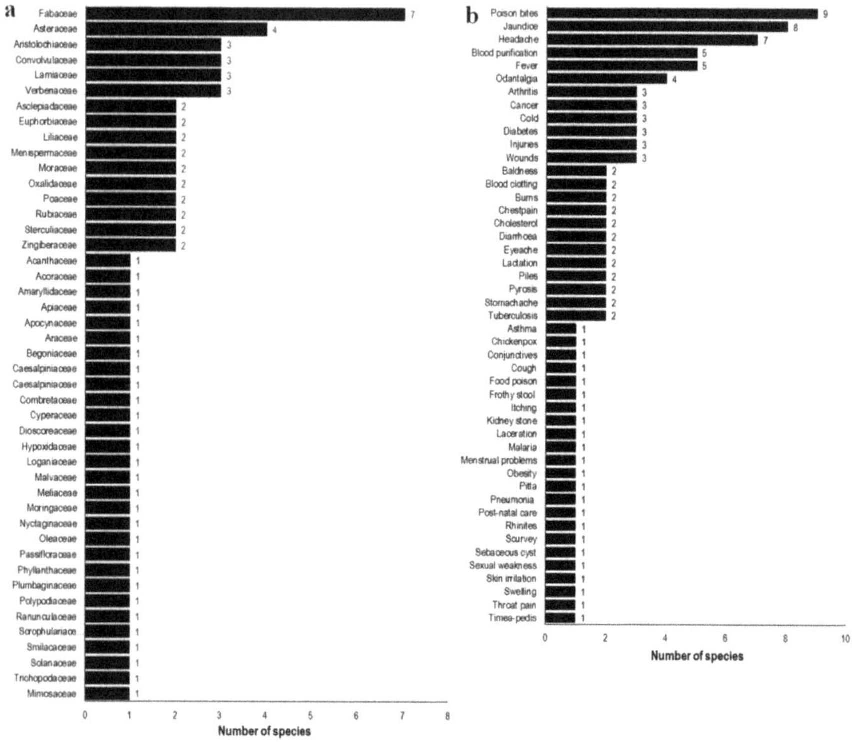

FIGURE 4.3 Family-wise distribution of medicinal plants used by the Kani tribes in Kerala state (a) and their uses to treat different diseases (b).

Literature analysis has revealed the use of 142 medicinal plant species (in 123 genera and 58 families) by the Kani tribes of Tamil Nadu (Table 4.3). The most members of plants are represented by the family Fabaceae (14 plants) followed by the Asteraceae (nine plants), Solanaceae, Euphorbiaceae (seven plants each), and Rubiaceae (five plants) (Figure 4.4a). Kani tribes in Tamil Nadu use the highest number of plant species for treating wounds (17 species) followed by treatment to improve the body strength, stomachache (16 species each), dermal diseases (11 species), fever, headache, and rheumatism (10 species each) (Figure 4.4b). Among the plant parts used by the Kani tribes in Tamil Nadu, leaves stand first (95 species) followed by stem, fruits, whole plant, root, and flowers (11–27 species) (Figure 4.2c).

TABLE 4.3 Details of Ethnomedicinal Plant Species Used by the Kani Tribes Residing in Tamil Nadu State.

	Family	**Parts used**	**Disease**	**Preparation**	**Mode of administration**
Abutilon indicum G. Don.	Malvaceae	Leaves stem and bark	Venereal diseases and over bleeding	Paste	Oral
Acacia nilotica (L.) Del.	Fabaceae	Stem and bark	Oral foul odor	Decoction	Mouthwash
Acalypha indica L.	Euphorbiaceae	Leaves	Itching and wounds	Paste	Oral
Achyranthes aspera L.	Amaranthaceae	Leaves	Tooth ache	Paste	Tooth powder
Adhatoda vasica Medicus	Acanthaceae	Leaves	Asthma, cold, headache, and earache	Paste	Oral
Aerva lanata Juss.	Amaranthaceae	Whole plant	Asthma, chest pain, and poison bites	Powder	Oral
Ageratum conyzoides L.	Asteraceae	Leaves	Diarrhea	Juice	Oral
Aglaia roxburghiana Hiern. var. *courtallensis*, Gamb.	Meliaceae	Leaves and seeds	Snake and scorpion bites	Decoction	Oral
A. cepa L.	Amaryllidaceae	Bulb	Rheumatism, headache, and baldness due to fungal infection	Juice	Oral and topical
Aloe vera (L.) Burm. f.	Asphodelaceae	Leaves	Stomach ache	Paste	Oral
Alpinia galanga Sw.	Amaranthaceae	Rhizome	Asthma, cold, cough, headache, and fever	Powder	Oral and topical
Alstonia scholaris R. Br.	Apocynaceae	Leaves, stem and latex	Swelling and latex for abortion	Paste	Topical and oral
Alternanthera sessilis (L.) R.Br. ex. DC.	Amaranthaceae	Leaves	Eye pain	Juice	Topical
Alysicarpus vaginalis DC.	Fabaceae	Leaves	Venereal disease	Decoction	Oral
Anacardium occidentale L.	Anacardiaceae	Fruits	Asthma, headache, and wounds	Juice	Oral

TABLE 4.3 *(Continued)*

	Family	Parts used	Disease	Preparation	Mode of administration
Ananus comosus (L.) Merr.	Bromeliaceae	Fruits	Venereal disease	Juice	Oral
Anotis monosperma B.andHk. f.	Rubiaceae	Leaves, root, and stem	Scorpion and insect bites	Paste	Topical
Areca catechu L.	Arecaceae	Fruits	Burns	Powder	Topical
Atalantia monophylla (L.) Corr.	Rutaceae	Leaves and fruits	Cold and poison bites	Decoction	Oral
Azadirachta indica A. Juss.	Meliaceae	Stem bark and leaves	Poison bites, stomachache, and scabies	Paste	Oral and topical
Bambusa arundinacea (Retz.) Willd.	Poaceae	Seeds	Rheumatism	Paste	Oral
B. malabarica Lam.	Begoniaceae	Leaves	Nasal infection	Paste	Topical
Bidens pilosa L.	Asteraceae	Leaves	Stomachache	Juice	oral
Biophytum candolleanum W.	Oxalidaceae	Leaves	Venereal disease	Paste	Topical
Borreria ocymoides DC	Rubiaceae	Leaves and stem	Wounds	Paste	Topical
Bridelia retusa (L.) Spreng.	Euphorbiaceae	Leaves	Wounds	Paste	Topical
Calophyllum inophyllum L.	Clusiaceae	Seeds, leaves, and seed oil	Baldness due to fungal infection and skin irritation	Paste	Topical
C. frutescens L.	Solanaceae	Whole plant and fruits	Cholesterol control, postnatal care, and labor pain	Raw and paste	Oral and topical
Cardiospermum halicacabum L.	Sapindaceae	Leaves	Labor pain, body pain, and rheumatism	Juice	Oral
Carica papaya L.	Caricaceae	Fruits and latex	Constipation	Raw and paste	Oral
Carissa carandas L.	Apocynaceae	Fruits	Stomachache	As pickle	Oral

TABLE 4.3 *(Continued)*

	Family	Parts used	Disease	Preparation	Mode of administration
Carmona retusa (Vahl.) Masam.	Cordiaceae	Leaves	Toothache	Powder	Topical
Caryota urens L.	Arecaceae	Stem	Body strength	Paste	Oral
Cassia alata L.	Fabaceae	Flowers	Abortion	Juice	Oral
Cassia auriculata L.	Fabaceae	Flowers and leaves	Stomachache, skin irritation, and itching	Paste	Oral and topical
Cayratia pedata Juss.	Vitaceae	Leaves, fruits, and stem	Gastric complaints	Juice	Oral
Centella asiatica (L.) Urban.	Mackinlayaceae	Leaves	Memory power in children and hair growth	Powder	Oral
Ceropegia candelabrum L.	Asclepiadaceae	Leaves and stem	Headache	Decoction	Oral
Cipadessa baccifera Miq.	Meliaceae	Leaves	Insect and snakebites	Juice	Oral
Cissus quadrangularis L.	Vitaceae	Stem and leaves	Stomachache	Powder and paste	Oral
Cissus trilobata Lam.	Vitaceae	Leaves and root	Rheumatism	Paste	Topical
Citrus aurantifolia (Christm. and Panz.) Sw.	Rutaceae	Leaves	Indigestion	Juice	Oral
Cleome viscosa L.	Cleomaceae	Leaves	Wounds, swelling, headache, and fever	Paste and juice	Topical
Clitoria ternatea L.	Fabaceae	Leaves	Throat pain, Swellings	Paste	Oral and topical
Coccinia indica (L.) Voigt.	Cucurbitaceae	Leaves	Body strength and increase semen production	Paste	Oral
Commelina benghalensis L.	Commelinaceae	Pseudostem	Wounds	Juice	Topical

TABLE 4.3 *(Continued)*

	Family	Parts used	Disease	Preparation	Mode of administration
Costus speciosus Smith.	Costaceae	Rhizome	Diabetes	Paste	Oral
Crotalaria pallida Aiton. Hort.	Fabaceae	Leaves, root bark	Skin diseases	Paste	Topical
Cynodon dactylon (L.) Pers.	Poaceae	Leaves and whole plant	Wounds, itching, body pain, and asthma	Juice and decoction	Topical and oral
Datura metel L.	Solanaceae	Leaves	Earache	Juice	Topical
Desmodium triangulare (Retz.) Merr.	Fabaceae	Leaves	Hair loss	Paste	Topical
Diospyros ebenum Koen.	Ebenaceae	Whole plant	Strengthen body	Juice	Oral
Ecbolium viride (Forssk.) Alston in Trimen.	Acanthaceae	Leaves	Reduce body heat and cool the eyes	Juice	Oral
Elephantopus scaber L.	Asteraceae	Leaves and whole plant	Rheumatism and blood clotting	Paste	Topical and oral
Elettaria cardamomum (L.) Maton.	Zingiberaceae	Fruits	Headache, rheumatism, and asthma	Powder	Oral
Eupatorium odoratum L.	Asteraceae	Leaves	Wounds	Paste	Topical
Euphorbia hirta L. (Euphorbiaceae)	Euphorbiaceae	Latex and leaves	Wounds	Raw paste	Topical
Evolvulus alsinoides L.	Convolvulaceae	Whole plant	Venereal disease	Paste	Topical
Evolvulus nummularius L.	Convolvulaceae	Leaves, flowers and root	Dysentery	Paste	Oral
Ficus benghalensis L.	Moraceae	Leaves and tender twigs	Wounds and strengthen teeth	Raw	Toothbrush

TABLE 4.3 *(Continued)*

	Family	Parts used	Disease	Preparation	Mode of administration
Ficus religiosa L.	Moraceae	Leaves and stem bark	Stomachache, indigestion, and breast pain	Powder	Oral
Ficus retusa L.	Moraceae	Fruits	Cure sterility in men	Juice	Oral
Gymnema sylvestre (L.) R. Br.	Apocynaceae	Stem bark and leaves	Diabetes, scorpion sting, snakebite, and itching	Powder	Oral
Helicteres isora (L.) W and A.	Sterculiaceae	Unripe fruits, flower, and leaves	Hair growth, cold, fever and cancer	Decoction	Topical and oral
Hemidesmus indicus (L.) R.Br.	Asclepiadaceae	Root	Blood purifier	Decoction	Oral
Hemionitis arifolia (Burm.) Moore	Hemionitidaceae	Leaves	Rabies	Paste	Topical
Hibiscus rosa-sinensis L.	Malvaceae	Leaves and flowers	Strengthen the heart, venereal diseases and stomachache	Raw and powder	Oral
Hygrophila auriculata (Schum.) Heine.	Acanthaceae	Leaves	Cough	Juice	Oral
Ipomoea obscura K.Gawl.	Convolvulaceae	Stem, leaves, flowers, and root	Conception	Juice	Oral
Jatropha gossypifolia L.	Euphorbiaceae	Resin	Mount foul odor, wounds in lips and tongue	Powder	Tooth powder and topical
Kalanchoe pinnata (Lam.) Pers.	Crassulaceae	Leaves	Body cooling	Decoction	Oral
Kleinia grandiflora (DC) N. Rani	Asteraceae	Leaves and root bark	Gastric complaints	Juice	Oral

TABLE 4.3 *(Continued)*

	Family	Parts used	Disease	Preparation	Mode of administration
Lantana camara L.	Verbenaceae	Leaves and root bark	Cold and fever	Decoction	Oral
Lawsonia inermis L.	Lythraceae	Leaves	Heel cracks, rheumatism, and disease resistance in children	Paste	Topical
Leucas aspera (Willd.) Link	Lamiaceae	Leaves and flowers	Dysentery, fever, headache, eye pain, and color blindness	Juice and paste	Oral and topical
Maesa indica W. var. perrottetiana Cl.	Myrsinaceae	Leaves	Disease resistance	Juice	Topical
Mallotus philippinensis (Lam.) Muell. Arg.	Euphorbiaceae	Leaves and stem bark	Hydrocele and stomachache	Decoction	Oral
Mangifera indica L.	Anacardiaceae	Stem bark	Body pain and labor pain	Powder and paste	Oral
Melia azedarach L.	Meliaceae	Leaves, stem, and root bark	Stomach ache, skin irritation, body pain and sperm production	Juice and paste	Topical and oral
Memecylon gracilis Bedd.	Melastomataceae	Leaves	Improved fertility in men	Paste	Topical
Merremia hastata Hall.	Convolvulaceae	Laves, stem, and root	As tooth powder and to cure tooth disease	Paste	Oral
Michelia champaca L.	Magnoliaceae	Leaves	Eye pain	Decoction	Topical
Milletia pinnata (L.) Panigrahi.	Fabaceae	Stem bark	Wounds	Raw	Topical
Mimosa pudica L.	Fabaceae	Leaves	Pimples	Paste	Topical
Mimusops elengi L.	Sapotaceae	Flowers	Body shining	Juice	Oral

TABLE 4.3 *(Continued)*

	Family	Parts used	Disease	Preparation	Mode of administration
Mollugo nudicaulis Lam.	Molluginaceae	Leaves and whole plant	Fever, cough, headache, stomachache, and venereal diseases	Decoction and powder	Oral
Mollugo pentaphylla L.	Molluginaceae	Leaves	Eye disease	Juice	Oral
Momordica dioica Roxb.	Cucurbitaceae	Leaves	Stomachache	Decoction	Oral
Morinda pubescens Roxb.	Rubiaceae	Leaves	Rheumatism, indigestion and wounds	Decoction, paste and powder	Topical and oral
Moringa oleifera Lam.	Moringaceae	Flowers	Increase perm production	Powder	Oral
Mukia maderaspatana (L.) M. Roem.	Cucurbitaceae	Leaves	Body strength	Paste	Oral
Murraya koenigii (L.) Spreng.	Rutaceae	Leaves	Eye pain, dandruff and hair loss	Paste	Oral
Mussaenda hirsutissima Hutch.	Rubiaceae	Leaves and stem bark	Cure sterility in men, and women	Juice	Oral
Ocimum basilicum L.	Lamiaceae	Leaves, stem, inflorescence and root	Cold, fever, and cough	Juice	Oral
Ocimum canum Sims.	Lamiaceae	Leaves	Cold, fever, and cough	Decoction	Oral
Ocimum tenuiflorum L.	Lamiaceae	Leaves	Cold, fever, and cough	Juice	Oral
Opuntia dillenii Haw.	Cactaceae	Stem	Wounds	Paste	Topical
Osbeckia zeylanica Willd.	Melastomataceae	Whole plant	Enhancement of stamina and disease resistance	Paste	Oral
Oxalis corniculata L.	Oxalidaceae	Leaves	Reduce body heat	Paste	Topical

TABLE 4.3 *(Continued)*

	Family	Parts used	Disease	Preparation	Mode of administration
Pandanus fascicularis Lam.	Pandanaceae	Stem	Jaundice	Raw	Oral
Phoenix sylvestris (L.) Roxb.	Arecaceae	Tender twigs and leaves	Male fertility, body strength	Raw and juice	Oral
Phyllanthus amarus Schum and Thonn.	Phyllanthaceae	Fruits and whole plant	Jaundice	Juice	Oral
Phyllanthus emblica L.	Phyllanthaceae	Leaves	Body strength	Powder	Oral
Phyllanthus virgatus G.Forst.	Euphorbiaceae	Leaves	Jaundice and stomachache	Paste	Oral
Physalis minima L.	Solanaceae	Fruits	Venereal disease and increase lactation	Decoction	Oral
Piper betle L.	Piperaceae	Leaves	Itching and skin irritation	Paste	Topical
Piper nigrum L.	Piperaceae	Fruits	Cough, bronchitis and snakebite	Powder	Oral
Pothos scandens L.	Araceae	Leaves	Post-natal wound healing	Paste	Topical
Pseudarthria viscida W. and A.	Fabaceae	Leaves	Cold and cough	Paste	Oral
Punica granatum L.	Lythraceae	Fruits	Stomachache	Powder	Oral
Richardia scabra L.	Rubiaceae	Leaves	Skin disease	Paste	Topical
Ricinus communis L.	Euphorbiaceae	Seed and seed oil	Joint and muscle pain	Powder	Topical
Ruellia prostrata Poir.	Acanthaceae	Leaves	Prevent hair loss	Juice	Topical
Sansevieria roxburghiana Schult. f.	Agavaceae	Stem	Earache	Juice	Topical
Santalum album L.	Santalaceae	Stem	Pimples and body cooling	Paste	Topical

TABLE 4.3 *(Continued)*

	Family	Parts used	Disease	Preparation	Mode of administration
Scleropyrum pentandrum (Dennst.) Mabb.	Santalaceae	Stem bark and leaves	Skin disease	Paste	Topical
Sesamum indicum L.	Pedaliaceae	Seed and Seed oil	Skin irritation and itching	Paste	Topical
Sesbania grandiflora Pers.	Fabaceae	Leaves	Body cooling	Decoction	Oral
Solanum nigrum L.	Solanaceae	Leaves	Gastric ulcer	Decoction	Oral
Solanum surattense Burm. f.	Solanaceae	Fruits	Toothache	Raw	Mouth inhalation
Solanum trilobatum L.	Solanaceae	Flowers and leaves	Male fertility and constipation	Raw and paste	Oral
Solanum vagum Heyne.	Solanaceae	Leaves and root	Dry skin	Juice	Topical
Sphaeranthus indicus L.	Asteraceae	Whole plant	Skin irritation	Paste	Topical
Strychnos nux-vomica L.	Loganiaceae	Leaves	Rheumatism and eye infection	Paste and juice	Topical
Syzygium cumini Skeels.	Myrtaceae	Leaves and Fruits	Diabetes, indigestion, and stomachache	Juice and raw paste	Oral
Tabernaemontana heyneana Wall.	Apocynaceae	Leaves, stem bark, and latex	Leaves to skin disease and latex to induce abortion	Paste	Topical
Tamarindus indica L.	Fabaceae	Flower and leaves	Body cooling and eye cooling	Decoction and Paste	Oral and topical
Tectona grandis L.f.	Verbenaceae	Seeds and oil	Hair loss and dandruff	Paste	Topical
Tephrosia purpurea (L.) Pers.	Fabaceae	Leaves	Gastric problems	Paste	Oral
Terminalia chebula Retz.	Combretaceae	Fruits	Gastric ulcer and toothache	Raw and powder	Oral as tooth powder

TABLE 4.3 *(Continued)*

	Family	Parts used	Disease	Preparation	Mode of administration
Themeda triandra Forsk.	Poaceae	Whole plant	Wounds	Paste	Topical
Trianthema portulacastrum L.	Aizoaceae	Leaves and root	Disease resistance	Paste	Topical
Tribulus terrestris L.	Zygophyllaceae	Whole plant and fruits	Fever, headache and heel cracks	Paste and powder	Topical
Trichopus *zeylanicus* Gaertn.	Trichopodaceae	Unripe fruits and leaves	Asthma, venereal disease and body strength	Juice and paste	Oral
Tridax procumbens L.	Asteraceae	Leaves	Swelling	Paste	Topical
Urena lobata L. subsp. *lobata* (L.) Bross. Wal.	Malvaceae	Root	Snakebite	Decoction	Oral
Vernonia cinerea Less.	Asteraceae	Whole plant	Brest tumor	Paste	Topical
Vitex negundo L.	Verbenaceae	Leaves	Body pain and poison bites	Decoction and paste	Topical and Oral
Wedelia calendulacea Less.	Asteraceae	Leaves	Hair loss and greying of hair	Powder	Topical
Zehneria maysorensis (W and A) Arn.	Cucurbitaceae	Leaves	Kill stomach worms	Juice	Oral
Ziziphus zizyphus (L.) H.Karst.	Rhamnaceae	Fruit	Blood purifier and weight loss	Raw	Oral
Zornia diphylla Pers.	Fabaceae	Whole plant	Wounds and stomach ulcer	Paste	Topical and oral

Source: Ayyanar and Ignacimuthu (2005, 2011).

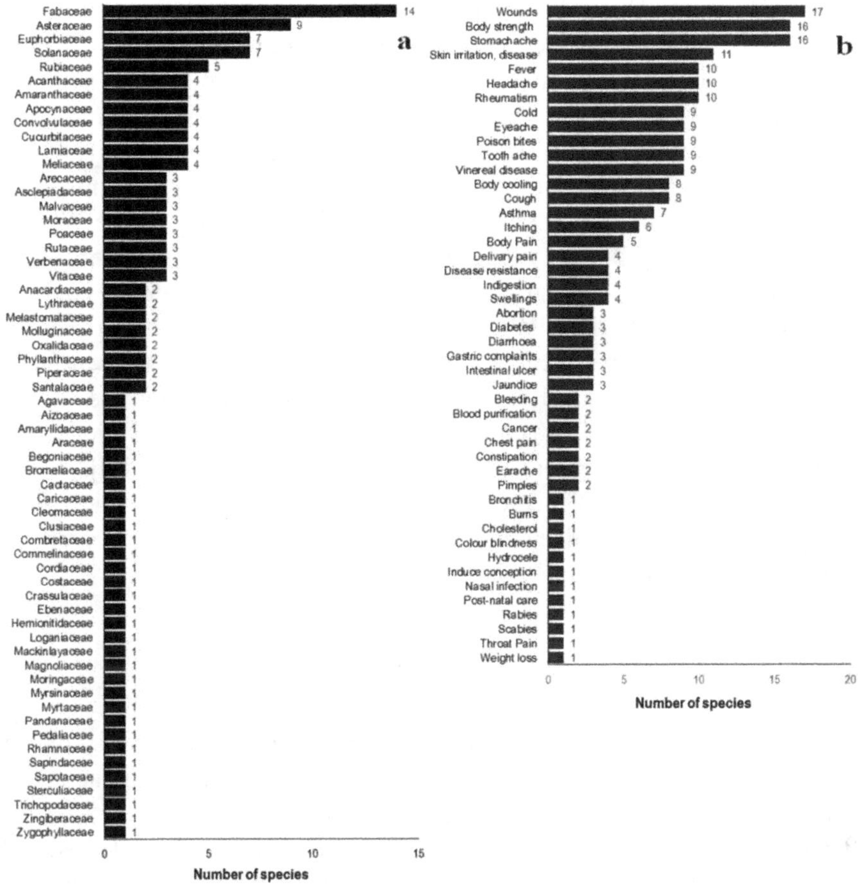

FIGURE 4.4 Family-wise distribution of medicinal plants used by the Kani tribes in Tamil Nadu state (a) and their uses to treat different diseases (b).

4.5 CONCLUSION

Although modern medicinal research has made substantial progress to treat several diseases, there exists a wide gap to find solution to combat many lifestyle diseases owing to lack of raw materials of specific plant species as precursor or to develop target oriented drug. Ethnobotanical exploration and documentation of medicinal plant species used by the tribes in different parts of India assumes importance to impart ethnic knowledge in to the modern medicine. Translation of tribal knowledge into modern medicine is one of the greatest challenges of the present century. However, the traditional knowledge is dwindling due to lack of tribal welfare as well as habitat loss leading to scarcity or extinction of preferred plant resources. The Western Ghats being one of the important biodiversity hotspots as well as world heritage center, the tribals living in such region and their folk knowledge on medicinal plants serve as a treasure to the modern medicine. This review brought out several interesting aspects of ethnobotanical and ethnomedicinal uses of plant resource by the tribals residing in the vicinity of the Western Ghats. As the tribal folk knowledge on medicinal applications of plant biodiversity is fast eroding, such studies or documentation from other parts of India particularly related to tribal knowledge will pave way to go forward toward total health care. It is pertinent to note that the leaves are extensively used for medication by the tribes of Karnataka, Kerala, and Tamil Nadu. Use of roots for medication by the tribes (range, 9–46 species) gives an indication to use such plants with caution and to provide preference for conservation. This documentation of use of medicinal plant diversity based on tribal folklore serve as a valuable baseline data toward conservation, further research and possible commercialization.

ACKNOWLEDGMENTS

Lokesh, S. acknowledges the SC-ST Special Cell, University of Mysore for the award of Senior Research Fellowship and Manjunath, B.R. acknowledges the University Grants Commission (UGC) for the award of UGC Post-Doctoral Fellowship. Council of Scientific and Industrial Research (CSIR), New Delhi awarded Research Associate Fellowship to Mahadevakumar, S.

KEYWORDS

- **conservation**
- **ethnomedicine**
- **medicinal plants**
- **traditional knowledge**
- **tribes**

REFERENCES

Aadhan, K.; Anand, S. P. Traditional Herbal Medicines for the Treatment of Snake Bite and Scorpion Sting by the Paliyar's Tribes of Sathuragiri Hills. *J. Med. Pl. Stud.* **2017,** *5*, 1–5.

Achar, S. G.; Rajkumar, N.; Shivanna, M. B. Ethno-Medico-Botanical Knowledge of Khare-Vokkaliga Community in Uttara Kannada District of Karnataka, India. *J. Compl. Integr. Med.* **2010,** *7*, 1–18.

Alagesaboopathi, C. Ethnomedicinal Plants and Their Utilization by Villagers in Kumaragiri Hills of Salem District of Tamil Nadu, India. *Afr. J. Trad. Compl. Alt. Med.* **2009,** *6*, 222–227.

Anuradha, R. V. Sharing with Kanis: A Case Study from Kerala, India. New Delhi, Kalpavriksha, Mimeo, 2000. https://www.cbd.int/financial/bensharing/india-kanis.pdf (accessed on Aug 07, 2021).

Arul-Manikandan, P. N. Folk Herbal Medicine: A Survey on the Paniya Tribes of Mundakunnu Village of the Nilgiri Hills, South India. *Anc. Sci. Life,* **2005,** *25*, 21–27.

Ayyanar, M.; Ignacimuthu, S. Ethnobotanical Survey of Medicinal Plants Commonly Used by Kani Tribals in Tirunelveli Hills of Western Ghats, India. *J. Ethnopharmacol.* **2011,** *134*, 851–864.

Ayyanar, M.; Ignacimuthu, S. Traditional Knowledge of Kani Tribals in Kouthalai of Tirunelveli Hills, Tamil Nadu, India. *J. Ethnopharmacol.* **2005,** *102*, 246–255.

Bhagya, B.; Sridhar, K. R. Ethnobiology of Coastal Sand Dunes of Southwest Coast of India. *Ind. J. Trad. Know.* **2009,** *8*, 611–620.

Bhandary, M. J.; Chandrashekar, K. R. Treatment of Poisonous Snake-Bites in the Ethnomedicine of Coastal Karnataka. *J. Med. Arom. Pl. Sci.* **2001,** *22*, 505–510.

Bhandary, M. J.; Chandrashekar, K. R.; Kaveriappa, K. M. Ethnobotany of Gawlis of Uttara Kannada District, Karnataka. *J. Econ. Taxon. Bot.* **1996,** *12*, 244–249.

Bhandary, M. J.; Chandrashekar, K. R.; Kaveriappa, K. M. Medical Ethnobotany of the Siddis of Uttarakannada District, Karnataka, India. *J. Ethnopharmacol.* **1995,** *47*, 149–156.

Bhandary, M. J.; Chandrashekar, K. R. Glimpses of Ethnic Herbal Medicine of Costal Karnataka. *Ethnobot.* **2002,** *14*, 1–12.

Bhandary, M. J.; Chandrashekhar, K. R. Herbal Therapy for Herpes in the Ethnomedicine of Coastal Karnataka. *Ind. J. Trad. Know.* **2011,** *10*, 528–532.

Bhat, P.; Hegde, G. R.; Hegde, G.; Mulgund, G. S. Ethnomedicinal Plants to Cure Skin Diseases—An Account of Traditional Knowledge in the Coastal Parts of Central Western Ghats, Karnataka, India. *J. Ethnopharmacol.* **2014,** *151*, 493–502.

Bhat, P.; Hegde, G.; Hegde, G. R. Ethnomedicinal Practices in Different Communities of Uttara Kannada District of Karnataka for Treatment of Wounds. *J. Ethnopharmacol.* **2012,** *143*, 501–14.

Bhat, S.; Mulgund, G. S.; Bhat, P. Ethnomedicinal Practices for the Treatment of Arthritis in Siddapur Region of Uttara Kannada District, Karnataka, India. *J. Her. Spic. Med. Pl.* **2019,** *25*, 316–329.

Binu, S. An Enumeration of Medicinal Plants Used by the Tribals in Pathanamthitta District of Kerala, India, Part–I. *J. Econ. Taxon. Bot.* **2012,** *36*, 280–312.

Binu, S.; Nayar, T. S.; Pushpangadan, P. An Outline of Ethnobotanical Research in India. *J. Econ. Taxon. Bot. (Add. Ser.),* **1992,** 405–428.

Calixto, J. B. Twenty-Five Years of Research on Medicinal Plants in Latin America: A Personal Review. *J. Ethnopharmacol.* **2005,** *100*, 131–134.

De, L. C. Bio-Diversity and Conservation of Medicinal and Aromatic Plants. *Adv. Pl. Agric. Res.* **2016,** *5*, 561–566.

Dilipikumar, E. K.; Janardhana, G. R. Ethno Botanical Polypharmacy of Traditional Healers in Wayanad (Kerala) to Treat Type 2 Diabetes. *Ind. J. Trad. Know.* **2012,** *11*, 667–673.

Dwarakan, P.; Diwarkar, P. G.; Ansari, A. A. Common Plants of the Krishna River Basin. *J. Econ. Taxon. Bot.* **1997,** *21*, 13–18.

Ernst, E. The Efficacy of Herbal Medicine—An Overview. *Fund. Clin. Pharmacol.* **2005,** *19*, 405–409.

Ganesh, T.; Ganesan, M.; Soubadra, D.; Davidar, P.; Bawa, K. A. Assessment of Plant Biodiversity at a Mid-Elevation Evergreen Forest of Kalakad—Mundanthurai Tiger Reserve, Western Ghats. *Curr. Sci.* **1996,** *71*, 379–392.

Gireesha, J. Studies on Diversity and Depletion of Medicinal Plants in Chamarajanagar District of Karnataka. Ph. D. Dissertation, University of Mysore, Mysore, 2019.

Gireesha, J.; Raju, N. S. Ethno Botanical Study of Medicinal Plants in BR Hills Region of Western Ghats, Karnataka. *Asian J. Plant Sci. Res.* **2013,** *3*, 36–40.

Gopakumar, K.; Vijayalakshmi, K. B.; Shantha, T. R.; Yoganarasimhan, S. N. Plants Used in Ayurveda from Chikmagalur District, Karnataka-II. *J. Econ. Taxon. Bot.* **1991,** *15*, 379–389.

Gunaga, S.; Rajeshwari, N.; Vasudeva, R. Documenting Angiosperm Diversity and Assigning Economic and Conservation Value of Kaan Forests: Traditionally Managed Climax Sacred Landscapes in Sagar Taluk of Central Western Ghats, India. *Asian J. Biol. Life Sci.* **2012,** *1*, 164–173.

Harihar, N. S.; Kotresha, K. Wild Medicinal Plants of Kappat Hills, Gadag District, Karnataka. Part-II. *Life Sci. Leaflets,* **2012,** *5*, 37–32.

Harsha, V. H.; Hebbar, S. S.; Hegde, G. R.; Shripathi, V. Ethnomedical Knowledge of Plants Used by Kunabi Tribe of Karnataka in India. *Fitoterapia* **2002,** *73*, 281–287.

Hathur, B.; Basavegowda, M.; Ashok, N. C. Hypertension: An Emerging Threat Among Tribal Population of Mysore; Jenu Kuruba Tribe Diabetes and Hypertension Study. *Int. J. Health Allied. Sci.* **2013,** *2*, 270–274.

Hebbar, S. S.; Harsha, V. H.; Hegde, G. R.; Shripathi, V. Ethno-Medicobotanical Survey in Dharwad-Plants Used for Jaundice. *Bull. Bot. Sur. India,* **2004a,** *46*, 268–272.

Hebbar, S. S.; Hegde, H. V.; Shripathi, V.; Hegde, G. R. Ethnomedicine of Dharwad District in Karnataka, India—Plants Used in Oral Health Care. *J Ethnopharmacol.* **2004b,** *94*, 261–266.

Hegde, H. V.; Hebbar, S. S.; Shripathi, V.; Hegde, G. R. Ethnomedicobotany of Uttara Kannada District in Karnataka, India—Plants in Treatment of Skin Diseases. *J. Ethnopharmacol.* **2003,** *84*, 37–40.

Hegde, H. V.; Hegde, G. R.; Kholkute, S. D. Herbal Care for Reproductive Health: Ethno-Medicobotany from Uttara Kannada district in Karnataka, India. *Compl. Ther. Clin. Pract.* **2007,** *13*, 38–45.

Heinrich, M. Ethnobotany and Its Role in Drug Development. *Phytother. Res.* **2000,** *14*, 479–488.

Hiremath, V. T.; Taranath, T. C. Traditional Phytotherapy for Snakebites by Tribes of Chitradurga District, Karnataka, India. *Ethnobot. Leaflets* **2010,** 2. https://opensiuc.lib.siu.edu/ebl/vol2010/iss2/2

Hoareau, L.; DaSilva, E. J. Medicinal Plants: A Re-Emerging Health Aid. *Elect. J. Biotechnol.* **1999,** *2*, 56–70.

Hosagoudar, V. B.; Henry, A. N. Plants Used in Birth Control and Reproductive Ailments by Soligas of B. R. Betta in Mysore District of Karnataka. *Ethnobot.* **1993,** *5*, 117–118.

Ignacimuthu, S.; Sankara Sivaraman, K.; Kesavan, L. Medicoethnobotanical Survey Among Kanikar Tribals of Mundanthurai Sanctuary. *Fitoterapia*, **1998,** *69*, 409–414.

Iwu, M. W.; Duncan, A. R.; Okunji, C. O. New antimicrobials of Plant Origin. In *Perspectives on New Crops and New Uses*. Janick, J., Ed., ASHS Press: Alexandria, **1999,** pp 457–462.

Janaki Ammal, E. K.; Prasad, P. N. Ethnobotanical findings on *Costus speciosus* among the Kanikkars of Tamil Nadu. *J. Econ. Taxon. Bot.* **1984,** *5*, 129–133.

Joy, P. P.; Thomas, J.; Mathew, S.; Skaria, B. P. *Medicinal Plants*. Kerala Agricultural University. Aromatic and Medicinal Plants Research Station. **1998,** p. 211.

Kattimani, K. N.; Munikrishnappa, P. M.; Hussain, S. A.; Reddy, P. N. Use Plants as Medicine Under Semi-Arid Tropical Climate of Raichur District of North Karnataka. *J. Med. Arom. Pl. Sci.* **2001,** *22−23*, 607–611.

Kosalge, S. B.; Fursule, R. A. Investigation of Ethnomedicinal Claims of Some Plants Used by Tribals of Satpuda Hills in India. *J. Ethnopharmacol.* **2009,** *121*, 456–461.

Kshirsagar, R. D.; Singh, N. P. Less Known Ethnomedicinal Uses of Plants in Coorg District of Karnataka State, Southern India. *Ethnobotany*, **2000a,** *12*, 12–16.

Kshirsagar, R. D.; Singh, N. P. Less Known Ethnomedicinal Uses of Plants Reported by Jenu Kuruba Tribe of Mysore District, Southern India. *Ethnobot.* **2000b,** *12*, 118–122.

Kshirsagar, R. D.; Singh, N. P. Some Less Known Ethnomedicinal Uses from Mysore and Coorg Districts, Karnataka State, India. *J. Ethnopharmacol.* **2001,** *75*, 231–238.

Madegowda, C. Traditional Knowledge and Conservation. *Econ. Polit. Wkly.* **2009,** *44*, 65–69.

Madegowda, C.; Usha, C. The Health Problems and Health Scenario of Soliga Tribals at Biligiri Rangaswamy Temple Wildlife Sanctuary, Karnataka, South India. *Int. J. Res. Soc. Sci.* **2015,** *5*, 443−458.

Maruthi, K. R.; Krishna, V.; Manjunatha, B. K.; Nagaraja, V. P. Traditional Medicinal Plants of Davangere District, Karnataka-with Reference to Cure Skin Diseases. *Environ. Ecol.* **2000,** *18*, 441–446.

Murthy, S. M. S. Traditional Knowledge on Edible Medicinal Plants of Harapanahalli Taluk in Davangere District of Karnataka, India. *World J. Pharm. Pharm. Sci.* **2015,** *4*, 494–504.

Murugeswaran, R.; Venkatesan, K.; Shahidar, B. T.; Aminuddin. Diversity of Unani Medicinal Plants in Chamarajanagar Wildlife Division Karnataka, India. *Int. J. Innov. Sci. Eng. Tech.* **2015,** *2*, 22–39.

Nair, N. C.; Daniel, P. Floristic Diversity of the Western Ghats and Its Conservation: A Review. *Proc. Ind. Acad. Sci.* (*Suppl.*), **1986,** 127–163.

Namsa, N. D.; Tag, H.; Mandal, M.; Kalita, P.; Das, A. K. Anethnobotanical Study of Traditional Anti-Inflammatory Plants Used by the Lohit Community of Arunachal Pradesh, India. *J. Ethnopharmacol.* **2009,** *125*, 234–245.

Nandini, N.; Shiddamallayya, N. Diversity of Medicinal Plants Flora of Old Mysore District, Karnataka, India. *Indo Am. J. Pharm. Res.* **2013,** *3*, 6248–6258.

Nanjunda, D. C. Ethno-Medico-Botanical Investigation of Jenu Kuruba Ethnic Group of Karnataka State, India. *Bangladesh J. Med. Sci.* **2010,** *9*, 161–169.

Parinitha, M.; Harish, G. U.; Vivek, N. C.; Mahesh, T.; Shivanna, M. B. Ethno-Botanical Wealth of Bhadra Wild Life Sanctuary in Karnataka. *Ind. J. Tradit. Know.* **2004,** *3*, 37–50.

Pattanaik, C.; Reddy, C. S.; Murthy, M. S. An Ethnobotanical Survey of Medicinal Plants Used by the Didayi Tribe of Malkangiri District of Orissa, India. *Fitoterapia*, **2008,** *79*, 67–71.

Poornima, G.; Manasa, M.; Rudrappa, D.; Prashith Kekuda, T. R. Medicinal Plants Used by Herbal Healers in Narasipura and Manchale Villages of Sagara Taluk, Karnataka, India. *Sci. Technol. Arts Res. J.* **2012,** *1*, 12–17.

Posey, D. A.; Plenderleith, K. *Kayapo Ethnoecology and Culture*; Routledge: New York, 2002.
Prakash, B. N.; Unnikrishnan, P. M. Ethnomedical Survey of Herbs for the Management of Malaria in Karnataka, India. *Ethnobot. Res. Appl.* **2013,** *11*, 289–298.
Prakasha, H. M.; Krishnappa, M. People's Knowledge on Medicinal Plants in Sringeri Taluk, Karnataka. *Ind. J. Tradit. Knowl.* **2006,** *5*, 353–357.
Prasad, A. G.; Kumar, K. J. Ethno–Botanical Potential of Medicinal Legumes in the Western Ghats of Karnataka. *Indo Am. J. Pharm. Res.* **2013,** *3*, 1300–1306.
Prasad, P. N.; Jabadhas, A. W.; Janaki Ammal, E. K. Medicinal Plants Used by the Kanikkars of South India. *J. Econ. Taxon. Bot.* **1987,** *11*, 149−155.
Prashantkumar, P.; Vidyasagar, G. M. Documentation of Traditional Knowledge on Medicinal Plants of Bidar District, Karnataka. *Indian J. Tradit. Know.* **2006,** *5*, 295–299.
Prashantkumar, P.; Vidyasagar, G. M. Traditional Knowledge on Medicinal Plants Used for the Treatment of Skin Diseases in Bidar District, Karnataka. *Ind. J. Tradit. Know.* **2008,** *7*, 273–276.
Pushpalata, H.; Sauthan, J. R.; Pattanshetty, J. K.; Holla, B. V. Folk Medicine from Some Rural Areas of Bangalore District. *Aryavaidyan*, **1990,** *12*, 215–219.
Rajakumar, N.; Shivanna, M. B. Ethno-Medicinal Application of Plants in the Eastern Region of Shimoga District, Karnataka, India. *J. Ethnopharmacol.* **2010a,** *126*, 64–73.
Rajakumar, N.; Shivanna, M. B. Traditional Herbal Medicinal Knowledge in Sagar Taluk of Shimoga District, Karnataka, India. *Ind. J. Nat. Prod. Res.* **2010b,** *1*, 102–108.
Rajasab, A. H.; Isaq, M. Documentation of Folk Knowledge on Edible Wild Plants of North Karnataka. *Ind. J. Tradit. Know.* **2004,** *3*, 419–429.
Ramana, P.; Patil, S. K.; Sankri, G. Floristic Diversity of Magadi Wetland Area in Gadag District, Karnataka. Proceedings of Taal **2007,** The 12th World Lake Conference, 2008; pp 424−429.
Ramesh, B. R.; Pascal, J. P. *Atlas of Endemics of the Western Ghats (India): Distribution of the Tree Species in Evergreen and Semi-Evergreen Forests*; Institut Françaiss de Pondichéry, 1997; p. 403.
Rao, R. R. Floristic Diversity in Western Ghats. *Sahyadri E-News*, **2012,** *38*, 2−38.
Rao, R. R.; Razi, B. A. *A synoptic Flora of Mysore District: With an Appendix of Unani, Ayurvedic, and Trade Names of Drugs*; Today and Tomorrow's Printers and Publishers: New Delhi. 1981.
Rates, S. M. K. Plants as Source of Drugs. *Toxicon.* **2001,** *39*, 603–613.
Roy, S.; Hegde, H. V.; Bhattacharya, D.; Upadhya, V.; Kholkute, S. D. Tribes in Karnataka: Status of Health Research. *Ind. J. Med. Res.* **2015,** *141*, 673–687.
Savithramma, N.; Sulochana, C.; Rao, K. N. Ethnobotanical Survey of Plants Used to Treat Asthma in Andhra Pradesh, India. *J. Ethnopharmacol.* **2007,** *113*, 54–61.
Shantamma, C.; Sudarshana, M. S.; Rachaih. *Flaveria trinervosa*—a New Herb to Cure Jaundice. *Ancient Sci. Life.* **1986,** *6*, 109–111.
Shiddamallayya, N.; Azra, Y.; Gopakumar, K. Hundred Common Forest Medicinal Plants of Karnataka in Primary Healthcare. *Ind. J. Trad. Know.* **2010b,** *9*, 90−95.
Shiddamallayya, N.; Azra, Y.; Gopakumar, K. Medico–Botanical Survey of Kumar Parvatha Kukke Subramanya, Mangalore, Karnataka. *Ind. J. Trad. Know.* **2010a,** *9*, 96–99.
Shivanna, M. B.; Rajakumar, N. Ethno-Medico-Botanical Knowledge of Rural Fold in Bhadravathi Taluk of Shimoga District, Karnataka. *Ind. J. Trad. Know.* **2010,** *9*, 158–162.
Sivakamasundari; Karuppusamy, S.; Parthipan, R. Survey on the RET-listed Medicinal Plants in Thadagamalai Range of Kanyakumari District, Tamil Nadu. *J. Biodiv. Endang. Spe.* **2015,** *3*, 151.

Sivaperumal, R.; Ramya, S.; Veera Ravi, A.; Rajasekaran, C.; Jayakumararaj, R. Ethnopharmacological Studies on the Medicinal Plants Used by Tribal Inhabitants of Kottur hills, Dharmapuri, Tamilnadu, India. Environ. *We Int. J. Sci. Tech.* **2010,** 5, 57–64.

Srinivas, V.; Manjunatha, B. R.; Anjaneya, S. Traditional Knowledge on Medicinal Plants of Tribals Residing in Heggadadevanakote and Hunsur Taluks of Mysore District, Karnataka, India. *Int. J. Agri. Sci.* **2019,** *11*, 7966–7970.

Subbaiyan, B.; Samydurai, P.; Karthik P. M.; Ramakrishnan, R.; Thangapandian, V. Inventory of Rare, Endangered and Threatened (RET) Plant Species in Maruthamalai Hills, Western Ghats of Tamilnadu, South India. *Our Nat.* **2014,** *12*, 37–43.

Subitha, K.; Ayyanar, T.; Udayakumar, M.; Sekar, T. Ethnomedicinal Plants Used by Kani Tribals in Pechiparai Forests of Southern Western Ghats, Tamil Nadu, India. *Int. Res. J. Plant Sci.* **2011,** *2* (12), 349–354.

Sudeesh, S. Ethnomedicinal Plants Used by Malayaraya Tribes of Vannapuram Village in Idukki, Kerala, India. *J. Sci. Res. Tech.* **2012,** *1*, 7–11.

Sushma, K. S.; Jayashankar, M.; Ali, S. M. Traditional Ayurvedic Practices of Ethnobotanical Plants by Tribal Communities of BR Hills, Karnataka. *Progr. Agricul.* **2019,** *19*, 1–13.

Upadhya, V.; Hegde, H. V.; Bhat, S.; Hurkadale, P. J.; Kholkute, S. D.; Hegde, G. R. Ethno-Medicinal Plants Used to Treat Bone Fracture from North- Central Western Ghats of India. *J Ethnopharmacol.* **2012,** *142*, 557–562.

Upadhyay, B.; Parveen; Dhaker, A. K.; Kumar, A. Ethnomedicinal and Ethnopharmaco-Statistical Studies of Eastern Rajasthan, India. *J. Ethnopharmacol.* **2010,** *129*, 64–86.

Vidyasagar, G. M.; Prashantkumar, P. Traditional Herbal Remedies for Gynecological Disorders in Women of Bidar District, Karnataka, India. *Fitoterapia.* **2007,** *78*, 48–51.

Vijayan, A.; Liju, V. B.; John, J. V. R.; Parthipan, B.; Renuka, C. Traditional Remedies of *Kani* Tribes of Kottoor Reserve Forest, Agasthyavanam, Thiruvananthapuram, Kerala. *Ind. J. Tradit. Knowl.* **2007,** *6*, 589–594.

Viswanathan, M. B.; Premkumar, E. H.; Ramesh, N. Ethnomedicines of Kanis in Kalakad Mundanthurai Tiger Reserve, Tamil Nadu. *Ethnobot.* **2001,** *13*, 60–66.

Xavier, T. F.; Kannan, M.; Lija, L.; Auxillia, A.; Rose, A. K. F.; Kumar, S. S. Ethnobotanical Study of Kani Tribes in Thoduhills of Kerala, South India. *J. Ethnopharmocol.* **2014,** *152*, 78–90.

Yoganarasimhan, S. N.; Togunashi, V. S.; Murthy, K. R. K.; Govindaiah. Medicobotany of Tumkur District, Karnataka. *J. Econ. Taxon. Bot.* **1982,** *3*, 391–406.

CHAPTER 5

Ethnomedicinal Flora in Sacred Groves of Jhargram of West Bengal, India

UDAY KUMAR SEN and RAM KUMAR BHAKAT

Ecology and Taxonomy Laboratory, Department of Botany and Forestry, Vidyasagar University, Midnapore, West Bengal, India

ABSTRACT

From ancient times application of plant species in indigenous medicine is well documented worldwide. The present study encompasses the traditional heritage of therapeutic uses of plant species in sacred groves of South West Bengal in India. A total of 146 plant species of 44 families were studied through interviews, questionnaires, and group discussion. Members of the family Fabaceae were leading among the plant species used for medicinal purposes (17.1%). Use of plant species among the 23 diseases, digestive disorders stand first (20.3%). Use of decoction is the principal mode of administration to cure the disease (38.3%). The informant consensus factor (Fic) was highest for liver disorders (0.98). The highest number of plant species are employed against digestive diseases, while it is the lowest for an insect bite. The highest-fidelity value (FL) was found for *Aegle marmelos* and *Azadirachta indica*, while it was the lowest for *Eucalyptus tereticornis*. This study has identified and documented traditional uses of medicinal plant species used in indigenous medicine or drugs. Some of the medicinal plant species are dwindling owing to overexploitation as well as injudicious utilization.

Ethnic Knowledge and Perspectives of Medicinal Plants, Volume 1: Curative Properties and Treatment Strategies. Munir Ozturk, Kandikere R. Sridhar, Maryam Sarwat, Volkan Altay, & Francisco Martín Huerta-Martínez (Eds.)

5.1 INTRODUCTION

Sacred groves are virgin forests that vary in plant species those are shielded by the ethnic communities for centuries as their cultural heritage, spiritual rituals, and taboos are protected by the local villagers (Merritt, 2010). Every grove has its folklore, mythology, and myths that are an important component of its culture. In terms of biodiversity, history, religious, and ethnic heritage, an inextricable link between modern society and the past persists in sacred groves (Thorley and Gunn, 2008). Sacred groves can be found all around the world, and different cultures recognize them in different ways, encoding different norms for their maintenance (Berkes et al., 2000). Many portions of India, including the Western Ghats, Central India, Northeast India, and other regions, have sacred groves, particularly where indigenous tribes live. These are recognized by distinct names given by the ethnic people to them. It acts as a model center for the conservation of biodiversity (Sharma and Kumar, 2020). Certain plants that are endangered in the forest are still well-conserved in some of the sacred groves. It has been noted that the sacred groves abound with many medicinal plant species that are not found in the forests (Doffana, 2017). Further, uncommon, vulnerable, endangered, and endemic species are sometimes clustered in these groves. Sacredness, religious activities, and taboos all have a role in promoting sustainable flora use and care (Mgaya, 2020). However, significant changes have taken place in the extent of the sacred groves in the recent past in composition with their vegetation, perception of people, religious beliefs, and taboos (Kossi et al., 2021). To evaluate the ecological position and formulate strategies for sacred grove protection, a comprehensive understanding of the current state, structure, and function are important (Adom et al., 2019).

In the rural location, sacred groves are treasure houses characteristic of the Jhargram district for flora and fauna. Because of the locals' faith and respect, they have been left alone. They believe that cutting down plant species, plucking flowers or fruits, or harassing or killing animals in sacred groves will insult the forest spirit or deities in question. There are religious beliefs and reverence for sacred groves among the villagers and tribals of Jhargram district. Different flora components are meant to be under the protection of the forest grove's local deity, as Indians are accustomed to dedicating forest pockets to different deities. These committed activities have led to plant species and forest products being protected and preserved. In sacred groves, the well-maintained vegetation is different from the surrounding areas. The conclusion of vegetation rich in plant species, herbs, shrubs, and climbers, including various birds and wild animals, is promoted by well-preserved sacred groves. In such groves, ecosystem components and their entirety play a significant role in conserving as well as providing ecosystem services. Sacred groves serve as critical safeguarding of plant species that are rare or endangered elsewhere. They display optimal vegetation growth that is important to the local terrain and climatic conditions. In addition to the lofty and majestic plant species, sacred groves are also associated with many uncommon and endemic species, they serve as a value-added source of medicinal plants (Mandal and Sarkar, 2013).

Despite their illiteracy, village inhabitants knew that destroying nearby forest regions invites disaster, scarcity of drinking water, fodder and fuel-wood, and wild edible and medicinal plants. If a man wants to chop plant species from the reserve forests in general, and groves in particular, tribes will fight back vehemently (Immanuel et al., 2018). In Jhargram district, the tribal such as *Kora*, *Munda*, *Sabar,* and *Santal* usually reside in remote, inaccessible areas. Poor economic situations, hygienic conditions, and malnutrition, as well as a lack of modern healthcare facilities, are also sources of concern for these tribal people. Residents and animals are completely reliant on "traditional barefoot doctors" and their time-tested treatments. They consider various illnesses to be God's punishment for their wrongdoings. A traditional tribal medicine man checks the patient and advises them on good behavior, offering to their God, and prescribing the same plant-based treatments (Kumar, 2011). Sacred groves nearby contain a variety of therapeutic plants that are rarely seen outside. The efficacy of these plants will be determined through botanical and pharmacological research. Systematic study and protection of sacred groves have become crucial for these reasons, as well as for the preservation of the natural ecosystem (Bodeker, 1995). The terrain, edaphic, and climatic variables of Jhargram district encourage lush plant growth, resulting in the formation of dense vegetation patches. Even now, because the area under cultivation is sparse and the majority of people believe in deities, the number of sacred groves in this zone is higher than in the rest of South West Bengal.

Because medicinally essential plant species are not found growing in a single location or a single season, the current inquiry focused on following the ethno-medico-botanical perspective on the sacred groves that are well kept by the local people. The research of sacred groves in the Jhargram district concerning the aforesaid element is relatively limited. There is more room for documenting medicinally essential plant species, as well as their use and research. Given documentation and the addition of new scientific information, the current study is envisaged. Briefly, this survey reviews the studies on sacred grove vegetation throughout the Jhargram district, in situ conservation of medicinal plant species and highlights the community empowerment with an intention of preservation and conservation of sacred groves.

5.2 STUDY AREA

Jhargram is the 22nd district of West Bengal in India (22.45°N, 86.98°E; 81 m asl) (Figure 5.1). It has a total area of 3038 km^2 and a population of about 1.14 million (2011 census). The rural population is about 96.5% and the urban population is about 3.5%. The population of scheduled caste is about 20.1% and scheduled tribe is about 29.4% (Anon, 2011). Jhargram is famous for its wooded beauty and topography culminating in the hilly ranges to the north and River Subarnarekha to the south. The climatic conditions are similar to most of the Bengal-like hot and humid. It is one of the popular destinations for those who venture to study forest ecosystems.

5.3 QUANTITATIVE ETHNOBOTANY

5.3.1 *FIDELITY LEVEL (FL)*

As several plant species could be considered to treat a single condition, we identified the most commonly used species for each ailment by FL (Friedman et al., 1986):

$$FL=Np/N$$

Where, Np is the number of use reports noted for a specific condition for a given species, while N is the overall number of use reports cited for that species.

High FL value (100%) is found for plant species for which practically all usage reports pertain to the same method, but low FL value obtained for plant species utilized for various purposes.

5.3.2 *INFORMANT CONSENSUS FACTOR*

The informant consensus factor (Fic) value has been considered to analyze the level of agreement between plant applications for distinct disease groups

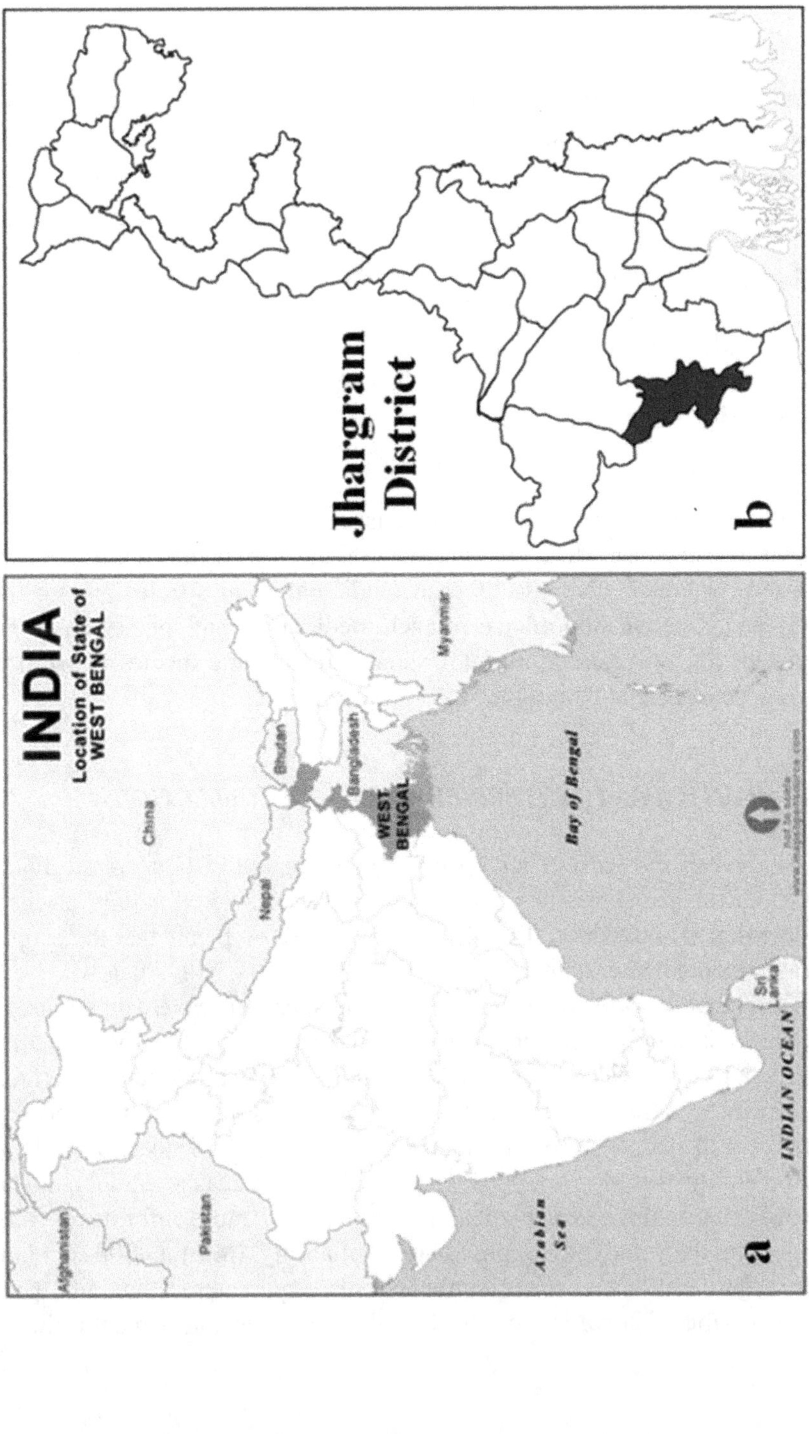

FIGURE 5.1 Location of West Bengal in India (**a**) and Jhargram district in West Bengal (**b**).

and study region respondents. It is calculated by the formula proposed by Phillips et al. (1994) and Muhammad et al. (2019):

$$Fic = Nur - Nt/(Nur - 1)$$

Where, Nur is the number of use citations of a certain disease group, while Nt is the total number of plant species utilized by all respondents for a specific use group.

5.3.3 USE-VALUE (UV) FOR SINGLE SPECIES

The UV index proposed by Phillips and Gentry (Phillips et al., 1994) has been adapted by Albuquerque et al. (2008) to estimate the citation of plant species during interviews:

$$UVc = \sum U\ is/ns$$

Where, U is the total number of usage citations made by all the informants for a specific species, while the *ns* is the total number of informants.

Based on the relative use of each medicinal plant species among the informants, Relative Importance of each medicinal plant species has been calculated. This indicator is useful for analyzing a single species' utilization and comparing plants within the same sample.

5.3.4 PARTICIPANTS, INTERVIEW, AND DATA COLLECTION

This study was carried out for up to 4 years (March 2017 to April 2021) throughout the year's seasons. Participants were considered mainly on their ethnomedicinal knowledge. The discussion focused on plants that the people used as ethnomedicine. With the help of the village elders, individuals who were identified locally as knowledgeable about plant species use were determined.

The questionnaire selection was reported as being done methodically and using the method of Participatory Rural Appraisal. A semistructured questionnaire with open and closed-ended questions was used to interview a total of 120 people. The questionnaire consisted of 18 questions, all of which were answered in the local Bengali dialect. Because ethnobotanical knowledge is complicated, plants cited by three or more informants were included in this study to improve data reliability (Martin, 2004). Plant species, their families, voucher numbers of plant specimen, habits, life span, nativity, period of flowering and fruiting, IUCN status, part/s plant utilized, route of administration, diseases treated, total citation, and ethnobotanical indices are all noted in a data sheet. After learning about the medicinal plants' unique uses, informants were taken out into the field to identify the plants using local (vernacular) names. For the voucher sheet preparation, plant photograph, habit, and reproductive components were considered, and the common plants were gathered. The herbarium receives the voucher sheet (Department of Botany, Vidyasagar University, Midnapore, West Bengal). Plant species that are rare or endangered were left alone. Plants were collected, compared with the literature, and recognized using conventional keys to the specimens (Prain, 1903; Haines, 1921–1925; Bennet, 1979; Pakrashi and Mukhopadhya, 2004). Scientific names of every plant's name were examined using www.wcvp.science.kew.org website and confirmed only accepted names (WCVP, 2021).

5.4 DISCUSSION

5.4.1 DEMOGRAPHIC FEATURES

Up to a total of 120 people were interviewed, including 51 men and 69 women ranging in age group from 30 to 80 years (the mean age was about 50 years). The age group of 51–60 was the most well-represented (up to 35%). In terms of ethnomedicinal knowledge, this age group was the most important. Traditional healers, herbalists, and knowledgeable villagers were questioned to obtain a wide range of information on the medicinal plants. Owing to seasonal visits for accessibility of plant species, several of the informants were questioned many times; 600 interviews were conducted with a total of 120 informants for up to 146 medicinal plant species. The interviews revealed that the elderly are particularly capable and have a far greater understanding of native plants than the younger ones. Younger people in the Jhargram district, on the other hand, tended to migrate to urban areas in search of work and were less involved in traditional medicine. Our findings were consistent with prior reports from other parts of India, where the indigenous knowledge on use of medicinal plants is still prevalent among the elderly (Kala et al., 2006; Upadhyay et al., 2007). The amount of education of the interviewed respondents was negatively associated with their knowledge of medicinal plants: illiterates (7.5%), primary education (50.8%), secondary education (20%), and University education (7.5%) (Table 5.1). This is consistent with earlier ethnobotanical studies on the usage of therapeutic plants in the Jhargram district (Chaudhury et al., 2017; Sen and Bhakat, 2018, 2020,

2021). Medicinal plant knowledge had mostly been passed down orally from generation to generation. The majority of interviewees learned traditional medical knowledge from family members, primarily from their parents and grandparents; however, such folk knowledge is not well documented. Quick strides with the informants were made throughout the study region to identify and gather the precise plant samples used for treatments. Wherever possible, photographs of medicinal plant species were acquired during field visits were exhibited to the informants. A short excursions with the informants in the study region also enabled the collection of the exact plant species used for a given condition (Albuquerque et al., 2008).

TABLE 5.1 Demographic Characteristics of Informants Helped to Follow the Ethnic Knowledge on Medicinal Value of Plant Species in Forests of Jhargram District.

	Categories	Number of the informants	Per cent
Sex	Male	51	42.5
	Female	69	57.5
Profession	Government employee	3	2.5
	Teacher	5	4.2
	Farming/Fishing	30	25.0
	Housewife	29	24.2
	Unemployed	14	11.7
	Professional herbalist	39	32.5
Age	≥30	3	2.5
	31–40	17	14.2
	41–50	33	27.5
	51–60	42	35.0
	≥61	25	20.8
Education	Illiterate	9	7.5
	Primary	61	50.83
	Secondary	24	20.00
	Higher secondary	17	14.17
	University/technical degree	9	7.50

5.4.2 FLORISTIC ANALYSIS OF MEDICINAL PLANT SPECIES

The sacred groves yielded a total of 146 plant species (116 taxa in 44 families) in this study. Species-by-species, the plants were arranged in alphabetical order. Each species was given information such as its name, voucher specimen, nativity, seasonal occurrence, IUCN Red List Status, used part/s, method of administration, disease treated with citation, and ethnobotanical indicators like FL and UV (Table 5.2).

The nine well-represented families in terms of species (≥5 species) quantity were the Fabaceae 25 (17.1%), Moraceae 11 (7.5%), Lamiaceae 7 (4.8%), Malvaceae 7 (4.8%), Rubiaceae 7 (4.8%), Combretaceae 6 (4.1%), Ebenaceae 5 (3.4%), Meliaceae 5 (3.4%), and Annonaceae 5 (3.4%) (Fig. 5.2a). Anacardiaceae, Apocynaceae, Bignoniaceae, Euphorbiaceae, Myrtaceae, Phyllanthaceae, and Sapindaceae contained four species each. Three families Arecaceae, Rutaceae, and Sapotaceae contained three species, whereas Boraginaceae, Burseraceae, Dilleniaceae, Lecythidaceae, Lythraceae, and Salicaceae held only two species. Another 19 families each carried only a single species. In India's sacred groves, Ray and Ray (2020) discovered the same type of dominant families.

The eleven prominent plant families consist of over 57% genera with falling numbers (≥4 species) belongs to the Fabaceae 22 (19%), Rubiaceae 7 (6%), and Malvaceae 6 (5.2%). The remaining families like Anacardiaceae, Annonaceae, Apocynaceae, Bignoniaceae, Lamiaceae, Meliaceae, Phyllanthaceae, and Sapindaceae carried only four species each. Such a type of dominance of plant families in ethnomedicine in the sacred grove was observed by Sen and Bhakat (2020). The 11 well-represented genera were *Ficus* (8 species), *Terminalia* (6 species), *Diospyros*, and *Premna* (3 species each), and *Albizia, Annona, Artocarpus, Bauhinia, Mallotus, Swietenia,* and *Vitex* (2 species each). In the other 82 genera, there were only one species. The existence of such rich traditional medicinal knowledge was primarily determined by cultural diversity and rich folklore (Tynsong et al., 2020).

More commonly utilized plant species in traditional medicine are due to their accessible availability, as well as their medicinal and healing potential due to a large spectrum of bioactive chemicals (Singh et al., 2020). There were 119 native species (81.5%) and 27 exotic species (18.5%) in total.

5.4.3 THE IUCN CATEGORIES

Sixty-four plant species are currently classified as not evaluated (NE) out of a total of 146. There were seventy-one species that were least concerned (LC), four that were vulnerable (VU), four that were near threatened (NT), one that was endangered (EN), and two that were data deficient (DD) (Figure 5.2b). According to the above community analysis and the ecological data regarding IUCN red listed species, it was discovered that the plants were still extant

TABLE 5.2 Database of Dominant Medicinal Trees with Part (s) Used, Mode of Administration, Ailments Treated, Fidelity Value and Use Value.

	Voucher number	Nativity	Seasonal availability	IUCN t Status	Plant part/s used	Mode of administration	Ailment treated with citation in parenthesis	Fidelity level (FL)	Use value (UV)
Acacia auriculiformis A.Cunn. ex Benth./Fabaceae	UKFA1	E	Feb.–Oct.	LC	Ro, Sb	Decoction	Astringent (12), Digestive disorder (20)	28.57	0.27
Adenanthera pavonina L./Fabaceae	UKFA2	N	Mar.–Jan.	LC	Le,Sb,Se	Decoction	Rheumatic disorder (12)	40.00	0.10
Adina cordifolia (Roxb.) Brandis/ Rubiaceae.	UKRB1	N	Jun.–Dec.	NE	Ro,Sb	Decoction	Digestive disorder (14), Febrifuge (9), Worm infection (22)	50.00	0.38
Aegle marmelos (L.) Corrêa/Rutaceae	UKRT1	N	May-Jul.	NT	Fr,Le	Raw	Digestive disorder (120), Respiratory disorder (50), Sexual disease (71)	100.00	2.01
Ailanthus excelsa Roxb./ Simaroubaceae	UKSI1	N	Jan.–Jun.	NE	Gu,Le,Sb	Paste	Child birth (8), Digestive disorder (14), Febrifuge (11), Respiratory disorder (9)	36.84	0.35
Alangium salviifolium (L.f.) Wangerin/Cornaceae	UKCR1	N	Mar.–Jul.	LC	Fr,Le,Rb, Sb,Se	Paste	Liver disorder (22), Rheumatism (14), Sexual disease (11), Wound healing (32)	61.54	0.66
Albizia odoratissima (L.f.) Benth./ Fabaceae	UKFA3	N	Apr.–Mar.	LC	Sb	Decoction	Rheumatism (13)	31.71	0.11
Albizia lebbeck (L.) Benth./Fabaceae	UKFA4	N	Mar.–Feb.	LC	Sb,Se	Powder	Respiratory disorder (11), Skin disease (23)	37.10	0.28
Alstonia scholaris (L.) R. Br./ Apocynaceae	UKAP1	N	Nov.–Aug.	LC	La,Le,Ro,Sb	Infusion	Astringent (14), Digestive disorder (22), Skin disease (32), Snake bite (8)	76.19	0.63
Anacardium occidentale L./ Anacardiaceae	UKAA1	E	Mar.–Jun.	NE	Fr,Le,Rb,Sb	Infusion	Dental problem (14), Digestive disorder (22), Skin disorder (21)	51.16	0.48
Annona reticulata L./Annonaceae	UKAN1	E	Jul.–Dec.	LC	Fr,Le,Sb	Paste	Digestive disorder (14), Febrifuge (16), Liver disorder (11), Worm infection (23)	56.10	0.53

TABLE 5.2 (*Continued*)

	Voucher number	Nativity	Seasonal availability	IUCN t Status	Plant part/s used	Mode of administration	Ailment treated with citation in parenthesis	Fidelity level (FL)	Use value (UV)
Annona squamosa L./Annonaceae	UKAN2	E	Mar.–Sep.	LC	Fr,Le,Ro,Se	Infusion	Astringent (22), Dental problems (18), Respiratory disorder (16), Rheumatic disorder (9)	68.75	0.54
Antidesma acidum Retz./ Phyllanthaceae	UKPH1	N	Jun.–Dec.	LC	Fr,Le,Ro	Juice	Digestive disorder (32), Insect bite (11)	55.17	0.36
Aphanamixis polystachya (Wall.) R.Parker/Meliaceae	UKME1	N	Mar.–Nov.	LC	Fr,Le,Sb	Raw	Astringent (9), Liver disorder (21), Metabolic disorder (28), Rheumatic disorder (9)	71.79	0.56
Artocarpus lacucha Buch.-Ham./ Moraceae	UKMO1	N	Feb.–Sep.	NE	Fl,Fr,Sb,Se	Vegetable	Astringent (11), Wound healing (22)	36.07	0.28
Artocarpus heterophyllus Lam./ Moraceae	UKMO2	N	Jan.–Aug.	NE	Fr,La,Le, Ro,Se	Pulp	Analgesic (24), Sexual disease (8), Skin disease (4)	64.86	0.30
Averrhoa carambola L./ Oxalidaceae	UKOX1	N	Feb.–Sep.	NE	Fl,Fr,Le,Se	Raw	Diabetes (25), Liver disorder (21), Respiratory disorder (20), Skin disease (11)	56.82	0.64
Azadirachta indica A.Juss./Meliaceae	UKME2	N	Mar.–Jul.	LC	Fr,Le,Sb, Se,St	Juice	Diabetes (72), Metabolic disorder (63), Skin disease (120), Wound healing (92)	100.00	2.89
Bambusa bambos (L.) Voss/Poaceae	UKPO1	N		NE	Le,Ro	Juice	Astringent (8), Immune system disorder/buster (11), Worm infection (14)	28.00	0.28
Barringtonia acutangula (L.) Gaertn./ Lecythidaceae	UKLE1	N	Jan.–Apr.	LC	Fr,Le,Sb,Se	Decoction	Digestive disorder (22), Menstrual disorder (11), Restorative (9)	53.66	0.35

TABLE 5.2 (*Continued*)

	Voucher number	Nativity	Seasonal availability	IUCN t Status	Plant part/s used	Mode of administration	Ailment treated with citation in parenthesis	Fidelity level (FL)	Use value (UV)
Bauhinia purpurea L./Fabaceae	UKFA5	N	Sep.–Mar.	LC	Fl,Le,Ro,Sb	Raw	Digestive disorder (18), Skin disease (14)	29.51	0.27
Bauhinia variegata L./Fabaceae	UKFA6	N	Feb.–Jun.	LC	Fl,Ro,Sb	Paste	Metabolic disorder (14), Skin disease (13), Snake bite (9), Worm infection (10)	29.17	0.38
Bixa orellana L./Bixaceae	UKBX1	E	Feb.–Jun.	LC	Fl,Gu,Le	Decoction	Digestive disorder (58), Metabolic disorder (72), Skin 24.disease (48)	80.00	1.48
Bombax ceiba L./Malvaceae	UKMA1	N	Jan.–May.	LC	Fl,Gu,Le, Ro,Sb	Decoction	Astringent (8), Digestive disorder (17), Menstrual disorder (32), Neurological disorder (28)	40.00	0.71
Borassus flabellifer L./Arecaceae	UKAR1	E	Mar.–Oct.	NE	Fr,Ro	Sap	Immune system disorder/buster (11), Liver disorder (48), Urinary disorder (45)	53.33	0.87
Boswellia serrata Roxb./Burseraceae	UKBU1	N	Dec.–Jun.	NE	Gu,Se	Paste	Liver disorder (38), Respiratory disorder (33), Rheumatic disorder (18)	50.00	0.74
Bridelia retusa (L.) A.Juss./ Phyllanthaceae	UKPH2	N	Mar.–Dec.	LC	Fr,Sb	Pulp	Analgesic (14), Astringent (22)	43.14	0.30
Careya arborea Roxb./Lecythidaceae	UKLE2	N	Jan.–Apr.	NE	Fr,Le,Sb,Se	Juice	Astringent (18), Respiratory disorder (22)	35.48	0.33
Cascabela thevetia (L.) Lippold/ Apocynaceae	UKAP2	E	All	LC	Fr,Gu,La,Le, Sb,Se	Decoction	Antitumor (11), Dental problems (8), Rheumatic disorder (12), Snake bite (17)	41.46	0.40
Casearia tomentosa Roxb./Salicaceae	UKSL1	N	Jan.–Mar.	NE	La,Le,St	Raw	Diabetes (14), Snake bite (8), Urinary disorder (28)	50.91	0.42

TABLE 5.2 (*Continued*)

	Voucher number	Nativity	Seasonal availability	IUCN t Status	Plant part/s used	Mode of administration	Ailment treated with citation in parenthesis	Fidelity level (FL)	Use value (UV)
Cassia fistula L./Fabaceae	UKFA7	N	Feb.–Dec.	LC	Fr,Se	Infusion	Antitumor (17), Immune system disorder/buster (14), Rheumatic disorder (32)	51.61	0.53
Casuarina equisetifolia L./ Casuarinaceae	UKCS1	N	Apr.–Oct.	LC	Ro,Sb	Decoction	Digestive disorder (11), Skin disease (21)	30.00	0.27
Catunaregam spinosa (Thunb.) Tirveng./Rubiaceae	UKRB2	N	Apr.–Oct.	NE	Fr,Ro,Sb	Juice	Analgesic (16), Digestive disorder (32), Febrifuge (28), Neurological disorder (34)	65.38	0.92
Ceiba pentandra (L.) Gaertn./ Malvaceae	UKMA2	E	Apr.–Sep.	LC	Fl,Fr,Gu,Ro, Sb,Se	Decoction	Astringent (9), Digestive disorder (8), Respiratory disorder (7), Skin disease (11), Wound healing (17)	34.69	0.43
Citrus maxima (Burm.) Merr./ Rutaceae	UKRT2	N	Feb.–Apr.	LC	Fr,Le	Raw	Digestive disorder (92), Respiratory disorder (82)	90.20	1.45
Cleistanthus collinus (Roxb.) Benth. ex Hook.f./Phyllanthaceae	UKPH3	N	Apr.–Sep.	VU	Fr,Le,Ro,Sb	Juice	Metabolic disorder (81), Urinary disorder (78)	88.04	1.33
Cocos nucifera L./Arecaceae	UKAR2	N	Apr.–Mar.	NE	Fr	Raw	Analgesic (44), Child birth (11), Digestive disorder (102), Respiratory disorder (48), Restorative (11)	85.00	1.80
Cordia dichotoma G.Forst./ Boraginaceae	UKBO1	N	Feb.–Apr.	LC	Fr,Le,Sb,Se	Decoction	Antitumor (9), Digestive disorder (11), Skin disease (14)	43.75	0.28
Crateva magna (Lour.) DC./ Capparaceae	UKCP1	E	Mar.–Jul.	NE	Le,Ro,Sb	Decoction	Digestive disorder (17), Metabolic disorder (16), Sexual disease (21)	41.18	0.45
Croton caudatus Geiseler/ Euphorbiaceae	UKEU1	N	Apr.– Jun.	NE	Fr,Ro,Se	Powder	Antitumor (9), Dental problems (13), Skin disease (18)	56.25	0.33

TABLE 5.2 (*Continued*)

	Voucher number	Nativity	Seasonal availability	IUCN t Status	Plant part/s used	Mode of administration	Ailment treated with citation in parenthesis	Fidelity level (FL)	Use value (UV)
Dalbergia sissoo Roxb. ex DC./ Fabaceae	UKFA8	N	Feb.–Aug.	LC	Le,Ro,Sb,St	Decoction	Digestive disorder (11), Liver disorder (14), Worm infection (32)	53.33	0.48
Delonix regia (Bojer ex Hook.) Raf./ Fabaceae	UKFA9	N	Apr.–Jun.	LC	Fl,Le,Sb,Se	Powder	Analgesic (8), Digestive disorder (14), Liver disorder (18), Rheumatic disorder (17)	27.69	0.48
Dillenia indica L./Dilleniaceae	UKDL1	N	Jun.– Dec.	LC	Fl,Fr,Le	Raw	Astringent (11), Digestive disorder (18), Respiratory disorder (14)	37.50	0.36
Dillenia pentagyna Roxb./ Dilleniaceae	UKDL2	N	Apr.–Nov.	NE	Fl,Fr,Le	Raw	Astringent (11), Digestive disorder (20), Respiratory disorder (13)	62.50	0.37
Dimocarpus longan Lour./ Sapindaceae	UKSP1	N	Apr.–Jul.	NT	Fr,Le,Rl,Sb	Decoction	Neurological disorder (18), Snake bite (4)	31.03	0.18
Diospyros malabarica (Desr.) Kostel./ Ebenaceae	UKEB1	N	Mar–Jun.	NE	Fl,Fr,Le,Sb	Juice	Antitumor (11), Astringent (12), Digestive disorder (44), Worm infection (52), Wound healing (32)	65.00	1.26
Diospyros melanoxylon var. *tupru* (Buch.-Ham.) V.Singh/Ebenaceae	UKEB2	N	Apr.–Jul.	NE	Fl,Fr,Sb,Se	Raw	Digestive disorder (46), Immune system disorder/buster (21), Neurological disorder (16), Urinary disorder (18)	65.71	0.84
Diospyros melanoxylon Roxb./ Ebenaceae	UKEB3	N	Apr.–Jul.	NE	Fr,Sb	Raw	Digestive disorder (39), Immune system disorder/buster (21), Neurological disorder (23), Urinary disorder (14)	75.00	0.81
Diospyros montana Roxb./Ebenaceae	UKEB4	N	Apr.–Jan.	NE	Fr,Sb	Paste	Restorative (11)	34.38	0.09
Diospyros sylvatica Roxb./Ebenaceae	UKEB5	N	May-Jun.	NE	Fr,Sb	Juice	Antitumor (9), Wound healing (17)	44.74	0.22

TABLE 5.2 (*Continued*)

	Voucher number	Nativity	Seasonal availability	IUCN t Status	Plant part/s used	Mode of administration	Ailment treated with citation in parenthesis	Fidelity level (FL)	Use value (UV)
Ehretia aspera Willd./Boraginaceae	UKBO2	N	Jan.–Apr.	NE	Fr,Sb	Juice	Digestive disorder (32)	61.54	0.27
Elaeodendron glaucum (Rottb.) Pers./ Celastraceae	UKCE1	N	Feb.–Aug.	DD	Gu,Le,Rb,Sb	Infusion	Menstrual disorder (15), Neurological disorder (17), Snake bite (11)	35.42	0.36
Erythrina variegata L./Fabaceae	UKFA10	E	Feb.–Jul.	LC	Le,Sb,Se	Decoction	Metabolic disorder (21), Neurological disorder (17), Respiratory disorder (18), Snake bite (9)	47.73	0.54
Eucalyptus tereticornis Sm./ Myrtaceae	UKMY1	E	Mar.–May	LC	Gu,Le,Sb	Decoction	Astringent (8), Metabolic disorder (12)	17.65	0.17
Euphorbia antiquorum L./ Euphorbiaceae	UKEU2	E	Jan.–Apr.	NE	La,WP	Raw	Dental problems (11), Metabolic disorder (9), Neurological disorder (14), Rheumatic disorder (15)	46.88	0.41
Ficus rumphii Blume/Moraceae	UKMO3	N	May-Jun.	NE	Fr,La,Le,Ro, Sb,Se	Juice	Skin disease (12), Worm infection (17)	39.53	0.24
Ficus virens Aiton/Moraceae	UKMO4	N	Sep.–Mar.	LC	Fr,La,Le,Ro, Sb,Se	Decoction	Antitumor (9), Febrifuge (12)	28.57	0.18
Ficus benghalensis L./Moraceae	UKMO5	N	Mar.–Sep.	NE	Fr,La,Le,Ro, Sb,Se	Infusion	Dental problems (18), Digestive disorder (22), Metabolic disorder (35), Rheumatic disorder (26), Sexual disease (8)	67.31	0.91
Ficus grossularioides Burm.f./ Moraceae	UKMO6	E	Jul.–Nov.	LC	La,Le	Decoction	Insect bite (7), Metabolic disorder (14)	29.17	0.18
Ficus hispida L.f./Moraceae	UKMO7	E	Feb.–Jun.	LC	Le,Ro,Sb,Se	Juice	Immune system disorder/buster (18), Liver disorder (49), Menstrual disorder (21)	70.00	0.73

TABLE 5.2 (*Continued*)

	Voucher number	Nativity	Seasonal availability	IUCN t Status	Plant part/s used	Mode of administration	Ailment treated with citation in parenthesis	Fidelity level (FL)	Use value (UV)
Ficus mollis Vahl./Moraceae	UKMO8	N	May.–Jun.	NE	Fr,La,Le,Ro, Sb,Se	Paste	Skin disease (4), Wound healing (14)	34.15	0.15
Ficus racemosa L./Moraceae	UKMO9	N	Mar.–Aug.	LC	Fr,La,Le,Sb	Decoction	Febrifuge (11), Menstrual disorder (18), Neurological disorder (22), Sexual disease (14)	62.86	0.54
Ficus religiosa L./Moraceae	UKMO10	N	Jun.–Aug.	NE	Fr,La,Le,Ro, Sb,Se	Decoction	Antitumor (21), Diabetes (28), Metabolic disorder (33), Neurological disorder (28), Sexual disease (8), Skin disease (11)	73.33	1.08
Gardenia gummifera L.f./Rubiaceae	UKRB3	N	Mar.–Aug.	LC	Fl,Gu,La	Raw	Skin disease (22)	64.71	0.18
Gliricidia sepium (Jacq.) Steud./ Fabaceae	UKFA11	E	Feb.–May	LC	Wp	Raw	Neurological disorder (23), Skin disease (11), Wound healing (18)	44.23	0.43
Gmelina arborea Roxb. ex Sm./ Lamiaceae	UKLA1	N	Feb.–Jun.	LC	Fr,Le,Ro, Sb,St	Infusion	Antitumor (8), Digestive disorder (12), Sexual disease (7), Wound healing (9)	27.27	0.30
Grewia asiatica L./Malvaceae	UKMA3	N	Feb.–Jun.	LC	Fr,Le,Ro, Sb,St	Juice	Febrifuge (8), Sexual disease (14), Urinary disorder (22)	53.66	0.37
Guazuma ulmifolia Lam./Malvaceae	UKMA4	E	Jun.–Aug.	LC	Fr,Le,Sb	Pulp	Digestive disorder (11), Respiratory disorder (14), Sexual disease (11), Urinary disorder (22), Wound healing (9)	44.90	0.56
Holarrhena pubescens Wall. ex G.Don/Apocynaceae	UKAP3	N	Apr.–Feb.	LC	Le,Ro,Sb,Se	Juice	Antitumor (8), Digestive disorder (92), Metabolic disorder (75), Sexual disease (22)	76.67	1.64

TABLE 5.2 (*Continued*)

	Voucher number	Nativity	Seasonal availability	IUCN † Status	Plant part/s used	Mode of administration	Ailment treated with citation in parenthesis	Fidelity level (FL)	Use value (UV)
Holoptelea integrifolia (Roxb.) Planch./Ulmaceae	UKUL1	N	Jan.–Jun.	NE	Le,Sb	Pulp	Diabetes (8), Digestive disorder (12), Menstrual disorder (13), Rheumatic disorder (22), Worm infection (21), Wound healing (18)	31.43	0.78
Huberantha cerasoides (Roxb.) Chaowasku/Annonaceae	UKAN3	N	Mar.–Aug.	NE	Ro,Sb	Infusion	Worm infection (14)	45.16	0.12
Lagerstroemia parviflora Roxb./ Lythraceae	UKLY1	N	Apr.–Jan.	NE	Fr,Le,Ro, Sb,Se	Boiled	Antitumor (11), Diabetes (9), Febrifuge (8), Immune system disorder/buster (7)	61.11	0.29
Lagerstroemia speciosa (L.) Pers./ Lythraceae	UKLY2	N	Feb.–Oct.	NE	Fr,Le,Ro, Sb,Se	Boiled	Antitumor (11), Diabetes (14), Febrifuge (9), Metabolic disorder (18), Urinary disorder (8)	41.86	0.50
Lannea coromandelica (Houtt.) Merr./ Anacardiaceae	UKAA2	N	Feb.–Jun.	NE	Fr,Sb	Powder	Antitumor (10), Metabolic disorder (22), Wound healing (9)	38.60	0.34
Lepisanthes rubiginosa (Roxb.) Leenh./Sapindaceae	UKSP2	N	Jan.–Jun.	LC	Fr,Le,Ro, Se	Decoction	Febrifuge (8), Neurological disorder (14)	48.28	0.18
Leucaena leucocephala (Lam.) de Wit/Fabaceae	UKFA12	E	Aug.–Mar.	NE	Fr,Se	Decoction	Diabetes (11), Digestive disorder (22), Restorative (9), Sexual disease (4)	31.43	0.38
Limonia acidissima Groff/Rutaceae	UKRT3	N	Jan.–Dec.	NE	Fr,Se	Raw	Diabetes (32), Digestive disorder 38), Respiratory disorder (28)	55.88	0.82
Litsea glutinosa (Lour.) C.B.Rob./ Lauraceae	UKLA1	N	Apr.–Sep.	LC	Gu,La,Sb	Powder	Astringent (14), Digestive disorder (18), Rheumatic disorder (29)	67.44	0.51

TABLE 5.2 (*Continued*)

	Voucher number	Nativity	Seasonal availability	IUCN t Status	Plant part/s used	Mode of administration	Ailment treated with citation in parenthesis	Fidelity level (FL)	Use value (UV)
Madhuca longifolia var. *latifolia* (Roxb.) A.Chev./Sapotaceae	UKSA1	N	Mar.–Jul.	NE	Fl,Fr	Vegetable	Antitumor (9), Diabetes (8), Febrifuge (11), Liver disorder (42), Sexual disease (11), Skin disease (18), Worm infection (22), Wound healing (11)	45.65	1.10
Mallotus repandus (Rottler) Müll. Arg./Euphorbiaceae	UKEU3	N	Nov.–Apr.	NE	Fr,Rb,Sb	Decoction	Metabolic disorder (38), Rheumatic disorder (30)	63.33	0.57
Mallotus nudiflorus (L.) Kulju & Welzen/Euphorbiaceae	UKEU4	N	Nov.–Apr.	LC	Fr,Rb,Sb	Decoction	Metabolic disorder (30), Rheumatic disorder (32)	52.46	0.52
Mangifera indica L./Anacerdiaceae	UKAA3	N	Feb.– Jun.	DD	Fr,Le	Vegetable	Dental problems (32), Digestive disorder (38), Rheumatic disorder (28), Urinary disorder (31), Worm infection (18)	86.36	1.23
Manilkara zapota (L.) P.Royen/ Sapotaceae	UKSA2	E	Apr.–Mar.	NE	Fl,Fr,Le,Ro, Sb,Se	Decoction	Antitumor (9), Diabetes (18), Digestive disorder (32), Febrifuge (21), Urinary disorder (24)	65.31	0.87
Melia azedarach L./Meliaceae	UKME3	N	Feb.–Nov.	LC	Fr,Le,Sb	Boiled	Diabetes (42), Digestive disorder (40), Rheumatic disorder (32), Urinary disorder (30)	82.35	1.20
Miliusa velutina (DC.) Hook.f. & Thomson/Annonaceae	UKAN4	N	Apr.–Jul.	NE	Ro,Sb	Paste	Antitumor (11), Worm infection (22)	35.48	0.28
Mimusops elengi L./Sapotaceae	UKSA3	N	Apr.–Sep.	LC	Fr,Ro,Sb	Raw	Antitumor (8), Digestive disorder (32), Liver disorder (38), Metabolic disorder (28), Urinary disorder (30), Wound healing (21)	73.08	1.31

TABLE 5.2 (*Continued*)

	Voucher number	Nativity	Seasonal availability	IUCN ŧ Status	Plant part/s used	Mode of administration	Ailment treated with citation in parenthesis	Fidelity level (FL)	Use value (UV)
Mitragyna parvifolia (Roxb.) Korth./ Rubiaceae	UKRB4	N	May-Apr.	NE	Fr,Ro,Sb	Juice	Metabolic disorder (28), Respiratory disorder (22), Sexual disease (9)	38.89	0.49
Monoon longifolium (Sonn.) B.Xue & R.M.K.Saunders/Annonaceae	UKAN5	N	Mar.–Jul.	NE	Le,Sb	Powder	Antitumor (21)	23.33	0.18
Morinda citrifolia L./Rubiaceae	UKRB5	N	Feb.–May	NE	Fr,Le,Ro,Sb	Juice	Diabetes (14), Worm infection (29)	82.86	0.36
Moringa oleifera Lam./Moringaceae	UKMR1	N	Feb.–Apr.	LC	Fl,Fr,Le,Ro, Sb,Se	Vegetable	Antitumor (32), Diabetes (38), Urinary disorder (35)	90.48	0.88
Neolamarckia cadamba (Roxb.) Bosser/Rubiaceae	UKRB6	N	Jul.–Nov.	NE	Le,Sb	Decoction	Digestive disorder (44), Skin disease (11), Urinary disorder (29)	84.62	0.70
Nyctanthes arbor-tristis L./Oleaceae	UKOL1	N	Sep.–Jan.	NE	Fl,Le,Ro	Paste	Digestive disorder (72), Liver disorder (85), Respiratory disorder (30), Skin disease (14), Snake bite (11)	94.44	1.77
Oroxylum indicum (L.) Kurz/ Bignoniaceae	UKBI1	N	Jun.–Jul.	NE	Fl,Fr,Le,Ro, Sb,Se	Powder	Digestive disorder (22), Immune system disorder/buster (28), Liver disorder (21), Metabolic disorder (24)	40.58	0.79
Parkinsonia aculeata L./Fabaceae	UKFA13	E	Oct.–Jun.	LC	Fr,Le,Sb	Decoction	Febrifuge (12), Rheumatic disorder (22)	32.84	0.28
Peltophorum pterocarpum (DC.) Backer ex K.Heyne/Fabaceae	UKFA14	E	Mar.–Jan.	NE	Sb	Decoction	Digestive disorder (21), Skin disease (24)	33.80	0.38
Phoenix sylvestris (L.) Roxb./ Arecaceae	UKAR3	N	Feb.–Jun.	NE	Fr,Sap	Raw	Analgesic (28), Dental problems (18), Restorative (42), Sexual disease (62)	86.11	1.25
Phyllanthus emblica L./ Phyllanthaceae	UKPH4	N	Mar.–Dec.	LC	Fr,Ro,Sb	Raw	Diabetes (72), Digestive disorder (68), Immune system disorder/buster (70)	96.00	1.75

TABLE 5.2 (*Continued*)

	Voucher number	Nativity	Seasonal availability	IUCN t Status	Plant part/s used	Mode of administration	Ailment treated with citation in parenthesis	Fidelity level (FL)	Use value (UV)
Pithecellobium dulce (Roxb.) Benth./ Fabaceae	UKFA15	E	Feb.–Jul.	LC	Fr,Le,Rb,Sb	Pulp	Astringent (22), Dental problems (20), Menstrual disorder (28)	41.18	0.58
Plumeria rubra L./Apocynaceae	UKAP4	E	Oct.–May	LC	Fl,La	Juice	Antitumor (22), Digestive disorder (28), Respiratory disorder (30)	76.92	0.67
Pongamia pinnata (L.) Pierre/ Fabaceae	UKFA16	N	Apr.–Feb.	LC	Fr,Le,Rb,Sb	Raw	Antitumor (32), Digestive disorder (30), Respiratory disorder (28), Sexual disease (21)	69.57	0.93
Premna pubescens Blume/Lamiaceae	UKLA2	N	Mar.–Jun.	NE	Le,Sb,St	Decoction	Digestive disorder (22), Metabolic disorder (24)	46.15	0.38
Premna mollissima Roth/Lamiaceae	UKLA3	N	May-Jul.	NE	Le,Sb,St	Decoction	Digestive disorder (28), Metabolic disorder (20)	51.85	0.40
Premna tomentosa Willd./Lamiaceae	UKLA4	N	Mar.–Jun.	LC	Le,Sb,St	Decoction	Digestive disorder (27), Metabolic disorder (18)	47.37	0.38
Prosopis juliflora var. *horrida* (Kunth) Burkart/Fabaceae	UKFA17	N	Apr.–Feb.	LC	Fr,Le,Rb,Sb	Powder	Astringent (9), Digestive disorder (11), Skin disease (9)	26.19	0.24
Protium serratum (Wall. ex Colebr.) Engl./Burseraceae	UKBU2	N	Apr.–Jun.	NE	Le,Fr	Raw	Antitumor (17)	41.46	0.14
Psidium guajava L./Myrtaceae	UKMY2	N	Apr.–Oct.	LC	Fr	Raw	Antitumor (11), Diabetes (62), Digestive disorder (78), Liver disorder (75), Neurological disorder (70), Respiratory disorder (62)	97.50	2.98
Pterocarpus indicus Willd./Fabaceae	UKFA18	E	Jul.–Dec.	EN	Gu,Le,Sb	Decoction	Antitumor (22), Restorative (18), Sexual disease (11)	62.86	0.43

TABLE 5.2 (*Continued*)

	Voucher number	Nativity	Seasonal availability	IUCN t Status	Plant part/s used	Mode of administration	Ailment treated with citation in parenthesis	Fidelity level (FL)	Use value (UV)
Pterocarpus marsupium Roxb./ Fabaceae	UKFA19	N	Oct.–Jan.	NT	Gu,Le,Sb	Infusion	Digestive disorder (22), Metabolic disorder (18), Rheumatic disorder (32), Skin disease (11)	88.89	0.69
Pterospermum suberifolium (L.) Raeusch./Malvaceae	UKMA5	N	Mar.–Sep.	NE	Fl,Le,Sb	Decoction	Antitumor (12), Menstrual disorder 13), Respiratory disorder (18), Wound healing (28)	68.29	0.59
Pterospermum acerifolium (L.) Willd./Malvaceae	UKMA6	N	Jan.–Aug.	LC	Fl,Le,Sb	Decoction	Antitumor (11), Digestive disorder (14), Urinary disorder (21)	46.67	0.38
Putranjiva roxburghii Wall./ Putranjivaceae	UKPU1	N	Mar.–Oct.	NE	Fr,Le,Se	Boiled	Astringent (14), Neurological disorder (28), Restorative (32), Rheumatic disorder (22), Sexual disease (42)	84.21	1.15
Salix tetrasperma Roxb./Salicaceae	UKSL2	N	Dec.–Feb.	LC	Le,Sb	Powder	Diabetes (32), Digestive disorder (38), Neurological disorder (21), Respiratory disorder (20), Wound healing (12)	86.36	1.03
Samanea saman (Jacq.) Merr./ Fabaceae	UKFA20	E	Mar.–Feb.	LC	Fr,Sb,Se	Decoction	Digestive disorder (8), Neurological disorder (14), Skin disease (22)	32.84	0.37
Santalum album L./Santalaceae	UKSN1	N	Oct.–Apr.	VU	Fl,Ro,Sb	Paste	Liver disorder (22), Respiratory disorder (21), Sexual disease (24), Skin disease (90), Urinary disorder (23)	91.84	1.50
Sapindus trifoliatus L./Sapindaceae	UKSP3	N	Dec.–May	NE	Fr,Le,Sb,Se	Boiled	Antitumor (8), Neurological disorder (14), Skin disease (38), Worm infection (28)	73.08	0.73

TABLE 5.2 (*Continued*)

	Voucher number	Nativity	Seasonal availability	IUCN t Status	Plant part/s used	Mode of administration	Ailment treated with citation in parenthesis	Fidelity level (FL)	Use value (UV)
Saraca asoca (Roxb.) J.J.de Wilde/ Fabaceae	UKFA21	N	Mar–Oct.	VU	Fl,Le,Sb,Se	Paste	Astringent (21), Digestive disorder (32), Menstrual disorder (43), Skin disease (14), Urinary disorder (32)	84.31	1.18
Schleichera oleosa (Lour.) Merr./ Sapindaceae	UKSP4	N	Mar.–Jul.	LC	Fr,Oi,Sb	Powder	Antitumor (14), Astringent (22), Skin disease (48), Wound healing (32)	80.00	1.42
Semecarpus anacardium L.f./ Anacardiaceae	UKAA4	N	Jul.–Dec.	NE	Fr	Raw	Antitumor (22), Immune system disorder/buster (18), Sexual disease (14)	36.07	0.45
Senegalia polyacantha (Willd.) Seigler & Ebinger/Fabaceae	UKFA22	N	Feb.–Oct.	NE	Ro,Sb	Raw	Digestive disorder (15)	26.32	0.13
Senna siamea (Lam.) H.S.Irwin & Barneby/Fabaceae	UKFA23	E	Sep.–Dec.	LC	Sb	Infusion	Diabetes (11), Digestive disorder (25), Menstrual disorder (18), Sexual disease (11)	59.26	0.54
Shorea robusta C.F.Gaertn./ Dipterocarpaceae	UKDP1	N	Mar.–Jun.	LC	Gu,Oi	Decoction	Antitumor (32), Astringent (22), Liver disorder (28), Menstrual disorder (25), Neurological disorder (23), Sexual disease (22), Skin disease (18)	80.00	1.42
Spathodea campanulata P.Beauv./ Bignoniaceae	UKBI2	N	Aug.–Feb.	LC	Fl,Fr,Le,Ro, Sb,Se	Juice	Antitumor (18), Digestive disorder (42), Liver disorder (54), Sexual disease (14), Skin disease (11), Wound healing (18)	67.50	1.31
Stereospermum chelonoides (L.f.) DC./Bignoniaceae	UKBI3	N	Aug.–Feb.	NE	Fl,Fr,Le,Sb	Infusion	Digestive disorder (22)	32.84	0.18
Streblus asper Lour./Moraceae	UKMO11	N	Feb.–Jun.	LC	Fr,La,Le,Ro, Sb,Se	Decoction	Skin disease (22), Urinary disorder (18), Worm infection (32)	55.17	0.60

TABLE 5.2 (*Continued*)

	Voucher number	Nativity	Seasonal availability	IUCN ŧ Status	Plant part/s used	Mode of administration	Ailment treated with citation in parenthesis	Fidelity level (FL)	Use value (UV)
Strychnos nux-vomica L./Loganiaceae	UKLO1	N	Mar.–Jan.	NE	Fr,Le,Rb,Se	Boiled	Digestive disorder (110), Menstrual disorder (22), Metabolic disorder (105), Neurological disorder (92), Restorative (80)	91.67	3.41
Swietenia mahagoni (L.) Jacq./ Meliaceae	UKME4	N	Mar.–Oct.	NT	Fr,Le,Sb	Infusion	Astringent (5), Sexual disease (9), Wound healing (11)	29.73	0.21
Swietenia macrophylla King/ Meliaceae	UKME5	E	Mar.–Oct.	VU	Fr,Le,Sb	Infusion	Astringent (6), Sexual disease (8), Wound healing (7)	25.81	0.18
Symplocos racemosa Roxb./ Symplocaceae	UKSY1	N	Feb.–Jun.	NE	La,Ro,Sb	Juice	Antitumor (9), Digestive disorder (8), Worm infection (11), Wound healing (18)	32.35	0.38
Syzygium cumini (L.) Skeels/ Myrtaceae	UKMY3	N	Mar.–Jul.	LC	Fr,Rb,Sb,Se	Decoction	Menstrual disorder (28), Sexual disease (22)	53.85	0.42
Syzygium samarangense (Blume) Merr. & L.M.Perry/Myrtaceae	UKMY4	N	Mar.–Jul.	LC	Fr,Rb,Sb,Se	Decoction	Menstrual disorder (30), Sexual disease (18)	71.43	0.40
Tamarindus indica L./Fabaceae	UKFA24	N	Apr.–Jan.	LC	Fl,Le,Ro,Se	Raw	Digestive disorder (52), Respiratory disorder (41), Worm infection (45), Wound healing (38)	86.67	1.47
Tamilnadia uliginosa (Retz.) Tirveng. & Sastre/Rubiaceae	UKRB7	N	Apr.–Oct.	NE	Fl,Fr,Le,Sb	Vegetable	Sexual disease (22), Skin disease (18), Urinary disorder (28)	59.57	0.57
Tecoma stans (L.) Juss. ex Kunth/ Bignoniaceae	UKBI4	N	Nov.–Mar.	LC	Le	Infusion	Diabetes (8), Digestive disorder (14), Urinary disorder (18), Worm infection (21)	36.84	0.51

TABLE 5.2 (*Continued*)

	Voucher number	Nativity	Seasonal availability	IUCN t Status	Plant part/s used	Mode of administration	Ailment treated with citation in parenthesis	Fidelity level (FL)	Use value (UV)
Tectona grandis L. f./Lamiaceae	UKLA5	N	Jul.–Jan.	NE	Fl,Fr,Ro,Sb, Se,St	Powder	Dental problems (22), Digestive disorder (18), Restorative (16), Urinary disorder (9)	33.85	0.54
Terminalia anogeissiana Gere & Boatwr./Combretaceae	UKCO1	N	Aug.–Jan.	NE	Fr,Gu,Le,Sb	Decoction	Digestive disorder (28)	87.50	0.23
Terminalia elliptica Willd./ Combretaceae	UKCO2	N	Mar.–Feb.	NE	Gu,Sb	Juice	Astringent (9), Digestive disorder (42), Wound healing (28)	87.50	0.61
Terminalia arjuna (Roxb. ex DC.) Wight & Arn./Combretaceae	UKCO3	N	Apr.–Feb.	NE	Fr,Gu,Le,Sb	Juice	Digestive disorder (52), Metabolic disorder (92), Snake bite (9)	89.66	1.28
Terminalia bellirica (Gaertn.) Roxb./ Combretaceae	UKCO4	N	Apr.–Feb.	NE	Fr,Gu,Le,Sb	Powder	Dental problems (18), Liver disorder (91), Respiratory disorder (65)	91.00	1.45
Terminalia catappa L./Combretaceae	UKCO5	N	Apr.–Feb.	LC	Fr,Gu,Le,Sb	Powder	Antitumor (9), Skin disease (12), Wound healing (14)	40.00	0.29
Terminalia chebula Retz./ Combretaceae	UKCO6	N	Apr.–Mar	NE	Fr,Gu,Le,Sb	Powder	Astringent (18), Diabetes (32), Digestive disorder (92), Restorative (26)	92.00	1.40
Thespesia populnea (L.) Sol. ex Corrêa/Malvaceae	UKMA7	N	Aug.–Jan.	LC	Le,Ro,St	Decoction	Astringent (11), Diabetes (18), Digestive disorder (22), Sexual disease (18), Skin disease (13)	44.90	0.68
Trema orientale (L.) Blume/ Cannabaceae	UKCN1	N	All	LC	Le,Ro,Sb	Boiled	Dental problems (11), Digestive disorder (22), Respiratory disorder (18), Worm infection (23)	40.35	0.62

TABLE 5.2 (*Continued*)

	Voucher number	Nativity	Seasonal availability	IUCN ŧ Status	Plant part/s used	Mode of administration	Ailment treated with citation in parenthesis	Fidelity level (FL)	Use value (UV)
Vachellia nilotica (L.) P.J.H.Hurter & Mabb./Fabaceae	UKFA25	E	Jun.–Sep.	LC	Ro,Sb	Decoction	Antitumor (28), Astringent (21), Digestive disorder (27), Immune system disorder/buster (25)	68.29	0.84
Vitex glabrata R.Br./Lamiaceae	UKLA6	N	Apr.–Sep.	LC	Fl,Fr,Le,Rb, Ro,Sb,Se	Infusion	Astringent (10), Digestive disorder (22), Worm infection (52)	67.53	0.70
Vitex negundo L./Lamiaceae	UKLA7	N	Mar.–Jun.	LC	Fl,Fr,Le,Rb, Ro,Sb,Se	Infusion	Astringent (12), Digestive disorder (28), Worm infection (110)	91.67	1.25
Ziziphus jujuba Mill./Rhamnaceae	UKRH1	N	Sep.–Mar.	LC	Fr,Ro,Sb,St	Raw	Liver disorder (58), Skin disease (11), Wound healing (13)	63.74	0.68

Abbreviations: Habit: C, Climber; H, Herb; S, Shrub; T, Tree; Lifespan: A, Annual; B, Biennial; P, Perennial; Nativity: E, Exotic; N, Native; IUCN Status: CR, Critically Endangered; DD, Data Deficient; EN, Endangered; LC, Least Concern; NE, Not evaluated; NT, Near Threatened; VU, Vulnerable; Part used: Ba, Bark; Fl, Flower; Fr, Fruit; Gu, Gum; In, Inflorescence; La, Latex; Le, Leaf; Rb, Root bark; Rh, Rhizome; Ro, Root; Sb. Stem bark; Se, Seed; St, Stem; Tu, Tuber; Wp, Whole Plant).

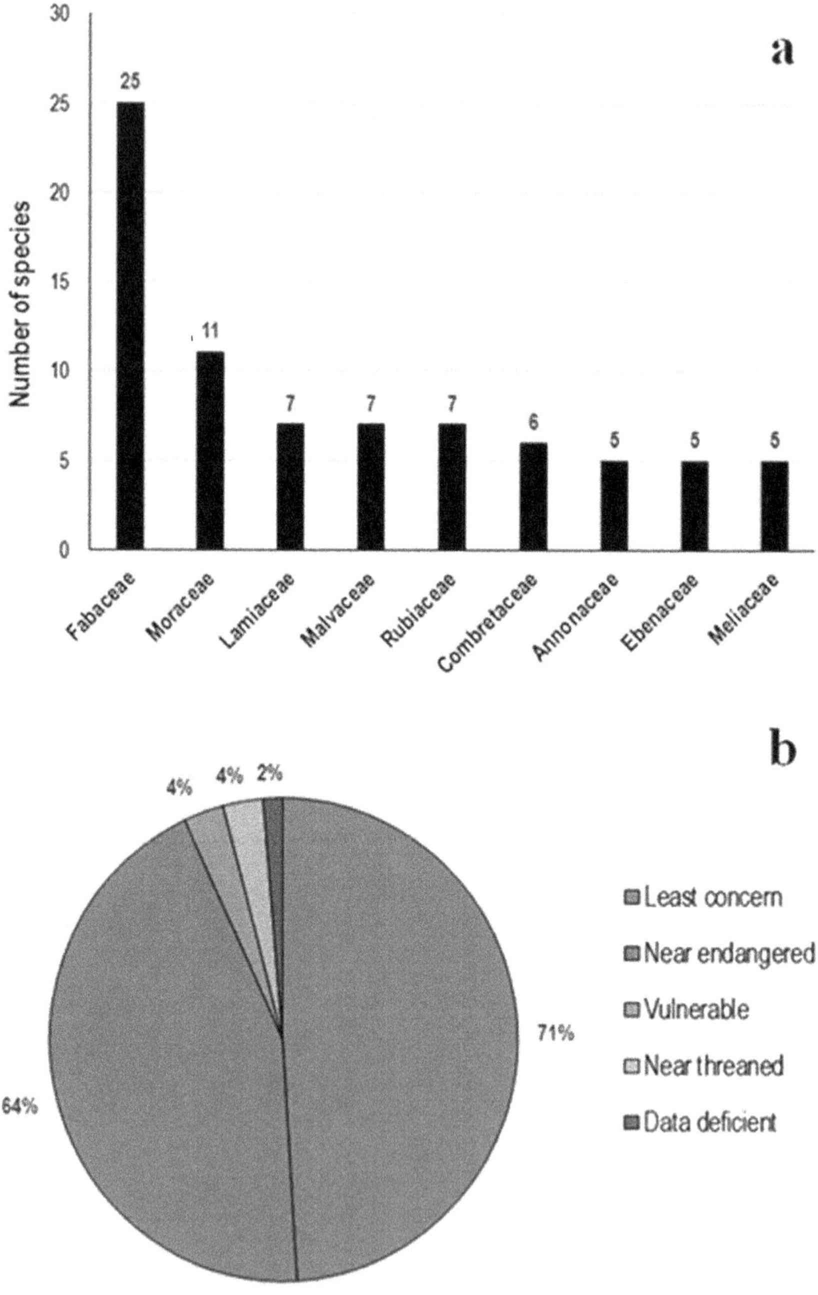

FIGURE 5.2 Dominant plant families (5 spp.) used to treat or cure different diseases (**a**) and the IUCN status of the medicinal plants studied (**b**).

and redeveloped in the sacred grove, but that they were locally vanishing in surrounding forests. Thus, highlights the status as well as distribution of the plant species in the research area and the climatic or ecological conditions necessary for their existence, as well as the risks posed by some of the species recognized using IUCN (2021) criteria. The vulnerable species number in this area has increased due to a variety of circumstances. Cattle overgrazing was a major factor in the devastation of seedlings. Restricted population as well as poor natural reproduction were found to be the main effective variables in reducing species vulnerability. The number of vulnerable species in this area has increased due to a variety of circumstances. Cattle overgrazing was a major factor in the destruction of seedlings. Restricted population and poor natural reproduction, on the other hand, were found to be the most effective variables in reducing species vulnerability.

5.4.4 APPLICATION OF MEDICINAL PLANT SPECIES

One hundred and forty-six medicinal plant species were identified as being used by the residents to treat 23 different diseases, according to 120 informants. One hundred forty-six medicinal plant species found were utilized by the inhabitants as conveyed by the 120 informants to treat 23 ailments. As mentioned in Table 5.3 digestive disorder cured by the maximum number of citations (2354), followed by metabolic disorders (948 citations), liver disorders (756 citations), skin diseases (745 citations), respiratory disorders (740 citations), worm infections (618 citations), diabetes (568 citations), urinary disorders (563 citations), wound healing (540 citations), sexual diseases (534 citations), neurological disorders (516 citations), antitumor (501 citations), rheumatic disorders (399 citations), astringents (391 citations), menstrual disorders (317 citations), restorative (254 citations), immune system disorders/busters (244 citations), dental problems (189 citations), febrifuges (164 citations), analgesics (134 citations), snake bite (80 citations), childbirth (19 citations), and insect bite (18 citations) (Fig. 5.3a). Digestive disorders, liver disorders, skin diseases, respiratory disorders, and worm infections are the most frequent disorders (Utzinger et al., 2012; Khan and Ahmad, 2015).

5.4.5 PART PLANT SPECIES USED IN MEDICATION

All part/s of different plant species were utilized against different diseases. The most used plant parts to treat different aliments were stem bark 109

TABLE 5.3 The informant consensus factor (Fic) values of use category of multiple plant species claimed as having medicinal values by informants of the ethnic communities.

	Plant species with citation (in parenthesis)	**Number of plant species used**	**Number of use citation**	**Percent of all citations**	**Fic value**
Analgesic	*Artocarpus heterophyllus* (24), *Bridelia retusa* (14), *Catunaregam spinosa* (16), *Cocos nucifera* (44), *Delonix regia* (8), *Phoenix sylvestris* (28)	6	134	1.16	0.96
Antitumor	*Cascabela thevetia* (11), *Cassia fistula* (17), *Cordia dichotoma* (9), *Croton caudatus* (9), *Diospyros malabarica* (11), *Diospyros sylvatica* (9), *Ficus virens* (9), *Ficus religiosa* (21), *Gmelina arborea* (8), *Holarrhena pubescens* (8), *Lagerstroemia parviflora* (11), *Lagerstroemia speciosa* (11), *Lannea coromandelica* (10), *Madhuca longifolia* var. *latifolia* (9), *Manilkara zapota* (9), *Miliusa velutina* (11), *Mimusops elengi* (8), *Monoon longifolium* (21), *Moringa oleifera* (32), *Plumeria rubra* (22), *Pongamia pinnata* (32), *Protium serratum* (17), *Psidium guajava* (11), *Pterocarpus indicus* (22), *Pterospermum suberifolium* (12), *Pterospermum acerifolium* (11), *Sapindus trifoliatus* (8), *Schleichera oleosa* (14), *Semecarpus anacardium* (22), *Shorea robusta* (32), *Spathodea campanulata* (18), *Symplocos racemosa* (9), *Terminalia catappa* (9), *Vachellia nilotica* (28)	34	501	4.32	0.93
Astringent	*Acacia auriculiformis* (12), *Alstonia scholaris* (14), *Annona squamosa* (22), *Aphanamixis polystachya* (9), *Artocarpus lacucha* (11), *Bambusa bambos* (8), *Bombax ceiba* (8), *Bridelia retusa* (22), *Careya arborea* (18), *Ceiba pentandra* (9), *Dillenia indica* (11), *Dillenia pentagyna* (11), *Diospyros malabarica* (12), *Eucalyptus tereticornis* (8), *Litsea glutinosa* (14), *Pithecellobium dulce* (22), *Prosopis juliflora* var. *horrida* (9), *Putranjiva roxburghii* (14), *Saraca asoca* (21), *Schleichera oleosa* (22), *Shorea robusta* (22), *Swietenia mahagoni* (5), *Swietenia macrophylla* (6), *Terminalia elliptica* (9), *Terminalia chebula* (18), *Thespesia populnea* (11), *Vachellia nilotica* (21), *Vitex glabrata* (10), *Vitex negundo* (12)	29	391	3.37	0.93
Child birth	*Ailanthus excelsa* (8), *Cocos nucifera* (11)	2	19	0.16	0.94

TABLE 5.3 *(Continued)*

	Plant species with citation (in parenthesis)	Number of plant species used	Number of use citation	Percent of all citations	Fic value
Dental problems	*Annona squamosa* (18), *Cascabela thevetia* (8), *Croton caudatus* (13), *Euphorbia antiquorum* (11), *Ficus benghalensis* (18), *Mangifera indica* (32), *Phoenix sylvestris* (18), *Pithecellobium dulce* (20), *Tectona grandis* (22), *Terminalia bellirica* (18), *Trema orientale* (11)	11	189	1.63	0.95
Diabetes	*Averrhoa carambola* (25), *Azadirachta indica* (72), *Casearia tomentosa* (14), *Ficus religiosa* (28), *Holoptelea integrifolia* (8), *Lagerstroemia parviflora* (9), *Lagerstroemia speciosa* (14), *Leucaena leucocephala* (11), *Limonia acidissima* (32), *Madhuca longifolia* var. *latifolia* (8), *Manilkara zapota* (18), *Melia azedarach* (42), *Morinda citrifolia* (14), *Moringa oleifera* (38), *Phyllanthus emblica* (72), *Psidium guajava* (62), *Salix tetrasperma* (32), *Senna siamea* (11), *Tecoma stans* (8), *Terminalia chebula* (32), *Thespesia populnea* (18)	21	568	4.90	0.96
Digestive disorder	*Acacia auriculiformis* (20), *Adina cordifolia* (14), *Aegle marmelos* (120), *Ailanthus excelsa* (14), *Alstonia scholaris* (22), *Anacardium occidentale* (22), *Annona reticulata* (14), *Antidesma acidum* (32), *Barringtonia acutangula* (22), *Bauhinia purpurea* (18), *Bixa orellana* (58), *Bombax ceiba* (17), *Casuarina equisetifolia* (11), *Catunaregam spinosa* (32), *Ceiba pentandra* (8), *Citrus maxima* (92), *Cocos nucifera* (11), *Cordia dichotoma* (11), *Crateva magna* (17), *Dalbergia sissoo* (11), *Delonix regia* (14), *Dillenia indica* (18), *Dillenia pentagyna* (20), *Diospyros malabarica* (44), *Diospyros melanoxylon* var. *tupru* (46), *Diospyros melanoxylon* (39), *Ehretia aspera* (32), *Ficus benghalensis* (22), *Gmelina arborea* (12), *Guazuma ulmifolia* (11), *Holarrhena pubescens* (92), *Holoptelea integrifolia* (12), *Leucaena leucocephala* (22), *Limonia acidissima* (38), *Litsea glutinosa* (18), *Mangifera indica* (38), *Manilkara zapota* (32), *Melia azedarach* (40), *Mimusops elengi* (32), *Neolamarckia cadamba* (44), *Nyctanthes arbor-tristis* (72), *Oroxylum indicum* (22), *Peltophorum pterocarpum* (21), *Phyllanthus emblica* (68), *Plumeria rubra* (28), *Pongamia pinnata* (30), *Premna pubescens* (22), *Premna mollissima* (28), *Premna tomentosa* (27), *Prosopis juliflora* var. *horrida* (11), *Psidium guajava*	74	2354	20.31	0.97

TABLE 5.3 *(Continued)*

	Plant species with citation (in parenthesis)	Number of plant species used	Number of use citation	Percent of all citations	Fic value
	(78), *Pterocarpus marsupium* (22), *Pterospermum acerifolium* (14), *Salix tetrasperma* (38), *Samanea saman* (8), *Saraca asoca* (32), *Senegalia polyacantha* (15), *Senna siamea* (25), *Spathodea campanulata* (42), *Stereospermum chelonoides* (22), *Strychnos nux-vomica* (110), *Symplocos racemosa* (8), *Tamarindus indica* (52), *Tecoma stans* (14), *Tectona grandis* (18), *Terminalia anogeissiana* (28), *Terminalia elliptica* (42), *Terminalia arjuna* (52), *Terminalia chebula* (92), *Thespesia populnea* (22), *Trema orientale* (22), *Vachellia nilotica* (27), *Vitex glabrata* (22), *Vitex negundo* (28)				
Febrifuge	*Adina cordifolia* (9), *Ailanthus excelsa* (11), *Annona reticulata* (16), *Catunaregam spinosa* (28), *Ficus virens* (12), *Ficus racemosa* (11), *Grewia asiatica* (8), *Lagerstroemia parviflora* (8), *Lagerstroemia speciosa* (9), *Lepisanthes rubiginosa* (8), *Madhuca longifolia* var. *latifolia* (11), *Manilkara zapota* (21), *Parkinsonia aculeata* (12)	13	164	1.41	0.93
Immune system disorder	*Bambusa bambos* (11), *Borassus flabellifer* (11), *Cassia fistula* (14), *Diospyros melanoxylon* var. *tupru* (21), *Diospyros melanoxylon* (21), *Ficus hispida* (18), *Lagerstroemia parviflora* (7), *Oroxylum indicum* (28), *Phyllanthus emblica* (70), *Semecarpus anacardium* (18), *Vachellia nilotica* (25)	11	244	2.10	0.96
Insect bite	*Antidesma acidum* (11), *Ficus grossularioides* (7)	2	18	0.16	0.94
Liver disorder	*Alangium salviifolium* (22), *Annona reticulata* (11), *Aphanamixis polystachya* (21), *Averrhoa carambola* (21), *Borassus flabellifer* (48), *Boswellia serrata* (38), *Dalbergia sissoo* (14), *Delonix regia* (18), *Ficus hispida* (49), *Madhuca longifolia* var. *latifolia* (42), *Mimusops elengi* (38), *Nyctanthes arbor-tristis* (85), *Oroxylum indicum* (21), *Psidium guajava* (75), *Santalum album* (22), *Shorea robusta* (28), *Spathodea campanulata* (54), *Terminalia bellirica* (91), *Ziziphus jujuba* (58)	19	756	6.52	0.98

TABLE 5.3 *(Continued)*

	Plant species with citation (in parenthesis)	**Number of plant species used**	**Number of use citation**	**Percent of all citations**	**Fic value**
Menstrual disorder	*Barringtonia acutangula* (11), *Bombax ceiba* (32), *Elaeodendron glaucum* (15), *Ficus hispida* (21), *Ficus racemosa* (18), *Holoptelea integrifolia* (13), *Pithecellobium dulce* (28), *Pterospermum suberifolium* (13), *Saraca asoca* (43), *Senna siamea* (18), *Shorea robusta* (25), *Strychnos nux-vomica* (22), *Syzygium samarangense* (28), *Syzygium cumini* (30)	14	317	2.73	0.96
Metabolic disorder	*Aphanamixis polystachya* (28), *Azadirachta indica* (63), *Bauhinia variegata* (14), *Bixa orellana* (72), *Cleistanthus collinus* (81), *Crateva magna* (16), *Erythrina variegata* (21), *Eucalyptus tereticornis* (12), *Euphorbia antiquorum* (9), *Ficus benghalensis* (35), *Ficus grossularioides* (14), *Ficus religiosa* (33), *Holarrhena pubescens* (75), *Lagerstroemia speciosa* (18), *Lannea coromandelica* (22), *Mallotus repandus* (38), *Mallotus nudiflorus* (30), *Mimusops elengi* (28), *Mitragyna parvifolia* (28), *Oroxylum indicum* (24), *Premna pubescens* (24), *Premna mollissima* (30), *Premna tomentosa* (18), *Pterocarpus marsupium* (18), *Strychnos nux-vomica* (105), *Terminalia arjuna* (92)	26	948	8.18	0.97
Neurological disorder	*Bombax ceiba* (28), *Catunaregam spinosa* (34), *Dimocarpus longan* (18), *Diospyros melanoxylon* var. *tupru* (16), *Diospyros melanoxylon* (23), *Elaeodendron glaucum* (17), *Erythrina variegata* (17), *Euphorbia antiquorum* (14), *Ficus racemosa* (22), *Ficus religiosa* (28), *Gliricidia sepium* (23), *Lepisanthes rubiginosa* (14), *Psidium guajava* (70), *Putranjiva roxburghii* (28), *Salix tetrasperma* (21), *Samanea saman* (14), *Sapindus trifoliatus* (14), *Shorea robusta* (23), *Strychnos nux-vomica* (92)	19	516	4.45	0.97
Respiratory disorder	*Aegle marmelos* (50), *Ailanthus excelsa* (9), *Albizia lebbeck* (11), *Annona squamosa* (16), *Averrhoa carambola* (20), *Boswellia serrata* (33), *Careya arborea* (22), *Ceiba pentandra* (7), *Citrus maxima* (82), *Cocos nucifera* (48), *Dillenia indica* (14), *Dillenia pentagyna* (13), *Erythrina variegata* (18), *Guazuma ulmifolia* (14), *Limonia acidissima* (28), *Mitragyna parvifolia* (22), *Nyctanthes arbor-tristis* (30), *Plumeria rubra* (30), *Pongamia pinnata* (28),	26	740	6.38	0.97

TABLE 5.3 *(Continued)*

	Plant species with citation (in parenthesis)	Number of plant species used	Number of use citation	Percent of all citations	Fic value
	Psidium guajava (62), *Pterospermum suberifolium* (18), *Salix tetrasperma* (20), *Santalum album* (21), *Tamarindus indica* (41), *Terminalia bellirica* (65), *Trema orientale* (18)				
Restorative	*Barringtonia acutangula* (9), *Cocos nucifera* (11), *Diospyros montana* (11), *Leucaena leucocephala* (9), *Phoenix sylvestris* (42), *Pterocarpus indicus* (18), *Putranjiva roxburghii* (32), *Strychnos nux-vomica* (80), *Tectona grandis* (16), *Terminalia chebula* (26)	10	254	2.19	0.96
Rheumatic disorder	*Acacia auriculiformis* (12), *Annona squamosa* (9), *Aphanamixis polystachya* (9), *Boswellia serrata* (18), *Cascabela thevetia* (12), *Cassia fistula* (32), *Delonix regia* (17), *Euphorbia antiquorum* (15), *Ficus benghalensis* (26), *Holoptelea integrifolia* (22), *Litsea glutinosa* (29), *Mallotus repandus* (30), *Mallotus nudiflorus* (32), *Mangifera indica* (28), *Melia azedarach* (32), *Parkinsonia aculeata* (22), *Pterocarpus marsupium* (32), *Putranjiva roxburghii* (22)	18	399	3.44	0.96
Sexual disease	*Aegle marmelos* (71), *Alangium salviifolium* (11), *Artocarpus heterophyllus* (8), *Crateva magna* (21), *Ficus benghalensis* (8), *Ficus racemosa* (14), *Ficus religiosa* (8), *Gmelina arborea* (7), *Grewia asiatica* (14), *Guazuma ulmifolia* (11), *Holarrhena pubescens* (22), *Leucaena leucocephala* (4), *Madhuca longifolia* var. *latifolia* (11), *Mitragyna parvifolia* (9), *Phoenix sylvestris* (62), *Pongamia pinnata* (21), *Pterocarpus indicus* (11), *Putranjiva roxburghii* (42), *Santalum album* (24), *Semecarpus anacardium* (14), *Senna siamea* (11), *Shorea robusta* (22), *Spathodea campanulata* (14), *Swietenia mahagoni* (9), *Swietenia macrophylla* (8), *Syzygium cumini* (22), *Syzygium samarangense* (15), *Tamilnadia uliginosa* (22) *Thespesia populnea* (18)	29	534	4.61	0.95
Skin disease	*Albizia lebbeck* (23), *Alstonia scholaris* (32), *Artocarpus heterophyllus* (4), *Averrhoa carambola* (11), *Azadirachta indica* (120), *Bauhinia purpurea* (14), *Bauhinia variegata* (13), *Casuarina equisetifolia* (21), *Ceiba pentandra* (11), *Cordia dichotoma* (14), *Croton caudatus*(18), *Ficus rumphii* (12), *Ficus mollis* (4), *Ficus religiosa* (11), *Gardenia gummifera*	34	745	6.43	0.96

TABLE 5.3 *(Continued)*

	Plant species with citation (in parenthesis)	Number of plant species used	Number of use citation	Percent of all citations	Fic value
	(22), *Gliricidia sepium* (11), *Madhuca longifolia* var. *latifolia* (18), *Neolamarckia cadamba* (11), *Nyctanthes arbor-tristis* (14), *Peltophorum pterocarpum* (24), *Prosopis juliflora* var. *horrida* (9), *Pterocarpus marsupium* (11), *Samanea saman* (22), *Santalum album* (90), *Sapindus trifoliatus* (38), *Saraca asoca* (14), *Schleichera oleosa* (48), *Shorea robusta* (18), *Spathodea campanulata* (11), *Streblus asper* (22), *Tamilnadia uliginosa* (18), *Terminalia catappa* (12), *Thespesia populnea* (13), *Ziziphus jujuba* (11)				
Snake bite	*Alstonia scholaris* (8), *Bauhinia variegata* (9), *Cascabela thevetia* (17), *Casearia tomentosa* (8), *Dimocarpus longan* (4), *Elaeodendron glaucum* (11), *Erythrina variegata* (9), *Nyctanthes arbor-tristis* (11), *Terminalia arjuna* (9)	9	80	0.69	0.90
Urinary disorder	*Borassus flabellifer* (45), *Casearia tomentosa* (28), *Cleistanthus collinus* (78), *Diospyros melanoxylon* var. *tupru* (18), *Diospyros melanoxylon* (14), *Grewia asiatica* (22), *Guazuma ulmifolia* (22), *Lagerstroemia speciosa* (8), *Mangifera indica* (31), *Manilkara zapota* (24), *Melia azedarach* (30), *Mimusops elengi* (30), *Moringa oleifera* (35), *Neolamarckia cadamba* (29), *Pterospermum acerifolium* (21), *Santalum album* (23), *Saraca asoca* (32), *Streblus asper* (18), *Tamilnadia uliginosa* (28), *Tecoma stans* (18), *Tectona grandis* (9)	21	563	4.86	0.96
Worm infection	*Adina cordifolia* (22), *Annona reticulata* (23), *Bambusa bambos* (14), *Bauhinia variegata* (10), *Dalbergia sissoo* (32), *Diospyros malabarica* (52), *Ficus rumphii* (17), *Holoptelea integrifolia* (21), *Huberantha cerasoides* (14), *Madhuca longifolia* var. *latifolia* (22), *Mangifera indica* (18), *Miliusa velutina* (22), *Morinda citrifolia* (29), *Sapindus trifoliatus* (28), *Streblus asper* (32), *Symplocos racemosa* (11), *Tamarindus indica* (45), *Tecoma stans* (21), *Trema orientale* (23), *Vitex negundo* (52), *Vitex glabrata* (110)	21	618	5.33	0.97

TABLE 5.3 *(Continued)*

	Plant species with citation (in parenthesis)	Number of plant species used	Number of use citation	Percent of all citations	Fic value
Wound healing	*Alangium salviifolium* (32), *Artocarpus lacucha* (22), *Azadirachta indica* (92), *Ceiba pentandra* (17), *Diospyros malabarica* (32), *Diospyros sylvatica* (17), *Ficus mollis* (14), *Gliricidia sepium* (18), *Gmelina arborea* (9), *Guazuma ulmifolia* (9), *Holoptelea integrifolia* (18), *Lannea coromandelica* (9), *Madhuca longifolia* var. *latifolia* (11), *Mimusops elengi* (21), *Pterospermum suberifolium* (28), *Salix tetrasperma* (12), *Schleichera oleosa* (32), *Spathodea campanulata* (18), *Swietenia mahagoni* (11), *Swietenia macrophylla* (7), *Symplocos racemosa* (18), *Tamarindus indica* (38), *Terminalia elliptica* (28), *Terminalia catappa* (14), *Ziziphus jujuba* (13)	25	540	4.66	0.96

(74.7%), leaves 93 (63.7%), fruits 90 (61.6%), roots 53 (36.3%), seeds 47 (32.2%), flowers 30 (20.6%), gum 19 (13%), latex 17 (11.6%), root bark 13 (8.9%), stem 11 (7.5%), oil 2 (1.4%), sap 2 (1.4%), and whole plant 2 (1.4%) (Figure 5.3b). All the above-mentioned plant parts are used in medicines were administered externally as well as internally. Similar results were reported by Ozioma and Chinwe (2019) and Sadeer et al. (2019) who stated that the stem bark and leaves as the most used plants in medication, while Dogan and Ugulu (2013) and Abbas et al. (2017) reported that fruits, roots, and seeds are the major plant material utilized in the treatment of different ailments.

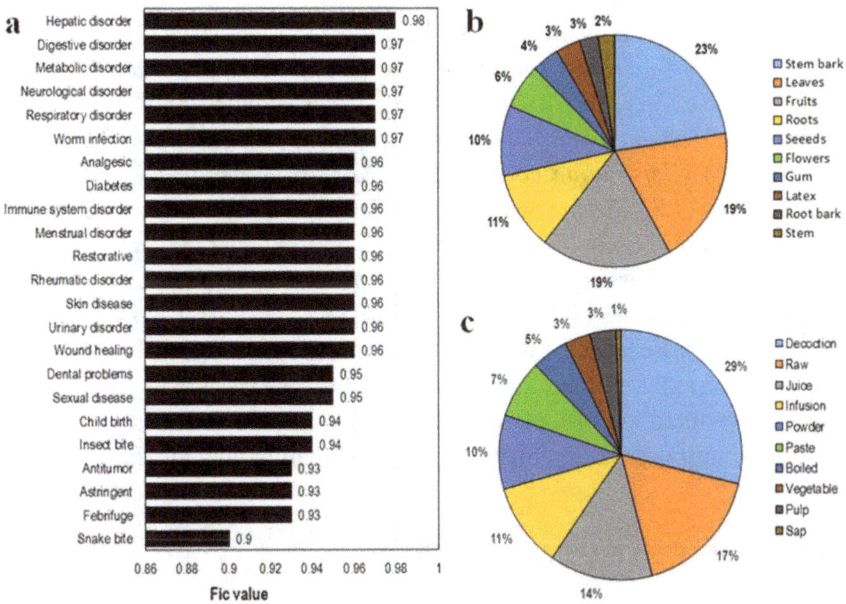

FIGURE 5.3 Uses of plant species to treat or cure diseases (**a**), plant part used (**b**) and mode of preparation or administration (**c**).

5.4.6 PREPARATION AND ADMINISTRATION

The most common form of preparation is whole plant decoction 42 (38.3%), followed by raw material 25 (17.1%), juice 20 (13.7%), infusion 16 (11%), powder 14 (9.6%), paste 11 (7.5%), boiled 7 (4.8%), vegetable 5 (3.4%), pulp 5 (3.4%), and the sap represented as the least used 1 (0.7%) (Figure 5.3c). In other words, the above 65% of the plant species were used as fresh and 35%

were heated processed. To cure various disorders, a variety of internal as well as external administration procedures were employed. External application has the advantage of being safe due to indirect but immediate effects on the area allowed for easy dosage management based on the amounts of helpful or harmful substances (Sivasankari et al., 2014).

5.4.7 USED VALUE

Medicinal plant species' utilized values (Uvi) ranged from 0.1 to 3.4. The medicinal herbs that prevailed with the highest usage values (>1) were *Strychnos nux-vomica* (3.4), *Psidium guajava* (3), *A. indica* (2.9), *A. marmelos* (2), *Cocos nucifera* (1.8), *Nyctanthes arbor-tristis* (1.8), *Phyllanthus emblica* (1.8), *Holarrhena pubescens* (1.6), *Santalum album* (1.5), *Bixa orellana* (1.5), *Tamarindus indica* (1.5, *Citrus maxima* (1.5), *Terminalia bellirica* (1.5), *Schleichera oleosa* (1.4), *Shorea robusta* (1.4), *Terminalia chebula* (1.4), *Cleistanthus collinus* (1.3), *Mimusops elengi* (1.3), *Spathodea campanulata* (1.3), *Terminalia arjuna* (1.3), *Diospyros malabarica* (1.3), *Phoenix sylvestris* (1.3), *Vitex negundo* (1.3), *Mangifera indica* (1.2), *Melia azedarach* (1.2), *Saraca asoca* (1.2), *Putranjiva roxburghii* (1.2), *Madhuca longifolia* var. *latifolia* (1.1), *Ficus religiosa* (1.1), and *Salix tetrasperma* (1) (see Table 5.2). Because of their extensive distribution and cultural drivers' responsiveness, the maximum usage values of the stated medicinal species may have resulted in those plant species being the preferred choice for pharmaceutical purposes (Rahman et al., 2016; Muhammad et al., 2020).

5.4.8 FIDELITY LEVEL (FL)

The fidelity level (FL%) was a standard ethnobotanical index used to classify organisms that were most commonly used by the locals to treat specific ailments/diseases. The current investigation found that FLs varied from 17.7 to 100%. The plant species with highest level of fidelity were *A. marmelos* and *A. indica* each cited 100% for diabetes, digestive disorder, metabolic disorder, respiratory disorder, sexual disease, skin disease, and wound healing. Some other species with the highest level of fidelity (>90%) were *P. guajava* (97.5%), *P. emblica* (96%), *Nyctanthes arbor-tristis* (94.4%), *T. chebula* (92%), *S. album* (91.8%), *Strychnos nux-vomica* (91.7%), *V. negundo* (91.7%), *T. bellirica* (91%), *Moringa oleifera* (90.5%), and *C. maxima* (90.2%) for various ailments (see Table 5.2). Further examination and evaluation of phytochemical, biological, and pharmacological activities may confirm these plant species as valuable therapeutic plants (Wangchuk et al., 2011). The FL% of 70 medicinal plant species lied in the range of <90 to ≥50, the remaining 64 species had a rate of less than 50%. *Eucalyptus tereticornis* (17.8%), on the other hand, had the lowest level of loyalty among these plants. Furthermore, plants with a low level of fidelity should not be abandoned, as failing to record them for future generations may result in the threat of gradual loss of traditional cultural or ethnic knowledge (Rahman et al., 2016).

5.4.9 INFORMANT CONSENSUS FACTOR

The informant consensus factor (Fic) was employed to highlight plants of special ethnic value and agreement of use of plant species for the study of common use of plant species. It identifies the plants that were commonly used within a population and amongst the ethnic groups, aiding with plant selection for pharmacological and phytochemical research (Giday et al., 2007; Ullah and Muhammad, 2018; Muhammad et al., 2019). In our study, the range of Fic was 0.98 for the liver disorders, and 0.90 for the snake bite (see Table 5.3) (see Fig. 5.3a). All the clusters had a Fic value greater than 0.9 and thus all of them could be considered to validate the bioactivity, isolate and characterize the active principles by the potential researchers in each cluster.

The following were the most commonly mentioned and cited disease categories: digestive disorders, metabolic disorders, neurological disorders, respiratory disorders, and worm infections (Fic, 0.97 each). The nine use category includes analgesic, diabetes, immune system disorder/booster, menstrual disorders, restorative, rheumatic disorders, skin diseases, urinary disorders, and wound healing showed 0.96 Fic value. The dental problems and sexual diseases showed 0.95 Fic, the childbirth and insect bite, 0.94 Fic, and antitumor, astringent, and febrifuge with each 0.93 Fic value. The Fic ranged from 0.90 to 0.98, while their use reports from 18 to 2354 in this study. The highest number of citations or plant species were found in various disease classes, however, their Fic values differed according to the Fic formula's basic indices, as consensus of the informers on usage of medicinal plant species against various health problems was principally characterized by the computed index. Many investigators described analgesic, diabetes, digestive disorders, liver disorders, metabolic disorders, neurological disorders, respiratory disorders, rheumatic disorders, and worm infections being the most often mentioned disease types (Tardio and Pardo-de-Santayana, 2008; Giday et al., 2009; Khan and Ahmad, 2015; Rahman et al., 2016; Ullah and Muhammad, 2018; Muhammad et al., 2019, 2020).

5.5 CONCLUSION AND OUTLOOK

The ethno-medico-botanical investigations of medicinally important plant species in sacred groves of Jhargram district are detailed in this paper. This area is noted for its biodiversity, as well as sacred groves and ethnic societies. As a result, efforts have been undertaken to investigate and identify the status of this research field from an ethno-medico-botanical standpoint, which will be useful for future research. Villagers and tribals in these locations use a range of plant species for various purposes, indicating that they are linked to sacred plant species and plants in the area. The current study gave significant and valuable information regarding ethnic medicinal knowledge of local plant species against various ailments, which included 146 plant species from 44 different families. Traditional oral information is with the elder generation, and the majority of that may perish soon after their deaths, resulting in the obliteration of such vital knowledge from society. As a result, the ethnic folk asset relating to the natural habitat of these remote sacred forests has been rather well preserved. Antimicrobial, antiviral, and pharmacological investigations will be needed in the future to confirm the medicinal plant species' efficacy and safety.

A majority of the plant species recorded in this study is restricted to the current geographic region as the study area is housed in a remote part of West Bengal, according to a comparative assessment of previously published research related to ethnomedicinal uses for the treatment of various diseases. Medicinal uses have been recorded for several exotic plant species around the world. Most of these plant species presently need scientific validation through experiments for safe and suggested dosages, as well as varied lethal and hazardous toxicities. To validate their present traditional usage, the reported plant species of inaccessible areas could be examined for antibacterial, antiviral, and pharmacological properties. When comparing this investigation to the literature, we discovered that the same plant species described for medicinal use in linked regions and other countries prompted us to consider its value by validating the pharmacological values. As a result, it is expected that such research will pave way to research not only to spread ethnic medicinal knowledge, but also to track the ingredients in medicinal plant species for commercial purposes. Due to the promotion of such knowledge by the locals or tribals, sacred groves have been serving society, religion, and culture in India and delivering environmental, ecological, economic, and health-promoting services since ancient times. The sacred groves in India are threatened by development and industrialization, thus their preservation depends on the creation and execution of new regulations, as well as teaching people about their importance so that they may participate in the maintenance and management of the sacred groves.

ACKNOWLEDGMENTS

Special thanks from the authors go to all informants who generously shared their knowledge of local plants and traditional medicinal uses. We are grateful for the explicit identification of plant species by Dr. G.G. Maity, Professor, Kalyani University. The authors declare that there are no conflicts of interest to publish this research in the form of a book chapter.

KEYWORDS

- **ethnic people**
- **fidelity level**
- **informant consensus factor**
- **medicinal plant species**
- **use value**

REFERENCES

Abbas, Z.; Khan, S. M.; Alam, J.; Khan, S. W.; Abbasi, A. M. Medicinal Plants Used by Inhabitants of the Shigar Valley, Baltistan Region of Karakorum Range, Pakistan. *J. Ethnobiol. Ethnomed.* **2017,** *13*, 1–15.

Adom, D.; Umachandran, K.; Sawicka, B.; Boamah, D.; Ziarati, P. The Concept, State, Roles and Management of Protected Areas in Ghana: A Review. *Acta Sci. Agric.* **2019,** *3*, 68–76.

Albuquerque, U. P.; Siva, V. A.; Cabral, M. C.; Alencar, N. L.; Andrade, L. H. C. Comparisons Between the Use of Medicinal Plants in Indigenous and Rural Caatinga (Dryland) Communities in NE Brazil. *Bol. Latinoam. Carib. Pl. Med. Aromat.* **2008,** *7*, 156–170.

Anon. *District Human Development Report, Paschim Medinipur*; Development and Planning Department, Government of West Bengal, Kolkata, 2011. file:///C:/Users/User1/Downloads/13_21062017103239.pdf.

Bennet, S. S. R. *Flora of Howrah District;* International Book Distributors, Dehradun, India, 1979; p 406.

Berkes, F.; Colding, J.; Folke, C. Rediscovery of Traditional Ecological Knowledge as Adaptive Management. *Ecol. Appl.* **2000,** *10*, 1251–1262.

Bodeker, G. Traditional Health Systems: Policy, Biodiversity, and Global Interdependence. *J. Alt. Compl. Med.* **1995,** *1*, 231–243.

Chaudhury, S.; Singh, H.; Bharati, K. A. Quantitative Analyses on Ethnogynecological Remedies Used by Lodhas of Paschim Medinipur District, West Bengal, India. *Ind. J. Trad. Know*. **2017,** *16*, 325–332.

Doffana, Z. D. Sacred Natural Sites, Herbal Medicine, Medicinal Plants and Their Conservation in Sidama, Ethiopia. *Cogent Food Agric.* **2017,** *3*, 1365399.

Dogan, Y.; Ugulu, I. Medicinal Plants Used for Gastrointestinal Disorders in Some Districts of Izmir Province, Turkey. *Stud. Ethno-Med.* **2013,** *7*, 149–161.

Friedman, J.; Yaniv, Z.; Dafni, A.; Palewitch, D. A Preliminary Classification of the Healing Potential of Medicinal Plants, Based on a Rational Analysis of an Ethnopharmacological Field Survey Among Bedouins in the Negev Desert, Israel. *J. Ethnopharmacol.* **1986,** *16*, 275–287.

Giday, M.; Asfaw, Z.; Woldu, Z.; Teklehaymanot, T. Medicinal Plant Knowledge of the Bench Ethnic Group of Ethiopia: An Ethnobotanical Investigation. *J. Ethnobiol. Ethnomed.* **2009,** *5*, 34.

Giday, M.; Teklehaymanot, T.; Animut, A.; Mekonnen, Y. Medicinal Plants of the Shinasha, Agew-awi and Amhara Peoples in Northwest Ethiopia. *J. Ethnopharmacol.* **2007,** *110*, 516–525.

Haines, H. H. *The Botany of Bihar and Orissa*, Vol. 1–6; Botanical Survey of India: Calcutta, India, 1921–1925.

Immanuel, R. R.; Thiruppathi, M.; Balasubramanian, A. *Social Forestry and Agroforestry: Past Triumphs and Future Horizons*; Impyreal Publishing House, India, 2018; p 218.

IUCN. The IUCN Red List of Threatened Species. Version 2021–1, 2021. https://www.iucnredlist.org (accessed on May 2, 2021).

Kala, C. P.; Dhyani, P. P.; Sajwan, B. S. Developing the Medicinal Plants Sector in Northern India: Challenges and Opportunities. *J. Ethnobiol. Ethnomed.* **2006,** *2*, 1–15.

Khan, M. P. Z.; Ahmad, M. Traditional Preference of Wild Edible Fruits (WEFs) for Digestive Disorders (DDs) Among the Indigenous Communities of Swat Valley, Pakistan. *J. Ethnopharmacol.* **2015,** *174*, 339–354.

Kossi, A.; Mazalo, K. P.; Novinyo, S. K.; Kouami, K. Impacts of Traditional Practices on Biodiversity and Structural Characteristics of Sacred Groves in Northern Togo, West Africa. *Acta Oecol.* **2021,** *110*, 103680.

Kumar, V. *Integrated Rural Development Program and Its Impact on the Socio-Economic Condition of the Rural Poor of Sitamarhi District*; Xlibris Corporation, USA, 2011; p 206.

Mandal, H.; Sarkar, A. *Traditional Wisdom and Sustainable Living: A Study on the Indian Tribal Societies*; Raj Publications: New Delhi, 2013; p 560.

Martin, G. J. *Ethnobotany: A Methods Manual*; Taylor and Francis, London, 2004; p 296.

Merritt, C. H. *Reframing Hope: Vital Ministry in a New Generation*; Rowman & Littlefield Publishers, USA, 2010; p 147.

Mgaya, E. *Traditional Institutions' Management of Sacred Forests in Tanzania: History, Narratives, and Evidence from Njombe Region, 1880s–2019*; Ph.D. Dissertation, Victoria University: New Zealand, 2020; p 245.

Muhammad, N.; Uddin, N.; Khan, M. K. U.; Mengjun, L.; Xuan, Z. et al. Ethnomedicinal and Cultural Uses of *Ziziphus* Species in Flora of Malakand Division, KP, Pakistan. *Singapore J. Sci. Res.* **2020,** *10*, 1–7.

Muhammad, N.; Uddin, N.; Xuan, Z.; Umer, M.; Liu, M. et al. Genetic Diversity Encourages Conservation of Threatened Ethno Medicinally Important Plant Species in Koz Abakhel District Swat, KP, Pakistan. *Int. J. Bot. Stud.* **2019,** *4*, 151–161.

Ozioma, E. O. J.; Chinwe, O. A. N. Herbal Medicines in African Traditional Medicine. *Herb. Med.* **2019,** *10*, 191–214.

Pakrashi, S. C.; Mukhopadhya S. *Medicinal and Aromatic Plants of Red Laterite Region of West Bengal (Bankura, Medinipore and Purulia).* West Bengal Academy of Science and Technology, Kolkata, India, 2004.

Phillips, O. L.; Hall, P.; Gentry, A. H.; Sawyer, S. A.; Vasquez, R. Dynamics and Species Richness of Tropical Forests. *Proc. Natl. Acad. Sci.* **1994,** *91*, 2805–2809.

Prain, D. *Bengal Plants*, Vol. 2; Botanical Survey of India: Calcutta, India, 1903.

Rahman, I. U.; Ijaz, F.; Afzal, A.; Iqbal, Z.; Ali, N.; Khan, S. M. Contributions to the Phyto-therapies of Digestive Disorders; Traditional Knowledge and Cultural Drivers of Manoor Valley, Northern Pakistan. *J. Ethnopharmacol.* **2016,** *192*, 30–52.

Ray, R.; Ray, A. Medicinal Practices of Sacred Natural Site: A Socio-Religious Approach for Successful Implementation of Primary Healthcare Services. *Ethnobot. Res. Appl.* **2020,** *20*, 1–46.

Sadeer, N. B.; Llorent-Martínez, E. J.; Bene, K.; Mahomoodally, M. F.; Mollica, A. et al. Chemical Profiling, Antioxidant, Enzyme Inhibitory and Molecular Modelling Studies on the Leaves and Stem Bark Extracts of Three African Medicinal Plants. *J. Pharm. Biomed. Anal.* **2019,** *174*, 19–33.

Sen, U. K.; Bhakat, R. K. Conservation of Resources by Religious and Social Prohibitions by Santal Communities in South West Bengal, India. *Time and Mind* **2021,** *14*, 332.

Sen, U. K.; Bhakat, R. K. Assessment of Psammophytic Medicinal Plant Diversity Used Among the Rural Communities in Coastal East Midnapore, West Bengal, India. *J. Herbs, Spices Med. Pl.* **2020,** *26*, 219–247.

Sen, U. K.; Bhakat, R. K. Ethnobotanical Study on Sand-Dune Based Medicinal Plants and Traditional Therapies in Coastal Purba Medinipur District, West Bengal, India. *Eur. J. Med. Pl.* **2018,** *26*, 119.

Sharma, S.; Kumar, R. Sacred Groves of India: Repositories of a Rich Heritage and Tools for Biodiversity Conservation. *J. For. Res.* **2020,** *32*, 899–916.

Singh, B.; Singh, B.; Kishor, A.; Singh, S.; Bhat, M. N. et al. Exploring Plant-Based Ethnomedicine and Quantitative Ethnopharmacology: Medicinal Plants Utilized by the Population of Jasrota Hill in Western Himalaya. *Sustainability* **2020,** *12*, 7526.

Sivasankari, B.; Anandharaj, M.; Gunasekaran, P. An Ethnobotanical Study of Indigenous Knowledge on Medicinal Plants Used by the Village Peoples of Thoppampatti, Dindigul District, Tamil Nadu, India. *J. Ethnopharmacol.* **2014,** *153*, 408–423.

Tardio, J.; Pardo-de-Santayana, M. Cultural Importance Indices: A Comparative Analysis Based on the Useful Wild Plants of Southern Cantabria (Northern Spain). *Econ. Bot.* **2008,** *62*, 24–39.

Thorley, A.; Gunn, C. M. *Sacred Sites: An Overview*; The Gaia Foundation: London, 2008; p 39.

Tynsong, H., Dkhar, M., Tiwari, B. K. Traditional Ecological Knowledge of Tribal Communities of North East India. *Biodiversitas* **2020,** *21,* 3209–3224.

Ullah, S.; Muhammad, N. Evaluation of Informant Consensus Factor of Medicinal Plants Used in Shamozai Valley Swat, KPK, Pakistan. *Int. J. Med. Pl. Nat. Prod.* **2018,** *4*, 1–7.

Upadhyay, B.; Roy, S.; Kumar, A. Traditional Uses of Medicinal Plants Among the Rural Communities of Churu District in the Thar Desert, India. *J. Ethnopharmacol.* **2007,** *113*, 387–399.

Utzinger, J.; Becker, S. L.; Knopp, S.; Blum, J.; Neumayr, A. L. et al. Neglected Tropical Diseases: Diagnosis, Clinical Management, Treatment and Control. *Swiss Med. Wkly.* **2012,** *142*, w13727.

Wangchuk, P.; Keller, P. A.; Pyne, S. G.; Taweechotipatr, M.; Tonsomboon, A. et al. Evaluation of an Ethnopharmacologically Selected Bhutanese Medicinal Plants for Their Major Classes of Phytochemicals and Biological Activities. *J. Ethnopharmacol.* **2011,** *137*, 730–742.

WCVP. *World Checklist of Vascular Plants*, Version 2.0. Facilitated by the Royal Botanic Gardens, Kew, 2021. http://wcvp.science.kew.org/ (accessed on April 28, 2021)

PART III

Indigenous Flora and Human Health

CHAPTER 6

Indigenous Medicinal Knowledge of the Common Medicinal Plants of Coastal Karnataka, India

KAKEKOCHI KESHAVACHANDRA[1], MUNDAMOOLE PAVITHRA[2], and KANDIKERE R. SRIDHAR[2,3]

[1]*Post-Graduate Department of Botany, Moodbidre, Karnataka, India*

[2]*Department of Biosciences, Mangalore University, Mangalagangotri, Mangalore, Karnataka, India*

[3]*Centre for Environmental Studies, Yenepoya (Deemed to be University), Mangalore, Karnataka, India*

ABSTRACT

The story of drugs and use of medicinal plants dates back to the prehistoric era. There are well known remedies of chronic ailments in classical texts as well as in indigenous knowledge. In the present study, an effort is made to document some simple remedies of 12 commonly used medicinal plants of the coastal Karnataka of India for chronic ailments (asthma, bronchitis, and furuncle). These plants have the capacity to increase the immunity, helpful as antidotes with unique formulations and processes using either whole plant or part of plant or part along with other plants. Majority of such plants recorded are climbers. Their applications are mainly documented according to use as

Ethnic Knowledge and Perspectives of Medicinal Plants, Volume 1: Curative Properties and Treatment Strategies. Munir Ozturk, Kandikere R. Sridhar, Maryam Sarwat, Volkan Altay, & Francisco Martín Huerta-Martínez (Eds.)

home remedies and there is an urgent need to optimise their use by modern investigation methods.

6.1 INTRODUCTION

The story of drugs and use of medicinal plants dates back to prehistoric era (Ozturk et al., 2020, 2021a, b). The Indian sages invented drugs and their therapeutic uses, which are well documented and the modern world recognises them as codified system of medicines such as Ayurveda and Siddha. A long association between the people of a specific region with ethnic knowledge and the plants in their locality has been more intimate. Use of medicinal plant products could be traced toward beginning of the human civilization. The oldest documentation of medicinal plants in Hindu culture or in Indian subcontinent is recorded in "*Rigveda,*" which is said to have been drafted during 4500 BC and 1600 BC, which seems to be the oldest repository of the human knowledge (Malla and Shakya, 1984). Traditional medicinal systems have been practiced to treat various human ailments in many countries like as China, India, and Japan (Ram et al., 2009). The "*Atharvaveda*" describes applications of a large number of drugs. In ancient India, two important classical texts are known: (1) "*Charaka-Samhita*" written by Charaka who was an ancient healer; (2) "*Susruta-Samhita*" written by Susruta an ancient surgeon as well as healer. These documents deal with about 700 Indian medicinal plants used in ethnic therapy. "*Vrikshayurveda*" is the science of medicinal plants, it was written by Parasara.

According to the WHO, over 80% of the world's population in the developing countries depend primarily on plant-based medicines for their basic wellbeing and healthcare requirements. A systematic survey, data gathering, specific documentation are *sine qua none* for success in the ethnobotanical studies. Similar trend of documentation center has also involved to gather all such information that will be helpful to identify to proper drug mentioned in Ayurvedic texts and lexicons (Raghunathan, 2010). In the recent times, due to high rate of anthropogenic disturbances (e.g., cattle grazing, fuel wood extraction, fire menace, and pollution), several medicinal flora are facing danger of extinction and loss of diversity. Recognition of suitable herbal plant species easily available and ethnic knowledge toward their therapeutic use are important in human wellbeing (Kaur and Vashistha, 2014). There was always exchange of views between Indian and foreign medical practitioners, which is evident by addition of new drugs into pharmacopoeia of other countries and addition of several unknown drugs to their own pharmacopoeia (Sharma, 2010). With an increased pressure on the popular or common edible and medicinal plants, it is absolutely essential to discover new sources. It is evident that documentation of traditional knowledge contributes toward such effort in many ways (Jain, 1995). Ayurvedic medical management of human ailments is multidimensional especially cumulative impacts rather than relying on a single molecule (Payyappallimana et al., 2020). According to Camara-Leret and Bascompto (2021), extinction of regional/vernacular languages causes the loss of traditional knowledge on medicinal plants.

Treating common ailments with naturally and easily available plant sources near the residence is known as home remedy. Many remedies are having years of history and some might have been standardized by the trial and error basis. Although traditional medicine and home remedies are two different aspects, they were all derived from Ayurveda (Santhosh and Amritha, 2020). The present study deals with the cumulative efforts of the documentation of traditional knowledge gained in different localities by experienced elders of the family, which is practicing herbal therapies based on the classical texts. Emphasis is given on the diseases and problems related to the diseases of respiratory tract, promotion of immunity and remedies to cure wounds using the most commonly occurring medicinal plants widely used in home remedies in coastal Karnataka state of India.

6.2 COMMON MEDICINAL PLANTS

Although climbers are neglected compared to other herbs, they are highly medicinal. Table 6.1 provides a list of eight climbers along with two herbs, and one each of shrub and tree used in home remedy toward treating ailments and also to boost the immunity (Figure 6.1).

6.2.1 CISSUS QUADRANGULARIS

It aids in recovery of the strength of the bones up to 90% in 6 weeks. In classical texts of Ayurveda, it is mentioned as "*Asthisamhaara*" toward rejuvenation of good health of bone (Kharre, 2007). According to the holistic concept of drug administration in Ayurveda, this plant is a doctrine of signatures, that is, the morphologically quadrangular stem resembles the

TABLE 6.1 Details of Common Plant Species in Medications in the Coastal Karnataka, India.

Plant species	Family	Vernacular name (Kannada)	Part used	Administration*
Cissus quadrangularis L. (C)	Vitaceae	Sandu balli	Stem	Paste for topical application
Cyclea peltata (Lam.) Hook.f. & Thomson (C)	Menispermaceae	Hade balli	Fresh leaves	Paste for topical application
Dregea volubilis (L.f.) Benth. ex Hook.f. (C)	Apocynaceae	Kadu hale balli/Hegalu balli	Leaves	Paste for topical application
Hemidesmus indicus (L.) R.Br. ex Schult. (C)	Apocynaceae	Nama sogade/Sogade beru	Root	Juice for oral consumption
Ichnocarpus frutescens (L.) W.T.Aiton (C)	Apocynaceae	Gowri balli	Root	Juice for oral consumption
Justicia adhatoda L. (S)	Acanthaceae	Adusoge	Leaves	Juice with ginger for oral consumption
Macaranga peltata (Roxb.) Muell. Arg. (T)	Euphorbiaceae	Uppalige	Gum of the petiole	Paste for topical application
Phyllanthus amarus Schumach. & Thonn. (H)	Phyllanthaceae	Nela nelli	Whole plant and root	Juice for oral consumption
Plectranthus amboinicus (Lour.) Spreng. (H)	Lamiaceae	Doddapatre/Sambrani soppu	Whole plant and root	Juice for oral consumption
Pothos scandens L. (C)	Aeraceae	Adikebeelu soppu	Stem	Root crushed with coconut oil for topical application
Tinospora cordifolia (Willd.) Miers (C)	Menispermaceae	Amruta balli	Stem	Juice for oral consumption
Tylophora indica (Burm. F.) Merr. (C)	Apocynaceae	Adumuttada balli	Leaves	Consumption of fresh leaves

Abbreviation: C, climber; H, herb; S, shrub; T, tree.

**See more details on remedy of each plant species.*

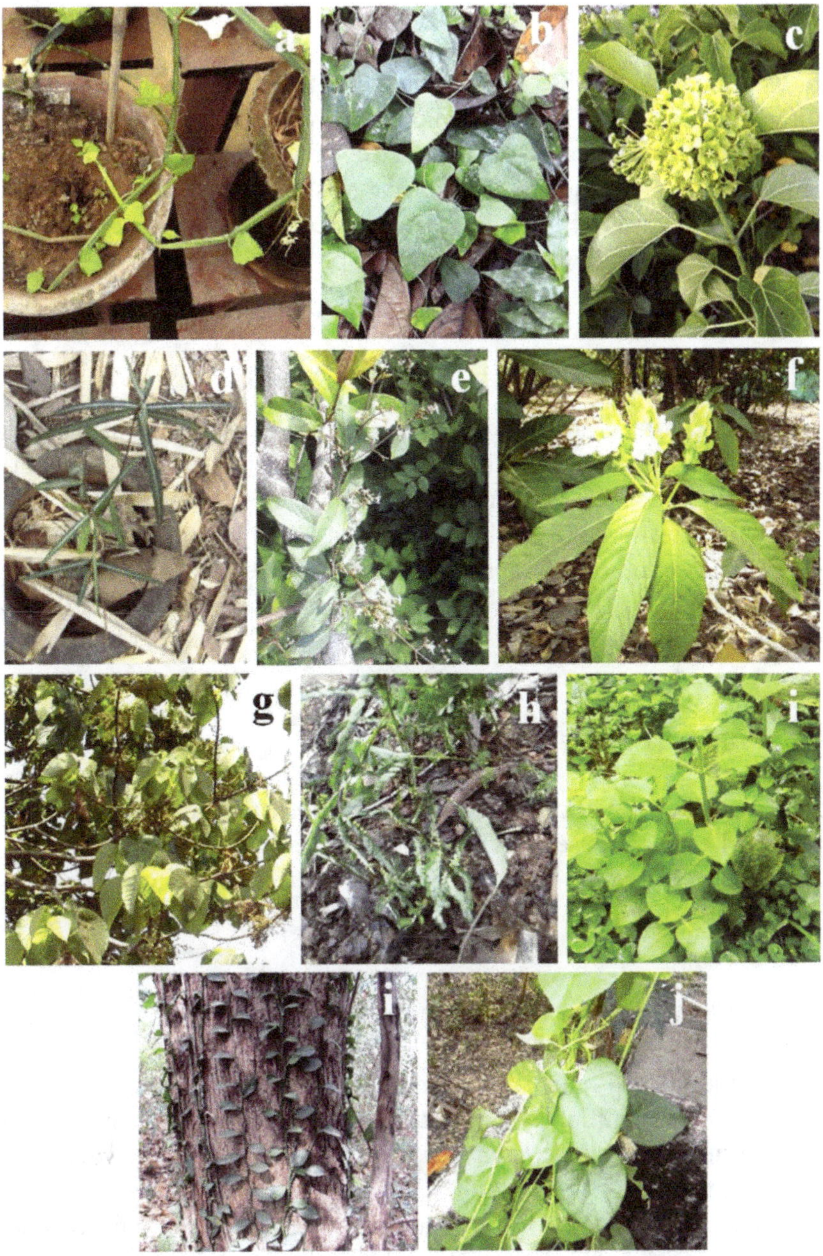

FIGURE 6.1 Indigenous common ethnic medicinal plants of coastal Karnataka: *Cissus quadrangularis* (a), *Cyclea peltata* (b), *Dregea volubilis* (c), *Hemidesmus indicus* (d), *Ichnocarpus frutescens* (e), *Justicia adhatoda* (f), *Macaranga peltata* (g), *Phyllanthus amarus* (h), *Plectranthus amboinicus* (i), *Pothos scandens* (j), and *Tinospora cordifolia* (k).

bone. The stem juice of this plant is useful in treating scurvy, menstrual disorders, otorrhoea (ear, nose, and throat ailments), and epistaxis (nose bleed). The herb is fed to cattle to induce easy milk flow (Sen and Dash, 2012). Paste prepared from the whole plant could be bandaged over bone fractured area with support of sticks. Decoction of plant also be applied on the wounds for quick healing (Panda and Mishra, 2016). The juice obtained from the stem could be used drop by drop to nostrils as remedy to cure the nose bleeding (Gurudeva, 2014).

6.2.2 CYCLEA PELTATA

Peoples of coastal Karnataka use this plant as a cooling agent (Bhandary and Chandrashekar, 2011). This also serve as herbal shampoo: about 20 leaves are crushed added to a mug full of water (~250 ml) to get viscous fluid for application over scalp and eyes as coolant (Hullatti et al., 2011). For burning sensation of chest, the paste of leaves can be applied to get relief from the pain (Bhandary et al., 1995). It is also useful to cure the fever (Kingston et al., 2007).

6.2.3 DREGEA VOLUBILIS

It is a very common climber and traditionally used in treating cold and eye diseases. Leaves are used in curing boils and abscesses (Shahla, 2011). In Ayurveda, it is used as sternutatory (having effect on sneezing) and eye-related disorders.

6.2.4 HEMIDESMUS INDICUS

Popularly known as Indian Sarsaparilla and it is a common twining under shrub. It can be identified by variegated elongated leaves with white conspicuous marking. This plant is having broad spectrum activity and two important formulations called "*Sarivadyasava*" and "*Sarivadyarishta*" containing many other herbs with *Hemidesmus* as the main ingradient can cure rheumatic pain (Shetty et al., 2002; Nandy et al., 2020). Traditionally the roots are also used as remedy for scorpion stings, snakebites, abdominal pain, anorexia, cough, diabetes, diarrhea, dyspnea (shortness of breath), dysentery, fever, menorrhagia, oligospermia rheumatism, and urinary disorders. Traditional medicine and home remedies use this plant in the preparation of "Panaka" (juice with jaggary). Its dried roots are boiled along with *Chrysopogon zizanioides* (bunch grass) to use in drinking water to get pleasant aroma and believed to be a coolant rejuvenates or improves blood circulation. Ethanol extract of the roots contain an alkaloid called "hindicusine," which serve as a good antioxidant (Sethi et al., 2010; Gurudeva, 2014).

6.2.5 *ICHNOCARPUS FRUTESCENS*

This is commonly known as the Black Sariva, an important medicinal plant found throughout India. In Ayurveda, it serves as a substitute for *H. indicus* (Shetty et al., 2002; Chowdhary et al., 2012). Decoction prepared from leaves and stem is used to cure fever and skin diseases.

6.2.6 *JUSTICIA ADHATODA*

Traditionally used from time immemorial as an expectorant and respiration related disorders like asthma. Phrmacognostically its leaf provides bronchodilator drug. Many tribes in India chew leaf buds alone or with ginger to clear respiratory passages (Yadav and Yadav, 2018). In Indian families, the leaf is dried over a hot plate or by the side of the flame (without exposing to flame directly). The primary alkaloid constituents of *Justiciaa* (vasicine and vasicinone) are well established therapeutic respiratory agents (Dorsch and Wagner, 1991). These alkaloids in equal ratio (1:1) showed the bronchodilatory activity in vitro as well as in vivo (Atal, 1980).

6.2.7 *MACARANGA PELTATA*

It is a common plant in Southeast Asia. In coastal Karnataka, people traditionally use this plant as a wound healer for sores and wounds especially to treat furuncle (boils) (Nehete and Tatke, 2016). Application of petiole gum externally twice a day up to 3–4 days will burst the furuncle and cures without any other medication.

6.2.8 PHYLLANTHUS AMARUS

A popular hepato-protective herb common in coastal Karnataka. It is used to traditionally to treat the jaundice. Its roots are bruised with raw milk and consumed orally for empty stomach daily in the morning. Kashaya (juice) prepared from the whole plant with a few fruits of *Piper nigrum* (pepper), a small piece of ginger (*Zingiber officinale*) and a few pieces of stem of *Tinospora sinensis*. Ingredients taken in ~200 ml water, boiled to reduce the volume up to 100 ml and consumed orally to improve or boost the immunity. Bhattacharya et al. (2003) reported that this plant has antihepatitis B virus property. In majority of the Ayurvedic or medicinal plant literature published in India give the nomenclature of this species as *Phyllanthus niruri*. But, this species does not exist in India, thus the same name could be synonymized as *P. niruri* auct. non L. (meaning: this species is not the Linnaeus account of *P. niruri* and it is different one), hence the correct name is *Phyllanthus amarus* Schumach. & Thonn.

6.2.9 P. AMBOINICUS

It is a common herb found in home gardens and its leaves serve as a good expectorant. Generally, the Lamiaceae members are good expectorants (Raja, 2012). Leaves dried around the flame, juice prepared by squeezing and addition of equal amount of honey. On mixing and administration orally will be very effective for children to expel the cough. The juice will be mixed with sugar is also serve as powerful carminative (relieving flatulence) (Prajapati et al., 2006). The leaf juice will also applied to treat the skin to cure the allergic skin thickening, insect bites, irritaton, itching and to overcome "*kapha*" (mucus or phlegm) (Wadikar and Patki, 2016). On chewing two to three leaves thrice a day affectively cures tonsils (Gurudeva 2001).

6.2.10 P. SCANDENS

P. scandens is traditionally used to treat small pox and wound caused by snake bite (Sojeethra and Acharya, 2020). Its roots are crushed and fried in oil (preferably in coconut oil) for application to abscesses. Its smoked stem with camphor and inhalation serve as a best medicine for asthma (Shetty et al., 2002).

6.2.11 *TINOSPORA CORDIFOLIA*

A climbing shrub largely used as an antipyretic drug. In Ayurveda, it is used as an antipyretic (for the treatment of fever) in a proprietary medicine called "*Amrutarishta.*" Pharmacognostically, it is popularly regarded as the stem drug (Gokhlae et al., 2013). In home remedies, it is used for dengue and chikungunya. Small pieces of raw stem (45 pieces) boiled in one glass of water, reduced the volume to one-third and oral administration after cooling twice a day will be effective against fever. The Kashaya prepared from this plant mixed with gum or resin of *Commiphora mukul* (2 g) and on oral administration twice a day cures arthritis (Gurudeva, 2001).

6.2.12 *TYLOPHORA INDICA*

This herb is especially effective in the treatment of bronchial asthma. Various studies have shown that alkaloids present in *T. indica* suppress cellular immune response. The fresh leaves of this plant chewed and swallowed daily along with water during the early morning to empty stomach for a week gives moderate or complete relief from asthma.

6.3 CONCLUSIONS

Harnessing the plant medicinal potential is very important and valuable especially to those countries lack of basic medical facilities. The present study has documented 12 most commonly available and ethnically used plant species for medicinal purposes in the southwest region of Karnataka. These consists of nine climbers, two herbs and one each of shrub and tree. In Ayurveda, currently several studies have been carried out on poly herbal formulations (herbs with similar properties) having curative effects on several aliments (e.g., antiviral formulations). The composition of ingredients and mode of preparation (or formulation) assumes importance in tackling specific ailment. Nowadays it is absolutely necessary to practice poly herbal remedies toward effective curing of one or more ailments and toward immunomodulation. In this context, five species (*P. amarus, P. amboinicus, P. scandens, Justicia adhathoda,* and *T. indica*) are useful as immunity boosters and they have the potential to cure the respiratory related ailments. Specific combination of these plant species may provide immunity against viral diseases including the corona and related viruses.

KEYWORDS

- **Ayurveda**
- **home remedies**
- **human ailments**
- **immunity boosters**
- **medicinal plants**
- **traditional knowledge**

REFERENCES

Atal, C. K. *Chemistry and Pharmacology of Vasicine—A New Oxytocic and Abortifacient*; Regional Research Laboratory: Jammu Tawi, India, 1980; p 37.

Bhandary, M. J.; Chandrashekar, K. R.; Kaveriappa, K. M. Medical Ethnobotany of the Siddis of Uttara Kannada District, Karnataka, India *J. Ethnopharmacol.* **1995,** *47*, 149–158.

Bhandary, M. J.; Chandrashekar K. R. Herbal Therapy for Herpes in the Ethno-Medicine of Coastal Karnataka. *Ind. J. Trad. Know.* **2011,** *10*, 528–532.

Bhattacharyya, R.; Bhattacharya, S.; Wenzel-Mothers, M.; Buckwold, V. E. *Phyllanthus amarus* Root Clone with Significant Activity Against Bovine Viral Diarrhoea Virus—a Surrogate Model of Hepatitis C Virus. *Curr. Sci.* **2003,** *84*, 529–533.

Camara-Leret, R.; Bascompto, J. Language Extinction Triggers the Loss of Unique Medicinal Knowledge. *Proc. Nat. Sci. Acad.* **2021,** *118*, e2103683118.

Chowdhary, K.; Agarwal, B.; Rajiv, S. K. *Ichnocarpus Frutescens*: A Medicinal Plant with Broad Spectrum. *Indo Glob. J. Pharma. Sci.* **2012,** *2*, 63–69.

Dorsch, W.; Wagner, H. New Antiasthmatic Drugs from Traditional Medicine. *Int. Arch. Aller. Immunol.* **1991,** *94*, 262–265.

Gokhlae, S. B.; Kokate, C. K.; Purohit, A. P. *Pharmacognosy*—III, Nirali Prakashan, Pune, India, 2013; p 880.

Gurudeva, R. M. *Karnatakada Aushadeeya Sasyagalu*, Vol. 2; Divyachandra Prakashana: Basaveshwaranagar, Bangalore, India, 2001; p 472.

Gurudeva, R. M. *Karnatakada Aushadeeya Sasyagalu*, Vol. 3; Divyachandra Prakashana: Basaveshwaranagar, Bangalore, India, 2014; p 1352.

Hullatti, K.; Gopikrishna, U.; Kuppast, I. Phytochemical Investigation and Diuretic Activity of *Cyclea peltata* Leaf Extracts. *J. Adv. Pharma. Technol. Res.* **2011,** *2*, 241–244.

Jain, S. K. *A Manual of Ethnobotany*; Scientific Publishers: Jodhpur, India, 1995; p 242.

Kaur, R.; Vashistha, B. D. Ethnobotanical Studies on Karnal District, Haryana, India. *Int. Res. J. Biol. Sci.* **2014,** *3*, 46–55.

Kharre, C. P. *Indian Medicinal Plants—An Illustrated Dictionary*; Springer-Verlag: New York, 2007; p 900.

Kingston C.; Nisha B. S.; Kiruba S.; Jeeva. S. Ethnomedicinal Plants by INDIGENOUS COMMUNITY in Traditional Health Care System. *Ethnobot. Leaflets*, 2007. https://opensiuc.lib.siu.edu/ebl/vol2007/iss1/7

Malla, S. B.; Shakya, P. R. *Medicinal Plants of Nepal*. In: *Nepal Nature's Paradise*; Majupuria, T. C., Ed.; Bangkok, Thailand, 1984; pp 261–297.

Nandy, S.; Mukherjee, A.; Pandey, D. K. et al. Sarsaparilla (*Hemidesmus indicus*): Recent progress in research on Ethnobotany, Phytochemistry and Pharmacology *J. Ethnopharmacol.* **2020,** *254*, 112609.

Nehete, M.; Tatke, P. Antioxidant, Antimicrobial and Wound Healing Potential of *Macaranga peltata* Bark Extracts. *Eur. J. Pharma. Med. Res.* **2016,** *3*, 313–320.

Ozturk, M.; Egamberdieva, D.; Milica, P. *Biodiversity and Biomedicine-Our Future*; Academic Press; Elsevier Inc, 2020.

Ozturk, M.; Altay, V.; Efe, R. *Biodiversity, Conservation and Sustainability in Asia: Volume I: Prospects and Challenges in West Asia and Caucasus*; Springer Nature: Switzerland AG, 2021a. DOI: 10.1007/978–3-030–59928–7.

Ozturk, M.; Khan, S. M.; Altay, V.; Efe, R.; Egamberdieva, D.; Khassanov, F. *Biodiversity, Conservation and Sustainability in Asia: Volume II: Prospects and Challenges in South and Middle Asia*; Springer Nature Switzerland AG, 2021b. DOI: 10.1007/978–3-030–73943–0.

Panda, T.; Mishra, N. Indigenous Knowledge on Animal Health Care Practices in Kendrapara District of Odisha, India. *Int. Lett. Nat. Sci.* **2016,** *53*, 10–27.

Payyappallimana, U.; Patwardhan, K.; Mangalath, P. et al. The COVID-19 Pandemic and the Relevance of Ayurveda's Whole Systems Approach to Health and Disease Management. *J. Alt. Complem. Med.* **2020,** *26*, 1089–1092.

Prajapati, N. D.; Purohit, S. S.; Sharma, A. K.; Kumar, T. *A Handbook of Medicinal Plants: A Complete Source Book.* Agrobios: Jodhpur, India, 2006; p 928.

Raghunathan, K. Medico-Ethno-Botanical Survey and Their Role in Research in Ayurveda In *A Manual of Ethnobotany*; Jain, S. K., Ed.; Scientific Publishers: Jodhpur, India, 2010; pp 86–101.

Raja, R. R. Medicinally Potential Plants of Labiatae (Lamiaceae) Family: An Overview. *Res. J. Med. Pl.* **2012,** *6*, 203–213.

Ram, A.; Duraisamy, A. J.; Selvakumar, B.; Singh, V. P. Medicinal Plants from Siddha System of Medicine Useful for Treating Respiratory Diseases. *Int. J. Pharma. Anal.* **2009,** *1*, 20–30.

Santhosh, C.; Amritha, M. S. Home Remedies-a Scientific Analysis. *World J. Pharma. Res.* **2020,** *9*, 1288–1294.

Sen, M. K.; Dash, B. K. A Review on Phytochemical and Pharmacological Aspects of *Cissus quadrangularis* L. *Int. J. Green Pharm.* **2012,** *6*, 169–173.

Sethi, A.; Bhatia, A.; Srivastava, S. et al. Pregnane Glycoside from *Hemidesmus indicus* as a Potential Anti-Oxidant and Anti-Dyslipidemic Agent. *Nat. Prod. Res.* **2010,** *24*, 1371–1378.

Shahla, N. Studies on *Wattakaka volubilis* (L.F.) Stap. A Medicinally Important Plant. *Res. J. Pharma. Biol. Chem. Sci.* 2011, *2*, 1964–1969.

Sharma P. V. *Introduction to Dravyaguna (Indian Pharmacology)*; Chaukamba Publishers: Varanasi, 2010; p 226.

Shetty B. V.; Kaveriappa K. M.; Bhat, G. K. *Plant Resources of Western Ghats and Lowlands of Dakshina Kannada and Udupi Districts*; Pilikula Nisarga Dhama Society: Mangalore, India, 2002; p 264.

Sojeetra, N. H.; Acharya, R. A Review on Ethnomedicinal Claims and Spread of *Pothos scandens* L. *Eur. J. Med. Pl.* **2020,** *31*, 22–28.

Wadikar, D. D.; Patki E. P. *Coleus aromaticus*: A Therapeutic Herb with Multiple Potentials *J. Food Sci. Technol.* **2016,** *53*, 2895–2901.

Yadav, S.; Yadav, V. K. Ethnomedicinal Value and Pharmacognosy of the Member of Acanthaceae: *Adhatoda vasica* (Linn.). *Asian Pac. J. Health Sci.* **2018,** *5*, 40–43.

CHAPTER 7

The Genus *Phyllanthus:* A Rich Source of Pharmacologically Active Compounds Useful in Traditional and Modern Medicines

K. K. SAMPATH KUMARA[1], S. SHISHUPALA[2], and H. S. PRAKASH[1]

[1]*Department of Studies in Biotechnology, University of Mysore, Manasagangothri, Mysore, Karnataka, India*

[2]*Department of Microbiology, Davangere University, Shivagangothri, Davangere, Karnataka, India*

ABSTRACT

The genus *Phyllanthus* (Family, Phyllanthaceae) includes more than 1200 species. *Phyllanthus amarus, Phyllanthus debilis, Phyllanthus emblica, Phyllanthus fraternus*, and *Phyllanthus urinaria* are found to be useful in Ayurvedic medicine to treat liver and kidney diseases. Although *Phyllanthus* species closely resemble each other, their ethnomedical uses and pharmacological activities are quite different. *Phyllanthus* species produce alkaloids, coumarins, flavonoids, lignans, and terpenes that are attributed to antioxidant, anticancer, hepatoprotective, antidiabetic, hypotensive, anti-inflammatory, and antiviral activities. Corilagin, ellagic acid, and gallic acid isolated from *Phyllanthus* species are considered to be natural antioxidants and used in the preparation of cosmeceutical products. The hypotensive and analgesic effects were attributed to specific phytochemical compounds geraniin

Ethnic Knowledge and Perspectives of Medicinal Plants, Volume 1: Curative Properties and Treatment Strategies. Munir Ozturk, Kandikere R. Sridhar, Maryam Sarwat, Volkan Altay, & Francisco Martín Huerta-Martínez (Eds.)

and ellagitannin. The hepatoprotective and antiviral activities have been attributed to lignans called phyllanthin and hypophyllanthin. Repandusinic acid A and niruriside produced by *Phyllanthus niruri* demonstrated significant reverse transcriptase inhibition. The current chapter discusses the use of different *Phyllanthus* species in traditional and modern medicinal system.

7.1 INTRODUCTION

Medicinal plants and their products constitute a treasury of immense value to mankind as they provide the most important ingredients for essential drugs both in traditional and modern system of medicine (Younessi-Hamze-khanlu et al., 2020; Ozturk et al., 2020, 2021a, b). The herbal medicines not only form the basis of primary health care in developing countries but also gained importance in developed countries as they are considered to be natural alternatives to synthetic drugs (Ozturk and Hakeem, 2018, 2019a, b; Plevkanovskaya et al., 2019; Masoodi et al., 2020). Use of traditional medicine over several generations by the practitioners of indigenous systems of medicine proved the sustained therapeutic value of medicinal plants. Traditional system of medicine is still widely practiced due to rise in population, inadequate drugs supply, and expensive cost of treatments and serious side effects associated with several allopathic drugs. Many plant species are being used as a source of traditional medicines for many human diseases (Petrovska, 2012; Ozturk et al., 2014, 2016, 2017a, b, c, 2018a, b, c, d, e, f, g). Medicinal plants are also rich sources of a large number of pharmacologically active therapeutic compounds used in different systems of medicine. Medicinal plants belong to a wide range of plant taxa and closely related species. More than 72,000 medicinal plants have been reported. *Phyllanthus* is one of the closely related taxa are being commonly used in traditional system of medicine. Many *Phyllanthus* species are being in use for the treatments of chronic dysentery, diabetes, jaundice, gonorrhea, hepatitis B, kidney-related ailments, pain, skin ulcers, and urinary bladder ailments (Calixto et al., 1998).

Linnaeus described the genus *Phyllanthus* for the first time in 1753. This genus belongs to family Phyllanthaceae. *Phyllanthus* is known as one of the largest genera among angiosperms with 1270 species with distribution spread over tropics and subtropics (Hoffmann et al., 2006). Among the herbaceous species of genus *Phyllanthus*: *Phyllanthus amarus*, *Phyllanthus debilis*, *Phyllanthus fraternus*, and *Phyllanthus urinaria* have been used for over 2000 years in Ayurvedic system of medicine. *Phyllanthus* is useful to treat Jaundice and other liver disorders in Burma, China, India, Pakistan, Philippines, South America, West Indies, and Africa (Unander et al., 1990; Calixto et al., 1998). *Phyllanthus niruri* is the major species used in different systems of medicine. It is known as "*Chanca Piedra*" (Spanish) and "*Quebra Pedra*" (Brazil), meaning "stone breaker," as it is effective treatment against gall and kidney stones. It also has a major role in treating diabetes, hepatitis, and kidney disorders (Santos et al., 1995). Webster (1957) reported that *P. niruri* is one of the natives of New World being endemic to America and not present in India. However, publications from India and other Asian countries reported *P. niruri*. This highlights the confusion in identification of *Phyllanthus* species (Dnyaneshwar et al., 2006). In India, *Phyllanthus* spp.: *P. amarus*, *P. debilis*, *P. fraternus*, and *P. urinaria* forms a complex group collectively known as "*Bhumyamalaki*" or "*Bhuiamla*"" and wrongly identified as *P. niruri*, often referred as "niruri complex." Even *Phyllanthus maderaspatensis*, *Phyllanthus tenellus*, and *Phyllanthus virgatus* are used as substitutes for "Bhumyamalaki." In Thailand, *P. amarus*, *P. debilis*, *P. urinaria*, and *P. virgatus* are collectively known as "*Luk-tai-bai*" or "*Ya-tai-bai*." Mitra and Jain (1987) critically examined Indian herbarium specimens of *Phyllanthus* species which are often misidentified with *P. niruri* and clearly stated that *P. niruri* described in Flora of British India actually consist of three closely related but distinct species such as *P. amarus*, *P. debilis*, and *P. fraternus*. Therefore, research publications from India having the name *P. niruri* are actually related to any one member of the "niruri complex" and not exactly on the *P. niruri* (Dnyaneshwar et al., 2006). Although, *P. niruri* is closely resembles *P. amarus* in morphology and phytochemical constituents, cladistic analysis indicated that *P. niruri* and *P. amarus* are distinct species (Lee et al., 2006a). Another *Phyllanthus* species, *Phyllanthus emblica*, widely used in traditional medicine in India, China, and Tibet is commonly known as "Amla" or "Indian gooseberry" and the fruits of this plant are considered as powerful rejuvenator (Yang and Liu, 2014).

Phytochemical investigation had shown that *Phyllanthus* produces lignans, alkaloids, terpenoids, flavonoids, and tannins. Mao et al. (2016) have listed over 500 phytochemicals isolated from different species of *Phyllanthus*. Many of the chemical compounds were unique to *Phyllanthus* and were highly bioactive. However, available phytochemical data represent less than 10% of the *Phyllanthus* species. Therefore, detailed phytochemical studies are needed covering other *Phyllanthus* species, owing to their diverse traditional medicinal uses (Nahar et al., 2011). Many studies have been conducted on pharmacological activities of *Phyllanthus* due to the extensive therapeutic applications in traditional medicine and diverse secondary metabolites they produce. Compounds isolated from *Phyllanthus* species are shown to have antioxidant, hepatoprotective, antidiabetic, hypotensive, and antiviral activities (Kalidas and Mohan, 2009). The main objective of the present chapter is to provide a comprehensive account on traditional medicinal uses of *Phyllanthus* species along with bioactive compounds, the pharmacological properties, and their utilization as phytomedicine.

7.2 *PHYLLANTHUS* IN TRADITIONAL MEDICINE

Phyllanthus species are used throughout the world in different traditional systems of medicine, especially in India, China, Brazil, and the Southeast Asian countries since ancient times (Mao et al., 2016). "Ayurveda" is an important traditional system of medicine practiced in Indian subcontinent in which about 15 *Phyllanthus* species are useful in the treatment of genitourinary, hepatic, digestive, and respiratory ailments. In Chinese and Tibetan system of traditional medicine, five *Phyllanthus* species have been used to treat hypertension and hepatitis B (Nain et al., 2012). *Phyllanthus acidus, P. amarus, P. debilis, P. emblica, P. fraternus, P. maderaspatensis, P. myrtifolius, P. niruri, P. reticulatus, P. tenellus, P. urinaria,* and *P. virgatus* are the most important source of traditional medicine in different parts of the world (Figure 7.1). Use of these *Phyllanthus* species in traditional system of medicines practiced in different countries is described here.

7.2.1 *P. ACIDUS*

P. acidus (L.) Skeels is commonly known as "star gooseberry" and distributed mainly in India and other Asian countries. The edible fruits are employed in Ayurveda as a liver tonic and a blood purifier. Root, stem, leaves, and fruits are used to treat jaundice, bronchitis, constipation, and piles. Star gooseberry fruit is used for improvement of eyesight and memory. It is also a remedy for diabetes and cough (Unander et al., 1990; Kirtikar and Basu, 1993). *P. acidus* is used in the treatment of hypertension and malarial fever in Thailand. In other parts of Asia and South America, it is used in the treatment of inflammation, rheumatism, respiratory diseases, liver diseases, and diabetes (Nain et al., 2012; Tan et al., 2020).

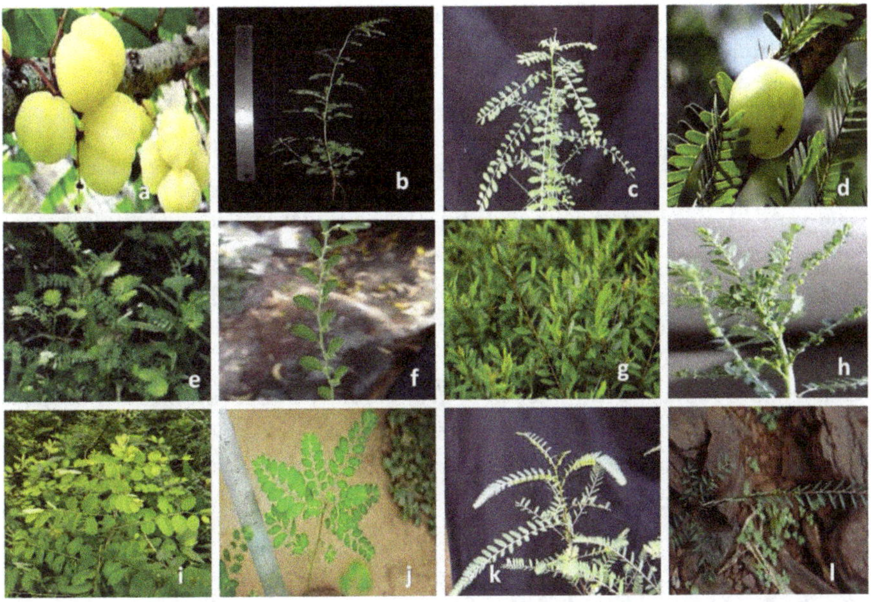

FIGURE 7.1 Major *Phyllanthus* species used in traditional medicine: *Phyllanthus acidus* (a), *P. amarus* (b), *P. debilis* (c), *P. emblica* (d), *P. fraternus* (e), *P. maderaspatensis* (f), *P. myrtifolius* (g), *P. niruri* (h), *P. reticulatus* (i), *P. tenellus* (j), *P. urinaria* (k), and *P. virgatus* (l).

7.2.2 *PHYLLANTHUS AMARUS*

In Ayurvedic system of medicine in India, *P. amarus* Schum. & Thonn. is known as "*Bhumyamalaki.*" Whole plant decoction is administered as a popular remedy for jaundice, stomach and genito-urinary system problems, and liver and kidney disorders. It is also used to treat flu, dropsy, diabetes, asthma, and other respiratory disorders. The aerial parts of *P. amarus* are mainly used in the ethnomedicine of Thailand for treating gonorrhea, diabetic, jaundice, and hepatic disorders (Nain et al., 2012). In Indonesia decoction of this herb is employed to cure liver and kidney problems. Aerial parts of the *P. amarus* are used to cure smallpox and venereal diseases in Nigeria and diabetes in Tanzania. In Peruvian traditional medicine *P. amarus* is known as "*Chanca Piedra*" and the leaves of this plant are used as sedative and astringent and also for diabetes and jaundice treatment (Bagalkotkar et al., 2006). In Brazil and other Latin American countries, African traditional medicine whole plant is used to cure jaundice, renal calculus, and malaria (Poompachee and Chudapongse, 2011). *P. amarus* known as "*Dukung Anak*" in Malaysia, has been traditionally used to treat viral infections, liver, and kidney-related disorders (Masturah et al., 2006).

7.2.3 PHYLLANTHUS DEBILIS

The uses of *P. debilis* Kleni ex Wild. (also known as "*Bhumyamalaki*") are similar to that of *P. amarus* in Ayurvedic medicine of India. Whole plant is employed as traditional remedy for diabetes, dysentery, jaundice, gonorrhea, headache, and skin ulcers. *Phyllanthus debilis* leaf juice is used for eye washing, sore throat, and wound dressing (Calixto et al., 1998). The tribes of Chattisgarh, India use leaf juice of *P. debilis* orally to treat problems associated with sickle-cell anemia. In Thiruvarur District of Tamil Nadu, India, the fresh leaf juice of this plant is taken to cure jaundice and diuresis (Renugadevi and Madhavan, 2016).

7.2.4 PHYLLANTHUS EMBLICA

P. emblica L., commonly known as "*Amla*" or "Indian gooseberry," plays an important role in different traditional systems of Chinese, Indian, Sri Lankan, and Tibetan systems of medicine as a powerful rejuvenator to delay aging. Fruit of Amla is an integral component of Ayurvedic formulation "Triphala" used to promote human health, immunity, and longevity. The Triphala consists of dried and powdered fruits of three plants (*P. emblica, Terminalia bellirica*, and *T. chebula*). It is an excellent laxative and antidiarrheal agent. Therefore, it is consumed as a health tonic by the people (Kumar et al., 2012). The fruits of *P. emblica* are edible and used to treat anemia. The fresh juice of the fruit is diuretic and antibilious. It is also used to overcome thirst, dyspepsia, burning sensation, and digestive problems such as anorexia, jaundice, diarrhea, and ulcers. In Malaysia, *P. emblica* leaves are used to treat fever and in Indonesia fruit pulp is applied on the head to relieve headache and dizziness (Liu et al., 2008).

7.2.5 PHYLLANTHUS FRATERNUS

Whole plant of *P. fraternus* Webster, also known as "*Bhuiamla,*" has astringent, deobstruent, diuretic, febrifugal, and antiseptic properties. In Indian traditional medicine, decoction of this herb is employed as laxative and anthelmintic drugs. The plant extract is employed to cure liver disorders and to expel kidney and gallbladder stones. The roots are considered to be beneficial in the treatment of jaundice. *P. fraternus* is used to cure gastrointestinal problems and diabetes (Kirtikar and Basu, 1993). The plant is reported to be analgesic, carminative, digestive, laxative, stomachic, and vermifuge in West African traditional medicine. In Thiruvarur District, Tamil Nadu, India, the leaf extract is used to treat jaundice and the root decoction for fever, hypertension, and body pain (Renugadevi and Madhavan, 2016).

7.2.6 *P. MADERASPATENSIS*

In Indian traditional medicine, the whole plant of *P. maderaspatensis* L. is used as a laxative and diuretic. The leaves are expectorant and diaphoretic and are used to relieve headache in South India. The seeds are useful in bronchitis, earache, griping, ophthalmia, and ascites, and are also employed in the preparation of liver tonic. The aerial plant parts act as a hepatoprotective agent and also useful in treating cough, blindness, sores, ulcers, stomachache, inflammations, intestinal spasms, fever, burns, and gonorrhea (Kirtikar and Basu, 1993; Khatoon et al., 2006; Renugadevi and Madhavan, 2016).

7.2.7 *PHYLLANTHUS MYRTIFOLIUS*

P. myrtifolius (Wight.) Mull. Arg. is an endemic plant of Sri Lanka and aerial parts are mainly used to treat genitourinary infections. Gastrointestinal diseases, diabetes, skin ulcers, headache, and respiratory ailments are also treated with this plant in traditional medicine (Calixto et al., 1998).

7.2.8 *PHYLLANTHUS NIRURI*

P. niruri, commonly known as "*Chanca Piedra*" or "*Quebra Pedra*" (Spanish) has a long history in traditional Chinese, Indonesian Jamu, Malayan, and Indian Ayurvedic system of medicine. It has a great impact on the health care system of tropical countries where it grows abundantly. In Brazilian and other South American countries, whole plant decoction is used effectively to remove gall stones and kidney stones. It is also used to treat cardiovascular problems, kidney and liver disorders, diabetes, stomachache, asthma, fever, inflammations, malaria, uterine complaints, and intestinal parasites (Santos et al., 1995). In Ayurveda, *P. niruri* is known as "*Bhumyamalaki*" and is extensively used as remedy for jaundice. *Phyllanthus niruri* is known as "*Dukung Anak*" in Malaysia which has been traditionally used to treat diarrhea, viral infections, liver and kidney problems, gonorrhea, and cough. Indonesian popular medicine "*Jamu*" employs aerial parts of this herb to treat viral infections and liver diseases (Khatoon et al., 2006; Masturah et al., 2006). The whole plant is used in treatment of hypertension, constipation, malaria, skin, and urinary disorders in Thailand. In Traditional Chinese Medicine, this herb is used in the treatment of inflammatory diseases, urinary infections, and ophthalmic problems (Nain et al., 2012).

7.2.9 PHYLLANTHUS RETICULATUS

P. reticulatus Poir. is widely used in Tropical Africa and South East Asian traditional medicine. In India, *P. reticulatus* is known as "*Pancoli*" or "*Karinelli*" and the leaves are reported to be bitter, diuretic, refrigerant, and astringent, and are used to treat diabetes and diarrhea. In Africa, dried bark decoction of this plant is a household remedy for gonorrhea, dysmenorrhea, diarrhea, sores, burns, and eye disorders. Dried root bark of *P. reticulatus* promotes fertility, stops anal bleeding, kills the hook worm, and cures smallpox. In South East Asian countries like China, Sri Lanka, Malaysia, and Philippines, the leaves and bark infusion of the plant is used to treat rheumatism, pinworms, syphilis, bowel inflammations, ophthalmic diseases, and bleeding gums. In Thailand, decoction of the above ground plant parts is used to cure constipation, malarial fever, skin, and urinary infections (Unander et al., 1990; Kirtikar and Basu, 1993; Nain et al., 2012).

7.2.10 P. TENELLUS

Health benefits and usage of *P. tenellus* Roxb. is very similar to *P. niruri* in traditional medicine. Aerial part of this herb is mainly used to treat diabetes, hepatitis B, urolithiasis, and bowel inflammations (Silva et al., 2012).

7.2.11 PHYLLANTHUS URINARIA

P. urinaria L. is widely distributed across the globe, mainly in China, South India, and South America, and is used as ethnic medicine to cure diverse ailments. In Ayurveda, it is often referred as "*Bhumyamalaki*" and considered as diuretic and used for treating dysentery. *P. urinaria* is known as "*Dukung Anak*" in Malaysian traditional medicine and whole plant is employed in treating viral infections, liver, and kidney disorders. In Thailand, it is known as "*Look Tai Bai*" and aerial parts are widely used to treat diabetes, gonorrhea, jaundice, and hepatic disorders. In the traditional Chinese and Taiwanese medicines, this herb is used to alleviate conjunctivitis, dropsy, diarrhea, edema, and jaundice. Decoction of the whole plant is used to expel kidney stones in South America. In African traditional medicine, whole plant is used as a remedy for asthma, bronchitis, chest pain, dysentery, and malaria (Kirtikar and Basu, 1993; Calixto et al., 1998; Lee et al., 2006b; Nain et al., 2012).

7.2.12 P. VIRGATUS

In Chinese, Indian, and Thailand traditional medicinal systems whole plant of *P. virgatus* G. Forst. is used to manage diabetes, gonorrhea, hepatic disorders, inflammation, rheumatism, and urinary infection. This herb is considered as an antiseptic and used to give wash for itches. In Tamil Nadu, India, the whole plant powder is used to cure dysentery and liver diseases (Kirtikar and Basu, 1993; Nain et al., 2012; Renugadevi and Madhavan, 2016).

7.3 PHARMACOLOGICAL PROPERTIES

The genus *Phyllanthus* has been the main target for pharmacological studies in recent times because of broad therapeutic use in traditional medicine and production of diverse secondary metabolites. Potential anticancer and antiviral properties of *Phyllanthus* species especially against hepatitis B virus have increased the interest in pharmacological research on this genus manifold. *P. amarus, P. emblica,* and *P. niruri* are the most widely studied species which have shown maximum biological activities (Kalidas and Mohan, 2009; Mao et al., 2016; Asmilia et al., 2020). Major pharmacological properties of genus *Phyllanthus* are discussed here.

7.3.1 ANTIOXIDANT ACTIVITY

Antioxidants interfere with the oxidative damage due to free radicals through radical scavenging and chelating metal ions. They play a major role in hepatoprotection and degenerative disorders. *Phyllanthus* species have shown antioxidant activity both in vitro and in vivo experiments. The hepatoprotective action of *Phyllanthus* species is attributed to anti-inflammatory or antioxidant properties. Indian *Phyllanthus* species have shown antioxidant property in experiments in vitro (Kumaran and Karunakaran, 2007; Kumara et al., 2012; Srirama et al., 2012). The species like *P. amarus, P. debilis, P. emblica, P. maderaspatensis*, and *P. virgatus* have shown greater antioxidant potential compared to other *Phyllanthus* species. The aqueous extract of *P. niruri* increased the activity of hepatic antioxidant enzymes (catalase glutathione and superoxide dismutase) and reduced lipid peroxidation against acetaminophen- and nimesulide-induced oxidative stress thus demonstrating its antioxidant potential (Bhattacharjee and Sil, 2006). *Phyllantus niruri, P. amarus,* and *P. urinaria* are useful in the preparation of natural products fit for human consumption with antioxidant properties (Liu et al., 2008; Poompachee and Chudapongse, 2011). Fruits of *P. emblica* used in the Ayurvedic formulation Triphala exhibited potent antioxidant activity (Yang and Liu, 2014).

7.3.2 ANTIVIRAL ACTIVITY

Suppressing the growth and replication of the virus is one of the main mechanisms behind antiviral therapy. *P. amarus* suppressed the activity of hepatitis B virus and improved the overall health of liver. Administration of 200 mg powder of aerial parts of *P. amarus* three times a day for one month to hepatitis B patients had shown that 59% of the patients were negative to Hepatitis B surface Antigen (HBsAg) (Thyagarajan et al., 1988). The aqueous extract of *P. niruri* suppresses enzyme Human Immunodeficiency Virus (HIV)-1 reverse transcriptase. *P. urinaria* acetone extract effectively inhibited herpes simplex virus infection (Zhong et al., 2013). *P. urinaria* and *P. myrtifolius* have shown activity against Epstein-Barr virus DNA polymerase which is attributed to the presence of novel ellagitannins (Liu et al., 1999). The fruits of *P. emblica* have also shown antiviral and antibacterial activity (Yang and Liu, 2014). These studies clearly indicated the effectiveness of *Phyllanthus* species in curing viral infections in human beings.

7.3.3 HEPATOPROTECTIVE ACTIVITY

The liver being an important organ of the body digests food, removes waste products or foreign substances from the bloodstream, regulates blood sugar levels, and produces essential nutrients. Toxic chemicals and alcohol cause severe damage to liver causing progressive dysfunction. The genus *Phyllanthus* has potential therapeutic benefits by managing hepatitis B, nephrolitis, and pain-related disorders (Calixto et al., 1998). Hepatoprotective activity of the genus *Phyllanthus* has been established through clinical research. *P. amarus* and *P. niruiri* were effective against hepatitis and other disorders of liver. The hepatoprotective effect of *Phyllanthus* species is largely attributed to the presence of two lignans, namely phyllanthin and hypophyllanthin (Thyagarajan et al., 1988; Lee et al., 2006b). Bioactive compounds like Phyllanthin, hypophyllanthin, triacontanal, and tricontanol have been reported from the hexane extract of *P. niruri*. A protein isolated from *P. niruri* exhibited hepatoprotective activity in acetaminophen- and nimesulide-induced liver damage in mice. The hepatoprotective activity of *P. niruri* protein is attributed to antioxidant property as evident from reduced lipid peroxide, increased activity of GSH levels, and other antioxidant enzymes in intoxicated mice (Bhattacharjee and Sil, 2006). The other *Phyllanthus* species (*P. emblica, P. fraternus, P. maderaspatensis, and P. urinaria)* also showed dose-dependent hepatoprotective activity and thus promising a potential therapeutic treatment for liver damage induced by chemicals (Sailaja and Setty, 2006; Yang and Liu, 2014).

7.3.4 ANTICANCER ACTIVITY

Many foreign chemical substances and the reactive oxygen species produced during aerobic respiration in cells are responsible for causing the different types of cancer. *Phyllanthus* species have long been used as traditional anti-cancer treatments throughout the globe due to their well-known bioactive chemicals. Among them, *P. emblica* is one of the potent medicinal plants commonly used in Indian and Chinese traditional medicine with strong anticancer properties (Joseph and Kuttan, 2011). *P. amarus* and *P. niruri* had shown promising antitumor and antineoplastic effect in both in vitro and in vivo. *Phyllanthus niruri* extract has greater role in treating colorectal cancer (Sawitri, 2016; Paul et al., 2019). *P. urinaria* extracts also showed encouraging cytotoxic and anticancer activities (Geethangili and Ding, 2018).

7.3.5 HYPOTENSIVE AND ANTIDIABETIC ACTIVITY

Hypertension is a major cause of chronic diseases like cardiovascular disease, renal disease, stroke, and diabetes. *P. amarus* leaf powder given to humans significantly reduced systolic blood pressure, increased urine volume, and sodium excretion in urine and serum. It also reduced the blood glucose levels effectively (Srividya and Periwal, 1995). Antidiabetic activity of *P. amarus* is attributed to increased utilization of glucose due to amelioration of damaged liver or kidney glycolysis and reduced gluconeogenic activity. In alloxan-induced diabetic albino rats, ethanolic extract of *P. fraternus* significantly decreased the blood sugar levels. The aqueous extract also showed considerable antidiabetic activity during the first 2 weeks, however, the effect did not sustain later (Garg et al., 2008). In Sri Lanka, aqueous extract of *P. debilis* on oral administration lowered the fasting blood glucose level in normoglycemic mice. Further, it improved the tolerance levels for oral glucose and sucrose up to five hours after treatment and inhibited significantly the glucose absorption in small intestine (Wanniarachchi et al., 2009). Pharmacological studies also showed antidiabetic activity of ethanolic and water extracts of aerial parts of *P. niruri* (Beidokhti et al., 2017).

P. emblica is reported to have antidiabetic and cardioprotective properties along with hypolipidemic, gastroprotective, antiulcerogenic, and chemoprotective properties (Yang and Liu, 2014; Majeed et al., 2020). Petroleum ether and ethanolic extract of *P. reticulatus* leaves had shown antidiabetic activity in alloxan-induced diabetic mice. In diabetic rat models also methanolic and aqueous extracts of *P. virgatus* showed antihyperglycemic effect. The bioactive fractions normalized the antioxidant enzyme levels and antioxidant markers in liver and kidney. Lipid and glycogen levels are also reduced to normal levels (Shabeer et al., 2009). These studies proved the hypoglycemic potential of *Phyllanthus* species.

7.3.6 ANTI-INFLAMMATORY ACTIVITY

Pharmacological studies have also proved the anti-inflammatory, pain-relieving, and antinociceptive potential of *Phyllanthus* species. Inflammation though is a defense mechanism, an uncontrolled inflammation is a sign of many chronic diseases. Administration with water or alcohol extracts of *Phyllanthus* species through oral, intragastric, or intraperitoneal route had shown analgesic effect in laboratory-induced pain models of mice. Hydro-alcoholic extract of *Phyllanthus* species at 35 mg/kg body weight showed significant analgesic effect. This analgesic effect might be the reason for people taking *Phyllanthus* species for kidney stones to relieve pain very quickly (Santos et al., 1995). Methanolic fraction of *P. amarus* suppressed paw edema formation in rat models caused by carrageenan, bradykinin, serotonin, and prostaglandin E1 (PGE1) (Mahat and Patil, 2007). The anti-inflammatory activity of *P. debilis* was evaluated in two different models. *Phyllanthus debilis* extract (50–400 mg/kg) markedly decreased the carrageenan-induced edema formation. The treatment also decreased the weight of cotton pellet-induced granuloma (Chandrashekar et al., 2005). Studies have also proved the anti-inflammatory potential of *P. emblica,* which is well known for its rejuvenation properties in Ayurvedic system of medicine (Bhattacharjee and Sil, 2006; Li et al., 2020).

P. urinaria inhibited the paw edema in adjuvant-induced arthritic mice model (Kang et al., 2008). Extract of *P. urinaria* prevented the myeloperoxidase activity and neutrophil migration into inflamed tissue. Enhanced production of nitric oxide (NO) was observed in both in vivo and in vitro models treated with acetone or aqueous extract of *P. tenellus* dried plant. *Phyllanthus niruri* is a pharmacologically well-studied species in this genus and has shown potent anti-inflammatory, analgesic, and antinociceptive effects (Santos et al., 1995; Bagalkotkar et al., 2006). *Phyllanthus reticulatus* methanolic extract of leaves fed to mice have exhibited marked antinociceptive effect in acetic acid-induced gastric pain writhing tests. Inhibition of writhing by *P. reticulatus* extract was very much comparable to the standard drug aspirin (Saha et al., 2007). These studies have shown the potential of *Phyllanthus* species in reducing inflammatory responses.

7.4 PHYTOCHEMICALS

Development of plant-based medicines depends on phytochemical constituents of selected plant species. *Phyllanthus* species are rich sources of diverse phytochemicals and many phytochemicals have shown potent ethnomedicinal and pharmacological properties (Table 7.1). Secondary metabolites belonging to alkaloids, flavonoids, lignans, polyphenols, sterols, tannins, and terpenoids have been reported and more than 500 compounds have been derived from different *Phyllanthus* species. These metabolites showed unique structural diversity and many of them have shown potent biological activity (Calixto et al., 1998; Nahar et al., 2011; Mao et al., 2016; Geethangili and Ding, 2018). *P. amarus*, *P. emblica, P. flexuosus, P. niruri, P. sellowianus,* and *P. urinaria* have been subjected to extensive phytochemical investigation.

Terpenoids, lignans, tannins, and flavonoids are considered as the major classes of compounds reported from *Phyllanthus*. So far, more than 90 lignans were isolated from different *Phyllanthus* species. Hypophyllanthin,

TABLE 7.1 Major Phytochemicals Isolated from Phyllanthus Species.

Class	Phytochemical compound	Phyllanthus species
Lignans	Phyllanthin, hypophyllanthin, niranthin, 5-demethoxy niranthin, demethylenedioxyniranthin, nirphyllin, nirtetralin, nirtetralin A, isonirtetralin, phyllanthusmin B, C, D, E, and F, phyllamyricin A, B, C, D, E, and F, phyllamyricoside A, B, and C, phyltetralin, phyllnirurin, linnanthin, lintetralin, isolintetralin, 2,3-demethoxy-seco-isolintetralin diacetate, seco-4-hydroxylintetralin, isolariciresinol, seco-isolariciresinol trimethyl ether, demethylenedioxy-niranthin, 5-demethoxy-niranthin, hydroxyniranthin, bursehernin, 2S,3S-bursehernin, dextrobursehernin, 3-(3,4-Dimethoxy-benzyl)-4-(7-methoxy benzo[1, 3] dioxol-5-yl-methyl)-dihydrofuran-2-one, 4-(3,4-dimethoxy-phenyl)-1-(7-methoxybenzol[1, 3]dioxol-5-yl)-2,3-bis methoxymethyl-butan-1-ol, lactone, 3,4-methylenedioxybenzyl-3',4'-dimethoxybenzylbutyrolactone, (+)-8-3,4-methylenedioxybenzyl-8'-(3',4'-dimethoxybenzyl)-butyrolactone, dibenzylbutyrolactone 3,4-methylenedioxybenzyl-3',4'-dimethoxybenzylbutyrolactone, cubebin dimethyl ether, (+)-dihydrocubebin, episyringaresinol, evofolin B, hinokinin, heliobuphthalmin, heliobuphthalmin lactone, (7R,7′R,8S,8′S)-icariol A2, (+)-lyoniresiol, 7′-hydroxy-3′,4′,5,9,9′-pentamethoxy-3,4-methylenedioxy lignin, lirioresinol A, isofraxidin, justicidin A and B, 4-ketopinoresinol, medioresinol, neolignan, 4,9,9′-Trihydroxy-3,4′-dimethoxy-8-O-3′-neolignan, norlignan, sesquineolignan, 4-oxopinoresinol, reticulatuside A and B, scopoletin, (-)-syringaresinol, turpenionoside A and B, urinatetralin, urinaligran, and virgatusin.	*P. amarus, P. debilis, P. emblica, P. flexuosus, P. fraternus, P. glaucus, P. maderaspatensis, P. myrtifolius, P. niruri, P. reticulatus, P. sellowianus, P. tenellus P. urinaria* and *P. virgatus*
Alkaloids	Epi-bubbialine, indole-3-carboxylic acid, E,Z-2,4-decadienamide, E,Z-2,4-octadienamide, isobubbialine, 3-(3-methylbut-2-en-1-yl) isoguanine, 5-hydroxy-isoquinoline, methyl (2S)-1-[2-(furan-2-yl)-2-oxoethyl]-5-oxopyrrolidine-2-carboxylate, nirurine, nitidine. Phyllanthidine, phyllanthine, phyllanthimide, phyllochrysine, phyllurine, phenazine, phenazine derivatives, securinine, allosecurinine, dihydrosecurinine, tetrahydrosecurinine, 4-methoxytetrahydrosecurinine, norsecurinine, 4-methoxy-nor-securinine, securinol A and B, (+)-allonorsecurinine, and simplexine.	*P. amarus, P. emblica, P. fraternus, P. niruri, P. sellowianus, P. reticulatus, P. urinaria* and *P. virgatus*

TABLE 7.1 *(Continued)*

Class	Phytochemical compound	Phyllanthus species
Flavonoids	Apigenin, apigenin-7-O-(6"-butyryl-β-glucopyranoside), astragalin, avicularin, catechin, chebulic acid, chibulinic acid, cyanidin glucoside, cyanidin malonylglucoside, emblirol A and B, (−)-epiafzelechin, gallocatechin, galangin-8-sulfonate, galangin-3-O-β-D-glucoside-8-sulfonate, fisetin-4-O-beta-d-glucoside, leucodelphinidin, kaempferol, kaempferol-3-O-β-D-glucopyranoside, kaempferol glycosides, kaempferol hexoside, kaempferol-4'-rhamnopyranoside, kaempferol-8-sulfonate, 4′-methoxyscutellarein, 6-metoxykaempferol-3-O-hexose-O-pentose, myricetrin, myricetin-rhamnoside, naringin, niruriflavone, nirurin, nirurin (5,6,7,4'-tetrahydroxy-8-(3-methylbut-2-enyl) flavanone-5-O-rutinoside), nirurinetin, pelargonidin glucoside, quercetin, quercetin-3-O-glucoside, quercetin-3-O-β-D-glucopyranoside, quercetin 3-O-a-L-(2,4-di-O-acetyl) rhamnopyranoside-7-O-a-L rhamnopyranoside, quercetin 3-O-a-L-(3,4-di-O-acetyl) rhamnopyranoside-7-O-a-L rhamnopyranoside, quercetin 3-O-a-L-rhamnopyranoside, quercetin 7-methyl ether, quercetol, quercitoside, quercitrin, isoquercitrin, rhamnocitrin, rutin, and urinariaflavone.	*P. acidus*, *P. amarus*, *P. caroliniensis*, *P. debilis*, *P. emblica*, *P. maderaspatensis*, *P. muellerianus*, *P. niruri*, *P. reticulatus*, *P. sellowianus*, *P. tenellus*, *P. urinaria* and *P. virgatus*
Tannins	Amariin, amariinic acid, amarulone, carpinusnin, castalin, castalagin, chebulagic acid, chebulanin, corilagin, elaeocarpusin, ellagic acid, epicatechin-(4β →8)-epigallocatechin, excoecarianin, furosin, gallic acid, geraniin, acetonylgeraniin D, geraniinic acid B, glucopyranoside, gallocatechin, gallotannin, 1-galloyl-2,3- dehydrohexahydroxydiphenoyl-glucose, 1,3,4,6-tetra-O-galloyl-β-Dglucose, 1-galloyl-2,4-(acetonyl dehydrohexahydroxydiphenoyl)-3,6 hexahydroxydiphenoyl geraniinic acid, hippomanin A, isocorilagin, isostrictinin, macatannin B, mallotinin, mallotusinin, isomallotusinin, neochebulagic acid, phyllanemblinin A, B, C, D, E, and F, phyllanthunin, phyllanthusiin A, B, C, D, G, and U, phyllemtannin, pinocembrin-7-O-[4′,6′-(S)-hexahydroxydiphenoyl]-β-D-glucose, prodelphinidin B1 and B2, punicafolin, putranjivain A and B, pyrogallol, pyrogallic acid, repandinin A and B, repandusinic acid A and B, strictinin, terchebin, tercatain, trimethyl ester 3,4-dehydrochebulic acid, virganin, and virgatyne.	*P. amarus*, *P. caroliniensis*, *P. debilis*, *P. emblica*, *P. flexuosus*, *P. muellerianus*, *P. myrtifolius*, *P. niruri*, *P. reticulatus*,

TABLE 7.1 *(Continued)*

Class	Phytochemical compound	Phyllanthus species
		P. sellowianus, *P. tenellus*, *P. urinaria* and *P. virgatus*
Terpenoids and Triterpenes	β-amyrin, amarosterol A and B, betulin, betulinic acid, (E)-coumaroyltaraxerol, (Z)-coumaroyltaraxerol, 2Z, 6Z, 10Z, 14E, 18E, 22E-farnesyl farnesol, flexuosoids A and B, friedelin, 21-α-hydroxy-friedelin, friedelanol, 3-oxofriedelan-28-oic acid, epifriedelinol, glochidiol, glochidonol, lupeol, lupeol acetate, 28-norlup-20(29)-ene-3,17β-diol, ocotillol-II, olean-18-en-3α-ol, oleanolic acid, phainanolide A, phainanoid G, H, and I, phyllanoside, phyllanthol, phyllanthenol, phyllanthenone, phyllantheol, and ursolic acid.	*P. acidus*, *P. amarus*, *P. emblica*, *P. flexuosus*, *P. fraternus*, *P. niruri*, *P. reticulatus*,
Diterpenes	Cleistanthol, ent-3β-hydroxykaur-l6-ene, 19-hydroxyspruceanol 19-O-β-D-glucopyranoside, orthosiphol G and I, phyllaciduloid A, B, C, and D, phyllanes A and B, phyllanflexoid A, B, and C, spruceanol, zeatin, zeatin nucleotide, and zeatin riboside.	*P. sellowianus*, *P. urinaria*.
Monoterpenes	*p*-Cymene, limonene, loliolide, (3S,5R,6S,9R)-megastigmane-3,9-diol 3-O-α-L-arabinofuranosyl-(1,6)-β-D-glucopyranoside, 7-megastigmen-3-ol-9-one 3-O-α-L-arabinofuranosyl-(1,6)-β-D-glucopyranoside, (6R)-menthiafolic acid, *trans*-phytol, turpenionoside A and B.	*P. acidus*, *P. emblica*, *P. flexuosus*, *P. niruri*, *P. reticulatus*, *P. urinaria*.
Sesquiterpenes	β-Bourbonene, β-caryophyllene, cloven-2β,9α -diol, dendranthemoside B,4′ hydroxyphyllaemblicin B, dihydrophaseic acid-4′-O-β-D-glucopyranoside, glochicoccin D, phyllaemblicin A, B, C, D, E, F, and G, phyllaemblic acid A, B, and C, phyllaemblinol, phyllanthusol A and B	*P. niruri*, *P. reticulatus* and *P. urinaria*

TABLE 7.1 *(Continued)*

Class	Phytochemical compound	Phyllanthus species
Steroids, sterols, and steroidal hormones	Estradiol, 7α-acetoxysitosterol, amarosterol A and B, campesterol, β-daucosterol, 7β-ethoxysiterol, fraternusterol, glochidonol, 7α-hydroxysitosterol, 7-ketositosterol, octacosanol, phyllanthosecosteryl ester, phyllanthosterol, phyllanthostigmasterol, β-sitosterol, 5α,6β-dihydroxysitosterol, 5α,6β,7α-trihydroxysitosterol, β-sitosterol-3-O-b-d-glucopyranoside, stigmasterol, (3 β,22E)-stigmasta-5,22-diene-3,25-diol, stigmast-4-en-3-one, stigmast-4-en-3,6-dione, stigmast-4-en-6β-ol-3-one, stigmast-4-ene-3β,6α-diol, stigmast-5-en-3-ol, oleate, taraxerone, taraxeryl acetate, 21-α-hydroxyfriedelan-3-one	*P. amarus, P. debilis, P. emblica, P. flexuosus, P. fraternus, P. muellerianus, P. reticulatus, P. sellowianus* and *P. urinaria*
Simple phenolics and benzene derivatives	Caffeic acid, caffeoylmalic acid, coumaric acid, chlorogenic acid, cinnamic acid, ferulic acid, 4-O-galloylquinic acid, 1,6-digalloylglucopyranose, 1β,6-di-O-galloylglucose, methyl caffeate, methyl gallate, ethyl gallate, mucic acid 2-O-gallate, mucic acid 3-O-gallate, mucic acid dimethyl ester 2-O-gallate, mucic acid 6-methyl ester 2-O-gallate, mucic acid 1,4-lactone methyl ester 5-O-gallate, mucic acid 1-ethyl 6-methyl ester 2-O-gallate, phyllangin, quinic acid, 2,4,5-trimethoxy propenylbenzene, 11-octadecenoic acid, 9,12-octadecadienoic acid, hexadecanoic acid, benzenedicarboxylic acid, and tridecyl ester, 6-octadecynoic acid	*P. amarus, P. emblica, P. muellerianus, P. myrtifolius, P. niruri, P. reticulatus, P. urinaria, P. sellowianus, P. tenellus* and *P. virgatus*

TABLE 7.1 *(Continued)*

Class	Phytochemical compound	Phyllanthus species
Lactones	Brevifolin, brevifolin carboxylic acid, debelalactone phyllantutinolactone, trimethyl-3,4-dehydrochebulate	*P. amarus,* *P. debilis,* *P. niruri,* *P. tenellus,* *P. urinari* and *P. virgatus*

Source: Calixto et al., 1998; Bagalkotkar et al., 2006; Sarin et al., 2014; Mao et al., 2016; Geethangili and Ding, 2018; Nisar et al., 2018; Jusoh et al., 2019.

niranthin, nirtetralin, phyllanthin, and phyltetralin are the prominent lignans reported from *P. amarus*, *P. maderaspatensis*, *P. niruri*, *P. urinaria*, and *P. virgatus*, having multiple biological activities. Rutin, astragin, astragalin, quercitrin, quercetin, and kaempferol are the prominent flavonoids reported in the genus *Phyllanthus*. Ellagic acid, gallic acid, geraniin, corilagin, and phyllanthusiins are the most prevalent tannins isolated from *Phyllanthus* species. Most of the sterols reported in this genus belong to *P. emblica*. Terpenoids are the most abundant phytochemicals found in the genus *Phyllanthus*, which includes triterpenoids, diterpenoids, monoterpenes, and sesquiterpenes. About 125 terpenoids were been reported from various *Phyllanthus* species (Mao et al., 2016).

7.5 BIOACTIVE POTENTIAL OF MAJOR PHYTOCHEMICALS

Many secondary metabolites of plants are commercially used as therapeutic agents to cure various disorders affecting the mankind. Different pharmacological properties of *Phyllanthus* species have been attributed to their diverse secondary metabolites (Kalidas and Mohan, 2009; Nisar et al., 2018). Phytochemicals isolated from various *Phyllanthus* species are shown to have multiple biological activities. Terpenoids, lignans, and tannins have been attributed with most biological activities since they are the abundant phytochemicals in this genus (Mao et al., 2016). Such an array of phytochemicals found in the genus *Phyllanthus* may act as lead molecules to develop new drugs with known biological activity.

Antihepatotoxic activity of *Phyllanthus* species is mainly credited to the two major lignans namely, hypophyllanthin and phyllanthin (Khatoon et al., 2006). Phyllanthin has been shown to have a number of pharmacological properties like hepatoprotective, hypotensive, immunomodulatory, anticancer, antiaging, antioxidant, and anti-inflammatory. The highest concentration of phyllanthin was recorded in *P. amarus*. Another lignan namely, niranthin, along with phyllanthin and hypophyllanthin is shown to have both antitumor and antiviral properties. Niranthin, nirtetralin, and phyltetralin isolated from *P. amarus* exhibited anti-inflammatory activities (Santos et al., 1995; Calixto et al., 1998; Sarin et al., 2014). Such molecules need to be considered for the development of modern medicine.

Corilagin, ellagic acid, gallic acid, and geraniin are the tannins present in different *Phyllanthus* species. Being natural antioxidants, these compounds have potential use in cosmetic industries as skin antiaging, sun-blocking, and whitening agents. Most widely obtained ellagitannins from the *Phyllanthus* species like corilagin and geraniin had shown multiple biological activities including antioxidant, anti-HIV, antitumor, and antihyperalgesic activities. The hypotensive and analgesic effects are also attributed to geraniin. Amariin, repandusinic acid, and phyllanthusiin showed antioxidant and radioprotective property. Ellagic acid was attributed to antidiabetic and aldose reductase inhibitory activity. Ellagic acid and gallic acid were known to be effective against viral diseases and different tumors. The tannins emblicanin A, emblicanin B, pedunculagin, phyllaemblicin B, and punigluconin present in *P. emblica* were shown to possess antioxidant activity. Ellagic acid, gallic acid, chebulagic acid, corilagin, and pyrogallol isolated from *P. emblica* fruits have shown cancer-preventive and antitumor effects in vitro and in in vivo animal models. Repandusinic acid A and niruriside obtained from *P. niruri* inhibited reverse transcriptase and cytotoxic activity to HIV-1 (Souza, 2000; Mahdi et al., 2011; Sarin et al., 2014; Zhao et al., 2015; Mao et al., 2016; Haddad et al., 2020; Li et al., 2020). Such properties of phytochemicals found in *Phyllanthus* species provide ample opportunity in biotechnological applications. It will be interesting to evaluate cell/tissue cultures of *Phyllanthus* species for phytochemical production.

Glochidone and lupeol are members of lupine triterpenoids, mainly isolated from *Phyllanthus* species and shown to have antitumor properties. The pentacyclic oleanane-type triterpenoid, β-amyrin is a potent analgesic, antinociceptive, anti-inflammatory, anticancer, and antimicrobial agent isolated from various *Phyllanthus* species. Oleanolic acid and its derivatives obtained from this genus have shown bioactive potential against many types of tumors. A monoterpenoid lactone, loliolide isolated from acetone extract of *P. urinaria* showed anti-HCV (Hepatitis C Virus) activity by inactivating virus particles, blocking HCV attachment, and preventing viral fusion. Monoterpenoids like *p*-cymene and limonene are known to possess antimicrobial, antioxidant, anticancer, and wound-healing properties (Bagalkotkar et al., 2006; Sarin et al., 2014; Chung et al., 2016; Mao et al., 2016; Geethangili and Ding, 2018). Multiple biological activities of chemical constituents of *Phyllanthus* species could be major advantage in phytomedicine development.

The flavonoids like rutin, quercetin, quercitrin, and quercetin-3-O-glucoside have demonstrated antioxidant, anti-inflammatory, and radioprotective properties. Quercetin is one of the potent flavonoid isolated from *Phyllanthus* species that had shown different pharmacological activities like antioxidant, antimicrobial, anti-inflammatory, antidiabetic, and chemoprotective activities. It exhibited anticancer activity in cancer cell lines, transgenic murine model of breast cancer, xenograft for leukemia in clinical trials. Rutin and quercetin are the most widely studied flavonoids in the genus *Phyllanthus* and they are considered as effective antiviral agents (Sarin et al., 2014; Zhao et al., 2015; Mao et al., 2016; Nisar et al., 2018). Chemical diversity and diverse array of biological activity would be interesting to explore for the development of modern medicines.

Securinine and norsecurinine are the alkaloids obtained from different *Phyllanthus* species that possess strong antispasmodic activity. Securinine also exhibits antimalarial and antibacterial activities. β-sitosterol isolated from genus *Phyllanthus* possesses anti-inflammatory activity (Bagalkotkar et al., 2006; Sarin et al., 2014; Geethangili and Ding, 2018). Although more than 500 chemicals have been isolated from genus Phyllanthus, biological activities are heavily focused only on a few of the phytochemicals like ellagic acid, gallic acid, geraniin, hypophyllanthin, niranthin, phyllanthin, quercetin, and rutin. Structural details of these bioactive phytochemical are provided in Figure 7.2.

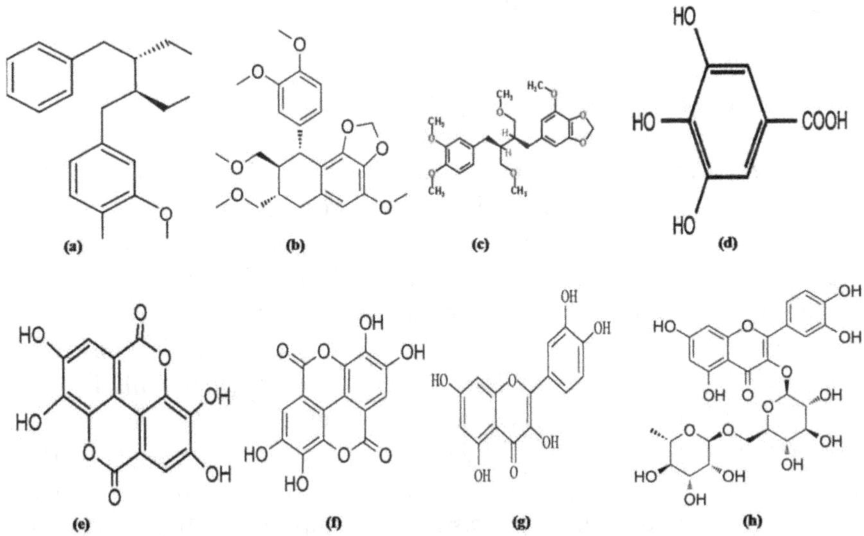

FIGURE 7.2 Major bioactive phytochemicals isolated from Phyllanthus species: Phyllanthin (a), hypophyllanthin (b), niranthin (c), gallic acid (d), ellagic acid (e), geraniin (f), quercetin (g), and rutin (h)

Source: www.chemsrc.com; www.medchemexpress.com; www.researchgate.net.

7.6 THERAPEUTIC PRODUCTS

Phyllanthus species forms a major ingredient in traditional as well as modern medicinal products. Crude, semipurified, and purified extracts of these plants are used to make capsules and tablets for treating various human ailments. Some of the *Phyllanthus* products are in the form of powders and syrups (Table 7.2). Among the *Phyllanthus* species that are used to obtain therapeutic products, *P. amarus, P. emblica,* and *P. niruri* are the prominent species either as a single herb or polyherbal preparations. *P. emblica* is a major component of Ayurvedic formulation Triphala, meaning three fruits. Triphala consists of dried powdered fruits of *P. emblica, Terminalia bellirica,* and *Terminalia chebula* in equal quantities. It is one of the important drugs "*Rasayana*" promoting health, immunity, and longevity. Several drugs have been prepared by using the constituents of *P. emblica* (Rai et al., 2012). The "*Diabet*" is a polyherbal formulation for treating diabetes having *P. reticulatus* as one of the major ingredients (Umamaheswari et al., 2012). "*Chanca Piedra*" is an herbal supplement for liver and kidney health prepared from *P. niruri* or *P. amarus.* The PHYLLPRO™ is one of the standardized ethanol extracts of leaves of *P. amarus* for protection against oxidative stress as well as recovery from the symptoms hangover (George et al., 2019).

7.7 CONCLUSION

Use of herbal drugs to treat various human diseases is commonly practiced throughout the world, especially in the third world countries due to the easy availability and low cost. The genus *Phyllanthus* includes many species that are reported to have high medicinal value. *Phyllanthus* species are extensively used in traditional systems of medicines especially for ailment for liver diseases and kidney stones. *P. amarus* and *P. niruri* are the most widely used species of this genus in different regions globally, especially in South-East Asia as well as South America. Wide acceptance of *Phyllanthus* species in traditional medicine has laid the foundation for screening the species for modern drugs. *Phyllanthus* species had shown antipyretic, diuretic, antimicrobial, antioxidant, antiparasitic, anticontraceptive, hepatoprotective, immunomodulatory, antidiabetic, anticancer, anti-inflammatory, hypotensive, and antiviral activities were attributed to plants of genus *Phyllanthus*. This genus has a reservoir of phytochemicals belonging to different classes of secondary metabolites like alkaloids, flavonoids, lignans, sterols, tannins, terpenoids, and other polyphenols. The major bioactive phytochemicals such as ellagic acid, gallic acid, geraniin, hypophyllanthin, niranthin, phyllanthin, quercetin, and rutin are known to possess multiple pharmacological properties. These multitude biological activities rendered by lead phytochemicals make the genus Phyllanthus as an integral part in biopharmaceutical drug

TABLE 7.2 Therapeutic Products Obtained from the *Phyllanthus* Species.

Product	Description of the product	Manufacturer
Chanca Piedra capsules	Herbal supplement for liver and kidney support prepared from the leaves and stems of *Phyllanthus niruri*	Swanson Health Products
Phyllanthus Complex capsules	Hypoallergenic dietary supplement prepared from the *Phyllanthus amarus* leaves, Milk Thistle seeds and Dandelion root extracts	NutriCology
Phyllanthus niruri capsules	Effective herbal remedy for liver and kidney diseases and these capsules are prepared from pure and standardized extract of the herb Bhumi amalaki	Planet Ayurveda
Phyllanthus tincture	Herbal dietary supplement prepared from *Phyllanthus amarus.*	Amazon Herbs
Bhuiamalaki powder	Ayurvedic product prepared from whole plant of *Phyllanthus niruri* for healthy liver	Herbal Hills
Amla capsules	Immune booster herbal supplement prepared from the fruits of *Phyllanthus emblica*	Shraddha Exports, Ahmedabad
Triphala churna	It is a combination of three plants dried fruit powder (*Phyllanthus emblica, Terminalia bellirica,* and *Terminalia chebula*) for fast relief from constipation, gas, and constipation	Baidyanath
Amla juice	Immunity booster prepared from the fruits of *Phyllanthus emblica*	Dabur India Limited

Source: https://swansoneurope.com; https://foodpharmacy.blog; https://www.planetayurveda.com; https://tropilab.com; https://www.indiamart.com; https://www.exportersindia.com; https://www.baidyanath.com; https://www.dabur.com

development. Although large number of phytochemicals were isolated in the genus Phyllanthus, biological activities are heavily focused only on few of the phytochemicals. Comprehensive pharmacological screening of all the phytochemicals in this genus is need of the hour and that will help in creating a library of novel bioactive compounds for the development of potential pharmaceutical drugs to treat various human disorders. Despite the wide traditional usage and greater biological activities attributed to genus Phyllanthus, nutraceutical studies are lacking except for *P. acidus* and *P. emblica*. Greater thrust in this area may be helpful in exploiting nutraceutical potential of Phyllanthus species. The genus Phyllanthus provide unique bioactive phytochemicals with greater impact in modern medicines. Among the various sources of phytomedicines, *Phyllanthus* stands apart with an array of biological activities. The characterized compounds can be used as the lead molecules in drug development in future.

KEYWORDS

- ***Phyllanthus***
- **Ayurveda**
- **traditional medicine**
- **phytochemicals**
- **therapeutic products**
- **phyllanthin**

REFERENCES

Asmilia, N.; Fahrimal, Y.; Abrar, M.; Rinidar, R. Chemical Compounds of Malacca Leaf (*Phyllanthus emblica*) After Triple Extraction with N-Hexane, Ethyl Acetate, and Ethanol. *Sci. World J.* **2020**. https://doi.org/10.1155/2020/2739056

Bagalkotkar, G.; Sagineedu, S. R.; Saad, M. S.; Stanslas, J. Phytochemicals from *Phyllanthus niruri* Linn. and Their Pharmacological Properties: A Review. *J. Pharm. Pharmacol.* **2006,** *58*, 1559–1570.

Beidokhti, M. N.; Andersen, M. V.; Eid, H. M.; Villavicencio, M. L. S.; Staerk, D.; Haddad, P. S.; Jager, A. K. Investigation of Antidiabetic Potential of *Phyllanthus niruri* L. Using Assays for α-Glucosidase, Muscle Glucose Transport, Liver Glucose Production, and Adipogenesis. *Biochem. Bioph. Res. Comm.* **2017,** *493*, 869–874.

Bhattacharjee, R.; Sil, P. C. The Protein Fraction of *Phyllanthus niruri* Plays a Protective Role Against Acetaminophen Induced Hepatic Disorder Via Its Antioxidant Properties. *Phytother. Res.* **2006,** *20*, 595–601.

Calixto, J. B.; Santos, A. R. S.; Cechinel, V.; Yunes, R. A. A Review of the Plants of the Genus *Phyllanthus*: Their Chemistry, Pharmacology, and Therapeutic Potential. *Med. Res. Rev.* **1998,** *18*, 225–258.

Chandrashekar, K. S.; Joshi, A. B.; Satyanarayana, D.; Pai, P. Analgesic and Anti–Inflammatory Activities of *Phyllanthus debilis* Whole Plant. *Pharm. Biol.* **2005,** *43*, 586–588.

Chung, C. Y.; Liu, C. H.; Burnouf, T.; Wang, G. H.; Chang, S. P.; Jassey, A.; Tai, C. J.; Tai, C. J.; Huang, C. J.; Richardson, C. D; Yen, M. H.; Lin, C. C.; Lin, L. T. Activity-Based and Fraction-Guided Analysis of *Phyllanthus urinaria* Identifies Loliolide as a Potent Inhibitor of Hepatitis C Virus Entry. *Antivir. Res.* **2016,** *130*, 58–68.

Dnyaneshwar, W.; Preeti, C.; Kalpana, J.; Bhushan, P. Development and Application of RAPD-SCAR Marker for Identification of *Phyllanthus emblica* L. *Biol. Pharm. Bull.* **2006,** *29*, 2313–2316.

Garg, M.; Dhar, V. J.; Kalia, A. N. Antidiabetic and Antioxidant Potential of *Phyllanthus fraternus* in Alloxan Induced Diabetic Animals. *Pharmacogn. Mag.* **2008,** *4*, 138–143.

Geethangili, M.; Ding, S. A review of the Phytochemistry and Pharmacology of *Phyllanthus urinaria* L. *Front. Pharmacol.* **2018,** *9*, 1–20.

George, A.; Udani, J. K.; Yusof, A. Effects of *Phyllanthus amarus* PHYLLPRO™ Leaves on Hangover Symptoms: A Randomized, Double-Blind, Placebo-Controlled Crossover Study. *Pharm. Biol.* **2019,** *57*, 145–153.

Haddad, J. G.; Grauzdyte, D.; Koishi, A. C.; Viranaicken, W.; Venskutonis, P. R.; Santos, C. N. D.; Despres, P.; Diotel, N.; Kalamouni C. E. The Geraniin-Rich Extract from Reunion Island Endemic Medicinal Plant *Phyllanthus phillyreifolius* Inhibits Zika and Dengue Virus Infection at Non-Toxic Effect Doses in Zebrafish. *Molecules* **2020**. https://doi.org/10.3390/25102316.

Hoffmann, P.; Kathriarachchi, H.; Wurdack, K. J. A Phylogenetic Classification of Phyllanthaceae. *Kew. Bull.* **2006,** *61*, 37–53.

Joseph, J.; Kuttan, R. Anticancer Activity of *Phyllanthus emblica.* In *Phyllanthus Species: Scientific Evaluation and Medicinal Applications*; Kuttan, R., Harikumar, K. B., Eds.; CRC Press: Taylor and Francis Group, USA, 2011; p 183.

Jusoh, N. H. M.; Subki, A.; Yeap, S. K.; Yap, K. C.; Jaganath, I. B. Pressurized Hot Water Extraction of from *Phyllanthus tenellus* Roxb. *BMC Chem* **2019,** *13*, 1–10.

Kalidas, C.; Mohan, V. R. In Vitro Rapid Clonal Propagation of *Phyllanthus urinaria* Linn. (Euphorbiaceae)—A Medicinal Plant. *The Researcher* **2009,** *4*, 61–65.

Kang, M. H.; Kim, T. S.; Park, C. G.; Park, H. W.; Ju, Y. W.; Cho, Y. M.; Koh, S. B.; Seong, H. J. Preventive Effects of *Phyllanthus urinaria* Extract on Paw Edema in Adjuvant-Induced Arthritis Rats. *FASEB J.* **2008,** *22*, 889–895.

Khatoon, S.; Rai, V.; Rawat, A. K.; Mehrotra, S. Comparative Pharmacognostic Studies of Three *Phyllanthus* Species. *J. Ethnopharmacol.* **2006,** *104*, 79–86.

Kirtikar, K. R.; Basu, B. D. *Indian Medicinal Plants*, Vol. 3, 2nd ed.; Bishen Singh Mahendra Pal Singh: Dehra Dun, 1993; pp 2219–2228.

Kumar, K. P. S.; Bhowmik, D.; Dutta, A.; Yadav, A. P.; Paswan, S.; Srivastava, S.; Deb, L. Recent Trends in Potential Traditional Indian Herbs *Emblica officinalis* and Its Medicinal Importance. *J. Pharmacog. Phytochem.* **2012,** *1*, 24–32.

Kumara, K. K. S.; Chethan, J.; Manasa, N.; Ashadevi, J. S.; Prakash, H. S. Bioactive Potential of Herbaceous *Phyllanthus* Species. *IJPPS* **2012,** *4*, 457–461.

Kumaran, A.; Karunakaran, R. J. In Vitro Antioxidant Activities of Methanol Extracts of Five *Phyllanthus* Species from India. *LWT Food Sci. Tech.* **2007,** *40*, 344–352.

Lee, C. Y.; Peng, W. H.; Cheng, H. Y.; Chen, F. N.; Lai, M. T.; Chiu, T. H. Hepatoprotective Effects of *Phyllanthus* in Taiwan on Acute Liver Damage Induced by Carbon Tetrachloride. *Am. J. Chin. Med.* **2006b,** *34*, 471–482.

Lee, S. K.; Li, P. T.; Lau, D. T.; Yung, P. P.; Kong, R. Y.; Fong, W. F. Phylogeny of Medicinal *Phyllanthus* Species in China Based on Nuclear ITS and Chloroplast *atpB-rbcL* Sequences and Multiplex PCR Detection Assay Analysis. *Planta Med.* **2006a,** *72*, 721–726.

Li, W.; Zhu, H.; Chen, Y.; Xiao, H.; Ge, Y.; Hu, H.; Li, X.; Cao, Y. Bioactivity-Guided Isolation of Anti-Inflammatory Components from *Phyllanthus emblica. Food Sci. Nutr.* **2020,** *8*, 2670–2679.

Liu X, Zhao M, Wang J.; Yang, B.; Jiang, Y. Antioxidant Activity of Methanolic Extract of Emblica Fruit (*Phyllanthus emblica* L.) from Six Regions in China. *J. Food Compos. Anal.* **2008,** *21*, 219–228.

Liu, K. C.; Lin, M. T.; Lee, S. S.; Chiou, J. F.; Ren, S.; Lien, E. J. Antiviral Tannins from Two *Phyllanthus* Species. *Planta Med.* **1999,** *65*, 43–46.

Mahat, M. A.; Patil, B. M. Evaluation of Antiinflammatory Activity of Methanol Extract of *Phyllanthus amarus* in Experimental Animal Models. *Indian J. Pharm. Sci.* **2007,** *69*, 33–36.

Mahdi, E. S.; Noor, A. M.; Sakeena, M. H.; Abdullah, G. Z.; Abdulkarim, M.; Sattar, M. A. Identification of Phenolic Compounds and Assessment of In Vitro Antioxidants Activity of 30% Ethanolic Extracts Derived from Two *Phyllanthus* Species Indigenous to Malaysia. *Afr. J. Pharm. Pharmacol.* **2011,** *5*, 1967–1978.

Majeed, M.; Majeed, S.; Mundkur, L.; Nagabhushanam, K.; Armugam, S.; Beede, K.; Ali, F. Standardized *Emblica officinalis* Fruit Extract Inhibited the Activities of α-Amylase, α-Glucosidase, and Dipeptidyl Peptidase-4 and Displayed Antioxidant Potential. *J. Sci. Food Agric.* **2020,** *100*, 509–516.

Mao, X.; Wu, L. F.; Guo, H. L.; Chen, W. J.; Cui, Y. P.; Qi, Q.; Li, S.; Liang, W. Y.; Yang, G. H.; Shao, Y. Y. The Genus *Phyllanthus*: An Ethnopharmacological, Phytochemical, and Pharmacological Review. *Evid. Based Complem. Alt. Med.* **2016,** *2016*, 1–36.

Masoodi, K. Z.; Amin, I.; Mansoor, S. et al. Botanicals from the Himalayas with Anticancer Potential—An Emphasis on Kashmir Himalayas. In *Biodiversity and Biomedicine—Our Future*; Ozturk, M.; Egamberdieva, D.; Pešić, M., Eds.; Chapter 11, Academic Press, 2020; pp 189–234.

Masturah, M.; Masitah, M.; Ramli W. D. W. Extraction of Hydrosable Tannins from *Phyllanthus niruri* Linn.: Effects of Solvents and Extraction Method. *Sep. Purif. Technol.* **2006,** *52*, 487–498.

Mitra, R. L.; Jain, S. K. Concept of *Phyllanthus niruri* (Euphorbiaceae) in Indian Floras. *Bull. Bot. Surv. India* **1987,** *27*, 161–176.

Nahar, L.; Sarker, S. D.; Delazar, A. Phytochemistry of the Genus *Phyllanthus*. In *Phyllanthus Species: Scientific Evaluation and Medicinal Applications.* Kuttan, R.; Harikumar, K. B., Eds.; CRC Press: Taylor and Francis Group, USA, 2011; pp 120–137.

Nain, P.; Saini, V.; Sharma, S.; Nain, J. Antidiabetic and Antioxidant Potential of *Emblica officinalis* Gaertn. Leaves Extract in Streptozotocin-Induced Type-2 Diabetes Mellitus (T2DM) Rats. *J. Ethnopharmacol.* **2012,** *142*, 65–71.

Nisar, M. H.; He, J.; Ahmed, A.; Yang, Y.; Li, M.; Wan, C. Chemical Components and Biological Activities of the Genus *Phyllanthus*: A Review of the Recent Literature. *Molecules* **2018,** *23*, 1–25.

Ozturk, M.; Hakeem, K. R. *Plant and Human Health—Vol. 1—Ethnobotay and Physiology*; Springer Science + Business Media: New York, 2018.

Ozturk, M.; Hakeem, K. R. *Plant and Human Health—Vol. 2—Phytochemistry and Molecular Aspects*. Springer Science + Business Media: New York, 2019a.

Ozturk, M.; Hakeem, K. R. *Plant and Human Health—Vol. 3—Phytochemistry and Therapeutic Uses*; Springer Science + Business Media: New York, 2019b.

Ozturk, M.; Altay, V.; Gucel, S.; Guvensen, A. Halophytes in the East Mediterranean-Their Medicinal and Other Economical Values. In *Sabkha Ecosystems: Volume IV: Cash Crop Halophyte and Biodiversity Conservation Tasks for Vegetation Science*, Vol. 47; Springer: The Netherlands, 2014; pp 247–272.

Ozturk, M.; Altay, V.; Altundağ, E.; Gucel, S. Halophytic Plant Diversity of Unique Habitats in Turkey: Salt Mine Caves of Çankırı and Iğdır. In *Halophytes for Food Security in Dry Lands*; Khan, M. A., Ozturk, M., Gul, B., Ahmed, M. Z., Eds., Chapter 18; Elsevier, 2016. http://dx.doi.org/10.1016/B978-0-12-801854-5.00018-2.

Ozturk, M.; Altay, V.; Hakeem, K. R.; Akçiçek, E. *Liquorice from Botany to Phytochemistry*; SpringerBriefs in Plant Science, 2017a. https://doi.org/10.1007/978-3-319-74240-3.

Ozturk, M.; Altay, V.; Gonenç, T. M. Herbal from High Mountains in the East Mediterranean. In *Drug Discovery from Herbs-Approaches and Applications*; Bhojraj, S. et al., Eds.; NAM S & T Centre, DAYA Publishing House: New Delhi, India, Chapter 24, 2017b; pp 327–367.

Ozturk, M.; Altay, V.; Gucel, S.; Altundağ, E. Plant Diversity of the Drylands in Southeast Anatolia-Turkey: Role in Human Health and Food Security. In *Plant Biodiversity: Monitoring, Assessment and Conservation*; Ansari, A. A., Gill, S. S., Eds., Chapter 5; CABI UK, 2017c; pp 83–124.

Ozturk, M.; Altay, V.; Orçen, N. et al. A Little Known and a Little Consumed Natural Resource: *Salicornia*. In *Global Perspectives on Underutilized Crops*; Ozturk, M. et al., Eds., Chapter 3; Springer International Publishing AG, 2018a; pp 83–108.

Ozturk, M.; Altundağ, E.; Ibadullayeva, S. J.; Altay, V.; Aslanıpour, B. A Comparative Analysis of Medicinal and Aromatic Plants Used in the Traditional Medicine of Iğdır (Turkey), Nakhchivan (Azerbaijan), and Tabriz (Iran). *Pak. J. Bot.* **2018b**, *50* (1), 337–343.

Ozturk, M.; Altay, V.; Altundağ, E.; Ibadullayeva, S. J.; Aslanipour, B.; Gönenç, T. M. Herbals in Iğdır (Turkey), Nakhchivan (Azerbaijan), and Tabriz (Iran). In *Plant and Human Health*; Ozturk, M., Hakeem, K.R., Eds., Vol. 1; Springer: Cham, Chapter 6, 2018c; pp 197–266.

Ozturk, M.; Altay, V.; Latiff, A. et al. A comparative analysis of the Medicinal Pteridophytes in Turkey, Pakistan, and Malaysia. In *Plant and Human Health*; Ozturk, M., Hakeem, K. R., Eds., Vol. 1; Springer: Cham, Chapter 9; Springer International Publishing AG, 2018d; pp 349–390.

Ozturk, M.; Altay, V.; Latiff, A. et al. A Comparative Analysis of the Medicinal Plants Used for Diabetes Mellitus in the Traditional Medicine in Turkey, Pakistan, and Malaysia. In *Plant and Human Health*; Ozturk, M., Hakeem, K.R., Eds., Vol. 1; Springer: Cham, Chapter 11; Springer International Publishing AG, 2018e; pp 409–461.

Ozturk, M.; Altay, V.; Latiff, A. et al. Potential Medicinal Plants Used in the Hypertension in Turkey, Pakistan, and Malaysia. In *Plant and Human Health*; Ozturk, M., Hakeem, K. R., Eds., Vol. 1; Springer: Cham, Chapter 16; Springer International Publishing AG, 2018f; pp 595–618.

Ozturk, M.; Gökler, I.; Altay, V. Medicinal Bryophytes Distributed in Turkey. In *Plant and Human Health*; Ozturk, M., Hakeem, K. R., Eds., Vol. 1; Springer: Cham, Chapter 8; Springer International Publishing AG, 2018g; pp 323–348.

Ozturk, M.; Egamberdieva, D.; Milica, P. *Biodiversity and Biomedicine-Our Future*; Academic Press; Elsevier Inc, 2020.

Ozturk, M.; Altay, V.; Efe, R. *Biodiversity, Conservation and Sustainability in Asia: Volume I: Prospects and Challenges in West Asia and Caucasus*; Springer Nature Switzerland AG, 2021a. DOI: 10.1007/978-3-030-59928-7

Ozturk, M.; Khan, S. M.; Altay, V.; Efe, R.; Egamberdieva, D.; Khassanov, F. *Biodiversity, Conservation and Sustainability in Asia: Volume II: Prospects and Challenges in South and Middle Asia*; Springer Nature Switzerland AG, 2021b. DOI: 10.1007/978-3-030-73943-0.

Paul, S.; Patra, D.; Kundu, R. Lignan Enriched Fraction (LRF) of *Phyllanthus amarus* Promotes Apoptotic Cell Death in Human Cervical Cancer Cells In Vitro. *Sci. Rep.* **2019.** https://doi.org/10.1038/s41598-019-51480-7

Petrovska, B. B. Historical Review of Medicinal Plants' Usage. *Pharmacogn. Rev.* **2012,** *6*, 1–5.

Pleskanovskaya, S. A.; Mamedova, M. A.; Ashıralıyeva, M. A. et al. *Glycyrrhiza glabra* (Liquorice) in Turkmenistan—Medicinal and Biological Aspects. In *Plant and Human Health,—Pharmacology and Therapeutic Uses*; Ozturk, M., Hakeem, K. R., Eds., Vol. 3, Chapter 2; Springer Nature: Switzerland, 2019; pp 23–35.

Poompachee, K.; Chudapongse, N. Comparison of the Antioxidant and Cytotoxic Activities of *Phyllanthus virgatus* and *Phyllanthus amarus* Extracts. *Med. Princ. Pract.* **2011,** *21*, 24–29.

Rai, N.; Tiwari, L.; Sharma, R. K.; Verma, A. K. Pharmaco-Botanical Profile on *Emblica officinalis* Gaertn.-A Pharmacopoeial Herbal Drug. *Res. Rev. J. Bot.* **2012,** *1*, 29–41.

Renugadevi, M.; Madhavan, S. Ethno Botanical Resource of *Phyllanthus* Species from Paddy Field in Thiruvarur District, Tamil Nadu. India. *Der Pharmacia Lett.* **2016,** *8*, 229–232.

Saha, A.; Masud, A. M.; Bachar, C. S.; Kundu, K. J.; Datta, K. B.; Nahar, F. L.; Sarker, D. S. The Analgesic and Anti-Inflammatory Activities of Extracts of *Phyllanthus reticulatus* in Mice Model. *Pharm. Biol.* **2007,** *45*, 335–359.

Sailaja, R.; Setty, O. H. Protective Effect of *Phyllanthus fraternus* Against Allyl Alcohol-Induced Oxidative Stress in Liver Mitochondria. *J. Ethnopharmacol.* **2006,** *105*, 201–209.

Santos, A. R.; Filho, V. C.; Yunes, R. A.; Calixto, J. B. Analysis of the Mechanisms Underlying the Antinococeptive Effects of the Extracts of Plants from the Genus *Phyllanthus*. *Gen. Pharmacol.* **1995,** *26*, 1499–1506.

Sarin, B.; Verma, N.; Martin, J. P.; Mohanty, A. An Overview of Important Ethnomedicinal Herbs of *Phyllanthus* Species: Present Status and Future Prospects. *Sci. World. J.* **2014,** *2014*, 1–12.

Sawitri, E. Apoptosis of Colorectal Cancer Cell on Sprague-Dawley Rats Induced with 1, 2 Dimethylhidrazine and *Phyllanthus niruri* Linn. Extract. *Int. J. Sci. Eng.* **2016,** *10*, 45–50.

Shabeer, J.; Srivastava, R. S.; Singh, S. K. Antidiabetic and Antioxidant Effect of Various Fractions of *Phyllanthus simplex* in Alloxan Diabetic Rats. *J. Ethnopharmacol.* **2009,** *124*, 34–38.

Silva, T.; Veras, F. J.; Lucia, C. D. A. E.; Antonia, D. S.; Albuquerque, U.; Cavalcante, de A. E. Acute Toxicity Study of Stone-Breaker (*Phyllanthus tenellus Roxb.*). *Rev. Cienc. Farm.* **2012,** *33*, 205–210.

Souza, C. R. Compounds Extracted from *Phyllanthus* and *Jatropha elliptica* Inhibit the Binding of [3H] Glutamate and [3H] GMP–PNP in Rat Cerebral Cortex Membrane. *Neurochem. Res.* **2000,** *25*, 211–215.

Srirama, R.; Deepak, H. B.; Senthilkumar, U.; Ravikanth, G.; Gurumurthy, B. R.; Shivanna, M. B.; Chandrasekaran, C. V.; Agarwal, A.; Shaanker, R. U. Hepatoprotective Activity of Indian *Phyllanthus*. *Pharm. Biol.* **2012,** *50*, 948–953.

Srividya, N.; Periwal, S. Diuretic, Hypotensive and Hypoglycaemic Effect of *Phyllanthus amarus*. *Indian J. Exp. Biol.* **1995,** *33*, 861–864.

Tan, S. P.; Tan, E. N.; Lim, Q. Y.; Nafiah, M. A. *Phyllanthus acidus* (L.) Skeels: A Review of Its Traditional Uses, Phytochemistry, and Pharmacological Properties. *J. Ethnopharmacol.* **2020.** DOI: 10.1016/j.jep.2020.112610.

Thyagarajan, S. P.; Subramanian, S.; Thirunalasundari, T.; Venkateswaram, P. S.; Blumberg, B. S. Preliminary Study: The Effects of *Phyllanthus amarus* on Chronic Carriers of Hepatitis B Virus. *The Lancet* **1988,** *2*, 764–766.

Umamaheswari, S.; Joseph, L. D.; Srikanth, J.; Lavanya, R.; Chamundeeswari, D.; Reddy, C. U. Antidiabetic Activity of a Polyherbal Formulation (Diabet). *Int. J. Pharmaceut. Sci.* **2012,** *2910*, 18–22.

Unander, D. W.; Webster, G. L.; Blumberg, B. S. Records of Usage or Assays in *Phyllanthus* (Euphorbiaceae). I. The Subgenera *Isocladus, Kirganelia, Cicca* and *Emblica*. *J. Ethanopharmacol.* **1990,** *30*, 233–264.

Wanniarachchi, K. K.; Dinithi, L.; Peiris, C.; Ratnasooriya, W. D. Antihyperglycemic and Hypoglycemic Activities of *Phyllanthus debilis* Aqueous Plant Extract in Mice. *Pharm. Biol.* **2009,** *47*, 260–265.

Webster, G. L. A Monographic Study of the West Indian Species of *Phyllanthus*. *J. Arn. Arb.* **1957,** *38*, 51–64.

Yang, B.; Liu, P. Composition and Biological Activities of Hydrolysable Tannins of Fruits of *Phyllanthus emblica*. *J. Agric. Food Chem.* **2014,** *62*, 529–541.

Younessi-Hamzekhanlu, M.; Ozturk, M.; Altay, V. et al. Ethnopharmacological Study of Medicinal Plants from Khoy City of West Azerbaijan-Iran. *Ind J. Trad. Knowl.* **2020,** *19* (2), 251-267.

Zhao, T.; Sun, Q.; Marques, M.; Witcher, M. Anticancer Properties of *Phyllanthus emblica* (Indian Gooseberry). *Oxid. Med. Cell Longev.* **2015,** *2015*, 1–7.

Zhong, M.; Xiang, Y.; Qiu, X.; Liu, Z.; Kitazato, K.; Wang, Y. F. Natural Products as a Source of Anti-Herpes Simplex Virus Agents. *RSC Adv.* **2013,** *3*, 313–328.

CHAPTER 8

Unique Traditional Approach to Address Human Health Issues with *Ocimum sanctum*

PROSENJIT PRAMANICK[1], SUFIA ZAMAN[1], and ABHIJIT MITRA[2]

[1]*Department of Oceanography, Techno India University, West Bengal, Kolkata, India*

[2]*Department of Marine Science, University of Calcutta, Kolkatta, West Bengal, India*

ABSTRACT

Ocimum sanctum (family, *Lamiaceae*) is known as holy basil and commonly called "tulsi." This plant has been used in India from time immemorial to treat different human ailments. Extract of tulsi with honey is widely consumed as a remedial juice to combat the cough and cold. The extract of the tulsi leaf will be mixed with channa (a milk product) to prepare a famous traditional sweet called "rasgulla." On comparison of rasgulla prepared without and with tulsi extract showed a significant increase in total protein, carbohydrates, total lipids, vitamin C, and minerals (Ca, K, and Mg) in the latter. Rasgulla prepared from tulsi also showed overall acceptance (enhanced the flavor, texture, and mouth feel). The traditional sweet rasgulla is a nutritionally and medicinally valued health food that has immense potential in sweet industries.

Ethnic Knowledge and Perspectives of Medicinal Plants, Volume 1: Curative Properties and Treatment Strategies. Munir Ozturk, Kandikere R. Sridhar, Maryam Sarwat, Volkan Altay, & Francisco Martín Huerta-Martínez (Eds.)

8.1 INTRODUCTION

Plants are important sources of medicine and drugs owing to their secondary metabolites and antimicrobial potential. Different types of herb species have been used in Ayurveda and Siddha systems of medicine from ancient times; *Ocimum sanctum* (called tulsi or holy basil) is one of them, which is a common domesticated plant in India as a symbol of the Hindu religion (Pandey and Sharma, 2010). The word "tulsi" has a Sanskrit origin, which means "incomparable one" or "matchless one" (Ghosh, 1995). This plant species is grown throughout India, Malaysia, Australia, West Africa, and many Arabian countries. The leaves, seeds, and roots of tulsi are used in Ayurveda and Siddha medicine systems, and they have different designations in local languages in India and other counties (Table 8.1). Tulsi is an aromatic and highly branched herb that grows up to 30–80 cm with simple leaves, opposite, elliptic to oblong, obtuse, or acute with entire or sub serrate or dentate margins. Purplish or reddish flowers are found in compact clusters on cylindrical spikes, and in each cluster, heart-shaped bracts are present at the basal position. The flower tube is a hair-like structure and produces fruits with small seeds (yellowish to reddish) (Buddhadev et al., 2014).

Two types of tulsi (*O. sanctum*) are commonly available: (1) Krishna Tulsi (black) and (2) Ram Tulsi (green). Their chemical composition and medicinal properties are almost the same (Das and Vasudevan, 2006). Other species of *Ocimum* include *Ocimum americanum*, *O. basilicum*, *O. campechianum*, *O. centraliafricanum*, *O. citriodorum*, *O. gratissimum*, *O. kilimandscharicum*, *O. minimum*, *O. ovatum*, *O. suave*, *O. selloi*, *O. tenuiflorum*, and *O. viride* (Joshi et al., 2011). All of them have different living conditions, morphological characters, medicinal values, and secondary metabolites (Buddhadev et al., 2014). The present chapter emphasizes the chemical composition, medicinal uses of tulsi (*O. sanctum*), and its utility in the preparation of Indian dessert rasgulla.

8.2 CHEMICAL COMPOSITION

The aromatic properties of tulsi are attributed to volatile or essential oils containing phenols terpenes, and aldehydes in seeds. In addition, organic acids, alkaloids, glycosides, saponines, and tannins are present in leaves. Due to the presence of ascorbic acid and carotene in the leaves, it is used in the treatment of cough and cold. Various studies in different parts of the world have shown that chemical constituents differ between the species due to influences of edaphic and geographic factors (Bakkali et al., 2008; Kothari et al., 2004).

TABLE 8.1 Different Names of *Ocimum sanctum* in Local and International Languages.

Name	Language	Indian state/country
Tulasii	Assamese	Assam, India
Tulsi, Kural, and Kalotulsi	Bengali	West Bengal, India
Talasi and Sabje	Gujarati	Gujarat, India
Tulsi and Niyan Posh	Dogri	Himachal Pradesh, India
Karitulasi and Tulasiya	Kannada	Karnataka, India
Pachcha and Kunnakum	Malayalam	Kerala, India
Sabja and Tulasa	Marathi	Maharashtra, India
Tulsi and Janglitulsi	Urdu	Kashmir, India
Dhala tulasi and Karpura	Oriya	Orissa, India
Tulsi	Panjabi	Punjab, India
Bajiru and Kami-Meboki	Japanese	Japan
Basilie and Sweet Basil	English	England
Loh Lahk and Yu Heung Choi	Chinese	China
Naruk-Pul and Yanggajuk	Korean	Korea
Tulsi patta and Bavariphul	Nepali	Nepal
Alfabega and Albacar	Spanish	Spain
Horapa and Kaphrau	Thai	Thailand

Source: Adapted from Kadian and Parle (2012).

O. sanctum consist of different types of chemical compounds: α-pinene, α-thujene, nonane, octane, benzene, (Z)-3-hexanol, ethyl 2-methyl butyrate, β-pinene, toluene, camphene, citronellal, sabinene, dimethyl benzene, myrecene, ethyl benzene, limocene, cis-β-ocimene, 1,8,-cineole, *p*-cymene, allo-oc-imene, terpiniolene, butyl-benzene, linalool, α-cubebene, eugenol, methyl eugenol, β-elemene, (E)-cinnamy, iso-eugenol, lactate, isocaryophyllene, β-caryophyllene, α-guaiene, α-amorphene, α-humulene, γ-humulene, 4,11-carvacro, seinadiene, α-terpeneol, α-selinene, isoborneol, borneol, germacrene-D, β-selinene, myrtenylformat, geraneol, α-murolene, calamene, cadinene, δ-cuparene, nerolidol, iedol, caryophyllene oxide, elemol, tetradecanal, humulene oxide, α- guaiol, τ-cadinol, α-bisbolol, (EZ)-famesol, cissesquisainene hydrate, Selin-11-en-4-α-ol, 14-hydroxy-α-humulenem urosolic acid, luteolin, apigenin, apigenin-7-oglucuronide, vicenin-2, luteolin-7-*O*-glucuronide, isorientin, orientin, molludistin, stigmasterol, triacontanol ferulate, vitexin, aesculin, isovitexin, procatechuic acid, aesculetin, chlorgenic acid, galuteolin, circineol, gallic acid, gallic acid methyl ester, vallinin acid, 4-hydroxybenzoic acid, caffiec acid, chlorogenic acid, β-stigmasterol, phenylpropane glucosides, palmitric acid, linolenic acid, stearic acid, sitosterol, oleic acid, dilinoleno-linolins, linodilinolin, and hexourenic acid (Kelm and Nair, 1998; Jaggi et al., 2003; Anbarasu and Vijaylaxmi, 2007; Luthra, 2010; Rahman et al., 2011; Shisodia, 2003; Singh et al., 2012a, b; Summy and Patyal, 2016). In addition, proteins, carbohydrates, lipids, vitamin c, carotene, and different minerals are present in *O. sanctum* (Table 8.2).

TABLE 8.2 Nutritional Composition of *Ocimum sanctum*.

Component	Quantity/100 g dry mass
Protein	4.2 g
Carbohydrate	2.3 g
Total lipids	0.5 mg
Vitamin C	25 mg
Carotene	2.5 μg
Phosphorus	287 mg
Calcium	25 mg
Iron	15.1 mg
Zinc	0.15 μg
Copper	0.4 μg
Vanadium	0.54 μg
Chromium	2.9 μg
Nickel	0.73 μg

Source: Adapted from Luthra (2010); Nissen et al. (2010); Pattanayak (2010).

8.3 MEDICINAL VALUE

In Ayurveda and Siddha systems of medicine, every part of tulsi is utilized. In rural areas, people use the root of the tulsi to treat the malarial fever. In case of gastric disorder of the children, infusion of tulsi leaf is very useful as antispasmodic. Water extract from leaf (as juice) is used as a demulcent, stimulant, and expectorant. Common diseases like cough, cold, influenza, fever, pain, asthma, and other respiratory problems including heart problems are cured by tulsi leaf decoctions. It also serves as an antidote for snake bites as well as scorpion stings. Ulcer and mouth infections could be cured using tulsi. The scientific literature confirms the medicinal properties of the tulsi plant due to the presence of antimicrobial, antioxidant, anti-inflammatory, radioprotective, neuroprotective, antiallergic, and many other properties. In Ayurveda, tulsi is used for curing many diseases like common cold, headache, heart disease, inflammation, kidney stones, malaria, and stomach disorders. It also serves as one of the best remedies to boost immunity. It aids in inhibiting the action of HIV and cells affected by carcinogens. Major human health-related disorders that are cured and healed by tulsi are listed in Table 8.3.

8.4 RASGULLA FROM TULSI

India is one of the promising milk-producing countries; 50–55% of produced milk convert into food products like yogurt and sweets. Rasgulla is one of the traditional sweets of India and commonly consumed by people in various states (mainly in Bihar, Orissa, and West Bengal). After a long fight, rasgulla of West Bengal was assigned the tag of geographic indication (GI) in November 2017. Rasgulla is a white, spongy, spherical, and juicy sweet that resembles a ping pong ball. It is one of the highly nutritious products as it comprises proteins, lipids, minerals (calcium and phosphorus), and fat-soluble vitamins (Sahu and Tiwari, 2008). In 2017, tulsi rasgulla was prepared and marketed in and around Kolkata city, and this was prepared by a retail sweet shop named "Satyanarayan Mistanna Bhander" located at Singur in the Hooghly district of West Bengal.

Rasgulla is usually prepared in a nonmechanized process in local markets for business purposes. However, research progress has been made in the preparation of rasgulla in a mechanized way for bulk production in minimum duration. Six steps will be followed in the preparation of tulsi rasgulla: 1) preparation of tulsi leaf extract; 2) preparation of channa (an acid-coagulated milk product); 3) kneading and ball formation of channa; 4) preparation of tulsi-sugar syrup; 5) cooking of channa ball; and 6) preparation of final product (Figure 8.1). First, tulsi leaves were thoroughly washed and semidried overnight. The soaked leaves were boiled and filtered through a fine cloth and centrifuged using a cold centrifuge (5000 rpm, 20 min). The supernatant was collected and preserved (−20 °C) in clean containers (served as tulsi syrup). The materials on the cloth (called tulsi mud) were collected and kept in a container to use for the preparation of rasgulla.

TABLE 8.3 Uses of Tulsi to Combat Human Diseases.

Disease	Mode of preparation
Respiratory disorder	Tulsi leaves boiled with water and mixed with honey help to fight bronchitis, cough, and cold
Sore throat	Drinking boiled water with tulsi leaves is a remedy for the treatment of sore throat
Cough	Tulsi leaves help in the mobilization of the mucus in bronchitis and asthma. It also relieves cold and flu by chewing the leaves
Fever and common cold	Tulsi leaves boil with tea help to combat malaria and dengue; the tulsi extract (juice) is also used during fever
Headache	A mixture of pounded leaves and sandwood paste is applied on the forehead for getting relief from heat, headache, etc.
Healing power	Leaves are used as a nerve tonic and sharpen memory. They also help in the removal of catarrhal matter and phlegm from the bronchial tube
Heart disorder	Leaves reduce the level of blood cholesterol
Stress	Chewing leaves twice a day prevents some stresses; it even purifies the blood and helps in the prevention of several common psychological disorders
Skin disease	Tulsi extract is used to cure the treatment of dermal diseases like ringworm and leucoderma. In the case of chicken pox, tulsi leaves are taken with saffron to explore the disease
Mouth infection	Ulcer and other infections in the mouth are cured by chewing of tulsi leaves
Eye care	Ayurvedic eye drop that is prepared with tulsi leaf extract and *Triphala* is the best remedy for glaucoma, cataract, chronic conjunctivitis, and other painful eye diseases
Teeth disorder	Tulsi toothpaste prepared with mustard oil is very good for maintaining dental health, counteracting bad breath, and for massaging the gum
Renal disorder	Regularly taken of a tulsi extract with honey (for 6 months) expel the renal stone through the urinary tract; the fresh leaves and flower tops are used as an antispasmodic agent
Diabetes mellitus	The presence of various essential oils in tulsi leaves causes improving pancreatic beta cell function and thus enhancing insulin secretion to control the blood sugar level of the diabetic patient
Gastrointestinal disorder	Aqueous decoction of tulsi leaves acts as a laxative in the treatment of gastric and hepatic disorder

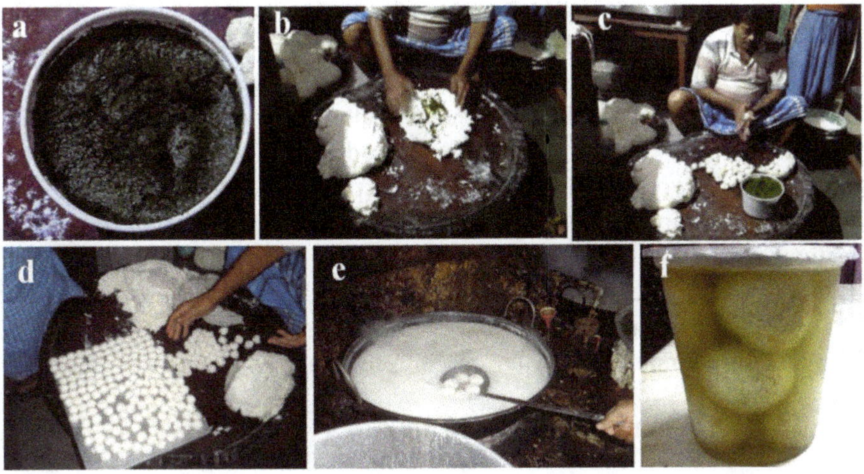

FIGURE 8.1 Steps followed in the preparation of rasgulla: Tulsi extract (tulsi mud) (a), kenading tulsi mud with channa (b), preparation of balls (c, d), cooking channa balls in sugar syrup (40% sugar syrup made from tulsi extract) (e), and packed rasgulla (f).

Channa is the main ingredient in preparing rasgulla; for its preparation, milk was boiled and cooled (to 70°C). Then, citric acid (as lemon juice) (or lactic acid could be used) was added to coagulate the milk (Rao, 1971; Iyer, 1978; Rajorhia and Sen, 1988). The coagulated mass called channa is off-white and mildly acidic in taste. The texture of rasgulla depends on the moisture content of channa. Excess moisture (>60%) causes the breakage of rasgulla in the sugar syrup, while due to less moisture (<50%), rasgulla becomes very hard. Thus, the optimum moisture content should be 55-58% to make a perfect and stable rasgulla (Bhattacharya and Des, 1980).

The important step of rasgulla preparation is the kneading of channa, which is nothing but a mixing and folding process by that rheological and textural properties change. Channa was kneaded, applying pressure until it became smooth and uniform. The desired pH of the channa ball is 6.6. Before starting the kneading process, the whole channa was divided into two parts. For assessment of quality, in the first part, tulsi leaf mud was not mixed, while in the second part, tulsi leaf mud was mixed and kneaded. After kneading, it was rolled into the size of ping pong balls.

The sweetness and shelf-life of a rasgulla depend on the strength and concentration of sugar syrup. The ratio of sugar and water 1:2 is perfect for an ideal rasgulla. In the case of tulsi rasgulla, water content was replaced with the tulsi extract. For the preparation of the syrup, first tulsi extract (water is used in control) was boiled in a container, and then a specific amount of sugar was added to it and boiled until dissolved and reached to standard concentration 50–55°Brix (Bhattacharya and Des, 1980). In this step (control and experimental), channa balls were added to the respective sugar syrup and boiled for 10 min in a closed container. Two types of syrups were used: 1) syrup with water and 2) syrup with tulsi extract. After 5 min, the syrup was stirred without disrupting the balls, and then a small amount of water was added. After 10 min, the balls swelled and their volume increased, and they were treated in low flame for 8–10 min. The balls were then soaked (one with plain water and the other with tulsi extract) and kept for 15–30 min at room temperature. After cooling, the final products were packed in containers.

8.5 COMPOSITION OF RASGULLA

The rasgulla samples (control and experimental) were analyzed for nutritional composition ($n = 5$). The total protein percentage was analyzed by the Lowry method (Lowry et al., 1951). The method of phenol-sulfuric acid (standard, D-glucose) was used to know the total carbohydrate content (Dubois et al., 1956). The variation in crude fat was analyzed by the Soxhlet method using petroleum ether (80°C) (AOAC, 2000). For the analysis of ascorbic acid, the standard protocol was followed (Nielsen, 1998; Zvaigzne et al., 2009). Concentrations of Ca, K, and Mg (mg/100g) were determined by flame photometry. The selected parameters exhibit considerable significant variations between the control and tulsi rasgulla. A comparison of the quality of rasgulla prepared without and with tulsi leaves is given in Table 8.4.

TABLE 8.4 Comparison of Nutritional Quality of Rasgulla Prepared Without and with Tulsi Leaves ($n = 5 \pm SD$).

Content	Rasgulla without tulsi	Rasgulla with tulsi
Protein (%)	6.8±0.28	7.7±0.24
Carbohydrates (%)	50.7±0.75	60.8±0.38
Total lipids (%)	4.2±0.11	5.7±0.25
Vitamin C (mg/100 g)	2.9±0.18	4.8±0.22
Ca (mg/100 g)	34.2±0.11	36.9±0.23
K (mg/100 g)	47.0±0.09	49.8±0.11
Mg (mg/100 g)	1.3±0.06	2.1±0.05

8.6 SENSORY EVALUATION

Sensory evaluation of rasgulla (control and experimental) was performed using nine-member panellists (Meilgaard et al., 2007). It was judged in terms of color, flavor, body and texture, mouth feel, sweetness, and overall acceptance using the nine-point hedonic scale (Piggott, 1984). The evaluation scale was according to Opawale et al. (2011) (Table 8.5).

TABLE 8.5 Sensory Evaluation of Both Types of Prepared Rasgulla.

Parameters	Rasgulla without tulsi	Rasgulla with tulsi
Color	8.5	7.0
Flavor	6.0	8.2
Body and texture	7.3	7.9
Mouth feel	8.0	8.2
Sweetness	8.7	8.0
Overall acceptance	8.2	8.8

Scale of Assessment:

1) Dislike Extremely; 2) Dislike Very Much; 3) Dislike Moderately; 4) Dislike Slightly; 5) Neither Dislike nor Acceptable; 6) Slightly Acceptable; 7) Moderately Acceptable; 8) Highly Acceptable; and 9) Extremely Acceptable.

Source: Adapted from Opawale et al. (2011).

Rasgulla is one of the most popular Indian desserts made from milk and is a special attraction for sweet lovers. This soft juicy milk product is a matter of concern to diabetic patients. This can be circumvented by replacing sucrose with low-calorie sweeteners. In the present pilot program, we observed a hike in the quality of tulsi rasgulla in terms of nutritional value. Tulsi rasgulla exhibited an increase in total protein than the control sample. The crude fat and total carbohydrates were also increased. An increase in minerals (Ca, K, and Mg) was seen. The ascorbic acid content was increased, which can fight against cough and cold being common health problem among the population in the tropics.

8.7 CONCLUSIONS

The nutritional profile of rasgulla made from tulsi leaves is better than milk alone and possesses dual benefits of nutrition and health. Rasgulla prepared with tulsi showed increased total protein, carbohydrates, total lipids, vitamin C, and minerals (Ca, K, and Mg). Sensory evaluation of rasgulla made from tulsi leaves also proved an overall acceptance (enhanced the flavor, texture, and mouth feel). The traditional sweet rasgulla made from tulsi leaves is popular and has wide potential in the sweet industry. The use of tulsi in the preparation for rasgulla provides an alternative livelihood for the farmers to grow tulsi in agricultural fields. With proven GI, rasgulla has ample export potential with precise shelf life and medicinal properties.

ACKNOWLEDGMENTS

The authors gratefully acknowledge the owners of Satyanarayan Mistanna Bhander, Singur, West Bengal for making provisions for carrying out experiments on rasgulla.

KEYWORDS

- ***Ocimum sanctum***
- **tulsi**
- **rasgulla**
- **nutritional value**
- **nonconventional sweets**

REFERENCES

Anbarasu, K.; Vijayalaxmi, G. Improve Shelf Life of Protein Rich Tofu Using *Ocimum sanctum* (Tulsi) Extract to Benefit Indian Rural Population. *J. Food Sci.* **2007**, *72*, M300–M305.

AOAC (Association of Official Analytical Chemists). *Official Method of Analysis*; 17th ed.; Washington, DC, 2000.

Bakkali, F.; Averbeck, S.; Averbeck, D.; Idaomar, M. Biological Effects of Essential Oils—A Review. *Food Chem. Toxicol.* **2008**, *46*, 446–475.

Bhattacharya, D. C.; Des, R. Studies on Production of Rasgulla. Part–II. Pressure Cooker Method. *Ind. J. Dairy Sci.* **1980**, *33*, 479–483.

Buddhadev, S. G.; Buddhadev, S. S.; Mehta, N. D. A Review Article on *Ocimum sanctum* Linn. *Punarna* **2014**, *2* (2), 1–6.

Das, S. K.; Vasudevan, D. M. Tulsi: The Indian holy power plant. *Nat. Prod. Radiance* **2006**, *5*, 279–283.

Dubois, M.; Gilles, K. A.; Hamilton, J. K.; Rebers, P. A.; Smith, F. Colorimetric Methods for Determination of Sugars and Related Substances. *J. Anal. Chem.* **1956**, *28*, 350–356.

Ghosh, G. R. Tulasi (N.O. Labiatae, Genus- *Ocimum*). New Approaches to Medicine and Health (NAMAH). 1995, Vol 3; pp 23–29.

Iyer, M. Physico-Chemical Studies on Chhana from Cow's and Buffalo's Milk. M.Sc. Dissertation, Kurukshetra University, Kuruskhetra, India, 1978.

Jaggi, R. K.; Maddan, R.; Singh, B. Anticonvulsant Potential of Holly Basal, *Ocimum sanctum* Linn. and Its Culture. *Ind. J. Exp. Biol.* **2003**, *41*, 1329–1333.

Joshi, B.; Sah, G. P.; Basnet, B. B.; Bhatt, M. R.; Sharma, D.; Subedi, K. Phytochemical Extraction and Antimicrobial Properties of Different Medicinal Plants: *Ocimum sanctum* (Tulsi), *Eugenia caryophyllata* (Clove), *Achyranthes bidentata* (Datiwan) and *Azadirachta indica* (Neem). *J. Microbiol. Antimicrob.* **2011**, *3* (1), 1–7.

Kadian, R.; Parle, M. Therapeutic Potential and Phytopharmacology of Tulsi. *Int. J. Pham. Life Sci.* **2012**, *3* (7), 1858–1867.

Kelm, M. A.; Nair, G. M. Mosquitocidal Compounds and Triglyceride 1, 3-dilinolenoeol-2-palmitin from *Ocimum sanctum*. *J. Agric. Food Chem.* **1998**, *40*, 3691–3693.

Kothari, S. K.; Bhattacharya, A. K.; Ramesh, S. Essential Oil Yield and Quality of Methyl Eugenol Rich *Ocimum tenuiflorum* L.f. (syn *Ocimum sanctum* L.) Grown in South India as Influenced by Method of Harvest. *J. Chromatogr. A.* **2004**, *1054*, 67–72.

Lowry, O. H.; Rosebrough, N. J.; Farr, A. L.; Randall, R. J. Protein Measurement with the Folin-Phenol Reagents. *J. Biol. Chem.* **1951**, *193*, 265–275.

Luthra, D. *Ocimum sanctum* (Tulsi): A Potent Medicinal Herb. *Webmed Cen Pharmacol.* **2010**, *1*, WMC001210.

Meilgaard, M. C.; Civille, G. V.; Carr, B. T. *Sensory Evaluation Techniques*, 4th ed.; CRC Press; Taylor and Francis Group, USA, 2007.

Nielsen, D. *Food Analysis*; Aspen Publishers, Inc.: Gaithersburg, MD; United State Department of Agriculture Nutrient Base (2004), 1998.

Nissen, L.; Zatta, A.; Stefanini, I.; Grandi, S.; Sgorbati, B.; Biavati, B.; Monti, A. Characterization and Antimicrobial Activity of Essential Oils of Industrial Hemp Varieties (*Cannabis sativa* L.). *Fitoterapia* **2010**, *81*, 413–48.

Opawale, B. O.; Giwa, O. E.; Jose, O. R.; Aladejimokun, O. A.; Aladenika, A. K. Physical Sensory and Microbial Attribute of Taro Flour Supplemented Cookies. National Conference Proceedings on Interdisciplinary Cooperation. *Panacea Food Secur.* **2011**, *1*, 6.

Pandey, G.; Sharma, M. Pharmacological Activities of *Ocimum sanctum* (Tulsi): A review. *Int. J. Pharm. Sci. Rev. Res.* **2010**, *5* (1), 61–66.

Pattanayak, P. *Ocimum sanctum* Linn. A Reservoir Plant for Therapeutic Applications: An Overview. *Pharmacogn. Rev.* **2010**, *4*, 95–105.

Piggott, J. R. *Sensory Analysis of Foods*, Vol. 250; Elsevier Applied Science Publishers: New York, 1984; pp 157–161.

Rahman, M. S.; Salehin, M. F.; Jamal, M. A. H. M.; Pravin, A.; Alam, M. K. Antimicrobial Activity of *Argimone Mexicana* L Against Water Born Microbs. *Res. J. Med. Pl.* **2011**, *5*, 621–626.

Rajorhia, G. S.; Sen, D. C. Technology of Chhana—A Review. *Ind. J. Dairy Sci.* **1988**, *41*, 141–148.

Rao, B. V. R. *Effect of Different Concentrations of Citric Acid Coagulant and Fat Levels of Milk from Crossbred Cows on Yield of Chhana, Fat Losses in Whey, Moisture Retained in Chhana and Quality Chhana*; Allahabad University: Allahabad, 1971.

Sahu, J. K.; Tiwari, A. Constraints and Solutions for Mechanization of Dairy Products Manufacturing in North Eastern India. *Ind. Dairyman.* **2008**, *60* (6), 17–29.

Shisodia, S. Urosolic acid Inhibits Nuclear Factor-Kapa B Activation Induced by Carcinogenic Agents Through Suppression of Ikappa B Alpha Kinase and p65 Phosphorylation: Correlation of Down Regulation of Cyclooxygenase 2, Matrix Metaloprotease 9 and Cyclin D1. *Canc. Res.* **2003**, *63*, 4375–4383.
Singh, E.; Sharma, S.; Dwivedi, J.; Sharma, S. Diversified Potentials of *Ocimum sanctum* Linn. (Tulsi): An Exhaustive Survey. *Scholars Res. Lib.* **2012a**, *2* (1), 39–48.
Singh, N.; Verma, P.; Pandey, B. R.; Bhalla, M. Therapeutic Potential of *Ocimum sanctum* in Prevention and Treatment of Cancer and Exposure to Radiation: An Overview. *Int. J. Pharm. Sci. Drug Res.* **2012b**, *4*, 97–104.
Summy, S.; Patyal, P. *Ocimum sanctum* (Tulsi) "Queen of All Medicinal Herbs": A Review. *Int. J. Innov. Pharm Sci. Res.* **2016**, *4*, 871–886.
Zvaigzne, G.; Karklina, D.; Seglina, D.; Krasnova, I. Antioxidants in Various Citrus Fruit Juices. *Chemine Technologija* **2009**, *3* (52), 56–61.

CHAPTER 9

Ethnomedicinal and Current Applications of Neem (*Azadirachta indica*)

S. SHISHUPALA

Department of Microbiology, Davangere University, Shivagangothri, Davangere, Karnataka, India

ABSTRACT

Neem (*Azadirachta indica*) is one of the important medicinal plants used in India and other countries owing to its medicinal potential. Over 140 bioactive compounds are being identified in neem with specific biological activities. Ethnomedically, neem is used to cure a wide range of human and animal ailments. It also serves in agriculture as one of the best known natural biopesticides. Metabolites of neem have shown a wide range of properties from insecticidal to anticarcinogenic. In modern medicine, neem and its products are used against various diseases. Some of the metabolites of neem have been produced by cell and tissue cultures (e.g., azadirachtin). Neem and its products are also useful in veterinary therapeutics and plant protection strategies. In biotechnological front, neem-based nanopesticides have been developed recently with several applications. Analysis of genome, transcriptome, and metabolome of neem further strengthened its precise applications. Ethnomedicinal uses, bioactive compounds, biopesticide potential, and biotechnological applications of neem have been discussed.

Ethnic Knowledge and Perspectives of Medicinal Plants, Volume 1: Curative Properties and Treatment Strategies. Munir Ozturk, Kandikere R. Sridhar, Maryam Sarwat, Volkan Altay, & Francisco Martín Huerta-Martínez (Eds.)

9.1 INTRODUCTION

Medicinal plants are gaining importance in view of phytotherapy in order to treat or cure many ailments. Ranges of herbs, shrubs, and trees have been used to exploit their medicinal values (Ugboko et al., 2020; Younessi-Hamzekhanlu et al., 2020; Ozturk et al., 2020, 2021a, b). Neem (*Azadirachta indica* A. Juss.; Meliaceae) is one of the common native trees in India used most extensively in ethnomedicine for many centuries owing to its broad medicinal properties. Besides India, it grows in many Asian countries, and due to its beneficial traits, it has been introduced into Africa as well as America. Currently, many compounds from neem have been extracted and are being used to tackle human, livestock, and plant health hazards. Neem grows prolifically in almost all soil conditions, produces compound leaves, small flowers in clusters attract insects, greenish fruits are favorable for birds, and seeds are filled with oil used extensively in medicine as well as biodiesel. Owing to diverse medicinal values, neem is used in dental treatments, Chagas disease (American trypanosomiasis), malaria, pain relief, fever reduction, contraceptive, veterinary ailments, and many human ailments (Pankaj et al., 2011; Alzohairy, 2016; Paula et al., 2019). An array of compounds like azadirachtin, meliantriol, salannin, nimbin, nimbidin, and others are being characterized from neem for their medical applications (Hashmat et al., 2012). A range of commercial products like oil, soap, cosmetics, lubricants, fertilizers, timber, fuel, and resin are being produced from neem (Chaudhary et al., 2017). Neem and neem products are used in crop protection (Paul et al., 2013; Campos et al., 2016). Neem has been intensely studied toward biopesticide research (Anonymous, 1992). Apart from agroforestry, neem has found a prominent place in afforestation and reforestation programs. In spite of well-known medicinal properties, neem also succumbs to pests and diseases. Efforts toward genetic improvement, as well as biotechnological applications, are underway. This chapter emphasizes the significance of neem in ethnomedicine, bioactive principles, biopesticide, and biotechnological applications.

9.2 NEEM AND ETHNIC PRACTICE

Neem is a moderate evergreen tree belonging to the dicotyledonous group and has more than 1400 species. It is a deep-rooted tree with thick furrowed bark that grows to a maximum height of 30 m; its trunk attains girth up to 2.5 m, and the bark is capable of exuding gum (Figure 9.1a). The leaves are lush green measuring 20–30 cm in length with 8–19 alternate or oppositely placed leaflets (ovate, glossy with serrate margin) (Figure 9.1b, c). Flowers are scented, bisexual, small, white to pale yellow, and in clusters on long axillary panicles. Honey-like substances are exuded from the flowers, which are attractive to many insects. Young fruits are green, ovoid or ellipsoidal, drupe, and change to yellow on maturity (Figure 9.1d, e). Each fruit has a thin epicarp enclosing the sweet pulp with a single seed. The flowering season of neem is January–May and fruits ripen in May–August. Seeds are oval with a hard coat. Usually, flowering occurs by 3–5 years after planting; it is capable of producing fruits for about 10 years (~50 kg/year), and the trees can survive for more than 200 years. In terms of distribution, neem is grown throughout the Indian subcontinent and other Asian countries, while it is an introduced tree in Africa and America. The other species of neem, *Azadirachta excels* is found in the Philippines and Indonesia (Anonymous, 1992; Pankaj, et al., 2011).

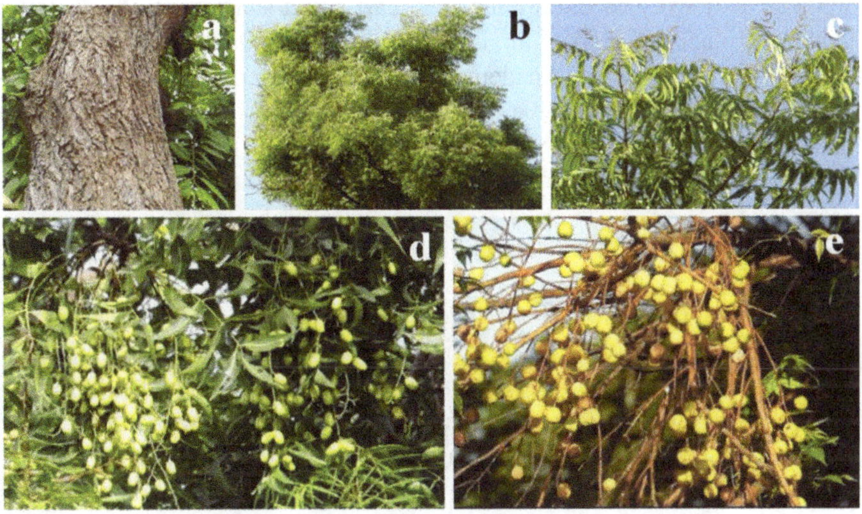

FIGURE 9.1 Characteristics of neem: bark (a), luxuriantly grown shoot (b), compound leaves (c), fresh fruits (d), and ripened fruits (e).

Traditional and complementary medicines are developed by the ethnic knowledge as well as the experience of native people. Such traditional practices need different plants and their parts for therapeutic purposes (Ozturk et al., 2017a, b, c, 2018a, b, c, d, e, f, g). With the development of modern medicine, ethnic medicinal knowledge has been sidelined. However, due to health consciousness, traditional and complementary medicines are receiving due weightage the world over. In particular, neem-based products are being used in India and in other Asian countries for curing various human ailments. Different religious documents mentioned the beneficial impacts of neem and other related plant species (Anonymous, 1992; Boeke et al., 2004; Brahmachari, 2004; Alzohairy, 2016; Kashif et al., 2019). The neem-based products are in traditional use in plant protection as well as in grain storage (Boursier et al., 2011; Gahukar, 2014; Doshi et al., 2018).

Ancient Indian documents like "*Charaka Samhita*" and "*Sushruta Samhita*" have provided ample information on the extensive medicinal properties and uses of neem (Pankaj et al., 2011). Neem has also been extensively used in Ayurveda, Unani, and Homeopathy, apart from traditional medicines. It has been one of the prominent components in Ayurvedic medicine of India for 4000 years. The name *Arista* in Sanskrit denotes neem as: "*perfect, complete and imperishable*". Neem is used in India for routine oral health care, especially to clean the teeth (by twigs), skin applicants (leaf and bark extract), decoction/tonic (leaf/bark), and against insect infestation in storage places (Kausik et al., 2002; Brahmachari, 2004; Girish and Bhat, 2008). The US National Academy of Sciences has considered neem as a "tree species capable to solve many global problems" (Anonymous, 1992; Pankaj et al., 2011).

9.3 BIOACTIVE METABOLITES

A wide range of substances has been identified in neem with a variety of biological activities, and these active principles exist as an admixture in different plant parts. The chief constituents of neem are grouped as limonoids under the triterpenes category, and the main insecticidal property is attributed to limonoids capable of inhibiting insect growth and metamorphosis. Among the various limonoids associated with the neem include azadirachtin, salannin, meliantriol, and nimbin (Anonymous, 1992; Paula et al., 2019; Ugboko et al., 2020). The details of the major bioactive metabolites of neem, their presence in plant parts, biological applications, and commercial products are given in Table 9.1. Hatti et al. (2014) developed a database to provide structural details of neem metabolites, and literature pertaining to them are accessible in the NeeMDB database. This database also provides information on the physicochemical properties of neem metabolites.

Azadirachtin is one of the most active ingredients of neem and possess insecticidal properties. This compound mainly acts as an insect repellent, capable of unbalancing insect reproduction on ingestion, and decreases the feeding practice of insect pests. Structurally, azadirachtin resembles that of insect molting hormones such as ecdysones, which are essential to control growth during metamorphosis. Azadirachtin interferes with insect ecdysones, hence interfering with insect development. The concentration of azadirachtin in neem seeds varies depending on the variety and region of cultivation (Koul et al., 1990; Anonymous, 1992; Gupta et al., 2017; Fernandes et al., 2019; Hodgson et al., 2019). Meliantriol is another compound of neem capable of reducing the feeding behavior of insects. Similarly, a triterpenoid called salannin is a powerful inhibitor of insect feeding.

TABLE 9.1 Bioactive Metabolites of Neem with Biological Activities and Commercial Products.

Metabolite	Plant part	Biological application		Commercial product
		Medicinal	Agricultural	
Azadirachtin	Seed oil, seed kernels, and leaves	Antimalarial, anticancer, and anti-inflammation	Insecticide, pesticide, and fertilizer	Bioneem oil, Foliar Parker Neem Coat, Neem Urea Guard, and Ozoneem Cake
Catechin and epicatechin	Bark	Immunomodulation	–	Used in various cosmetics, creams, soaps, and toothpastes
Gallic acid	Bark	Immunomodulation	–	
Gedunin	Seed oil	Antimicrobial	–	
Mahmoodin	Seed oil	Antibacterial	–	
Margolone, margolonone, and isomargolonone		Antimicrobial	–	
Nimbin	Seed oil	Spermicide	–	
Nimbindin	Seed oil	Antimicrobial, anti-inflammation, antipyretic, and antidiabetic	–	
Nimbolide	Seed oil	Antimicrobial, anticancer, and anti-inflammation	–	
Salannin	Leaves and seeds	–	Insecticide	

Nimbin and nimbidin produced by neem are capable of inhibiting many animal and plant viruses. Besides, many animals are also affected by these metabolites. A few minor constituents of neem are capable of paralyzing insect mouth parts causing difficulty in swallowing. Deacetylazadirachtin, gedunin, azadirone, quercetin, β-sitosterol, and flavanoids are other metabolites found in neem with potential biological activity (Koul et al., 1990; Kumar et al., 2013; Alzohairy, 2016; Balaji et al., 2018; Saleem et al., 2018). These compounds could be isolated by various extraction methods using water and solvents (hexane, pentane, and alcohol), and many protocols for isolation have also been developed (Fernandes et al., 2019; Suttiarporn and Choommongkol, 2020).

Evaluation of neem products and their biological activities in biotechnological applications are widely discussed (Alzohairy, 2016; Aneesa and Gayathri, 2016; Balaji et al., 2018; Alsanad et al., 2018; Hodgson et al., 2019; Thota et al., 2020; Braga et al., 2021). Antimicrobial effect of neem is well established, and such principles constitute a major ingredient in cosmetics, creams, and soaps (mainly to scavenge the free radicles). Neem metabolites are useful in combating several multi-drug-resistant bacterial strains (Okoh et al., 2019). The major metabolites involved in such properties are caryophyllene, phytol, elemene, and linoleic acid. Thus, the use of the traditional neem products is boosted using an appropriate concentration of essential oils from neem seeds. The metabolite nimbolide is present in neem leaf extracts and is known for anticancerous properties. Suttiarporn and Choomnogkol (2020) developed a microwave-assisted extraction procedure to get nimbolide yield of up to 98% purity. In addition, time required for solvent extraction and microwave protocols provide ease of purification of nimbolide within three hours. Another most common bioactive phytochemical belonging to limonoids is gedunin that has been detected in neem fruit epicarp. Series of biological activities like antimicrobial, anti-inflammatory, anticancer, insecticidal, and neuroprotective effects have been attributed to gedunin (Braga et al., 2020). Neem leaf extract is used as an antimicrobial agent by incorporation into seaweed biopolymer. This biocomposite film shows improved properties by mixing neem leaf extract (5%, w/w) followed by gamma irradiation. Improved hydrophobicity with changes in color and opacity of the product are noticed due to the combination of neem, and this product serves as packaging material (Kumar et al., 2020).

9.4 BIOPESTCIDE

Increased use of chemical pesticides in agriculture resulted in serious environmental pollution problems and health risks. There is a renewed interest in producing microbial or botanical insecticides in order to reduce the use of chemical pesticides. Biological pesticides are being foreseen as effective alternatives in sustainable agriculture. Neem and other members of Meliaceae have been identified as biopesticides owing to their effectiveness in controlling lepidopteran insects. The mechanisms involved in such control lie in their impact on insect digestive enzymes (e.g., amylases, glycosidases, lipases, and proteases). Neem metabolites are also reported to interfere with the alkaline and acid phosphatases of insects. Acetylcholine esterase, the enzyme involves in nerve impulses of insects, gets altered by neem metabolites, which qualifies neem as a potential bioinsecticide (Senthil-Nathan, 2013).

Biopesticide properties of neem and possible mode of action are discussed by Chaudhary et al. (2017). The major insecticidal activity of neem was attributed to azadirachtin, which acts as an insect repellent, reduces feeding activity, and also decreases the reproductive potential of target insects. Integration of neem along with bioinsecticidal fungus *Metarhizium anisopliae* was effective against the mosquito larvae. The insecticidal properties of neem enhanced the efficiency of entomopathogenic fungus *M. anisopliae* and helped to prolong the insecticidal property (Paula et al., 2019). Similarly, neem oil in combination with biocontrol fungus *Leptoleginia chapmanii* proved effective in controlling mosquito *Aedes aegypti*. At effective concentration, neem oil will not inhibit fungal growth, but the combination enhances the efficiency of mosquito management (Paramo et al., 2019). Neem oil has the property to reduce the immune response of agricultural pests like caterpillars of *Spodoptera frugiperda* (Duarte et al., 2020). The caterpillars exposed to neem oil showed a significant reduction in the hemocyte count and lysozyme-like enzyme activity. The biopesticidal activity of neem extracts could be enhanced by different additives. The use of sesame oil and pyrethrins (extracts of flowers of *Chrysanthemum* with insecticidal properties) has been shown to increase insecticidal properties up to 20-folds. The insecticidal activity was also improved instead of using the bacterial bioinsecticide *Bacillus thuringiensis* or other biological agents (Anonymous, 1992; Paramo et al., 2019; Paula et al., 2019; Petrikovszki et al., 2019). Targeted activity and efficiency of neem products have been well documented. This provides an excellent opportunity to commercialize neem products in agriculture and related fields.

Pest management of stored grains is one of the major concerns in saving the food source. Chemical pesticides are toxic or carcinogenic to humans as well as livestock; hence, neem botanicals are of great significance. Ahmad et al. (2019) compared different plant species against the pest *Tribolicum castaneum* (red flour beetle). Neem seed powder mixed with wheat successfully controlled this insect. A higher level of insecticidal properties of neem was proved even at a low concentration (1%, w/w). Another study showed promising neem essential oil as a bioinsecticide (Zaka et al., 2019). Macchioni et al. (2019) tested the efficacy of neem oil as a repellent against mosquitoes (*Aedes albopictus*) in multilocational field trials. The neem oil was found to be an effective repellant as tested over a period of six months. The efficacy was also dependent on climatic conditions like rainfall and temperature. Petrikovszki et al. (2019) tested neem-derived pesticides in combination with entomopathogenic slug-parasitic nematodes. The safe concentration of neem extract was as low as 0.1% without any side effects on insecticidal nematodes. Hence, it was shown to have no lethal effect on beneficial nematodes supporting the combination of neem with entomopathogenic nematodes in agricultural insect control programs.

9.5 MEDICINAL USES

9.5.1 HUMAN DISEASES

Traditional and ethnic uses of neem provided opportunities to evaluate its ingredients in human health care products. A wide range of biological activities and ethnomedicinal knowledge helped in the development of several products that serve as human medicines. Most of the toothpastes, creams, body lotions, soaps, and Ayurvedic products possess neem components.

Moga et al. (2018) reviewed the uses of compounds of neem with special reference to gynecological cancers. Over 140 compounds of neem have multiple biological activities; among them, as many as 35 compounds serve to suppress tumors. These compounds possessing anticarcinogenic potential have been localized in different parts of the neem tree. Nimbolide from neem was shown to be involved in autophagy and apoptosis in hamster/human cell lines. Molecular mechanisms involved in the anticancer properties of nimbolide were studied by Sophia et al. (2018). Inhibition of cytoprotective autophagy and activation of apoptosis are important characteristic features for potential use in oral cancer therapy. Morris et al. (2019) tested neem leaf extract against oral squamous cell carcinoma and found promising results. Both in vitro and in vivo experiments demonstrated that neem leaf extract interferes with tumor growth and metastasis. In mouse models, neem leaf extract significantly reduced pro-inflammatory cytokines responsible for tumor development. Nimbolide was shown to be a biologically active compound of neem with anticancerous property. The anticancerous property of neem leaf glycoprotein was proved on cell lines using different techniques (Ghosh et al., 2019; Saha et al., 2020). By modulating immune mechanisms, the glycoprotein from neem showed tumor growth restrictions. Downregulation of interleukin-10 along with other mechanisms was proved under cell culture conditions. Such precise mechanisms involved in neem extract provided ample evidence for antitumor activity. Significant reduction in vascular endothelial growth factor production was evident. Agrawala et al. (2020) discussed the possible use of neem as an anticancer agent with special reference to oral cancer. Neem and its products are known to modify the tumor environment and suppress tumor proliferation. At the same time, neem components can induce high cytotoxicity of monocytes against cancer cell. Thus, neem components have potential to become therapeutic agents in oral cancer. Regular intake of neem oil was found to significantly reduce breast cancer development in Wistar rat models (Zingue et al., 2019). Dose-dependent inhibition of tumor was noticed, and higher consumption of neem oil resulted in hepatotoxicity. Hence, the optimum dose and frequency of oral intake of neem oil were proved to be effective in reducing breast cancer. Neem oil was successfully used to reduce scleroderma skin ulcers in case of patients suffering from calcinoisis (calcium deposits on soft tissues) (Giuggioli et al., 2019).

Dental caries treatment, restorative, or filling up is an important process. The dental restorative materials comprise composite resins, and amalgam and atraumatic restorative materials are highly useful in dentistry. The anti-microbial property of neem in preventing dental diseases is well known in traditional literature. Multiple bacterial infections are responsible for dental cavities. The study conducted by Kumari et al. (2019) showed the effectiveness of neem extract with filling material to inhibit dental caries causing *Streptococcus mutans*. The effect of neem as an antibacterial agent was also evident by inhibition of bacterial growth in vitro. *Enterococcus faecalis* is the predominant bacterial species responsible for root canal infections. Hence, dentistry involves root canal treatment where an antimicrobial irrigant is used for flushing out the debris and also provide antibacterial action. Cinnamon and neem extracts are useful herbal considerations as an alternative to the harsh sodium hypochlorite (Panchal et al., 2020).

One of the factors for Alzheimer's disease is modifications of a phosphoprotein *Tau*. In this protein, change for binding to microtubules has been sighted as a mechanism for the disorder. Bioactive compounds of neem, the nimbin and salannin, have been considered to prevent Tau aggregation, thus potential to manage the disease. These compounds are limonoid derivatives found to be nontoxic to human cell lines (Gorantla et al., 2019). Control of tungiasis (female sand flea, *Tunga penetrans* causes skin disease) was achieved using a blend of neem oil and coconut oil. The oil mixture reduced acute pathological conditions and induced a reduction in pain in the children by the tungiasis (Elson et al., 2019). Neem is known to reduce sperm production and also has spermicidal properties. Hence, it is considered as a contraceptive in humans (Anonymous, 1992; Pankaj et al., 2011).

9.5.2 LIVESTOCK DISEASES

The properties of neem to cure many human ailments made it possible to use neem-based medicine as therapeutics in veterinary medicine (e.g., farm animals and poultry) (Sarkar et al., 2020). Neem as well as other medicinal plants is being used as phytotherapy for endometritis (inflammation of the uterus lining). In dairy animals, endometritis is one of the gynecological problems resulting in the reduction of efficiency in milk production as well as reproduction. A higher rate of success has been achieved using neem, garlic, turmeric, and *Ocimum sanctum* in traditional herbal medication of cattle owing to the antimicrobial properties of these herbs (Mandhwani et al., 2017). Poultry feed prepared by mixing neem seed oil as a supplement resulted in reduced feed intake and body weight. Interestingly, the LDL-cholesterol was significantly reduced providing an opportunity to produce low-cholesterol chicken meat (Sonhafouo et al., 2019). Natural insecticides obtained from different plants including neem may show toxic effects on animals. Hence, it is important to use a safe concentration of such products (Mossa et al., 2018). It was recommended to use neem extract in the food industry as a natural antioxidant (Ouerfelli et al., 2019). The natural antioxidant activity of neem in protecting raw beef patties during storage was found to be worthy. Lipid oxidation of beef patties was prevented by fresh neem leaves. The prominent antibacterial property of neem was proved against *Staphylococcus aureus* as well as *Micrococcus luteus*.

9.5.3 PLANT DISEASES

Neem cake and oil are mainly used to develop commercial products in crop management. Endophytic fungi from neem have been isolated, and their biological activities are reported. Some important genera of endophytic fungi include *Clasdosporium*, *Drechslera*, *Periconia*, *Phomopsis*, *Pestolotiopsis*,

Stenella, and *Trichoderma* (Chutulo and Chalannavar, 2018). The medicinal properties of neem have been complemented by these endophytic fungi.

Bioassay studies have been conducted to follow the efficacy of a blend of neem seed oil and *Pongamia pinnata* seed oil (also known as *Karanja* oil) as an insecticide against Colorado potato beetles (Kovarikova and Pavela, 2019). A mixture of these oils (1:1, v/v) was found to have a synergistic effect against the larvae of the pest compared to individual oils. The lethal dose of the mixture was less compared to individual oils indicating the efficacy of this combination. To follow the adverse effects of neem products, Doshi et al. (2018) carried out some experiments and confirmed that the nontarget soil isopod *Porcellionides pruinosus* was not affected by neem products.

Fungal growth inhibition and a drastic reduction in the production of mycotoxins are essential parameters in grain storage mold management. The antifungal activity of neem oil was well demonstrated against *Aspergillus carbonarius* by Rodrigues et al. (2019). A low concentration of neem oil (0.3%) showed an average growth inhibition of up to 97% of six strains of *A. carbonarius*, clearly establishing the neem oil's efficiency at the same concentration; production of ochratoxin A was almost stopped in all the fungal strains tested. Pre- as well as post-harvest pest management of plant diseases involves the use of neem-based products. Neem leaf extract and commercial neem products were found to be effective in the reduction of sporangial germination of *Plasmopara halstedii*. In vitro studies showed a reduction in downy mildew disease of sunflower with neem products. The possible systemic effect of neem is envisaged to prevent plant pathogens (Doshi et al., 2020). Neem-based products were found to be highly useful in protecting maize from fall armyworm (*Spodoptera frugiperda*). The cost-benefit ratio and efficiency favored neem products over other chemical treatments. Hence, in the field studies, neem was shown to be a potential biopesticide contributing to ecofriendly pest management strategies in maize (Babendreier et al., 2020). In India and USA, neem-based fertilizers are available under different trade names like Ozoneem Cake, Fortuneem Cake, Bioneem Oil Foliar, Neem Urea Guard, and Parker Neem Coat (see also Table 9.1). Many agrochemicals with trade names like Neemix 4.5, Fortune Aza, Azamax, Ecosense, Azatin XL, and NeemDrop are available as bioinsecticide formulations (Campos et al., 2016).

9.6 NEEM IN BIOTECHNOLOGY

Current trends in neem research revolve around genome analysis and the commercial production of metabolites. Developments in molecular biological techniques would provide further scope for exciting prosperity. Metabolite profiling with respect to identifying genes in neem was carried out by Kuravadi et al. (2015). Neem genomes and transcriptomes were analyzed to predict the occurrence of 44,495 genes in the genome. Additionally, neem genes showed phylogenetic relationships with *Citrus sinensis*. This study is expected to provide a genetic basis for metabolic pathways in neem.

Metabolite production in vitro is extremely important in the commercial exploitation of neem. Azadirachtin-producing capacities of neem cell and hairy root cultures were reviewed by Thakore and Srivastava (2017). Presently, most of the azadirachtin is produced from the seeds, which can be obtained only once a year. However, efficient plant cell culture technology can provide a continuous supply of azadirachtin. Successful applications of this process in industries may provide commercially viable technology for the production of azadirachtin by hairy root or cell cultures (Prakash et al. 2002). In view of this, Ashokhan et al. (2020) made successful attempts to generate callus formation of neem for the production of azadirachtin. Using different plant growth regulators in a culture medium, it was possible to produce colored callus of neem. Green callus was having a higher amount of azadirachtin compared to brown and cream-colored calli. Besides, the green callus was nontoxic to the zebra fish showing the successful establishment of callus for bioinsecticide production.

Neem seed oil has been used as a bioactive product having an antioxidant activity to produce nanoemulsions (Rinaldi et al., 2017). Such emulsions provide an opportunity to exploit pharmacologically active ingredients through nanodelivery systems. Iron oxide nanoparticles were prepared using leaf extracts of neem. The corresponding magnetite nanoparticles with neem as a stabilizing agent provided high-purity structures required for a drug delivery system. Various techniques employed for the analysis of nanoparticles clearly demonstrated the usefulness of neem extract in nano-biotechnology (Zambri et al., 2019). Patra et al. (2019) were successful in developing nanoparticles with the metabolite nimbolide for the treatment of breast and pancreatic cancers. These nanoparticles are referred to as Nim-nano showed up to threefold cytotoxicity against cancer cells. Such neem-based nanoparticles are found to be superior for the drug delivery system. Using neem leaf extract, silver and zinc nanoparticles were generated by Taha et al. (2020). Such nanocomposites showed antibacterial activities. Different methods of nanoparticle production were assessed to retain the efficiency of the antibacterial activity of neem in the production of stable nanoparticles.

These particles showed superparamagnetic properties and hence potential use for magnetic targeting in drug delivery.

Neem-based silver nanoparticles were prepared for biosensing as well as photocatalysis. Biosensors of such nanoparticles are capable of detecting an agrofungicide mancozeb (Alex et al., 2020). Apart from medicinal uses, neem has been applied in nanotechnology for bioremediation. Silver and copper nanoparticles prepared using neem were highly effective in the removal of naphthalene from wastewater. Nanoparticles produced from neem were found to be better compared to nanoparticles prepared using other plants (Abbas et al., 2020). Efficient neem-based nanopesticides have been developed. Chaudhary et al. (2017) used different neem extracts as well as neem oil for the successful production of nanoparticles with a wide size range between 20 and 500 nm, and they were tested for biopesticide potential. The neem extract was used as a stabilizing agent for the particles in preparation for linear low-density polyethylene (LLDPE). This material was used in textile industry wastewater treatment systems. The LLDPE showed an enhanced ability to remove the dye in the effluent and also reduce the biological and chemical oxygen demand contributing to bioremediation (Basiron et al., 2020). Water-in-oil emulsion formulation of neem oil was found to be effective in mosquito eradication. Composition process technology was developed to improve the efficacy of neem oil. Turbulence stirring was employed to decrease the particle size, which increased the efficacy (Iqbal et al., 2020).

Ever increasing demand for petroleum-based products laid constraints on the limited resource, and biodiesel production has been considered a useful alternative. Plant species like neem, *Pongamia* and *Jatropa* have the potential to produce biodiesel. Biodiesel produced from neem seed oil was found to be comparable to petrodiesel in terms of physicochemical characteristics. The volarization quality of neem oil was found to be satisfactory for the production of biodiesel (Hamadou et al., 2020). The performance of concrete buildings during fire outbreaks is a requirement in the structural designs of buildings. In an interesting study, neem seed husk ash was incorporated into the concrete mixture and exposed to high temperatures. The comprehensive strength of the concrete was better with neem seed husk supplement provided additional benefits of neem (Mwilongo et al., 2020).

In one of the recent studies, a computational approach was employed to predict the inhibition of structural proteins of corona virus by neem-derived compounds. Docking and simulation methods provided information on the potential neem compounds interacting with a spike as well as envelop proteins of SARS-CoV2. The study has also opened up the possible identification of neem compounds in modern medicine (Borkotoky and Banerjee, 2020). Home remedies including neem have been considered to combat COVID-19 (Orisakwe et al., 2020; Thota et al., 2020). One of the important characteristics of azadirachtin was its nontoxicity to mammals although it is toxic to arthropods. Azadirachtin is highly toxic to aquatic animals. Liu et al. (2021) assessed the azadirachtin stress against Chinese aquatic mitten crab (*Eriocheir hepuensis*). On cloning three genes of this crab coding for glutathione-S-transferase, studies were conducted to know the expression of these genes under azadirachtin stress. Interference of azadirachtin in animal physiology was evident by tissue-specific increase in the expression of these cloned genes. Neem leaf, bark, and seed extracts administered by injection were found to show acute toxicity in rats. However, oral administration showed no adverse effects in animals (Braga et al., 2021). Hence, Pasquoto-Stigliani et al. (2017) suggested using neem oil as a nanopesticide rather than directly.

9.7 AFFORESTATION

Neem has been considered as one of the favorite tree species in afforestation and reforestation programs. It is also a tree of choice in backyards, agroforestry, urban forestry, and even as an avenue tree. It can grow in tropical and subtropical regions up to 700 m ASL. Although it can withstand hot conditions, it will not withstand extended cold conditions. Neem can grow in all sorts of soils, but its growth is better in black cotton soils. Preferred rainfall necessary for neem growth ranges between 400 and 1200 mm. Good growth could be expected even in shallow, stony, and unfertile soils. It can withstand soil pH up to 10, and the fallen leaves are capable of neutralizing the acidity of the soil. Neem grows very fast and yields timber by about seven years. Naturally, seeds are distributed by birds, bats, and monkeys. Ever increasing demand for neem products makes it an ideal species for cultivation (Quandt et al., 2021).

9.8 PESTS AND DISEASES

In spite of its wide medicinal properties, neem is prone to several pests and pathogens (Schmutterer, 1990; Anonymous, 1992; Boa, 1995; Bhat et al.,

1998). Even though neem has biopesticide potential, it succumbs to mild to serious insect attacks as seen in Asia and Africa. The major insect pests of neem are trotricid moth (*Adoxophyes aurata*), phyralid moth (*Hypsipyla* sp.), scale insect (*Pinnaspis strachani*), leaf cutter ants (*Acromyrmex* spp.), and the bug (*Helopeltis theivora*). These pests can feed on different parts of the neem and may be responsible for severe damage (Schmutterer, 1990; Anonymous, 1992; Boa, 1995).

The neem is known to possess antifungal and antibacterial substances in different parts. Even then, the plant is attacked by several pathogens. Some major diseases reported in neem are root rot (*Ganoderma lucidum*), stem blight (*Corticium salmonicolor*), bleeding canker (*Botrydiplodia theobromae*), leaf spots (*Alternaria alternata*, *Cercospora meliae*, and *Colletotrichum capsici*), powdery mildew (*Oidium* sp.), bacterial blight (*Xanthomonas azadirachtae*), and bacterial wilt (*Pseudomonas solanacearum*). Seedlings also may show diseases like leaf blight (*Sclerotium rolfsi*), web blight (*Rhizoctonia solani*), damping-off (*Fusarium oxysporum*), and wilt (*Fusarium solani*). Such bacterial and fungal diseases of neem affect their quality and survival ability (Boa, 1995). It is extremely important to have proper control measures and effectively suppress such diseases. Comprehensive disease management strategies are required in order to monitor the growth and development of neem without affecting its medicinal qualities.

During the field survey in Southern India (Karnataka state), wide occurrence of new destructive die-back disease of neem was recorded by Bhat et al. (1998) and demonstrated severe loss of fruit production. A detailed investigation on isolation and characterization of the pathogen revealed a new fungal species *Phomopsis azadirachtae*. Once the tree gets infected, the twig blight occurs and the tips show die-back resulting in severe loss of growing tissue. This disease is also widespread in India and needs to be attended to for possible remedial measures (Sateesh et al., 1997; Bhat et al., 1998). In this disease, the tips of a tree show die-back symptoms (Figure 9.2a), and in severe cases, the whole tree appears to be dead (Figure 9.2b). However, relatively there will be a regeneration of growing tips.

The neem may also suffer from nutritional deficiencies such as zinc and potassium deficiencies, resulting in leaf chlorosis and older leaves may fall off. Forest fires also harm neem trees, but they can regrow once the dead parts are removed. Neem cannot withstand high winds and cyclones. Seedlings are highly sensitive to intense sunlight. Neem cultivation is highly essential considering the significance of its manifold benefits. Precise care of plants from the nursery to plantation necessitates the use of physical, chemical, and biological methods. Formulations of integrated pest and disease management practices may improve the growth and desired yields.

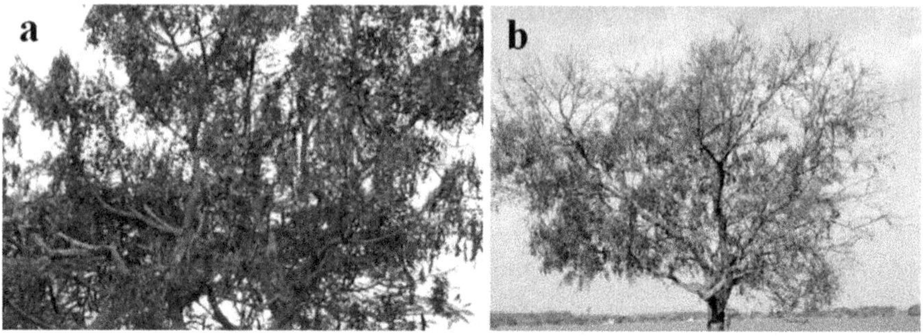

FIGURE 9.2 Die-back disease of neem caused by *Phomopsis azadirachtae*: Typical die-back symptoms on growing shoot tips (a) and severally infected tree (b).

9.9 CONCLUSIONS AND PROSPECTS

Products based on neem are increasing continuously with new information on beneficial effects. The multifaceted use of neem products makes it an essential plant species to solve several burning problems in health and agricultural sectors. Natural genetic variations contributing to differences in medicinal values have not been the subject of interest in most of the research. Available technologies in plant genetic improvement need to be applied to neem to enhance its potential. The information available on the neem genome must be upgraded, and different genes responsible for useful metabolites need to be characterized. Efforts are also required to make use of metabolic engineering to enhance the potential for the cellular production of useful compounds. Cell and tissue culture may provide an alternate and efficient methodology for special metabolite production by neem. Nanobiotechnology has opened up new avenues for the development of the efficient, target-oriented drug-delivery system. Transgenic research seems to be ignored in neem; however, this field promises its prospective returns by capturing the advantages of available germplasm. Identification of genes for useful metabolites and the use of recombinant DNA technology may provide improved methods for the commercial production of useful compounds. Traditional knowledge of medicinal values of neem should not be ignored to formulate modern medicines.

KEYWORDS

- **ethnomedicine**
- **bioactive metabolites**
- **biopesticide**
- **azadirachtin**
- **nimbin**
- **salannin**

REFERENCES

Abbas, S.; Nasreen, S.; Haroon, A.; Ashraf, M. A. Synthesis of Silver and Copper Nanoparticles from Plants and Application as Adsorbents for Naphthalene Decontamination. *Soudi J. Biol Sci.* **2020,** *27*. DOI: 10.1016/j.sjbs.2020.02.011

Agrawala, S.; Poplib, D. B.; Sircarb, K.; Chowdhry, A. A Review of the Anticancer Activity of *Azadirachta indica* (Neem) in Oral Cancer. *J. Oral Biol. Craniofacial Res.* **2020,** *10*, 206–209.

Ahmad, F; Iqbal, N.; Zaka, S. M.; Qureshi, M. K.; Saeed, Q. et al. Comparative Insecticidal Activity of Different Plant Materials from Six Common Plant Species Against *Tribolium castaneum* (Herbst) (Coleoptera:Tenebrionidae). *Saudi J. Biol. Sci.* **2019,** *26*, 1804–1808.

Alex, K. V.; Pavai, P. T.; Rugmini, R.; Prasad, M. S.; Kamakshi, K.; Sekhar, K. C. Green Synthesized Ag Nanoparticles for Bio-Sensing and Photocatalytic Applications. *ACS Omega* **2020,** *5*, 13123–13129.

Alsanad, S.; Aboushanab, T.; Khalil, M.; Alkhamees, O. A. A Descriptive Review of the Prevalence and Usage of Traditional and Complementary Medicine Among Saudi Diabetic Patients. *Scientifica* **2018,** 6303190. https://doi.org/10.1155/2018/6303190

Alzohairy, M. A. Therapeutics Role of *Azadirachta indica* (Neem) and Their Active Constituents in Diseases Prevention and Treatment. *Evid. Based Compl. Alt. Med.* **2016,** 7382506. DOI: 10.1155/2016/7382506

Aneesa, N.; Gayathri. Beneficial Effects of Neem Oil—An Updated Review. *J. Pharm. Sci. Res.* **2016,** *8*, 756–758.

Anonymous. *Neem: A Tree for Solving Global Problems*; National Research Council Report, National Academy Press: Washington DC, 1992; p 139.

Ashokhan, S.; Othman, R., Rahim, M. H. A.; Karsani, S. A.; Yaacob, J. S. Effect of Plant Growth Regulators on Coloured Callus Formation and Accumulation of Azadirachtin, an Essential Biopesticide in *Azadirachta indica. Plants*, **2020,** *9*, 352–368.

Babendreier, D.; Agboyi, L. K.; Beseh, P.; Osae, M.; Nboyine, J. et al. The Efficacy of Alternative, Environmentally Friendly Plant Protection Measures for Control of Fall Armyworm, *Spodoptera frugiperda*, in Maize. *Insects* **2020,** *11*, 240–261.

Balaji, K. T.; Shivaji, K. R.; Krishna, R. K.; Balasaheb, K. N. Medicinal Uses of Neem (*Azadirachta indica*) in Human Life: A Review. *Int. J. Life Sci.* **2018,** *A10*, 181–184.

Basiron, N.; Sreekantan, S.; Kang, L. J.; Akil, H. M.; Mydin, R. B. S. M. N. Coupled Oxides/LLDPE Composites for Textile Effluent Treatment: Effect of Neem and PVA Stabilization. *Polymers* **2020,** *12*, 394–408.

Bhat, S. S.; Sateesh, M. K.; Devaki, N. S. A New Destructive Disease of Neem (*Azadirachta indica*) Incited by *Phomopsis azadirachtae*. *Curr. Sci.* **1998,** *74*, 17–19.

Boa, E. R. A Guide to the Identification of Diseases and Pests of Neem (*Azadirachta indica*). Food and Agriculture Organization of the United Nations (FAO): Bangkok, 1995; p 75.

Boeke, S. J.; Boersma, M. G.; Alink, G. M.; Van Loon, J. J. A.; Van Huis, A. et al. Safety Evaluation of Neem (*Azadirachta indica*) Derived Pesticides. *J. Ethnopharmacol.* **2004,** *94*, 25–41.

Borkotoky, S.; Banerjee, M. A computational prediction of SARS-CoV-2 Structural Protein Inhibitors from *Azadirachta indica* (Neem). *J. Biomol. Str. Dyn.* **2020.** DOI: 10.1080/07391102.2020.1774419.

Boursier, C. M.; Bosco, D.; Coulibaly, A.; Negre, M. Are Traditional Neem Extract Preparations as Efficient as a Commercial Formulation of Azadirachtin A? *Crop Protect.* **2011,** *30*, 318–39.

Braga, T. M.; Rocha, L.; Chung, T. Y.; Oliveira, R. F.; Pinho, C. et al. Biological Activities of Gedunin- A Limonoid from Meliaceae Family. *Molecules* **2020,** *25*, 493–518.

Braga, T. M.; Rocha, L.; Chung, T. Y.; Oliveira, R. F.; Pinho, C. et al. *Azadirachta indica* A. Juss. In Vivo Toxicity—An Updated Review. *Molecules* **2021,** *26*, 252–272.

Brahmachari, G. Neem an Omnipotent Plant: A Retrospection. *Chem. Biochem.* **2004,** *5*, 408421.

Campos, E. V. R.; de Oliveira, J. L.; Pascoli, M.; Lima, R. D.; Fraceto, L. F. Neem Oil and Crop Protection: from Now to the Future. *Front. Plant Sci.* **2016,** *7*, 1494–1502.

Chaudhary, S.; Kanwar, R. K.; Sehgal, A.; Cahill, D. M.; Barrow, C. J. et al. Progress on Azadirachta Indica Based Biopesticides in Replacing Synthetic Toxic Pesticides. *Front. Plant Sci.* **2017,** *8*, 610.

Chutulo, E. C.; Chalannavar, R. K. Endophytic Mycoflora and Their Bioactive Compounds from *Azadirachta indica*: A Comprehensive Review. *J. Fungi* **2018,** *4*, 42.

Doshi, P.; Nisha, N.; Yousif, A. I. A.; Körösi, K.; Bán, R.; Turóczi, G. Preliminary Investigation of Effect of Neem-Derived Pesticides on *Plasmopara halstedii* Pathotypc 704 in Sunflower Under In Vitro and In Vivo Conditions. *Plants* **2020,** *9*, 535.

Doshi, P.; Póss, A. M.; Tóth, E.; Szalai, M.; Turóczi, G. Effect of Neem-Derived Plant Protection Products on the Isopod Species *Porcellionides pruinosus* (Brandt, 1833). *ZooKeys* **2018,** *801*, 415–425.

Duarte, J. P.; Redaelli, L. R.; Silva, C. E.; Jahnke, S. M. Effect of *Azadirachta indica* (Sapindales: Meliaceae) oil on the Immune System of *Spodoptera frugiperda* (Lepidoptera: Noctuidae) immatures. *J. Insect Sci.* **2020,** *20*, 17, 1–6.

Elson, L.; Randu, K.; Feldmeier, H.; Fillinger, U. Efficacy of a Mixture of Neem Seed Oil (*Azadirachta indica*) and Coconut Oil (*Cocos nucifera*) for Topical Treatment of Tungiasis. A Randomized Controlled, Proof-of-Principle Study. *PLoS Negl. Trop. Dis.* **2019,** *13*, e000789.

Fernandes, S. R.; Barrėiros, L.; Oliveira, R. F.; Cruz, A.; Prudêncio, C. et al. Chemistry, Bioactivities, Extraction and Analysis of Azadirachtin: State-of-the-Art. *Fitoterapia* **2019,** *134*, 141–150.

Gahukar, R. Factors Affecting Content and Bioefficacy of Neem (*Azadirachta indica* A. Juss.) Phytochemicals Used in Agricultural Pest Control: A Review. *Crop Protect.* **2014,** *62*, 93–99.

Ghosh, T.; Nandi, P.; Ganguly, N.; Guha, I.; Bhuniya, A.; Ghosh, S.; Sarkar, A.; Saha, A.; Dasgupta, S.; Baral, R.; Bose, A. NLGP Counterbalances the Immunosuppressive Effect of Tumor Associated Mesenchymal Stem Cells to Restore Effector T Cell Functions. *Stem Cell Res. Therapy* **2019,** *10*, 296–307.

Girish, K.; Bhat, S. S. Neem—A Green Treasure. *Electronic J. Biol.* **2008,** *4*, 102–111.

Giuggioli, D.; Lumetti, F.; Spinella, A.; Cocchiara, E.; Sighinolfi, G. et al. Use of Neem Oil and *Hypericum perforatum* for Treatment of Calcinosis-Related Skin Ulcers in Systemic Sclerosis. *J. Int. Med. Res.* **2019,** *48*, 300060519882176. DOI: 10.1177/0300060519882176

Gorantla, N. V.; Dasa, R.; Mulanib, F. A.; Thulasiramb, H. V.; Chinnathambia, S. Neem Derivatives Inhibits Tau Aggregation. *J. Alzheimer's Dis. Rep.* **2019,** *3*, 169–178.

Gupta, S. C.; Prasad, S.; Tyagi, A. K.; Kunnumakkara, A. B.; Aggarwal, B. B. Neem (*Azadirachta indica*): An Indian Traditional Panacea with Modern Molecular Basis. *Phytomedicine*, **2017,** *34*, 14–20.

Hamadou, B.; Djomdi; Falama, R. Z.; Delattre, C.; Pierre, G. et al. Influence of Physicochemical Characteristics of Neem Seeds (*Azadirachta indica* A. Juss) on Biodiesel Production. *Biomolecules* **2020,** *10*, 616.

Hashmat, I.; Azad, H.; Ahmed, A. Neem (*Azadirachta indica* A. Juss)—A Nature's Drugstore: An Overview. *Int. Res. J. Biol. Sci.* **2012,** *1*, 76–79.

Hatti, K. S.; Muralitharan, L.; Hegde, R.; Kush, A. NeeMDB: Convenient Database for Neem Secondary Metabolites. *Bioinformation* **2014,** *10*, 314–315.

Hodgson, H.; La Peña, R. D.; Stephenson, M. J.; Thimmappa, R.; Vincent, J. L. et al. Identification of Key Enzymes Responsible for Protolimonoid Biosynthesis in Plants: Opening the Door to Azadirachtin Production. *Proc. Natl. Acad. Sci. USA* **2019,** *116*, 17096–17104.

Iqbal, N.; Kumar, N.; Saini, M. K.; Dubey, S.; Agrawal, A.; Kumar, J. Role of High Shear Mixing in Improving Stability and Bio-Efficacy of Botanical Oil in Water Formulation for Early Stage Mosquito Eradication. *Heliyon*, **2020,** *6*, e03380.

Kashif, M.; Hwang, Y.; Kim, W. -J.; Kim, G. In Vitro Morphological Assessment of Apoptosis Induced by Nimbolide; A Limonoid from *Azadirachta indica* (Neem Tree). *Iran. J. Pharm. Res.* **2019,** *18*, 846–859.

Kausik, B.; Ishita, C.; Ranajit, B. K.; Uday, B. Biological Activities and Medicinal Properties of Neem (*Azadirchta india*). *Curr. Sci.* **2002,** *82*, 1336–1345.

Koul, O.; Murrary, I. B.; Ketkar, C. M. Properties and Uses of Neem, *Azadirachta indica*. *Can. J. Bot.* **1990,** *68*, 1–11.

Kovaríková, K.; Pavela, R. United Forces of Botanical Oils: Efficacy of Neem and Karanja Oil Against Colorado Potato Beetle Under Laboratory Conditions. *Plants* **2019,** *8*, 608.

Kumar, U. S. U.; Abdulmadjid, S. N.; Olaiya, N. G.; Amirul. A. A.; Rizal, S. et al. Extracted Compounds from Neem Leaves as Antimicrobial Agent on the Physico-Chemical Properties of Seaweed-Based Biopolymer Films. *Polymers* **2020,** *12*, 12051119.

Kumar, V. S.; Navaratnam, V. Neem (*Azadirachta indica*): Prehistory to Contemporary Medicinal Uses to Humankind. *Asian Pac. J. Trop. Biomed.* **2013,** *3*, 505–514.

Kumari, P. D.; Shenoy, S. M.; Khijmatgara, S.; Chowdhury, A.; Lynch, E,; Chowdhury, C. R. Antibacterial Activity of New Atraumatic Restorative Treatment Materials Incorporated with *Azadirachta indica* (Neem) Against *Streptococcus mutans*. *J. Oral Biol. Craniofacial Res.* **2019,** *9*, 321–325.

Kuravadi, N. A.; Yenagi, V.; Rangiah, K.; Mahesh, H. B.; Rajamani, A. et al. Comprehensive analyses of genomes, transcriptomes and metabolites of neem tree. *PeerJ* **2015,** *3*, e1066.

Liu, K.; Liu, J.; Ren, T.; Xu, Y.; Lu, M. et al. Cloning and analysis of three glutathione S-transferases in *Eriocheir hepuensis* and their expression in response to azadirachtin stress. *Aquacult. Rep.* **2021,** *19*, https://doi.org/10.1016/j.aqrep.2021.100635.

Macchioni, F.; Sfingi, M.; Chiavacci, D.; Cecchi, F. *Azadirachta indica* (Sapindales: Meliaceae) Neem Oil as a Repellent Against *Aedes albopictus* (Diptera: Culicidae) Mosquitoes. *J. Insect Sci.* **2019,** *12*, 1–4.

Mandhwani, R.; Bhardwaz, A.; Kumar, S.; Shivhare, M.; Aich, R. Insights Into Bovine Endometritis with Special Reference to Phytotherapy. *Veterinary World* **2017,** *10*, 1529–1532.

Moga, M. A.; Balan, A.; Anastasiu, C. V.; Dimienescu, O. G.; Neculoiu, C. D.; Gavris, C. An Overview on the Anticancer Activity of *Azadirachta indica* (Neem) in Gynecological Cancers. *Int. J. Mol. Sci.* **2018,** *19*, 3898.

Morris, J.; Gonzales, C. B.; La Chapa, J. J. D.; Cabang, A. B.; Fountzilas, C. et al. The Highly Pure Neem Leaf Extract, SCNE, Inhibits Tumorigenesis in Oral Squamous Cell Carcinoma Via Disruption of Pro-Tumor Inflammatory Cytokines and Cell Signaling. *Front. Oncol.* **2019,** *9*, 890–903.

Mossa, A. H.; Mohafrash, S. M. M.; Chandrasekaran, N. Safety of Natural Insecticides: Toxic Effects on Experimental Animals. *BioMed Res. Int.* **2018**. DOI: 10.1155/2018/4308054.

Mwilongo, K. P.; Machunda, R. L.; Jande, Y. A. C. Effect of Elevated Temperature on Compressive Strength and Physical Properties of Neem Seed Husk Ash Concrete. *Materials* **2020,** *13*, 1198.

Okoh, S. O.; Okoh, O. O.; Okoh, A. I. Inhibitory Effects of *Azadirachta indica* Secondary Metabolites Formulated Cosmetics on Some Infectious Pathogens and Oxidative Stress Radicals. *BMC Compl. Alter. Med.* **2019,** *19*, 123–135.

Orisakwe, O. E.; Orish, C. N.; Nwanaforo, E. O. Coronavirus Disease (COVID-19) and Africa: Acclaimed Home Remedies. *Sci. Afr.* **2020,** *10*, e00620.

Ouerfelli, M.; Villasante, J.; Kaâb, L. B. B.; Almajano, M. P. Effect of Neem (*Azadirachta indica* L.) on Lipid Oxidation in Raw Chilled Beef Patties. *Antioxidants* **2019,** *8*, 305–322.

Ozturk, M.; Altay, V.; Hakeem, K. R.; Akçiçek, E. *Liquorice from Botany to Phytochemistry.* SpringerBriefs in Plant Science, 2017a. https://doi.org/10.1007/978-3-319-74240-3.

Ozturk, M.; Altay, V.; Gonenç, T. M. Herbal from High Mountains in the East Mediterranean. In *Drug Discovery from Herbs-Approaches and Applications*; Bhojraj, S. et al., Eds.; NAM S & T Centre, DAYA Publishing House: New Delhi, India, Chapter 24, 2017b; pp 327–367.

Ozturk, M.; Altay, V.; Gucel, S.; Altundağ, E. Plant Diversity of the Drylands in Southeast Anatolia-Turkey: Role in Human Health and Food Security. In *Plant Biodiversity: Monitoring, Assessment and Conservation*; Ansari, A. A.; Gill, S. S., Eds.; Chapter 5; CABI UK, 2017c; pp 83–124.

Ozturk, M.; Altay, V.; Orçen, N. et al. A Little Known and a Little Consumed Natural Resource: *Salicornia.* In *Global Perspectives on Underutilized Crops*; Ozturk, M. et al., Eds., Chapter 3; Springer International Publishing AG, 2018a; pp 83–108.

Ozturk, M.; Altundağ, E.; Ibadullayeva, S. J.; Altay, V.; Aslanıpour, B. A Comparative Analysis of Medicinal and Aromatic Plants Used in the Traditional Medicine of Iğdır (Turkey), Nakhchivan (Azerbaijan), and Tabriz (Iran). *Pak. J. Bot.* **2018b**, *50* (1), 337–343.

Ozturk, M.; Altay, V.; Altundağ, E.; Ibadullayeva, S. J.; Aslanipour, B.; Gönenç, T. M. Herbals in Iğdır (Turkey), Nakhchivan (Azerbaijan), and Tabriz (Iran). In *Plant and Human Health*; Ozturk, M., Hakeem, K.R., Eds., Vol. 1; Springer: Cham, Chapter 6, 2018c; pp 197–266.

Ozturk, M.; Altay, V.; Latiff, A. et al. A Comparative Analysis of the Medicinal Pteridophytes in Turkey, Pakistan, and Malaysia. In *Plant and Human Health*; Ozturk, M., Hakeem, K. R.,

Eds., Vol. 1; Springer: Cham, Chapter 9; Springer International Publishing AG, 2018d; pp 349–390.

Ozturk, M.; Altay, V.; Latiff, A. et al. A Comparative Analysis of the Medicinal Plants Used for Diabetes Mellitus in the Traditional Medicine in Turkey, Pakistan, and Malaysia. In *Plant and Human Health*; Ozturk, M., Hakeem, K. R., Eds., Vol. 1; Springer: Cham, Chapter 11; Springer International Publishing AG, 2018e; pp 409-461.

Ozturk, M.; Altay, V.; Latiff, A. et al. Potential Medicinal Plants Used in the Hypertension in Turkey, Pakistan, and Malaysia. In *Plant and Human Health*; Ozturk, M., Hakeem, K. R., Eds.; Vol. 1; Springer: Cham, Chapter 16; Springer International Publishing AG, 2018f; pp 595–618.

Ozturk, M.; Gökler, I.; Altay, V. Medicinal Bryophytes Distributed in Turkey. In *Plant and Human Health*; Ozturk, M., Hakeem, K. R., Eds., Vol. 1; Springer: Cham, Chapter 8; Springer International Publishing AG, 2018g; pp 323–348.

Ozturk, M.; Egamberdieva, D.; Milica, P. *Biodiversity and Biomedicine-Our Future*; Academic Press, Elsevier Inc., 2020.

Ozturk, M.; Altay, V.; Efe, R. *Biodiversity, Conservation and Sustainability in Asia: Volume I: Prospects and Challenges in West Asia and Caucasus*; Springer Nature Switzerland AG. DOI: 10.1007/978-3-030-59928-7, **2021a**.

Ozturk, M.; Khan, S. M.; Altay, V.; Efe, R.; Egamberdieva, D.; Khassanov, F. *Biodiversity, Conservation and Sustainability in Asia: Volume II: Prospects and Challenges in South and Middle Asia*; Springer Nature Switzerland AG, 2021b. DOI: 10.1007/978-3-030-73943-0.

Panchal, V.; Gurunathan, D.; Muralidharan, N. P. Comparison of Antibacterial Efficacy of Cinnamon Extract, Neem Extract as Irrigant and Sodium Hypochlorite Against *Enterococcus fecalis*: An In Vitro Study. *Ind. J. Dent. Res.* **2020,** *31*, 124–128.

Pankaj, S.; Lokeshwar, T.; Mukuesh, B.; Vishnu, B. Review on Neem (*Azadirachta indica*): Thousand Problems One Solution. *Int. Res. J. Pharm.* **2011,** *2*, 97–102.

Paramo, M. E. R.; Falvoa, M.; Garcíaa, J.; Lastra, C. C. L. Compatibility Between *Leptolegnia chapmanii* and Diflubenzuron and Neem Oil for the Control of *Aedes aegypti*. *Rev. Argent. Microbiol.* **2019.** doi.org/10.1016/j.ram.2019.10.001

Pasquoto-Stigliani, T.; Campos, E. V. R.; Oliveira, J. L.; Silva, C. M. G.; Bilesky-José, N. et al. Nanocapsules Containing Neem (*Azadirachta indica*) Oil: Development, Characterization and Toxicity Evaluation. *Sci. Rep.* **2017,** *7*, 5929.

Patra, A.; Satpathy, S.: Hussain, M. D. Nanodelivery and Anticancer Effect of a Limonoid, Nimbolide, in Breast and Pancreatic Cancer Cells. *Int. J. Nanomed.* **2019,** *14*, 8095–8104.

Paul, S. C.; Miah, M. Y.; Bhattacharjee, S. *Neem Oil from Neem Seeds and Application*; LAP Lambert Academic Publishing: Germany, 2013; p 145.

Paula, A. R.; Ribeiro1, A.; Lemos, F. J. A.; Silva, C. P.; Samuels, R. I. Neem Oil Increases the Persistence of the Entomopathogenic Fungus *Metarhizium anisopliae* for the Control of *Aedes aegypti* (Diptera: Culicidae) Larvae. *Parasites Vectors* **2019,** *12*, 163–171.

Petrikovszki, R.; Doshi, P.; Turóczi, G.; Tóth, F.; Nagy, P. Investigating the Side-Effects of Neem-Derived Pesticides on Commercial Entomopathogenic and Slug-Parasitic Nematode Products Under Laboratory Conditions. *Plants* **2019,** *8*, 281–288.

Prakash, G.; Bhojwani, S. S.; Srivastava, A. K. Production of Azadirachtin from Plant Tissue Culture: State of the Art and Future Prospects. *Biotechnol. Bioproc. Eng.* **2002,** *7*, 185–193.

Quandt, A. Agroforestry Trees for Improved Food Security on Farms Impacted by Wildlife Crop Raiding in Kenya. *Trees, Forests People* **2021,** *4*, 100069.

Rinaldi, F.; Hanieh, P. H.; Longhi, C.; Carradori, S.; Secci, D. et al. Neem Oil Nanoemulsions: Characterisation and Antioxidant Activity. *J. Enz. Inhib. Med. Che.* **2017,** *32*, 1265–1273.

Rodrigues, M. P.; Astoreca, A. L.; de Oliveira, Á. A.; Salvato, L. A., Biscoto, G. L. et al. In Vitro Activity of Neem (*Azadirachta indica*) Oil on Growth and Ochratoxin A Production by *Aspergillus carbonarius* isolates. *Toxins* **2019,** *11*, 579–590.

Saha, A.; Nandi, P.; Dasgupta, S.; Bhuniya, A.; Ganguly, N. et al. Neem Leaf Glycoprotein Restrains VEGF Production by Direct Modulation of HIF1a-Linked Upstream and Downstream Cascades. *Front. Oncol.* **2020,** *10*, 260–270.

Saleem, S.; Muhammad, G.; Hussain, M. A.; Bukhari, S. N. A. A Comprehensive Review of Phytochemical Profile, Bioactives for Pharmaceuticals, and Pharmacological Attributes of Azadirachta Indica. *Phyther. Res.* **2018,** *32*, 1241–1272.

Sarkar, L.; Putchala, R. K.; Safiriyu, A. A.; Sarma, J. D. *Azadirachta indica* A. Juss Ameliorates Mouse Hepatitis Virus-Induced Neuroinflammatory Demyelination by Modulating Cell-to-Cell Fusion in an Experimental Animal Model of Multiple Sclerosis. *Front. Cell. Neurosci.* **2020,** *14*, 116–137.

Sateesh, M. K.; Bhat, S. S.; Devaki, N. S. *Phomopsis azadirachtae* sp nov from India. *Mycotaxon* **1997,** *65*: 517–520.

Schmutterer, H. Observations on Pests of *Azadirachta indica* (Neem Tree) and Some *Melia* Species. *J. App. Entomol.* **1990,** *109*, 390–400.

Senthil-Nathan, S. Physiological and Biochemical Effect of Neem and Other Meliaceae Plants Secondary Metabolites Against Lepidopteran Insects. *Front. Physiol.* **2013,** *4*. DOI: 10.3389/fphys.2013.00359.

Sonhafouo, V. M.; Kana, J. R.; Dongmo, K. N. Effects of Graded Levels of *Azadirachta indica* Seed Oil on Growth Performance and Biochemical Profiles of Broiler Chickens. *Vet. Med. Sci.* **2019,** *5*, 442–450.

Sophia, J.; Kowshik, J.; Dwivedi, A.; Bhutia, S. K.; Manavathi, B. et al. Nimbolide, a Neem Limonoid Inhibits Cytoprotective Autophagy to Activate Apoptosis via Modulation of the PI3K/Akt/GSK-3β Signalling Pathway in Oral Cancer. *Cell Death Dis.* **2018,** *9*, 1087–1104.

Suttiarporn, P.; Choommongkol, V. Microwave-Assisted Improved Extraction and Purification of Anticancer Nimbolide from *Azadirachta indica* (Neem) Leaves. *Molecules* **2020,** *25*, 2913–2027.

Taha, A.; Aissa, M. B.; Da'na, E. Green Synthesis of an Activated Carbon-Supported Ag and ZnO Nanocomposite for Photocatalytic Degradation and Its Antibacterial Activities. *Molecules* **2020,** *25*, 1586–1603.

Thakore, D.; Srivastava, A. K. Production of Biopesticide Azadirachtin Using Plant Cell and Hairy Root Cultures. *Eng. Life Sci.* **2017,** *17*, 997–1005.

Thota, S. M.; Balan, V.; Sivaramakrishnan, V. Natural Products as Home-Based Prophylactic and Symptom Management Agents in the Setting of COVID-19. *Phytotherapy Res.* **2020,** *34*, 3148–3167.

Ugboko, H. U.; Nwinyi, O. C.; Oranusi, S. U.; Fatoki, T. H.; Omonhinmin, C. A. Antimicrobial Importance of Medicinal Plants in Nigeria. *Sci. World J.* **2020,** 7059323. https://doi.org/10.1155/2020/7059323.

Younessi-Hamzekhanlu, M.; Ozturk, M.; Altay, V. et al. Ethnopharmacological Study of Medicinal Plants from Khoy City of West Azerbaijan-Iran. *Ind. J. Trad. Knowl.* **2020,** *19* (2), 251–267.

Zaka, S. M., Iqbal, N.; Saeed, Q.; Akrem, A.; Batool, M. et al. Toxic Effects of Some Insecticides, Herbicides, and Plant Essential Oils Against *Tribolium confusum* Jacquelin du val (Insecta: Coleoptera: Tenebrionidae). *Saudi J. Biol. Sci.* **2019,** *26*, 1767–1771.

Zambri, N. D. S.; Taib, N. I.; Latif, F. A.; Mohamed, Z. Utilization of Neem Leaf Extract on Biosynthesis of Iron Oxide Nanoparticles. *Molecules* **2019,** *24*, 3803–3814.

Zingue, S.; Silihe, K. K.; Bourfane, I. F.; Boukar, A.; Tueche, A. B. et al. Potential of Regular Consumption of Cameroonian Neem (*Azadirachta indica* L.) Oil for Prevention of the 7,12-dimethylbenz(a)anthracene-Induced Breast Cancer in High-Fat/Sucrose-Fed Wistar Rats. *Hindawi Evid. Based Compl. Alt. Med.* **2019.** http://dx.doi.org/10.1155/2019/2031460

PART IV

Perceptions of Ethnomedicine

CHAPTER 10

Plant-Based Medicinal Attributes in India

MUNDAMOOLE PAVITHRA[1] and KANDIKERE R. SRIDHAR[1,2]

[1]Department of Biosciences, Mangalore University, Mangalagangotri, Mangalore, Karnataka, India

[2]Centre for Environmental Studies, Yenepoya (deemed to be) University, Mangalore, Karnataka, India

ABSTRACT

Enormous ethnic knowledge is concentrated in the ethnic population of the Indian subcontinent, especially to meet the primary needs of nutrition, health, and shelter. Throughout the Indian subcontinent, several wild and cultivated plant species serve to cure many diseases. Plant species use for primary health care as well as specific aliments include dermal, gastrointestinal, respiratory, gynecological, and pediatric-related (new born, infants, and children). This is one of the main reasons to document ethnic knowledge on wild and cultivated plants with their geographic indications. To conserve and propagate economically viable wild plant species, exploration and cultivation of region-specific wild plant species need to be followed more scientifically. The current chapter discusses the ethnic knowledge of the application of plant species toward treating several human ailments across the Indian subcontinent.

Ethnic Knowledge and Perspectives of Medicinal Plants, Volume 1: Curative Properties and Treatment Strategies. Munir Ozturk, Kandikere R. Sridhar, Maryam Sarwat, Volkan Altay, & Francisco Martín Huerta-Martínez (Eds.)

10.1 INTRODUCTION

The ethnobotanical knowledge has been transferred from one generation to another similar to folklore without specific documentation. The rural folks and tribes depend on forest resources to meet their basic needs (food, medicine, and shelter) through inherited knowledge (Ozturk et al., 2021a, b). Wild plant species are immensely valuable for medicinal remedial purposes to tackle many diseases. Up to 85% of ethnic-based medicines worldwide are derived from plants useful in primary healthcare (Ignacimuthu et al., 2006). Similarly, several wild plant species meet the basic nutritional requirements. Interestingly, some of the wild plants have a dual role as nutraceuticals to combat nutritional as well as medicinal needs (e.g., Pavithra et al., 2017; Anita and Sridhar, 2020; Shreelalitha and Sridhar, 2021). Ethnically, wild plants (herbs, shrubs, and trees) are not only used for medicinal purposes but also for the preparation of several nutritional and nutraceutical benefits (Fig. 10.1). Several recent studies have projected the medicinal importance of herbs, shrubs, and tree species (Diaz-de-Cerio et al., 2017; Hirapara et al., 2017; Mikawlrawng et al., 2018, Navya and Anitha, 2018; Agarwal et al., 2019; Seriana et al., 2019; Ozturk et al., 2014, 2016, 2017a, b, c, 2018a, b, c, d, e, f, g, 2020, 2021a, b). Although different parts of some of the plant species are used mainly for nutritional purposes, they serve as a health food (e.g., beverages, fermented foods, and fruits) (Karun et al., 2014; Das et al., 2016; Anita and Sridhar, 2020; Shreelalitha and Sridhar, 2021).

Indian subcontinent being one of the 12 mega biodiversity countries endowed with a rich variety of wild plant species possessing medicinal value (Ignacimuthu et al., 2006). Indian subcontinent being endowed with 15 agro-climatic regions possess enormous plant species (18,000 spp.), and about one-third are therapeutically versatile (6000–7000 spp.). Plants have been used as herbal medicine in India since time immortal as they are inexpensive and easily accessible (Srivastav et al., 2011). The ethnic communities and rural folk from different parts of India utilize several plant species and their parts for the preparation of many indigenous medicines as well as delicacies. The plant parts used mainly include leaves, flowers, fruits, seeds, stems, roots, tubers, and whole-plant (Sridhar and Karun, 2017). Seeds are the significant source of oils of industrial, nutritional, and pharmaceutical value and such oils provide up to 85% of visible oil or fat necessary for human consumption (Ramadan et al., 2006, 2010, 2016). Owing to several applications of plant-based oils, it is necessary to invent oils in wild plant species those yield high quantities for nutritional, pharmaceutical, cosmetics, and other applications (Ramadan et al., 2006, 2016).

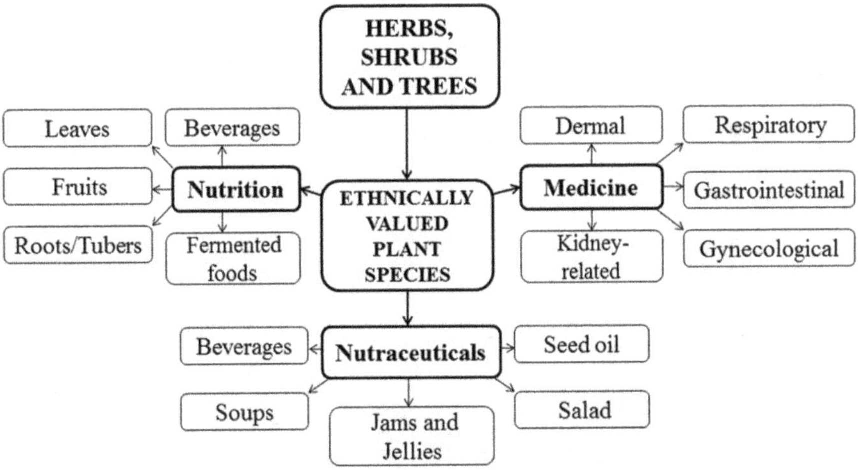

FIGURE 10.1 Medicinal, nutritional, and nutraceutical benefits of ethnically valued plant species (herbs, shrubs, and tree species).

In India, several wild plant seeds have been locally used traditionally for oil extraction for medicinal and edible purposes. Herbal and indigenous medicines have high-value fetching global market up to US$ 57 million in 2019; it is likely to elevate up to US$ 189 by 2026 (https://www.ibef.org/blogs/high-demand-for-medicinal-plants-in-india). Application of wild plant species increased drastically through ancient medicinal systems like Ayurveda, Unani, Siddha, Sowa-Rigpa, and homeopathy. Knowledge of plant folklore needs authentic documentation before it diminishes (Yadav et al., 2014). Documentation of indigenous knowledge should emphasize plant selection, season of use, parts used, and methods of processing for edible or medicinal purposes (Sridhar and Bhagya, 2007; Bhagya and Sridhar, 2009; Bhagya et al., 2013; Sridhar and Karun, 2017). Similar to biodiversity, the Indian subcontinent is also known for its enormous ethnic diversity and traditional knowledge. The ethnic healers, tribes, rural people, and forest dwellers from different parts of India relay on indigenous plantlore for primary health care. This review intends to document the heritage of the Indian subcontinent by pooling ethnic knowledge on the medicinal properties of wild and cultivated plant species. An innumerable number of plant species are used in indigenous medicine mainly to treat or cure skin diseases, gastrointestinal problems, respiratory diseases, kidney-related ailments, gynecological problems, and diseases pertaining to infants/children (Table 10.1). Dermal (30 diseases), gastrointestinal (20 diseases), respiratory (12 diseases), kidney

TABLE 10.1 Diversity of Plant Species Use to Cure Different Ailments in the Indian Subcontinent.

Nature of disease	Plant species
Dermal diseases (30 diseases)	*Abrus precatorius, Acacia catechu, Acacia farnesiana, Acalypha indica, chyranthes aspera, Aloe vera, Alstonia scholaris, Amaranthus viridis, Angallis arvensis, Areca catechu, Argemone mexicana, Arisaema intermedium, Arnebia euchorma, Arum dioscoridis, Azadirachta indica, Barleria cristata, Barleria prionitis, Bauhinia variegata, Begonia thomsonii, Berberis lycium, Bombax malabaricum, Brassica compestris, Butea frondosa, Calendula officinalis,*
	Callicarpa arborea, Calotropis gigantea, Calotropis procera, Cannabis sativa,
	Cassia alata, Cassia auriculata, Cassia fistula, Cassia occidentalis, Cassia tora,
	Celosia argentea, Centaurea iberica, Centella asiatica, Chenopodium album,
	Citrus assamensis, Cleome gynandra, Coccinia grandis, Colocasia esculenta,
	Commelina benghalensis, Coriandrum sativum, Cuscuta europaea, Cuscuta reflexa, Cyclea peltata, Cyperus rotundus, Datura metel, Datura stramonium,
	Daucus carota, Dioscorea bulbifera, Diospyros montana, Docynia indica,
	Duranta repens, Eclipta prostrata, Emblica officinalis, Eriobotrya bengalensis,
	Erythrina indica, Euphorbia helioscopia, Euphorbia hirta, Euphorbia ligularia,
	Ficus asperrima, Ficus benghalensis, Ficus religiosa, Fumaria indica, Gardenia gummifera, Gliricidia sepium, Gloriosa superba, Glycosmis pentaphylla, Gossypium harbaceum, Gynandropis pentaphylla, Heliotropium indicum, Holarrhena pubescens, Holoptelea integrifolia, Houttuynia cordata, Hyptis suaveolens, Impatiens balsamina, Ipomoea aquatica, Jasminum malabaricum,
	Jatropha gossypifolia, Leonotis nepetifolia, Lepidagathis cristata, Leucas aspera,
	Litsea glutinosa, Macaranga denticulata, Madhuca indica, Mangifera indica,
	Memecylon malabaricum, Michelia champaca, Mimosa pudica, Momordica charantia, Moringa oleifera, Mussaenda frondosa, Naravelia zeylanica, Nerium indicum, Nicotiana tabaeccum, Papaver dubium, Phaseolus aconitifolius, Phyllanthus emblica, Pinus wallichiana, Piper longum, Plumbago zeylanica, Plumeria rubra, Pongamia glabra, Pongamia pinnata, Pterocarpus marsupium,

TABLE 10.1 *(Continued)*

Nature of disease	Plant species
	Randia dumetorum, Rauvolfia serpentina, Santalum album, Saraca indica, Saussurea obvallata, Solanum myriacanthum, Solanum nigrum, Solanum surattense, Sonchus arvensis, Spilanthes paniculata, Swertia chirayita, Tamarindus indica, Taxillus tomentosus, Tectona grandis, Terminalia arjuna,
	Tinospora cordifolia, Tridax procumbens, Vitex negundo, Withania somnifera,
	Wrightia tinctoria, Xylia xylocarpa, and *Ziziphus mauritiana*
Gastrointestinal diseases (20 diseases)	*Acacia leucophloea, Acacia pennata, Acalypha indica, Achyranthes aspera, Adansonia digitata, Aegle marmelos, Amaranthus spinosus, Andrographis paniculata, Annona squamosa, Apama siliquosa, Artemisia vulgaris, Azadirachta indica, Bambusa vulgaris, Basella rubra, Bauhinia vahlii, Benincasa hispida, Butea monosperma, Calotropis procera, Cannabis sativa, Careya arborea,*
	Cassia tora, Cedrus deodara, Celosia argentea, Cissampelos pareira, Cyclea peltata, Dillenia indica, Ficus religiosa, Gloriosa superba, Gnaphalium affine,
	Helicteres isora, Hemidesmus indicus, Holarrhena antidysenterica, Holarrhena pubescens, Jatropha curcas, Leucas zeylanica, Macaranga indica, Madhuca longifolia, Mangifera indica, Nyctanthes arbor-tristis, Ocimum gratissimum,
	Oxalis corniculata, Oxalis latifolia, Pavonia zeylanica, Phyllanthus amarus,
	Piper nigrum, Pueraria tuberosa, Shorea robusta, Syzygium cumini, Urena lobata, Vernonia anthelmintica, Vitex negundo, Zanthoxylum armatum, and *Ziziphus oenopolia*
Respiratory diseases (12 diseases)	*Abrus precatorius, Acacia farnesiana, Acalypha indica, Aconitum heterophyllum,*
	Acorus calamus, Adhatoda vasica, Adhatoda zeylanica, Aeschynanthus sikkimensis, Allium sativum, Alpinia calcarata, Alstonia scholaris, Andrographis paniculata, Areca catechu, Aristolochia indica, Barleria cristata, Butea frondosa,
	Cassia alata, Cassia auriculata, Cinnamomum macrocarpum, Cinnamomum sulphuratum, Cinnamomum zeylanicum, Clerodendrum serratum, Clerodendrum viscosum, Cymbopogon nardus, Cynodon dactylon, Daemia extensa, Datura stramonium, Dipsacus inermis, Drymaria cordata, Embelia tsjeriam-cottam,
	Emblica ribes, Euphorbia neriifolia, Ficus religiosa, Flickingeria nodosa, Glycyrrhiza glabra, Hedyotis scandens, Helicteres isora, Justicia adhatoda,

TABLE 10.1 *(Continued)*

Nature of disease	Plant species
	Kaempferia galangal, Leucas cephalotus, Leucas indica, Leucas lanata, Litsea cubeba, Lychnis coronaria, Madhuca longifolia, Mangifera indica, Melia azedarach, Nyctanthes arbor-tristis, Ocimum basilicum, Ocimum sanctum, Ocimum tenuiflorum, Oroxylum indicum, Piper longum, Prunus persica, Pseudarthria viscida, Psidium guajava, Senna tora, Sisymbrium irio, Solanum torvum, Solanum viarum, Solanum violaceum, Spilanthus acmella, Tabernemontana divaricata, Tephrosia purpurea, Terminalia bellerica, Terminalia chebula, Thymus linearis, Trigonella foenum-graecum, Tylophora asthamatica, Tylophora indica, Vanda spathulata, Vanda testacea, Viola odorata,
	Vitex negundo, Withania somnifera, Zingiber officinale, and *Ziziphus mauritiana*
Kidney-related diseases (four diseases)	*Acalypha indica, Achyranthes aspera, Aerva javanica, Aerva lanata, Amaranthus spinosus, Asparagus racemosus, Boerhaavia diffusa, Bryophyllum calycinum, Bryophyllum pinnatum, Cardiospermum helicacabum, Celosia cristata, Coleus aromaticus, Costus speciosus, Cuscuta reflexa, Cyperus rotundus, Dolichos biflorus, Eclipta alba, Ensete superbum, Gmelina arborea, Helicanthes elastica, Hemidesmus indicus, Heracleum rigens, Justicia Adhatoda, Lawsonia inermis, Mimosa pudica, Moringa oleifera, Musa paradisiaca, Oryza rufipogon, Pongamia pinnata, Rotula aquatica, Saraca asoca, Scoparia dulcis, Sida acuta, Sonchus oleraceus, Tinospora cordifolia, Tribulus terrestris, Tridax procumbens, Typha domingensis*, and *Vitex negundo*
Gynecological diseases (14 diseases)	*Abutilon indicum, Acacia farnesiana, Achyranthes aspera, Achyranthes bidentata,*
	Adina cordifolia, Ailanthus excels, Albizia lebbeck, Amaranthus spinosus, Ananassa sativa, Argemone mexicana, Asparagus racemosus, Asparagus racemosus, Azadirachta indica, Bauhinia purpurea, Bauhinia recemosa, Belamcanda chinensis, Boerhavia diffusa, Borassus flabellifer, Butea monosperma, Calotropis procera, Cassia auriculata, Cassia occidentalis, Cassytha filiformis, Centratherum anthelminticum, Cocculus hirsutus, Coffea arabica, Coix lacryma-jobi, Crotalaria prostrata, Curculigo orchioides, Curcuma longa, Cycas circinalis, Cyclea peltata, Cynodon dactylon, Daucus carota,
	Dendrophthoe falcata, Desmodium pulchellu, Dichrostachys cinerea, Dioscorea alata, Dolichandrone falcata, Echinops echinatus, Emblica officinalis, Erythrina indica, Euphorbia hirta, Ficus benghalensis, Ficus religiosa, Gardenia latifolia, Gloriosa superba, Hibiscus rosa-sinensis, Holostemma ada-kodien, Hydrocotyle javanica, Hyptis suaveolens, Kaempferia galanga, Lagerstroemia speciosa, Leonurus sibiricus, Lycoperisicon esculenta, Madhuca indica, Mangifera indica,

TABLE 10.1 *(Continued)*

Nature of disease	Plant species
	Manihot esculenta, Maytenus senegalensis, Meiogyne pannosa, Melia azadirachta, Mesua ferrea, Murraya koenigii, Musa paradisiaca, Nothapodytes nimmoniana, Ochna obtusata, Ocimum tenuiflorum, Pedalium murex, Pergularia daemia, Phyllanthus emblica, Pseudarthria viscida, Pterocarpus marsupium,
	Raphanus sativus, Saraca asoca, Scoparia dulcis, Sesamum indicum, Sida cordifolia, Spondias pinnata, Syzygium cumini, Tephrosia purpurea, Terminalia paniculata, Thottea siliquosa, Tribulus terrestris, Turpinia malabarica, Urginea indica, Urtica diocia, Vernonia cinerea, Vinca rosea, Withania somnifera, Woodfordia fruticosa, and *Ziziphus xylopyrus*
Diseases of infants and children (14 diseases)	*Achyranthes aspera, Acorus calamus, Anisochilus carnosus, Anisochilus malabarica, Asparagus racemosus, Bacopa monnieri, Calendula officinalis, Chrozophora rottleri, Clitoria ternatea, Coccinia grandis, Corallocarpus epigaeus, Dryopteris barbigera, Elephantopus scaber, Gloriosa superba, Helicteres isora, Marrubium vulgare, Morinda pubescens, Oryza sativa, Pinus wallichiana, Prunus armeniaca, Ricinus communis, Ruellia patula, Ruta graveolens, Sauropus bacciformis, Sida rhombifolia, Sisymbrium irio, Spilanthes paniculata, Thymus linearis,* and *Zanthoxylum armatum*

(4 diseases), gynecological (14 diseases), and infant/children (14 diseases) diseases were treated or cured by 128, 53, 77, 39, 91, and 29 plant species, respectively.

10.2 DERMAL DISEASES

Dermal diseases are a major health concern, and many plant species have the potency to cure a variety of dermal ailments. Some of the general skin-related problems cured by plant species include swellings, rashes, blisters, allergies, wounds, boils, cuts, itching, rashes, abscess, and chilblains. Many plant species are capable of curing specific skin diseases like ringworm, blemishes (skin discoloration), leucoderma, dandruff, scabies, eczema, leprosy, alopecia, psoriasis, hair fall, and pimples. Other skin problems like burns, cracked heels, infection in toes, and cracks in heels are also cured by plant products. Bacterial (impetigo) and viral (chicken pox, small pox, and herpes) infections could also be treated by plant-derived products. Up to 30 dermal diseases can be treated or cured by 128 plant species (Table 10.1).

10.2.1 JAMMU AND KASHMIR

In Bandipora District of Jammu and Kashmir, *Angallis arvensis*, *Calendula officinalis*, *Centaurea iberica*, *Euphorbia helioscopia*, and *Fumaria indica* are useful in treating several skin-related problems (itching, boils, burns, rashes, and eruptions) (Lone et al., 2013). The herbal healers and tribes of this region use *Brassica compestris*, *Papaver dubium*, *Pinus wallichiana*, and *Sonchus arvensis* against skin-related ailments, especially eruption and boils (Lone and Bhardwaj, 2013). The villagers of Udhampur District use 49 plant species against dermatological problems (abscess, ringworm, acne, blemishes, leucoderma, dandruff, boils, and alopecia) (e.g., *Arnebia euchorma*, *Azadirachta indica*, *Berberis lycium*, *Calotropis procera*, and *Solanum nigrum*) (Bhatia et al., 2014).

10.2.2 UTTARAKHAND

In Uttarakhand, plant species like *Argemone mexicana*, *Solanum surattense*, and *Swertia chirayita* possess active ingredients against alopecia and scabies (Dangwal and Sharma, 2011). The local people of Rudraprayag District use

44 plant species against skin diseases (Chandra et al., 2013). The "*Gujjar*" tribe utilizes 109 angiosperms to cure skin ailments (mainly boils, blisters, allergies, eczema, ringworm, leprosy, and wounds) (Sharma et al., 2013). The "*Tharu*" community uses 90 plant species to treat 15 different skin diseases (e.g., boils, burns, chilblains, cracked heels, cuts, dandruff, eczema, hair fall, itching, leprosy, leucoderma, ringworm, infection in toes and wounds) (Sharma et al., 2014a). The medicinal preparations used for treatments include paste, juice, latex, seed oil, powder, gum, and ash. Herbal healers use *Ficus benghalensis* against burns and *Saussurea obvallata* for cut and wounds, *Nerium indicum* against eczema, *A. indica* for pimples, *Colocasia esculenta* against skin infections and *Chenopodium album* against white spots (Kala et al., 2005). Among 113 medicinal plant species of Garhwal Himalaya, many are used to treat skin diseases (burns, ringworm, wound, and skin infections) (e.g., *Aloe vera, Arisaema intermedium, Bauhinia variegata, Cannabis sativa, Centella asiatica, Coriandrum sativum, Cuscuta europaea,* and *Dioscorea bulbifera*) (Uniyal and Shiva, 2005).

10.2.3 NORTHEAST INDIA

The "*Mishing*" community inhabiting in Northeast India applies paste derived from the roots of two plant species (*Gossypium harbaceum* and *Houttuynia cordata*) separately to cure skin diseases (Shankar et al., 2012). Among the 17 threatened medicinal plant species from the Sonitpur District of Assam, *Citrus assamensis*, and *Piper longum* are used to cure pimples (Jyoti et al., 2013). The "*Jaintia*" tribes from North Cachar Hills District of Assam utilizes *Achyranthes aspera, Arum dioscoridis, Barleria cristata, Cassia tora, Cuscuta reflexa,* and *Nicotiana tabaeccum* against boils, skin infections, ringworms, and dandruff (Sajem and Gosai, 2006). The tribes from Cachar District also follow ethnic medicines prepared by many plants against allergies, abscesses, and small pox (e.g., *Alstonia scholaris, Amaranthus viridis, A. indica, Cassia alata, C. occidentalis, C. tora, Datura stramonium, Glycosmis pentaphylla, Hyptis suaveolens, Macaranga denticulata,* and *N. indicum*) (Das et al., 2008). The "*Chorei*" tribe from Assam uses several plant species against skin infections, boils, rashes, and ulcers (e.g., *Areca catechu, A. indica, Begonia thomsonii, Callicarpa arborea, C. tora, C. asiatica, Cleome gynandra, D. stramonium, Duranta repens, Docynia indica, Eriobotrya bengalensis, Euphorbia hirta, E. ligularia, F. benghalensis, Ipomoea aquatica, Leucas aspera, Litsea glutinosa, Mimosa pudica, Michelia champaca, Tinospora cordifolia,* and *Ziziphus mauritiana*)

(Choudhury et al., 2012). The ethnic tribes from Barpeta District of Assam use a few medicinal plants against skin diseases (e.g., *Acacia catechu*, *A. indica*, *Impatiens balsamina*, and *Solanum myriacanthum*) (Das, 2016). Among 66 medicinal plants reported from the North Garo Hills of Meghalaya, six are exclusively useful in treating skin diseases (Sharma et al., 2014b).

10.2.4 BIHAR, CHHATTISGARH, WEST BENGAL, AND ORISSA

About 26 plant species are used against skin diseases (ringworm, burns, boils, small pox, eczema, and scabies) in Bihar (Singh et al., 2013). The remote tribes from three selected districts of Chhattisgarh use 34 plant species against many skin diseases (e.g., abscess, boils, burns, eczema, itching, leprosy, ringworm, and sunstroke) (Tiwari, 2015). Three plant species from the Bankura District of West Bengal (*Eclipta prostrata*, *Pterocarpus marsupium*, and *Terminalia arjuna*) possess active ingredients against skin diseases (Sinhababu and Banerjee, 2013). A survey in the Bhadrak District of Orissa reported 57 plant species used to cure several skin-related ailments (e.g., boils, burns, chicken pox, eczema, itches, pimples, ringworm, and small pox) (Panda et al., 2016).

10.2.5 MADHYA PRADESH AND ANDHRA PRADESH

The tribal population from Central Narmada Valley in Madhya Pradesh utilizes several formulations or products (latex, paste, decoction, and juice) derived from 29 plant species to treat skin diseases (Choudhary et al., 2011). A survey in Panchmarhi Biosphere Reserve revealed a total 29 plant species active against skin diseases (Kadam and Sharma, 2013). The seed oil of *Celastrus paniculatus* is applied to cure skin diseases by "Bhil" tribe of Dhar District (Alawa et al., 2016).

A total of 36 plant species are helpful in curing skin diseases as reported from the Adilabad District, Andhra Pradesh (Madhu and Yarra, 2011). The "*Konda-Dora*" tribe from Visakhapatnam District uses 11 plant species against boils, burns, cuts, chicken pox, itching, leucoderma, leprosy, rashes, ringworm, scabies, and wounds (Padal et al., 2013). Up to 26 plant species are helpful in treating skin problems like boils, chicken pox, cuts, eczema, itching, wounds, and other skin ailments reported from East Godavari District (Raju et al., 2014). The "*Yanadi*" tribe and local villagers from Veyilingalakona (sacred groove) uses five plant species exclusively for skin diseases (*Gardenia gummifera*, *Lepidagathis cristata*, *Phaseolus aconitifolius*, *Randia dumetorum*, and

Taxillus tomentosus) (Savithramma et al., 2014). Five plant species reported from the Mahabubnagar District of Telangana are effective against skin diseases especially boils, burns, leprosy, mosquito-bite allergies, and ringworm (Singh and Singh, 2015). Another study from the Chityal Nalgonda District of Telangana resulted in exposing three plant species useful against skin diseases like itching (*Vitex negundo*), wrinkles in children (*Coccinia grandis*), and skin rashes (*Phyllanthus emblica*) (Prabhakar et al., 2015).

10.2.6 MAHARASHTRA AND KARNATAKA

Among 53 plant species reported from Bhandara District, many are used to cure skin diseases like itching, black spot, ringworm, acne, and wound by the "*Gond*" tribe (Gupta et al., 2010). More than 10 plant species are used by the tribal women from the Thane District to treat skin ailments (e.g., *Celosia argentea*, *Emblica officinalis*, *Ficus religiosa*, *Madhuca indica*, *Mangifera indica*, *Pongamia pinnata*, *P. marsupium*, and *Tectona grandis*) (Oak et al., 2015).

Six plant species (*Cassia fistula*, *Commelina benghalensis*, *Cyperus rotundus*, *Gloriosa superba*, *Leonotis nepetifolia*, and *Tridax procumbens*) are used to treat skin problems like cracks in heels, psoriasis, sores, and wounds in the Bidar District of Karnataka (Prashantkumar and Vidyasagar, 2006). Another survey from this region reported 26 plant species commonly used as a remedy against skin diseases (Prashantkumar and Vidyasagar, 2008). The *Acalypha indica* is helpful to cure scabies and eczema, *A. aspera* combat eczema, *A. mexicana* cures blisters, *Barleria prionitis* controls scabies, *Cassia auriculata* heels wounds, *Datura metel* controls dandruff, *Daucus carota* controls eczema, *Jatropha gossypifolia* prevents scabies and eczema, *T. procumbens* serves to treat cuts/bruises, and *Withania somnifera* prevents scabies as reported from the Gulbarga District (Ghatapanadi et al., 2011). The ethnobotanical study carried out in Hyderabad Karnataka reported 60 plant species used to combat skin problems. The main parts of plants used for treatment are leaves, followed by seeds (Policepatel and Manikrao, 2013). Another documentation from this region deals with plant species effective against different candidiasis (cutaneous, nail-plate fungal infection, oral, and vaginal infections) (Sharanappa and Vidyasagar, 2014).

A survey carried out in Harapanahalli Taluk of Davangere District resulted in the use of *Erythrina indica*, *G. superba*, and *Gynandropis pentaphylla* to treat skin-related disorders (Murthy, 2015). More than 15 plant species are effective against skin diseases (e.g., *Abrus precatorius*, *Acacia farnesiana*,

C. fistula, *Heliotropium indicum*, and *Spilanthes paniculata*) in Hassan District (Kumar and Siddamallayya, 2016). The local communities from some villages of Shimoga District utilize *Holoptelea integrifolia*, *Santalum album*, and *Tamarindus indica* to cure herpes; *Plumbago zeylanica* and *Pongamia glabra* against itching; *A. indica* and *Xylia xylocarpa* against leprosy; *Butea frondosa*, *L. aspera*, and *Momordica charantia* to treat skin diseases (dhobi's itch and ringworm); *P. zeylanica* against sore wounds; and *Bombax malabaricum* and *Diospyros montana* against boils, burns, and sores (Mahishi et al., 2005). A total of 48 plant species are reported from Sagar Taluk of Shimoga District (Rajakumar and Shivanna, 2010). Among them, *Rauvolfia serpentina* cures boils and sores; *Jasminum malabaricum* treats cuts and wounds; *Memecylon malabaricum* and *Moringa oleifera* against herpes; *Ficus asperrima*, *Holarrhena pubescens*, and *Mussaenda frondosa* against allergies; and *Gliricidia sepium*, *Naravelia zeylanica*, *Plumeria rubra*, and *T. cordifolia* against wounds. In another study, over 301 endemic herbal species were documented from the Western Ghats of Shimoga District with about 100 species active against many skin diseases (Kumar and Shivaraju, 2016). Among 25 plant species, only two were used by the herbal practitioners from Kadur Taluk, Chikmagalore District to cure skin diseases (*A. indica* and *V. negundo*) (Santhosh et al., 2014). About 22 plant species are effective against several skin-related problems (e.g., eczema, herpes, and skin allergies) used by tribes from the Kodagu District of Karnataka (Lingaraju et al., 2013). The survey in coastal Karnataka (Dakshina Kannada, Udupi, and Uttara Kannada districts) documented up to 342 medicinally useful plant species. Up to 22% of these plant species are useful against many skin diseases (herpes, scabies, eczema, leucoderma, skin ulcers/wounds, cuts, and burns) (Bhandary and Chandrashekar, 2014).

10.2.7 KERALA

Fourteen plant species are used against skin diseases, nine plant species against dandruff, six plant species against burns, seven plant species against leprosy, and five plant species to cure wounds by "*Mullu-Kuruma*" tribe from Wayanad District (Silja et al., 2008). The medicinal plants used by five tribes ("*Adiyan*," "*Kattunaika*," "*Kurichia*," "*Kuruma*," and "*Paniya*") of Mananthavady of Wayanad District documented 295 medicinal plants. Among them, 39 species are used in the treatment of skin-related problems (e.g., psoriasis, itching, and boils) (Shyma and Prasad, 2012). "*Malayaraya*" community from Idukki uses eight plant species to cure burns, dandruff, skin discoloration, and wounds (e.g., *Calotropis gigantea, D. stramonium*, and *Saraca indica*) (Sudeesh, 2012). A survey in the Malabar region (2008–2011) revealed 113 plant species (including two pteridophytes) useful in curing skin diseases (Deepthy and Remashree, 2014). A survey in a small village of Ernakulam District reported two plant species effective against psoriasis, leprosy, and other skin diseases (*C. tora* and *Wrightia tinctoria*) (Akhila et al., 2015). The ethobotanical survey from Malappuram District reported nine plants effective against leprosy and seven plants against skin diseases (Chithra et al., 2016). The study in Northern parts of Kerala revealed only two plant species useful against burns (*Cyclea peltata* and *P. emblica*) and one plant species against psoriasis (*R. serpentina*) (Jose et al., 2015).

10.2.8 TAMIL NADU

An exploration of indigenous knowledge of medicinal plant species useful in treating skin diseases in Kanyakumari District resulted in a total of 30 plant species to treat as many as 11 skin diseases (dandruff, eczema, impetigo, leprosy, parasite, psoriasis, rash, scabies, swellings, tinea cruris, and tinea versicolor) (Kingston et al., 2009). The study on medicinal plants used by the tribe "*Irula*" from the Erode District revealed a total of 70 plant species, and 29% of them are useful to cure skin diseases (Revathi and Parimelazhagan, 2010). The "*Kaani*" tribe from Kanyakumari District prefers 55 plant species to treat skin-related ailments. The main plant parts used were leaves (19 plants), whole-plant (11 plants), root (8 plants), and other parts (bark, seeds, flowers, rhizome, latex, woods, pods, shoots, and fruits) from the rest of the plants (Johnsy et al., 2012). A report on traditional medicinal plants against skin diseases from Nagapattinam District resulted in a total of 49 plant species (Sivaranjani and Ramakrishnan, 2012). These are used to cure skin problems, especially dandruff, eczema, itching, leucoderma, psoriasis, rashes, scabies, swelling, and many more. A survey conducted in Kolli Hills of the Eastern Ghats revealed 26 plant species useful to combat many dermatological problems (Xavier et al., 2015). The main route of administration of medicinal preparations is topical, followed by oral.

10.3 GASTROINTESTINAL AILMENTS

Gastrointestinal ailment is one of the major problems and needs immediate attention as first aid or treatment. Plant-based medicine is useful in treating many gastrointestinal diseases. Some of the common stomach-related ailments that are treated or cured by plant-based products include abdominal discomfort, stomachache, flatulence, indigestion, helminthiasis, loose motion, constipation, and stomach worms. Some of the specific gastrointestinal problems need special care; those ailments include acidity, blood dysentery, blood vomiting, diarrhea, dysentery, dyspepsia, gastric trouble, gastroenteritis, infantile diarrhea, oral ulcer, piles, and vomiting. Up to 20 gastrointestinal-related ailments are treated or cured by 53 plant species (Table 10.1).

10.3.1 JAMMU, KASHMIR, AND UTTARAKHAND

The traditional herbal healers and tribes from Bandipora District use 16 plant species to cure gastrointestinal ailments such as abdominal pain, acidity, constipation, dysentery, diarrhea, indigestion, and intestinal infections (Lone and Bhardwaj, 2013). Another report from the same region documented up to 18 plants used against gastrointestinal disorders (Lone et al., 2013). Bhatia et al. (2014) have recorded 64 plant species utilized to treat gastrointestinal ailments (appetizer, oral ulcer, constipation, piles, gastroenteritis, dyspepsia, dysentery, diarrhea, acidity, and flatulence) in Udhampur District.

In Uttarakhand, three plant species (*Cedrus deodara*, *Gnaphalium affine*, and *Shorea robusta*) were active against piles, diarrhea, and dysentery as recorded by Dangwal and Sharma (2011) from the Narendra Nagar Block. The local inhabitants from Rudraprayag District treat gastrointestinal ailments using powder formulations prepared from 70 plant species (constipation, colic pain, indigestion, vomiting, diarrhea, dysentery, gastric, and ulcer) (Chandra et al., 2013). The herbal healers use more traditional-based medicine to cure many gastrointestinal diseases using a dual mix of plant species or ingredients (dysentery, indigestion, piles, stomach worms, stomachache, and vomiting) (Kala et al., 2005). The rural women from Garhwal use up to 22 plant species to cure stomach diseases in children as well as adults (Uniyal and Shiva, 2005).

10.3.2 NORTHEAST INDIA

The "*Mishing*" community from Northeast India uses eight plant species against stomach-related disorders, especially digestion problems, gastric troubles, loose motion, and stomachache (e.g., *Acacia pennata*, *Amaranthus spinosus*, and *Macaranga indica*) (Shankar et al., 2012). Another study from Northeast India documented uses of 26 plant species against stomach disorders in Arunachal Pradesh followed by Manipur (23 spp.), Assam and Meghalaya (8 spp. each), Mizoram (6 spp.), and Sikkim and Tripura (3 spp. each) (Ramashankar et al., 2015). The traditional healers from Sikkim utilize 36 plant species to cure gastrointestinal diseases (Chanda et al., 2007). The "*Jaintia*" tribe from North Cachar Hills District of Assam employs 12 plant species against blood vomiting, diarrhea, dyspepsia, dysentery, piles, and stomachache (Sajem and Gosai, 2006). A total of 107 medicinal plant species are used by different tribes in the Cachar District of Assam (Das et al., 2008). Among them, 13 species are genuinely used against dysentery, 10 species against stomach disorders, and remaining few species are used to cure constipation, gastric troubles, diarrhea, piles, and also as digestive stimulants. Sixteen plant species are utilized by "*Chorei*" tribe from Southern Assam against constipation, diarrhea, digestive problems, dysentery, and tape-worm infection (Choudhury et al., 2012). Another survey in the Sonitpur District of Assam revealed the use of nine plant species against stomach and intestinal problems (diarrhea, dysentery, indigestion, stomach worms, and stomach infections) (Jyoti et al., 2013). Das (2016) has documented about 34 plant species used by tribal people from the Barpeta District of Assam in the treatment of stomach-related ailments. About 14 plant species are used by "Garo" tribe from North Garo Hills, Meghalaya, to treat gastrointestinal ailments (Sharma et al., 2014b). The tribal sect from the Bankura District of West Bengal follows traditional medicine prepared by 15 plant species against stomach disorders (constipation, diarrhea, dysentery, and intestinal worms) (e.g., *A. indica*, *F. religiosa*, *Ocimum gratissimum*, and *V. negundo*) (Sinhababu and Banerjee, 2013).

10.3.3 MADHYA PRADESH AND ANDHRA PRADESH

The tribal people from 30 remote locations of Madhya Pradesh utilize eight plants against intestinal problems (e.g., piles, infantile diarrhea, and dysentery) and also as a stomachic tonic (Dwivedi et al., 2008). The "*Bhil*" tribe from Madhya Pradesh utilizes *Adansonia digitata* and *Madhuca longifolia* against abdominal pain and *Annona squamosa* and *Butea monosperma* against intestinal worms (Alawa et al., 2016). Saheb et al. (2012) documented 29 plant species commonly use to cure gastrointestinal disorders by the tribal people of Nallamallais, Andhra Pradesh. The "*Konda-Dora*" tribe from Visakhapatnam uses many plant species against stomach and intestinal disorders; some examples include *Aegle marmelos*, *Nyctanthes arbor-tristis*, and *O. latifolia* for piles; *Basella rubra* and *Vernonia anthelmintica* for dyspepsia; *Bauhinia vahlii* for blood dysentery; *Benincasa hispida*, *Dillenia indica*, and *Urena lobata* for stomachache; *C. sativa* and *Pavonia zeylanica* for diarrhea; *C. argentea* for ulcers; *Cissampelos pareira* for diarrhea and piles; *Oxalis corniculata* for dysentery; and *Zanthoxylum armatum* for dysentery and vomiting (Padal et al., 2013). Approximately, 20 plant species are used in the East Godavari District to cure digestive and intestinal problems (Raju et al., 2014).

10.3.4 MAHARASHTRA AND KARNATAKA

The "*Gond*" tribe from the Bhandara District of Maharashtra depends on *Acacia leucophloea*, *A. marmelos*, *Andrographis paniculata*, *C. tora*, *Helicteres isora*, *Pueraria tuberosa*, and *Ziziphus oenopolia* to treat diarrhea, piles, and stomachache (Gupta et al., 2010). Twenty-five plant species are useful against gastrointestinal problems as used by the tribal women from Thane District (Oak et al., 2015). The ethnic groups from Bidar District of Karnataka use *A. indica*, *A. paniculata*, and *C. procera* to cure stomach pain and *G. superba* against piles (Prashantkumar and Vidyasagar, 2006). The folklore knowledge from villages of Bellary District revealed the utilization of 32 plant species to cure exclusively gastrointestinal disorders (Murthy and Vidyasagar, 2013a). The local healers from Gulbarga District depend on 13 medicinal plants to cure many stomach-related ailments (such as dysentery, piles, constipation, abdominal pain, gastric trouble, and vomiting) and also to improve digestion (Ghatapanadi et al., 2011). The villagers of Harapanahalli Taluk of Davangere District depend on 13 medicinal plants to treat digestive disorders (dysentery, piles, and stomachache) (Murthy, 2015). Ten medicinal plant species are used by "*Hakki-Pikki*" tribe from Hassan District to treat stomach and intestinal problems (Kumar and Siddamallayya, 2015). More than 50 plant species are reported from the Hassan District active against various gastrointestinal diseases (Kumar and Siddamallayya, 2016). The local communities of some villages of Shimoga District use *Holarrhena antidysenterica*, *Jatropha curcas*, *M. indica*, *Phyllanthus amarus*, and *Syzygium cumini* to treat chronic dysentery; *Careya arborea* against piles; and *A. indica* and *Hemidesmus indicus* to cure stomachache (Mahishi et al., 2005). The herbal healers from Sagar Taluk of Shimoga District use *A. aspera* to cure stomachache and *C. peltata* against dysentery (Rajakumar and Shivanna, 2010). More than 50 endemic plant species are very effective against stomach, intestine, and digestion-related diseases as reported from the Western Ghats region of Shimoga District (Kumar and Shivaraju, 2016). About 25 plant species are used by the herbal ethnic practitioners from Kadur Taluk of Chikmagalore District (8 spp. are useful exclusively against intestinal worms, dysentery, stomach pain, and stomach disorders) (Santhosh et al., 2014). About 35 plant species are effective against gastrointestinal diseases as reported from the tribal areas of Kodagu District (Lingaraju et al., 2013). A survey from the coastal region of Karnataka (Dakshina Kannada, Udupi, and Uttara Kannada districts) documented 342 species of medicinal plants used to treat many ailments with 15% of them against gastrointestinal problems (constipation or indigestion, dysentery, diarrhea, flatulence, intestinal worms, and piles) (Bhandary and Chandrashekar, 2014).

10.3.5 KERALA AND TAMIL NADU

The tribe "*Mullu-Kuruma*" of the Wayanad District of Kerala follows many ethnic medicines to cure several diseases (Silja et al., 2008). Ten plant species are useful to treat dysentery, six plants against piles, and four plants to treat constipation. The tribal people from Mananthavady of Wayanad District use 14 plant species to cure many stomach and intestine-related diseases (e.g., abdominal pain, diarrhea, dysentery, and piles) (Shyma and Prasad, 2012). The "*Adiayn*," "*Kattunaika*," "*Kurichia*," "*Kuruma*," and "*Paniya*" tribes from Wayanad District use 32 plant species to cure digestive ailments like abdominal pain, acidity, diarrhea, dysentery, pinworm, and stomachache (Prasad et al., 2013). Seven plant species are used to treat abdominal discomfort, indigestion, piles, intestinal worms, gastric problems, and constipation by "*Malayaraya*" community of Idukki (Sudeesh, 2012). Five plant species (angiospermic epiphytes and parasites) are also very effective against gastrointestinal diseases as reported from the Western Ghats region (Shanavaskhan et al., 2012). The *C. peltata* serves against constipation; *Apama siliquosa* and *H. pubescens* cure gastrointestinal disorders, which are in use by the local dwellers in Idamalayar, Ernakulam District (Akhila et al., 2015). Four plant species (*Artemisia vulgaris*, *Bambusa vulgaris*, *Leucas zeylanica*, and *Piper nigrum*) are used in the northern part of Kerala to treat dysentery, indigestion, and stomach problems (Jose et al., 2015).

The "*Irula*" tribe from Erode District of Tamil Nadu utilizes as many as 70 wild plant species against various diseases, of which 27% are useful to combat digestive problems (Revathi and Parimelazhagan, 2010). The villagers from Villupuram District utilize 28 plant species to treat gastrointestinal disorders (constipation, diarrhea, dysentery, indigestion, piles, and stomachache) (Muralidharan and Narasimhan, 2012).

10.4 RESPIRATORY DISEASES

Plant-based medicines treat or cure many respiratory diseases like asthma, bronchitis, common cold, cough, chronic cough, dry cough, whooping cough, catarrh (excessive blood loss in nose or throat), pneumonia, sore nose, throat infection, and tuberculosis. Up to 12 respiratory ailments are treated or cured by 77 plant species (Table 10.1).

10.4.1 JAMMU AND KASHMIR

The tribal people and herbal healers from Bandipora District utilize nine plant species against respiratory disorders like asthma, common cold, cough, pneumonia, chronic cough, and throat infection (*Allium sativum*, *Cynodon dactylon*, *Dipsacus inermis*, *Prunus persica*, *Trigonella foenum-graecum*, *Lychnis coronaria*, *Sisymbrium irio*, *Thymus linearis*, and *Viola odorata*) (Lone and Bhardwaj, 2013). Another report from the same region revealed the importance of 12 plant species to combat lung-related diseases (asthma, dry cough, cough, cold, pneumonia, and whooping cough) (Lone et al., 2013). The villagers of Udhampur District utilize 18 plant species against asthma, nose congestion, cough, cold, halitosis, suffocation, and whooping cough (Bhatia et al., 2014).

10.4.2 NORTH INDIA

Two plant species (*Adhatoda vasica* and *D. stramonium*) are effective against asthma, bronchitis, and tuberculosis in Narendra Nagar Block in Uttarakhand (Dangwal and Sharma, 2011). The local inhabitants or *Vaidya* from Rudraprayag District use many plant species against cough, throat problems, pneumonia, and respiratory ailments (Chandra et al., 2013). The main formulations use to treat these diseases are ash, powder, fresh juice, and tablets. The herbal healers use many medicinal plant species either single or in combination with other plant species to cure cough, cold, throat chock, pneumonia, and tuberculosis (Kala et al., 2005). The rural women from Garhwal utilize 15 plant species to treat respiratory ailments, especially asthma, breathing problems, bronchitis, cough, cold, and tuberculosis (Uniyal and Shiva, 2005).

10.4.3 NORTHEAST INDIA

The "*Mishing*" community uses five plant species against cough (*Acorus calamus*, *Adhatoda zeylanica*, *B. cristata*, *Glycyrrhiza glabra*, and *Tabernemontana divaricata*); *G. glabra* to cure throat pain; and *Leucas indica* and *T. divaricata* against pneumonia (Shankar et al., 2012). A study on medicinal plants in Assam revealed that 14 plant species are useful to cure respiratory disorders (Bhuyan and Baruah, 2015). Many plant species are used to cure respiratory problems (asthma, cough, cold, throat pain, and pneumonia) in Northeast India (Ramashankar et al., 2015). Two plant species are used in Arunachal Pradesh (*Litsea cubeba* and *Solanum torvum*); four plant species in Assam (*A. calamus*, *Euphorbia neriifolia*, *Justicia adhatoda*, and *Melia azedarach*); two plant species are used in Tripura (*Kaempferia galanga* and *Leucas lanata*); one plant species each in Manipur (*A. calamus*), Meghalaya (*Hedyotis scandens*), Mizoram (*Aeschynanthus sikkimensis*), and Sikkim (*Drymaria cordata*). The "*Jaintia*" tribes from the North Cachar District of Assam utilize two medicinal plants to cure asthma (*A. scholaris* and *Clerodendrum viscosum*) (Sajem and Gosai, 2006). Different tribes in the Cachar District of Assam utilize six plants against cough (Das et al., 2008). Three medicinal plants (*A. vasica*, *Ocimum basilicum*, and *Psidium guajava*) are active against cough and cold as used by the "*Chorei*" tribe in Southern Assam (Choudhury et al., 2012). A total of 17 threatened medicinal plant species are reported from the Sonitpur District of Assam with three species useful in treating cough, cold, and asthma (Jyoti et al., 2013). The traditional tribal people from the Barpeta District of Assam employ 19 plant species against respiratory problems (Das, 2016). A survey from the North Garo Hills of Meghalaya revealed a total of 11 plant species helpful in treating cough, throat infection, throat pain, and tuberculosis (Sharma et al., 2014b). The tribals from the Bankura District of West Bengal utilize nine medicinal plants to cure asthma, bronchitis, cough, and cold (Sinhababu and Banerjee, 2013).

10.4.4 MADHYA PRADESH AND ANDHRA PRADESH

The tribes of Madhya Pradesh use only three medicinal plants against respiratory problems (cough: *Leucas cephalotus*, *Ocimum sanctum*, and

Tephrosia purpurea; asthma: *T. purpurea*) (Dwivedi et al., 2008). "Bhil" tribe of Dhar District uses four plants to treat cough, cold, pneumonia, and other respiratory problems (*J. adhatoda*, *M. longifolia*, *N. arbor-tristis*, and *Z. mauritiana*) (Alawa et al., 2016).

The "*Konda-Dora*" tribe from Visakhapatnam District of Andhra Pradesh depends on five plant species against lung-related diseases (*A. precatorius*, *C. alata*, *Ocimum tenuiflorum*, *Oroxylum indicum*, and *Zingiber officinale*) (Padal et al., 2013). A survey on indigenous knowledge in Krishna District showed 23 plant species used to cure several respiratory diseases (e.g., asthma, bronchitis, cough, and cold) (Kumari et al., 2014). Up to five plants are utilized to treat lung-related problems in East Godavari District (Raju et al., 2014). Six medicinal plant species are effective against respiratory ailments (asthma, cough, and catarrh) as documented from the Mahabubnagar District of Telangana (Singh and Singh, 2015). Prabhakar et al. (2015) have reported the application of three plants to cure cough (*Aristolochia indica*, *Solanum viarum*, and *Senna tora*) and one species against lung diseases (*A. farnesiana*) in the Chityal Nalgonda District of Telangana.

10.4.5 MAHARASHTRA AND KARNATAKA

The "*Gond*" tribe from Bhandara District depends on five plants (*A. zeylanica*, *A. paniculata*, *M. indica*, *Spilanthus acmella*, and *Terminalia chebula*) to overcome lung problems, especially cough and asthma (Gupta et al., 2010). Up to 12 plant species are utilized by villagers of Nanded District against lung diseases (Shaikh et al., 2014). A total of eight plants are used by the tribal women of Thane District to treat cough, asthma, sore throat, and throat congestion (Oak et al., 2015).

The ethnic groups from different villages of the Bidar District of Karnataka utilize only one plant species (*A. indica*) to cure cough (Prashantkumar and Vidyasagar, 2006). A survey in 16 villages of Bellary District revealed that 26 plant species are useful against respiratory problems (majority of them are used in the treatment of asthma) (Murthy and Vidyasagar, 2013b). The herbal formulations use to treat lung diseases include decoction, juice, paste, and pills. Ghatapanadi et al. (2011) documented the use of six medicinal plants to treat cough, cold, and whooping cough in Gulbarga District. Ten traditional medicinal plants are used to treat asthma, cold, whooping cough, and other respiratory problems in Harapanahalli Taluk of Davangere District (Murthy, 2015). Only one less-known plant species (*Cymbopogon nardus*) is used to treat bronchitis by "*Hakki-Pikki*" tribes in Hassan District (Kumar and Siddamallayya, 2015). More than 30 plant species are used in traditional medicine to cure many lung-related diseases (e.g., asthma, cough, whooping cough, cold, and bronchitis) as reported from the Hassan District (Kumar and Siddamallyya, 2016). Local communities from some of the villages of Shimoga District depend on *A. catechu*, *B. frondosa*, *Daemia extensa*, and *O. sanctum* against cough and *F. religiosa*, *Terminalia bellerica*, *Tylophora asthamatica*, and *W. somnifera* to treat asthma (Mahishi et al., 2005). The locals of Sagar Taluk of Shimoga utilize *Clerodendrum serratum* against asthma; *C. auriculata* against cold; *C. auriculata*, *Emblica ribes*, and *H. isora* against cough; and *V. negundo* against sore nose (Rajakumar and Shivanna, 2010). More than 25 endemic plant species are used to cure respiratory ailments (asthma, cough, cold, and bronchitis) in the Western Ghats region of Shimoga District (Kumar and Shivaraju, 2016). The herbal healers from Kadur Taluk of Chikmagalore District depend on seven medicinal plants to cure asthma, cold, and cough (Santhosh et al., 2014). A survey on medicinal plants in tribal areas of Kodagu District reported 12 plant species used against respiratory problems (asthma, cough, and common cold) (Lingaraju et al., 2013). A study on ethnic medicinal plants in three coastal districts (Dakshina Kannada, Udupi, and Uttara Kannada) revealed the existence of 342 plant species, with 6% of them are useful in the treatment of respiratory diseases (cold, cough, and asthma) (Bhandary and Chandrashekar, 2014).

10.4.6 KERALA AND TAMIL NADU

"*Mullu-Kuruma*" tribe from Wayanad District utilizes 20 plant species to cure asthma, cough, and bronchial diseases, while only one plant species to treat tuberculosis (Silja et al., 2008). Five plants are very effective against respiratory problems in Mananthavady, Wayanad District (*Cinnamomum macrocarpum*, *C. sulphuratum*, *C. zeylanicum*, *Embelia tsjeriam-cottam*, and *Pseudarthria viscida*) (Shyma and Prasad, 2012). The "Malayaraya" community from Idukki depends on *Aconitum heterophyllum*, *Alpinia calcarata*, *D. stramonium*, *O. sanctum*, and *V. negundo* to treat asthma as well as cough (Sudeesh, 2012). Akhila et al. (2015) reported the importance of *P. longum*, *Solanum violaceum*, and *Tylophora indica* in curing asthma, cough, and bronchial problems in Ernakulam District. Three angiosperm epiphytes (*Flickingeria nodosa*, *Vanda spathulata*, and *V. testacea*) are effective against asthma reported from the Western Ghats of Kerala (Shanavaskhan et al., 2012). The tribal communities from Malappuram District utilize nine plant species to cure asthma and four plant species to treat tuberculosis (Chithra et al., 2016). The "*Irula*" tribe from Erode District of Tamil Nadu depends on six plant species to cure various lung-related disorders (cough, cold, breathing problems, and asthma) (Revathi and Parimelazhagan, 2010).

10.5 KIDNEY-RELATED DISORDERS

Plant-based medicines are useful to treat or cure many of the kindly related ailments. A remedy could be possible by several plant species, and the diseases that could be cured include urinary irritation, urinary calculi, kidney stones, and dysuria. Up to 39 plant species treat or cure about four kidney ailments (Table 10.1).

10.5.1 JAMMU AND KASHMIR

The rural herbal healers and tribes from Bandipora District use five medicinal plants to treat kidney-related diseases (kidney stones, dysuria, and urinary irritation) (Lone and Bhardwaj, 2013). Another survey in Bandipora District showed the importance of seven plant species to treat many kidney-related ailments like kidney stones, burning sensation, dysuria, and pus urination (Lone et al., 2013). The villagers in Udhampur District depend on eight plant species to cure diuresis and hematuria (Bhatia et al., 2014).

10.5.2 NORTH AND NORTHEAST INDIA

Up to five plant species are useful in treating kidney diseases in the Chamoli District of Uttarakhand (e.g., kidney stones) (Bisht et al., 2013). The herbal healers use four formulations prepare by medicinal plants to cure kidney stones (Kala et al., 2005). The rural women from Garhwal depend on four medicinal plants to treat kidney stones and other urinary problems (Uniyal and Shiva, 2005).

The "*Mishing*" community of Northeast India utilizes two plant species to cure urinary ailments like urinary trouble (*P. pinnata*) and kidney stones (*Sonchus oleraceus*) (Shankar et al., 2012). The "*Chorei*" tribe from Southern Assam uses *Gmelina arborea* against urinary infections (Choudhury et al., 2012). *T. cordifolia* is used in Sonitpur District to treat urinary problems (Jyoti et al., 2013). The tribals of Barpeta District depend on three plants against kidney stones and urinary problems (*A. indica*, *Bryophyllum pinnatum*, and *J. adhatoda*) (Das, 2016). Ramashankar et al. (2015) have reported the use of three plant species to cure urinary problems (*Asparagus racemosus, Bryophyllum calycinum*, and *Costus speciosus*) in Assam and one species (*C. speciosus*) in Manipur. A survey in the Muzaffarnagar District of Uttar Pradesh documented 15 plant species against problems of stones in the urinary tract as well as in kidney (Prachi et al., 2009).

10.5.3 MADHYA PRADESH, ANDHRA PRADESH, AND MAHARASHTRA

The tribes in Madhya Pradesh use six plant species against diuresis (Dwivedi et al., 2008). The traditional healers from the Nizamabad District of Andhra Pradesh utilize 18 plant species against kidney stones (Dinesh et al., 2013). *Aerva javanica* and *M. pudica* are useful in treating kidney stones in the Chityal Nalgonda District of Telangana (Prabhakar et al., 2015). The "*Gond*" tribe from the Bhandara District of Maharashtra utilizes two plant species to treat urological problems: *A. aspera* (to cure problems of burning micturition) and *Cardiospermum helicacabum* (against burning urination) (Gupta et al., 2010). The villagers from Nanded District depend on *C. rotundus* and *Sida acuta* against urinary disorders and *Celosia cristata* against kidney stones (Shaikh et al., 2014). The tribal women from Thane District employ nine plant species against urological problems (e.g., urinary calculi, concretions, kidney stones, and urinary tract infections) (Oak et al., 2015).

10.5.4 KARNATAKA

Many ethnic tribes of Bidar District use *T. procumbens* to treat kidney stones (Prashanthkumar and Vidyasagar, 2006). Ghatapanadi et al. (2011) from Gulbarga District have documented the use of *Coleus aromaticus, Lawsonia inermis, Saraca asoca, T. cordifolia*, and *V. negundo* against renal calculi and *A. indica* to cure urinary problems. The ethnic communities from Harapanahalli Taluk of Davangere District use *Dolichos biflorus* and *Tribulus terrestris* to eliminate stones in urinary tract and kidney, respectively (Murthy, 2015). The "Hakki-Pikki" tribe in Hassan District uses *Ensete superbum* to treat kidney stones; *M. oleifera, Musa paradisiaca*, and *Oryza rufipogon* for diuresis; and *Typha domingensis* against urinary calculi and dysuria (Kumar and Siddamallayya, 2015). A survey documented more than 30 plant species use to treat kidney-related diseases in Hassan District (Kumar and Siddamallayya, 2016). *A. racemosus* is useful in eliminating kidney stones as reported from the Sagar Taluk in Shimoga District (Rajakumar and Shivanna, 2010). Ten endemic plant species are used to cure kidney stones, and five species are used to treat other urinary disorders in Shimoga District (Kumar and Sivaraju, 2016). Traditional healers from Kadur Taluk in Chikmagalore District employ *V. negundo* as diuretic (Santhosh et al., 2014). Tribes from Kodagu District utilize *A. spinosus*, *H. indicus*, and *Heracleum rigens* as diuretics (Lingaraju et al., 2013). A study in three districts of coastal Karnataka revealed the usage of several plant species to treat urinary problems (polyuria, dysuria, and urinary stones) (Bhandary and Chandrashekar, 2014).

10.5.5 KERALA AND TAMIL NADU

The "*Mullu-Kuruma*" tribe of Wayanad District employs 12 medicinal plants to treat urinary complications and kidney stones (Silja et al., 2008). The "*Malayaraya*" community in Idukki uses *Aerva lanata*, *Boerhaavia diffusa*, and *Eclipta alba* as a remedy for kidney-related ailments (Sudeesh, 2012). The two angiospermic parasites are used as a remedy for urinary problems (Shanavaskhan et al., 2012). *C. reflexa* is used against hematuria and *Helicanthes elastica* against urinary bladder and kidney stones. The villagers from Idamalayar, Ernakulam District, use *Scoparia dulcis* against urinary diseases (Akhila et al., 2015). Different tribes from Malappuram District employ four plant species as a remedy for kidney stones and eight species for other urinary disorders (Chithra et al., 2016). Based on the indigenous knowledge of medicinal plants in Northern Kerala, people use two plant species (*S. dulcis* and *Rotula aquatica*) to treat kidney stones (Jose et al., 2015). "*Irula*" tribe from Erode District of Tamil Nadu uses *S. album* to treat urinary tract infections (Revathi and Parimelazhagan, 2010).

10.6 GYNECOLOGICAL PROBLEMS

Cures of many gynecological problems are dependent on plant-based medicines. Gynecological ailments cured by plant-based medicine include mucus discharge, leucorrhoea, postnatal complications, menorrhagia (prolonged menstruation), dysmenorrhea (painful menstrual periods), oligomenorrhea (infrequent menstrual periods), excessive menstrual flow, abortion, postdelivery uterus contraction, separation of umbilical cord, excessive bleeding during pregnancy, excessive menstrual bleeding, postdelivery bleeding, and regulation of menstrual cycle. Up to 91 plant species treat or cure about 14 gynecological ailments (Table 10.1).

10.6.1 JAMMU, KASHMIR, AND UTTARAKHAND

About 50 plant species are useful to combat menstrual disorders in the Udhampur District of Jammu and Kashmir (Bhatia et al., 2015). Administration of decoction of *O. tenuiflorum* seeds (twice a day) and decoction of tender twigs of *A. indica* (thrice a day) are advised by herbal healers to regularize the menstruation cycle in Uttarakhand (Kala et al., 2005). *A. racemosus* and *O. tenuiflorum* are also used to treat leucorrhoea (whitish/yellowish mucus discharge) (Kala et al., 2005). The rural women from Garhwal use leaves of *Urtica diocia* and bark of *S. cumini* against menstrual disorders and fruits of *F. religiosa* to overcome leucorrhoea (Uniyal and Shiva, 2005).

10.6.2 NORTHEAST INDIA

The *"Mishing"* community from Northeast India utilizes oral administration of plant extract prepared out of *Belamcanda chinensis* against menstrual disorders (Shankar et al., 2012). Different tribes from the Cachar District of Assam use six plant species against menstrual problems (leaf juice of *A. aspera*; bark juice of *Bauhinia purpurea*; juice made out of *C. dactylon* + juice of flowers of *Hibiscus rosa-sinensis* + sugar; flower extract of *H. rosa-sinensis* alone; seeds of *E. officinalis* and juice of *S. dulcis*) (Das et al., 2008). Two species are also useful in treating leucorrhoea (bark juice of *B. purpurea* and leaf juice of *Vernonia cinerea*). Up to 21 plant species in Assam are helpful in curing reproductive health-related ailments (Taid et al., 2014).

10.6.3 BIHAR, ORISSA, AND ANDHRA PRADESH

Five plant species (*Abutilon indicum*, *A. spinosus*, *F. benghalensis*, *Sida cordifolia*, and *W. somnifera*) in Bihar are used to treat menstrual problems and leucorrhoea (Singh et al., 2013). Tribals from the Mayurbhanj District of Orissa utilize 24 plant species against leucorrhoea, anemia, contraceptive, abdominal pain, postnatal complications, and other menstrual disorders (Behera, 2006). The "*Bhil*" tribe from Dhar District, Madhya Pradesh, uses the inflorescence of male plants of *Borassus flabellifer* against menstrual cycle problems (Alawa et al., 2016). The "*Konda-Dora*" tribe from Visakhapatnam District, Andhra Pradesh, consumes medicinal products prepared by three plant species to cure menstrual disorders (*M. azedarach*, *Urginea indica*, and *Woodfordia fruticosa*) (Padal et al., 2013). The stem bark of *Ailanthus excelsa* is used against leucorrhoea and menorrhagia (prolonged menstruation), while *S. asoca* against menorrhagia.

10.6.4 MAHARASHTRA AND KARNATAKA

The leaf juice of *Cassia occidentalis* and seeds of *Gardenia latifolia* along with the leaf of *Piper* are employed by the "*Gond*" tribe to set regularity in menstruation in Maharashtra (Gupta et al., 2010). The tribal women from Thane District consume fruits of *M. indica* to regularize menstrual irregularities (Oak et al., 2015). The villagers of Nanded District utilize three plants against menstrual problems (*Bauhinia recemosa, C. procera*, and *Ochna obtusata*) (Shaikh et al., 2014).

Documentation on medicinal plants in the Bidar District of Karnataka resulted in the use of five plant species (*B. monosperma*, *Crotalaria prostrata*, *Dolichandrone falcata*, *H. suaveolens*, and *Maytenus senegalensis*) and four plant species (*B. monosperma*, *D. falcata*, *H. suaveolens*, and *M. senegalensis*) to cure leucorrhoea and menorrhagia, respectively (Prashanthkumar and Vidyasagar, 2006). A survey from Bellary District reported that 26 plant species are helpful against menstrual disorders: menorrhagia, leucorrhoea; dysmenorrhea (painful menstrual periods); oligomenorrhea (infrequent menstrual periods); and other types of menstrual problems (Vidyasagar and Siddalinga, 2012). Documentation on ethnic knowledge of medicinal plants in Gulbarga District revealed that *Echinops echinatus*, *F. religiosa*, and *Vinca rosea* are helpful in curing leucorrhoea; *F. religiosa*, *S. asoca* against menorrhagia; and *T. purpurea* against abdominal pain during menstrual cycle (Ghatapanadi et al., 2011). About 35 plant species from the Hyderabad Karnataka region are found to be active against white discharge (Sharanappa and Vidyasagar, 2014). A report on medicinal plants in Davangere District detailed the use of *A. racemosus*, *Dichrostachys cinerea*, *F. religiosa*, and *Sesamum indicum* against menstrual disorders, while *A. farnesiana* against leucorrhoea (Murthy, 2015). The "*Hakki-Pikki*" tribes from Hassan District use flowers of *C. auriculata* against the excessive menstrual flow (Kumar and Siddamallayya, 2015). As reported by Kumar and Siddamallayya (2016) from Hassan District, *Dendrophthoe falcata*, *Pergularia daemia*, and *Ziziphus xylopyrus* are helpful to treat menstrual disorders, while *Achyranthes bidentata*, *Albizia lebbeck*, *A. mexicana*, *E. hirta*, and *F. benghalensis* are useful against leucorrhoea. *H. rosa-sinensis* and *Terminalia paniculata* are useful in treating menstrual disorders as reported from Sagar Taluk of Shimoga District (Rajakumar and Shivanna, 2010). Several medicinal plants from the Western Ghats of Shimoga region are useful in treating leucorrhoea (*Coffea arabica*, *E. indica*, *Pedalium murex*, and *Spondias pinnata*) and menstrual problems (*Ananassa sativa*, *C. arabica*, *Manihot esculenta*, *Meiogyne pannosa*, and *Turpinia malabarica*) (Kumar and Shivaraju, 2016). Among 25 plant species utilize by the traditional herbal healers from Kadur Taluk (Chikmagalore District), *D. carota*, *M. indica*, and *Raphanus sativus* are active against menstrual problems (Santhosh et al., 2014). The tribes of Kodagu District utilize *Desmodium pulchellu* and *Hydrocotyle javanica* against menorrhagia; *C. peltata*, *H. rosa-sinensis*, *Leonurus sibiricus*, and *M. paradisiaca* against leucorrhoea. *M. paradisiaca* is also active against dysmenorrhea (Lingaraju et al., 2013).

10.6.5 KERALA AND TAMIL NADU

The "*Adiyan*," "*Kattunaika*," "*Kurichia*," "*Kuruma*," and "*Paniya*" tribes from Wayanad District use the bark of *S. asoca* in the treatment of excessive menstrual bleeding; the "*Kurichia*" tribe uses tuberous roots of *G. superba* to cure white discharge; and leaf of *Nothapodytes nimmoniana* is used to cure headache during postdelivery (Shyma and Prasad, 2012). The "*Kurichia*" and "*Adiyan*" tribes from Wayanad depend on the root juice of *Centratherum anthelminticum* against obesity after delivery (Prasad and Shyma, 2013). Tubers of *Curculigo orchioides* are used by "*Malayaraya*" community from Idukki to cure stomach pain after delivery, while fresh leaves of the rare plant *Lycoperisicon esculenta* help to prevent menstruation (Sudeesh, 2012). The "*Urali*" tribe from Idukki uses 29 plant species to treat several gynecological disorders (abortion, anaemia, antifertility, lactation prevention, uterus clean after delivery, postdelivery uterus contraction, separation of umbilical cord, easy delivery, excessive bleeding during pregnancy and menopause, excessive menstrual bleeding, postdelivery bleeding, and regulation of menstrual cycle) (Ajesh and Kumuthakalavalli, 2012). The tribal communities from Malappuram District follow ethnic medicine to cure several ailments: five plants against menstrual problems (*A. indica*, *Curcuma longa*, *P. marsupium*, *Murraya koenigii*, and *A. racemosus*) and 13 plant species to restore postpartum health (*A. racemosus*, *Coix lacryma-jobi*, *C. longa*, *Cycas circinalis*, *C. peltata*, *Dioscorea alata*, *Holostemma ada-kodien, K. galanga, Lagerstroemia speciosa, Mesua ferrea, P. emblica, P. viscida*, and *Thottea siliquosa*) (Chithra et al., 2016). Two angiosperm parasites (*Cassytha filiformis* and *D. falcata*) of the Western Ghats of Kerala are in use against leucorrhoea (Shanavaskhan et al., 2012). A survey in 14 districts showed many plant species helpful against menstrual problems (19 spp. against menorrhagia, 26 spp. against dysmenorrhea, 25 spp. against oligomenorrhea; five spp. against hypomenorrhea; four spp. against amenorrhea) (Rajith et al., 2012). The decoction made from the leaves and stem of *Boerhavia diffusa* and *T. terrestris* are useful for easy delivery, while the juice from bark of *P. emblica* mixed with boiled rice is helpful to cure the wound due to child birth, reported from North Kerala (Jose et al., 2015).

"*Irula*" tribe from the Erode District of Tamil Nadu uses the bark of *Adina cordifolia* against uterus-related problems; combination of leaves + fruits of *E. hirta* and leaves of *Cocculus hirsutus* are used to treat leucorrhoea (Revathi and Parimelazhagan, 2010).

10.7 DISEASES OF INFANTS AND CHILDREN

Infants and children need immediate attention to their health problems. Plant-based medicine is an immediate remedy for many ailments, including abdominal pain, cold, cough, diarrhea, dysentery, fever, gastric troubles, helminthiasis, indigestion, pneumonia, skin infections, tongue-related ailments, measles, and mumps. Up to 29 plant species treat or cure about 14 ailments of infants and children (Table 10.1).

10.7.1 JAMMU AND KASHMIR

The tribal people and traditional healers from Bandipora District utilize many plant species against the ailments of children: *Dryopteris barbigera* and *P. wallichiana* against worms; *S. irio* to cure measles; and *T. linearis* to treat pneumonia (Lone and Bhardwaj, 2013). Another survey in Bandipora District revealed the use of medicinal plants against diseases in children: *Amaranthus retroflexus* to cure measles; *C. officinalis* to treat pneumonia; *Marrubium vulgare* against abdominal pain; and *Oryza sativa* to cure mumps (Lone et al., 2013). The villagers of Udhampur District depend on two ethnomedicinal plants against diseases and maintain the general health of infants as well as children (Bhatia et al., 2014). They are *A. aspera* (against cough) and *A. calamus* (as memory enhancer and for curing speech disorder).

10.7.2 UTTARAKHAND AND NORTHEAST

Traditional healers from the Narendra Nagar Block make use of *G. affine* against infants suffering from diarrhea (Dangwal and Sharma, 2011). The local inhabitants in Rudraprayag District utilize *A. calamus* against gastric troubles in infants (Chandra et al., 2013). The tribal communities from the Uttarakhand Himalayan region use *Rosa* sp. against urine infection in children (Prakash, 2015). *Sida rhombifolia* is active against stomachache in children as reported from Chamoli District (Bisht et al., 2013). The rural women of Garhwal employ *Prunus armeniaca* and *S. rhombifolia* to treat stomachache in children (Uniyal and Shiva, 2005).

The "*Chorei*" tribe from Southern Assam uses *C. viscosum* to cure dysentery in children (Choudhury et al., 2012). Ethnic tribes of Barpeta District utilize *Marsilea minuta* against worms and *S. paniculata* to cure skin and tongue-related ailments in children (Das, 2016). The tribals of Bankura District of West Bengal employ *Clitoria ternatea* as a tonic to improve mental status and *Mimusops elengi* to cure constipation problems (Sinhababu and Banerjee, 2013).

10.7.3 SOUTHERN INDIA

The "*Konda-Dora*" tribe in the Visakhapatnam District of Andhra Pradesh uses *Z. armatum* against dysentery and vomiting (Padal et al., 2013). The villagers from Chityal Nalgonda District of Telangana utilize *Anisomeles malabarica* for invulnerability; *C. grandis* to cure wrinkles in young children; and *Corallocarpus epigaeus* against constipation in young children (Prabhakar et al., 2015). The seed oil of *Ricinus communis* is used as massage oil for children by tribal people in the Mahabubnagar District of Telangana (Singh and Singh, 2015). The villagers in the Nanded District of Maharashtra use *Ruta graveolens* to cure indigestion in infants and *Anisochilus carnosus* and *Chrozophora rottleri* to cure cough in children (Shaikh et al., 2014). The tribal women of Thane District use *G. superba* to cure asthma and *H. isora* against digestive infections in children (Oak et al., 2015). *R. graveolens* is active against helminthic infestation, cold, cough, fever, and stomach pain in children as reported from Gulbarga District of Karnataka (Ghatapanadi et al., 2011). The documentation on medicinal plants from tribal areas of Kodagu District reveals the use of *Bacopa monnieri* against epilepsy and *L. aspera* to treat cough and fever in children (Lingaraju et al., 2013). Medicinal attributes of the indigenous flora of Southwest India have been documented by Pavithra et al. (2021). The "*Mullu Kuruma*" tribe in the Wayanad District of Kerala uses *Elephantopus scaber* to cure amoebic dysentery and stomachache in children (Silja et al., 2008).

The tribe "*Irula*" in the Erode District of Tamil Nadu employs *A. racemosus* to improve immunity and *Ruellia patula* to treat fever in children (Revathi and Parimelazhagan, 2010). The "*Kaani*" tribe of Kanyakumari District employs seeds of *R. communis* to cure skin diseases in children (Johnsy et al., 2012). *Morinda pubescens* is used against dysentery and *Sauropus bacciformis* to treat indigestion in children as documented from Villupuram District (Muralidharan and Narasimhan, 2012). The herbal healers, rural women, and senior citizens from Pudukkottai District opined that 97 plant species are useful to treat common health problems in children (e.g., diarrhea, dysentery, cough, cold, abdominal pain, fever, and skin diseases) (Sambath et al., 2015).

10.8 CONCLUSIONS

India is well known for its richness in diversity of ethnic knowledge. People from different parts of India follow traditional or ethnic knowledge for various purposes (e.g., nutritional, medicinal, and nutraceutical). Several ethnic herbal healers (e.g., "*Pandit*," "*Siddi*," and "*Vaidya*") tribals and rural older generation believe and depend on indigenous knowledge for management of primary nutrition and health care. Most of the native plant species are neglected, and many herbs and shrubs with medicinal values are treated as unwanted weeds. Thus, it is necessary to educate people on the beneficial uses and importance of native plant species in and around. In addition to drawing the attention of publics to the mere nutritional and medicinal uses of indigenous plant sources, the assessment of specific medicinal and nutritional versatilities further reinforces their usefulness by tagging their novel ingredients with geographic indications. Understanding supplementary benefits, especially the nutraceutical potential of indigenous plant species, is immensely valuable in disease resistance in ethnic groups.

According to the 2011 census, the tribal population of the Indian subcontinent is up to 8.6%. Enormous ethnic knowledge has concentrated in these populations especially to meet the primary needs of diet and health. Documentation of ethnic knowledge is of utmost importance to protect our biota, including their geographic indications. To conserve and propagate economically viable wild plant species, exploration and cultivation of region-specific plant species need to be followed more systematically. In most of the literature, methods necessary in the preparation, processing, and preservation of ethnic medicines are lacking. Thus, the scientific basis of such methodology needs to be validated for future economic growth. The scientific personnel need to follow integrated approaches to explore the scientific basis of ethnic knowledge toward remedy against lifestyle diseases like cancers, diabetes, and cardiovascular problems. Nevertheless, the tribal security and betterment of their livelihood should be given prime importance in return for disclosing ethnic knowledge.

KEYWORDS

- **diversity**
- **ethnic medicine**
- **remedial medicine**
- **traditional knowledge**
- **wild plants**

REFERENCES

Agarwal, P.; Gaur, P. K.; Tyagi, N., Puri, D.; Kumar, N.; Kumar, S. An Overview of Phytochemical, Therapeutic, Pharmacological and Traditional Importance of *Syzygium cumini*. *Asian J. Pharmacogn.* **2019,** *3*, 5–17.

Ajesh, T. P.; Kumuthakalavalli, R. Ethnic Herbal Practices for Gynaecological Disorders from Urali Tribes of Idukki District of Kerala, India. *Int. J. Pharm. Life Sci.* **2012,** *3*, 2213–2219.

Akhila, S.; Rajappan, A. V.; Sree, P. K.; Baby, L.; Pillai, P. G. An Ethno-Pharmacological Survey on Medicinal Plants from Idamalayar, Ernakulam (Dist.), Kerala. *World J. Pharm. Pharmaceut. Sci.* **2015,** *4*, 1254–1260.

Alawa, K. S.; Ray, S.; Dubey, A. Folklore Claims of Some Ethnomedicinal Plants Used by Bhil Tribes of Dhar District Madhya Pradesh. *Biosci. Disc.* **2016,** *7*, 60–62.

Anita, D. D.; Sridhar, K. R. Nutraceutical Potential of Ripened Beans of Mangrove Wild Legume *Sesbania speciosa*. In *Biotechnological Utilization of Mangrove Resources*, Patra, J. K., Mishra, R. R., Thatoi, H., Ed., Elsevier Inc., Academic Press, USA, **2020** pp 243–259.

Behera, K. K. Plants Used for Gynaecological Disorders by Tribals of Mayurbhanj District, Orissa, India. *Ethnobot. Leaflets* **2006,** *10*, 129–138.

Bhagya, B.; Ramakrishna, A.; Sridhar, K. R. Traditional Seasonal Health Food Practices in Southwest India: Nutritional and Medicinal Perspectives. *Nitte Uni. J. Health Sci.* **2013,** *3*, 30–34.

Bhagya, B.; Sridhar, K. R. Ethnobiology of Coastal Sand Dune Legumes of Southwest Coast of India. *Ind. J. Trad. Know.* **2009,** *8*, 611–620.

Bhandary, M. J.; Chandrashekar, K. R. Diversity and Use of Ethnomedicinal Plants in Coastal Karnataka, India. *Biodiversitas* **2014,** *15*, 89–93.

Bhatia, H.; Sharma, Y. P.; Manhas, R. K.; Kumar, K. Ethnomedicinal Plants Used by the Villagers of District Udhampur, J & K, India. *J. Ethnopharmacol.* **2014,** *151*, 1005–1018.

Bhatia, H.; Sharma, Y. P.; Manhas, R. K.; Kumar, K. Traditional Phytoremedies for the Treatment of Menstrual Disorders in District Udhampur, J & K, India. *J. Ethnopharmacol.* **2015,** *160*, 202–210.

Bhuyan, S. I.; Baruah, B. N. Medicinal Plants Used for the Treatment of Respiratory Disorders: A Study in Bongaigaon, North Eastern Himalayan Sub-Region of India. *Pharma Innov. J.* **2015,** *4*, 108–110.

Bisht, V. K.; Kandari, L. S.; Negi, J. S.; Bhandari, A. K.; Sundriyal, R. C. Traditional Use of Medicinal Plants in District Chamoli, Uttarakhand, India. *J. Med. Pl. Res.* **2013,** *7*, 918–929.

Chanda, R.; Mohanty, J. P.; Bhuyan, N. R.; Kar, P. K.; Nath, L. K. Medicinal Plants Used Against Gastrointestinal Tract Disorders by the Traditional Healers of Sikkim Himalayas. *Ind. J. Trad. Know.* **2007,** *6*, 606–610.

Chandra, K.; Nautiyal, B. P.; Nautiyal, M. C. Herbal-Based Traditional Medicinal Knowledge of Local Inhabitants in Rudraprayag District of Uttarakhand, India. *Ethnobot. Res. Appl.* **2013,** *11*, 299–313.

Chithra, M.; Kumar, P. K. M.; Geetha, S. P. A Comparative Study on Ethnobotanical Usage of Plants for Twenty Selected Diseases by Six Tribal Communities in Malappuram District. *Int. J. Herb. Med.* **2016,** *4*, 108–113.

Choudhary, M. S.; Mishra, N.; Upadhyay, S. T.; Upadhyay, R. Indigenous Knowledge of Using Medicinal Plants in Treating Skin Diseases by Tribal's in Central Narmada Valley of Madhya Pradesh (India). *Bull. Environ. Pharmacol. Life Sci.* **2011,** *1*, 60–63.

Choudhury, S.; Sharma, P.; Choudhury, M. D.; Sharma, G. D. Ethnomedicinal Plants Used by Chorei Tribes of Southern Assam, North Eastern India. *Asian Pac. J. Trop. Dis.* **2012,** *2*, S141–S147.

Dangwal, L. R.; Sharma, A. Indigenous Traditional Knowledge Recorded on Some Medicinal Plants in Narendra Nagar Block (Tehri Garhwal), Uttarakhand. *Ind. J. Nat. Prod. Resour.* **2011,** *2*, 110–115.

Das, A. K.; Dutta, B. K.; Sharma, G. D. Medicinal Plants Used by Different Tribes of Cachar District, Assam. *Ind. J. Trad. Know.* **2008,** *7*, 446–454.

Das, R. Biodiversity of Ethnomedicinal Plants Used by the Ethnic Tribal People of Barpeta District of Assam, North East India. *Asian J. Pharmaceut. Sci. Technol.* **2016,** *6*, 27–32.

Deepthy, R.; Remashree, A. B. Ethno Botanical Studies on Medicinal Plants Used for Skin Diseases in Malabar Region of Kerala. *Int. J. Herb. Med.* **2014,** *2*, 92–99.

Diaz-de-Cerio, E.; Verardo, V.; Gómez-Carvaca, A.; Fernández-Gutiérrez, A.; Segura-Carretero, A. Health Effects of *Psidium guajava* L. Leaves: An Overview of the Last Decade. *Int. J. Mol. Sci.* **2017,** *18*, 897. 10.3390/ijms18040897

Dinesh, V.; Bembrekar, S. K.; Sharma, P. P. Herbal Formulations Used in Treatment of Kidney Stone by Native Folklore of Nizamabad District, Andhra Pradesh, India. *Biosci. Disc.* **2013,** *4*, 250–253.

Dwivedi, S.; Dwivedi, A.; Dwivedi, S. N. Folk Lore Uses of Some Plants by the Tribes of Madhya Pradesh with Special Reference to Their Conservation. *Ethnobot. Leaflets* **2008,** *12*, 763–771.

Ghatapanadi, S. R.; Johnson, N.; Rajasab, A. H. Documentation of Folk Knowledge on Medicinal Plants of Gulbarga District, Karnataka. *Ind. J. Trad. Know.* **2011,** *10*, 349–353.

Gupta, R.; Vairale, M. G.; Deshmukh, R. R.; Chaudhary, P. R.; Wate, S. R. Ethnomedicinal Uses of Some Plants Used by Gond Tribe of Bandara District, Maharashtra. *Ind. J. Trad. Know.* **2010,** *9*, 713–717.

Hirapara, H.; Ghori, V.; Anovadiya, A.; Baxi, S.; Tripathi, C. Effects of Ethanolic Extract of *Jasminum grandiflorum* Linn. Flowers on Wound Healing in Diabetic *Wistar* Albino Rats. *Avicenna J. Phytomed.* **2017,** *5*, 401–408.

Ignacimuthu, S.; Ayyanar, M.; Sivaraman, S. K. Ethnobotanical Investigations Among Tribes in Madurai District of Tamil Nadu (India). *J. Ethnobiol. Ethnomed.* **2006,** *2*, 25. DOI: 10.1186/1746-4269-2-25

Johnsy, G.; Sargunam, S. D.; Kaviyarasan, V. Indigenous Knowledge of Medicinal Plants Used for the Treatment of Skin Diseases by the Kaani tribe of Kanyakumari District. *Int. J. Pharm. Pharmaceut. Sci.* **2012,** *4*, 309–313.

Jose, T.; Sebastian, A.; Antony, V. T. Ethnobotanical Study of Traditional Medicinal Plants Used by Indigenous People in North Kerala. *Ind. J. Appl. Res.* **2015,** *5*, 184–186.

Jyoti, D. A.; Rajesh, K.; Mohammad, A.; Singh, R. D.; Manoj, K.; Aqueel, K. M.; Jai, P. Ethno Medicinal Study of Threatened Plants of Sonitpur District in Assam, North east India. *Int. Res. J. Pharm.* **2013,** *4*, 146–149.

Kadam, D.; Sharma, A. Indigenous Knowledge of Using Medicinal Plants in Treating Skin Diseases in Panchmarhi Biosphere Reserve, Madhya Pradesh, India. *Int. J. Green Herb. Chem.* **2013,** *2*, 194–198.

Kala, C. P.; Farooquee, N. A.; Majila, B. S. Indigenous Knowledge and Medicinal Plants Used by Vaidyas in Uttaranchal, India. *Nat. Prod. Radiance* **2005,** *4*, 195–206.

Karun, N. C.; Vaast, P.; Kushalappa, C. G. Bioinventory and Documentation of Traditional Ecological Knowledge of Wild Edible Fruits of Kodagu-Western Ghats, India. *J. For. Res.* **2014,** *3*, 717–721.

Kingston, C.; Jeeva, S.; Jeeva, G. M.; Kiruba, S.; Mishra, B. P.; Kannan, D. Indigenous Knowledge of Using Medicinal Plants in Treating Skin Diseases in Kanyakumari District, Southern India. *Ind. J. Trad. Know.* **2009,** *8*, 196–200.

Kumar, A. K. M.; Shivaraju, H. P. A Study on Traditional Knowledge and Medicinal Applications of the Endemic Herbal Species in the Western Ghats of Shimoga Region, Karnataka, India. *Int. J. Res. Chem. Environ.* **2016,** *6*, 1–13.

Kumar, P. G. M.; Siddamallayya, N. Ethnobotanical Study of Less Known Wild Edible Plants of Hakki Pikki Tribes of Angadihalli, Hassan District, Karnataka. *J. Med. Pl. Stud.* **2015,** *3*, 80–85.

Kumar, P. G. M.; Siddamallayya, N. Survey of Wild Medicinal Plants of Hassan District, Karnataka. *J. Med. Pl. Stud.* **2016,** *4*, 91–102.

Kumari, B. S.; Prabhu, Y. T.; Pavani, T. Traditional Knowledge of Medicinal Plants Used to Cure Respiratory Diseases in Krishna District of Andhra Pradesh, India. *J. Med. Pl. Stud.* **2014,** *2*, 34–37.

Lingaraju, D. P.; Sudarshana, M. S.; Rajashekar, N. Ethnopharmacological Survey of Traditional Medicinal Plants in Tribal Areas of Kodagu District, Karnataka, India. *J. Pharm. Res.* **2013,** *6*, 284–297.

Lone, P. A.; Bhardwaj, A. K. Traditional Herbal Based Disease Treatment in Some Rural Areas of Bandipora District of Jammu and Kashmir, India. *Asian J. Pharmaceut. Clin. Res.* **2013,** *6*, 162–171.

Lone, P. A.; Bhardwaj, A. K.; Bahar, F. A. A Study of Some Locally Available Herbal Medicines for the Treatment of Various Ailments in Bandipora District of J & K, India. *Int. J. Pharma Biosci.* **2013,** *4*, 440–453.

Madhu, V.; Yarra, R. Investigations on Ethno-Medicinal Plants Used to Cure Skin Diseases in Adilabad District, Andhra Pradesh, India. *Int. J. Pharma. Life Sci.* **2011,** *2*, 742–745.

Mahishi, P.; Srinivasa, B. H.; Shivanna, M. B. Medicinal Plant Wealth of Local Communities in Some Villages in Shimoga District of Karnataka, India. *J. Ethnopharmacol.* **2005,** *98*, 307–312.

Mikawlrawng, K.; Rani, R.; Kumar, S.; Bhardwaj, A. R.; Prakash, G. Anti-Paralytic Medicinal Plants—Review. *J. Trad. Complem. Med.* **2018,** *8*, 4–10.

Muralidharan, R.; Narasimhan, D. Ethnomedicinal Plants Used Against Gastrointestinal Problems in Gingee Hills of Villupuram District, Tamil Nadu. *J. Appl. Pharmaceut. Sci.* **2012,** *2*, 123–125.

Murthy, S. S. M. Traditional Medicinal Plants Used to Treat Human Ailments in Harapanahalli Taluk of Davangere District, Karnataka. *J. Med. Pl. Stud.* **2015,** *3*, 27–31.

Murthy, S. S. M.; Vidyasagar, G. M. Medicinal Plants Used in the Treatment of Gastrointestinal Disorders in Bellary District, Karnataka, India. *Ind. J. Trad. Know.* **2013a,** *12*, 321–325.

Murthy, S. S. M.; Vidyasagar, G. M. Traditional Knowledge on Medicinal Plants Used in the Treatment of Respiratory Disorders in Bellary District, Karnataka, India. *Ind. J. Nat. Prod. Resour.* **2013b,** *4*, 189–193.

Navya, A. S.; Anitha, A. Antimicrobial Activities of *Careya arborea*: A Review. *J. Pharmacog. Phytochem.* **2018,** *7*, 3155–3157.

Oak, G.; Kurve, P.; Kurve, S.; Pejaver, M. Ethno-Botanical Studies of Edible Plants Used by Tribal Women of Thane District. *J. Med. Pl. Stud.* **2015,** *3*, 90–94.

Ozturk, M.; Altay, V.; Altundağ, E.; Gucel, S. Halophytic Plant Diversity of Unique Habitats in Turkey: Salt Mine Caves of Çankırı and Iğdır. In *Halophytes for Food Security in Dry Lands*; Khan, M. A., Ozturk, M., Gul, B., Ahmed, M. Z., Eds., Chapter 18; Elsevier, 2016. http://dx.doi.org/10.1016/B978-0-12-801854-5.00018-2

Ozturk, M.; Altay, V.; Altundağ, E.; Ibadullayeva, S. J.; Aslanipour, B.; Gönenç, T. M. Herbals in Iğdır (Turkey), Nakhchivan (Azerbaijan), and Tabriz (Iran). In *Plant and Human Health*; Ozturk, M., Hakeem, K. R., Eds., Vol 1; Springer: Cham, Chapter 6, 2018c; pp 197–266.

Ozturk, M.; Altay, V.; Efe, R. *Biodiversity, Conservation and Sustainability in Asia: Volume I: Prospects and Challenges in West Asia and Caucasus*; Springer Nature Switzerland AG, 2021a. DOI: 10.1007/978-3-030-59928-7

Ozturk, M.; Altay, V.; Gonenç, T. M. Herbal from High Mountains in the East Mediterranean. In *Drug Discovery from Herbs-Approaches and Applications*; Bhojraj, S. et al., Eds.; NAM S & T Centre, DAYA Publishing House: New Delhi, India, Chapter 24, 2017b; pp 327–367.

Ozturk, M.; Altay, V.; Gucel, S.; Altundağ, E. Plant Diversity of the Drylands in Southeast Anatolia-Turkey: Role in Human Health and Food Security. In *Plant Biodiversity: Monitoring, Assessment and Conservation*; Ansari, A. A., Gill, S. S., Eds., Chapter 5: CABI UK, 2017c; pp 83–124.

Ozturk, M.; Altay, V.; Gucel, S.; Guvensen, A. Halophytes in the East Mediterranean-Their Medicinal and Other Economical Values. In *Sabkha Ecosystems: Volume IV: Cash Crop Halophyte and Biodiversity Conservation Tasks for Vegetation Science*, Vol. 47; Springer: The Netherlands, 2014; pp 247–272.

Ozturk, M.; Altay, V.; Hakeem, K. R.; Akçiçek, E. *Liquorice from Botany to Phytochemistry*; SpringerBriefs in Plant Science, 2017a. https://doi.org/10.1007/978-3-319-74240-3

Ozturk, M.; Altay, V.; Latiff, A. et al. A Comparative Analysis of the Medicinal Pteridophytes in Turkey, Pakistan, and Malaysia. In *Plant and Human Health*; Ozturk, M., Hakeem, K.

R., Eds., Vol. 1; Springer: Cham, Chapter 9; Springer International Publishing AG, 2018d; pp 349–390.

Ozturk, M.; Altay, V.; Latiff, A. et al. A Comparative Analysis of the Medicinal Plants Used for Diabetes Mellitus in the Traditional Medicine in Turkey, Pakistan, and Malaysia. In *Plant and Human Health*; Ozturk, M., Hakeem, K. R., Eds., Vol. 1; Springer: Cham, Chapter 11; Springer International Publishing AG, 2018e; pp 409–461.

Ozturk, M.; Altay, V.; Latiff, A. et al. Potential Medicinal Plants Used in the Hypertension in Turkey, Pakistan, and Malaysia. In *Plant and Human Health*; Ozturk, M., Hakeem, K. R., Eds., Vol. 1; Springer: Cham, Chapter 16; Springer International Publishing AG, 2018f; pp 595–618.

Ozturk, M.; Altay, V.; Orçen, N. et al. A Little Known and a Little Consumed Natural Resource: *Salicornia*. In *Global Perspectives on Underutilized Crops*; Ozturk, M. et al., Eds., Chapter 3; Springer International Publishing AG, 2018a; pp 83–108.

Ozturk, M.; Altundağ, E.; Ibadullayeva, S. J.; Altay, V.; Aslanıpour, B. A Comparative Analysis of Medicinal and Aromatic Plants Used in the Traditional Medicine of Iğdır (Turkey), Nakhchivan (Azerbaijan), and Tabriz (Iran). *Pak. J. Bot.* **2018b,** *50* (1), 337–343.

Ozturk, M.; Egamberdieva, D.; Milica, P. *Biodiversity and Biomedicine-Our Future*; Academic Press, Elsevier Inc., 2020.

Ozturk, M.; Gökler, I.; Altay, V. Medicinal Bryophytes Distributed in Turkey. In *Plant and Human Health*; Ozturk, M., Hakeem, K. R., Eds., Vol. 1; Springer: Cham, Chapter 8; Springer International Publishing AG, 2018g; pp 323–348.

Ozturk, M.; Khan, S. M.; Altay, V.; Efe, R.; Egamberdieva, D.; Khassanov, F. *Biodiversity, Conservation and Sustainability in Asia: Volume II: Prospects and Challenges in South and Middle Asia*; Springer Nature Switzerland AG, 2021b. DOI: 10.1007/978-3-030-73943-0

Padal, S. B.; Raju, J. B.; Chandrasekhar, P. Traditional Knowledge of Konda Dora tribes, Visakhapatnam District, Andhra Pradesh, India. *IOSR J. Pharm.* **2013,** *3*, 22–28.

Panda, T.; Mishra, N.; Pradhan, B. K. Folk Knowledge on Medicinal Plants Used for the Treatment of Skin Diseases in Bhadrak District of Odisha, India. *Med. Arom. Pl.* **2016,** *5*, 4. DOI: 10.4172/2167-0412.1000262

Pavithra, M.; Sridhar, K. R.; Greeshma, A. A. Bioactive Attributes of Traditional Leafy Vegetable *Talinum triangulare*. In *Handbook of Nutrition in Heart Health*, Watson, R. R., Zibadi. S. Ed., Wageningen Academic Publishers: The Netherlands, 2017; pp 357–372.

Pavithra, M.; Sridhar, K. R.; Keshavachandra, K. Diverse Medicinal Attributes of Indigenous Flora of the Southwest India. In *Biodiversity, Conservation and Sustainability in Asia*, Vol. 2: *South and Middle Asia* (Part III: *Ethnobotany*), Öztürk, M. Khan, S. M., Altay, V., Efe, R., Egamberdieva, D., Ed.; Springer Nature: Switzerland, 2021.

Policepatel, S. S.; Manikrao, V. G. Ethnomedicinal Plants Used in the Treatment of Skin Diseases in Hyderabad Karnataka Region, Karnataka, India. *Asian Pac. J. Trop. Biomed.* **2013,** *3*, 882–886.

Prabhakar, G.; Kamalakar, P.; Shailaja, K. Indigenous Knowledge on Medicinal Plants Prevalent in Cure Chronic Disorders in Chityal Nalgonda District Telangana India. *Int. J. Sci. Res.* **2015,** *4*, 773–777.

Prachi; Chauhan, N.; Kumar, D.; Kasana, M. S. Medicinal Plants of Muzaffarnagar District Used in Treatment of Urinary Tract and Kidney Stones. *Ind. J. Trad. Know.* **2009,** *8*, 191–195.

Prakash, R. Medicinal Plants Used by Tribal Communities: A Study of Uttarakhand Himalayan Region. *Int. J. Human. Soc. Sci. Inven.* **2015,** *4*, 55–61.

Prasad, A. G. D.; Shyma, T. B. Medicinal Plants Used by the Tribes of Vythiri Taluk, Wayanad District (Kerala state) for the Treatment of Human and Domestic Animal Ailments. *J. Med. Pl. Res.* **2013,** *7*, 1439–1451.

Prasad, A. G. D.; Shyma, T. B.; Raghavendra, M. P. Plants Used by the Tribes for the Treatment of Digestive System Disorders in Wayanad District, Kerala. *J. Appl. Pharmaceut. Sci.* **2013,** *3*, 171–175.

Prashanthkumar, P.; Vidyasagar, G. M. Documentation of Traditional Knowledge on Medicinal Plants of Bidar District, Karnataka. *Ind. J. Trad. Know.* **2006,** *5*, 295–299.

Prashantkumar, P.; Vidyasagar, G. M. Traditional Knowledge on Medicinal Plants Used for the Treatment of Skin Diseases in Bidar District, Karnataka. *Ind. J. Trad. Know.* **2008,** *7*, 273–276.

Rajakumar, N.; Shivanna, M. B. Traditional Herbal Medicinal Knowledge in Sagar Taluk of Shimoga District, Karnataka, India. *Ind. J. Nat. Prod. Resour.* **2010,** *1*, 102–108.

Rajith, N. P.; Ambily, D. V.; Dan, V. M.; Devi, P. S.; George, V.; Pushpangadan, P. A Survey on Ethnomedicinal Plants Used for Menstrual Disorders in Kerala. *Ind. J. Trad. Know.* **2012,** *11*, 453–460.

Raju, Y. R.; Yugandhar, P.; Savithramma, N. Documentation of Ethnomedicinal Knowledge of Hilly Tract Areas of East Godavari District of Andhra Pradesh, India. *Int. J. Pharm. Pharmaceut. Sci.* **2014,** *6*, 369–374.

Ramadan, M. F.; Kinni, S. G.; Seshagiri, M.; Mörsel, J. T. Fat-Soluble Bioactives, Fatty Acid Profile and Radical Scavenging Activity of *Semecarpus anacardium* Seed Oil. *J. Am. Oil Chem. Soc.* **2010,** *87*, 885–894.

Ramadan, M. F.; Mohdaly, A. A. A.; Assiri, A. M. A.; Tadros, M.; Niemeyer, B. Functional Characteristics, Nutritive Value and Industrial Applications of *Madhuca longifolia* Seeds: An Overview. *J. Food Sci. Technol.* **2016,** *53*, 2149–2157.

Ramadan, M. F.; Sharanabasappa, G.; Parmjyothi, S.; Seshagiri, M.; Moersel, J. T. Profile and Levels of Fatty Acids and Bioactive Constituents in Mahua Butter from Fruit-Seeds of Buttercup Tree [*Madhuca longifolia* (Koenig)]. *Eur. Food Res. Technol.* **2006,** *222*, 710–718.

Ramashankar, Deb, S.; Sharma, B. K. Traditional Healing Practices in North East India. *Ind. J. Hist. Sci.* **2015,** *50*, 324–332.

Revathi, P.; Parimelazhagan, T. Traditional Knowledge on Medicinal Plants Used by the Irula Tribe of Hasanur Hills, Erode District, Tamil Nadu, India. *Ethnobot. Leaflets* **2010,** *14*, 136–60.

Saheb, S. T.; Rao, B. R. P.; Parveen, N.; Obaidullah, M. Medicinal Plants Used Against Gastrointestinal Disorders by the Tribal People of Nallamallais Andhra Pradesh. *Agrobios Res.* **2012,** *1*, 61–63.

Sajem, A. L.; Gosai, K. Traditional Use of Medicinal Plants by the Jaintia Tribes in North Cachar Hills District of Assam, Northeast India. *J. Ethnobiol. Ethnomed.* **2006,** *2*, 33. DOI: 10.1186/1746-4269-2-33

Sambath, G.; Komalavalli, N.; Ravikumar, R. Traditional Healthcare Practice for Common Ailments of Children in Pudukkottai District, Tamil Nadu—A Survey. *Ind. J. Nat. Sci.* **2015,** *6*, 10475–10483.

Santhosh, N. R.; Kumar, Y. R. G.; Krishnaswamy, K. Ethno Medicinal Plants Used by Traditional Herbal Practitioners of Kadur Taluk of Chikmagalore District of Karnataka, India. *J. Med. Pl. Stud.* **2014,** *2*, 69–72.

Savithramma, N.; Yugandhar, P.; Babu, R. H.; Prasad, K. S. Validation of Indigenous Knowledge of Yanadi Tribe and Local Villagers of Veyilingalakona—A Sacred Grove of Andhra Pradesh, India. *J. Pharmaceut. Sci. Res.* **2014,** *6*, 382–388.

Seriana, I.; Akmal, M.; Darjsman; Wahyuni, S. Neem Leaves Extract (*Azadirachta indica A. Juss*) on Male Reproductive System: A Mini-Review. *Earth Environ. Sci.* **2019,** *399*, 1–7. DOI: 10.1088/1755-1315/399/1/012106

Shaikh, R. U.; Dukare, D. D.; Sarwade, K. P.; Sarwade, P. P. Ethnobotanical Study of Folk Medicinal Plants Used by Villagers in Nanded District of Maharashtra (India). *Int. J. Ayur. Herb. Med.* **2014,** *4*, 1585–1595.

Shanavaskhan, A. E.; Sivadasan, M.; Alfarhan, A. H.; Thomas, J. Ethnomedicinal Aspects of Angiospermic Epiphytes and Parasites of Kerala, India. *Ind. J. Trad. Know.* **2012,** *11*, 250–258.

Shankar, R.; Lavekar, G. S.; Deb, S.; Sharma, B. K. Traditional Healing Practice and Folk Medicines Used by Mishing Community of North East India. *J. Ayur. Integr. Med.* **2012,** *3*, 124–129.

Sharanappa, R.; Vidyasagar, G. M. Documentation of Traditional Knowledge on Medicinal Plants Used in Treating Candidiasis in Hyderabad Karnataka Region, India. *World J. Pharm. Pharmaceut. Sci.* **2014,** *3*, 739–751.

Sharma, J.; Gairola, S.; Sharma, Y. P.; Gaur, R. D. Ethnomedicinal Plants Used to Treat Skin Diseases by Tharu Community of District Udham Singh Nagar, Uttarakhand, India. *J. Ethnopharmacol.* **2014,** *158*, 140–206.

Sharma, J.; Gaur, R. D.; Gairola, S.; Painuli, R. M.; Siddiqi, T. O. Traditional Herbal Medicines Used for the Treatment of Skin Disorders by the Gujjar Tribe of Sub-Himalayan Tract, Uttarakhand. *Ind. J. Trad. Know.* **2013,** *12*, 736–746.

Sharma, M.; Sharma, C. L.; Marak, P. N. Indigenous Uses of Medicinal Plants in North Garo Hills, Meghalaya, NE India. *Res. J. Rec. Sci.* **2014,** *3*, 137–146.

Shreelalitha, S. J.; Sridhar, K. R. Nutraceutical Perspectives of Coastal Sand Dune Wild Legume *Sesbania bispinosa*. In *Bioresource Technology: Solution to Future Sustainability*; Hakeem, K. R., Pirzadah, T. B., Malik, B., Ed.; Springer Nature: Switzerland, 2021.

Shyma, T. B.; Prasad, A. G. D. Traditional Use of Medicinal Plants and Its Status Among the Tribes in Mananthavady of Wayanad District, Kerala. *World Res. J. Med. Arom. Pl.* **2012,** *1*, 22–26.

Silja, V. P.; Varma, K. S.; Mohanan, K. V. Ethnomedicinal Plant Knowledge of the Mullu Kuruma Tribe of Wayanad District, Kerala. *Ind. J. Trad. Know.* **2008,** *7*, 604–612.

Singh, A.; Singh, M. K.; Singh, R. Traditional Medicinal Flora of the District Buxar (Bihar, India). *J. Pharmacog. Phytochem.* **2013,** *2*, 41–49.

Singh, S.; Singh, R. Documentation of Tribal's Traditional Knowledge of Medicinal Plants from Renlagadda Thanda, Kodangal Mandal, Mahabubnagar Dist. Telangana, India. *Int. Lett. Nat. Sci.* **2015,** *35*, 13–24.

Sinhababu, A.; Banerjee, A. Ethno-Botanical Study of Medicinal Plants Used by Tribals of Bankura Districts, West Bengal, India. *J. Med. Pl. Stud.* **2013,** *1*, 98–104.

Sivaranjani, R.; Ramakrishnan, K. Traditional Uses of Medicinal Plants in Treating Skin Diseases in Nagapattinam District of Tamil Nadu, India. *Int. Res. J. Pharm.* **2012,** *3*, 201–204.

Sridhar, K. R.; Bhagya, B. Coastal Sand Dune Vegetation: A Potential Source of Food, Fodder and Pharmaceuticals. *Livest. Res. Rural Develop.* **2007,** *19*, Article # 84: http://www.cipav.org.co/lrrd/lrrd19/6/srid19084.htm

Sridhar, K. R.; Karun, N. C. Plant-Based Ethnic Knowledge on Food and Nutrition in the Western Ghats. In *Ethnobotany of India: Western Ghats and West Coast of Peninsular India*; Pullaiah, T., Krishnamurty, K. V., Bahadur, B., Ed., Vol. 2; Apple Academic Press, Inc.: Canada, 2017; pp 255–276.

Srivastav, S., Singh, P.; Mishra, G.; Jha, K. K.; Khosa, R. L. *Achyranthes aspera*—An Important Medicinal Plant: A Review. *J. Nat. Prod. Pl. Resour.* **2011,** *1*, 1–14.

Sudeesh, S. Ethnomedicinal Plants Used by Malayaraya Tribes of Vannapuram Village in Idukki, Kerala, India. *Ind. J. Sci. Res. Technol.* **2012,** *1*, 7–11.

Taid, T. C.; Rajkhowa, R. C.; Kalita, J. C. A Study on the Medicinal Plants Used by the Local Traditional Healers of Dhemaji District, Assam, India for Curing Reproductive Health Related Disorders. *Adv. Appl. Sci. Res.* **2014,** *5*, 296–301.

Tiwari, A. K. Indigenous Knowledge for Treating Skin Diseases in Some Selected Districts of Chattisgarh (India). *Int. J. Rec. Sci. Res.* **2015,** *6*, 2654–2657.

Uniyal, B.; Shiva, V. Traditional Knowledge on Medicinal Plants Among Rural Women of the Garhwal Himalaya, Uttaranchal. *Ind. J. Trad. Know.* **2005,** *4*, 259–266.

Vidyasagar, G. M.; Siddalinga, S. M. M. Ethnomedicinal Plants Used to Treat Menstrual Disorders by Tribal People in Bellary District of Karnataka, India. *Int. J. Pharm. Life Sci.* **2012,** *3*, 1871–1876.

Xavier, T. F.; Kannan, M.; Auxilia, A. Traditional Medicinal Plants Used in the Treatment of Different Skin Diseases. *Int. J. Curr. Microbiol. Appl. Sci.* **2015,** *4*, 1043–1053.

Yadav, S.; Das, S.; Baruah, N. C.; Dubey, M. Preliminary Evaluation of Some Traditionally Used Medicinal Plants as Antidiarrhoeal in Assam. *Int. J. Herb. Med.* **2014,** *1*, 05–09.

CHAPTER 11

COVID-19 Treatment Strategies and Phytoprophylaxis

TAPTI SENGUPTA, SINCHITA BISWAS, SOUVIK NATH, ARIJIT MONDAL, and TIRTHANKAR SAHA

Department of Microbiology, West Bengal State University, Berunanpukuria, Malikapur, Barasat, West Bengal, India

ABSTRACT

The recently emerged pandemic of novel coronavirus (2019-nCoV) is threatening by causing mass mortalities worldwide. Viral isolates have recently been available and the world is fighting to find a vaccine. International spread through travelers and community spread of the infection poses a challenge. The primary causing factors for this zoonotic disease include anthropogenic stress, food habits, and irresponsible laboratory ethics. The 2019 n-CoV is a positive strand of RNA-based virus belonging to the SARS family causing COVID-19. Furin-like proteases present in the S-protein in CoV binds to the host. Pneumonia and flu-like symptoms are observed in COVID-19 patients. Diagnostic detection of m-RNA by RT-PCR techniques from nasal and oral swabs is recommended. The choice of drugs like hydroxychloroquine along with Remdesivir play a vital role in the treatment of infected population suggests studies. Antimalarial drugs and plasma therapy are also being used to combat the positive cases. Clinical trials of vaccines are now being carried out in several countries and some potential vaccine candidates like Covaxin, Covishield, and ones from Oxford are being administered countrywide.

Ethnic Knowledge and Perspectives of Medicinal Plants, Volume 1: Curative Properties and Treatment Strategies. Munir Ozturk, Kandikere R. Sridhar, Maryam Sarwat, Volkan Altay, & Francisco Martín Huerta-Martínez (Eds.)

Aesthetic medicines and plant-based biomolecules are known to be an effective alternative medication for various cardiovascular, renal, and respiratory diseases. Some herbal concoctions could be used to combat the side effects and associated symptoms in the COVID-19 in patents, if they are used judiciously.

11.1 INTRODUCTION

The world is facing a severe crisis at present which is related to chronic respiratory syndrome caused by a coronavirus strain. There was an increase in number of pneumonia-like cases during the month of December 2019 in the Wuhan province, China. As of 18th May 2020, a total of 82,954 people were affected in China itself. On 11th March 2020, the WHO declared novel coronavirus as a pandemic disease (Aljazeera, 2020). India saw its first case being reported on 30th January 2020. As of 12th July 2020, the Indian Council of Medical Research as well as the Ministry of Health and Family Welfare confirmed 133,086 active cases, 10,587,351 recoveries, migration and 155,484 deaths. Rate of infection is remarkably lower compared to the worst affected countries as per previously released data. Maharashtra has shown a significant number of confirmed cases, highest in India as of 12th February 2021 followed by Kerala and Karnataka (COVID-19 India). It was also reported that domestic ferrets and cats were able to cause infection that could be transferred to people causing symptoms like SARS and food habits of Chinese people might have been the primary cause, indicating COVID-19 to be a zoonotic disease. Conspiracy theories are also circulating relating this strain; some calling it an engineered bio-weapon since it is changing randomly and modifying itself, but concrete proof has not been available till date. The infected animals could also transmit the virus to uninfected animals suggesting horizontal transfer (Lun and Qu, 2004). Chinese Journal of Epidemiology identified about 72,000 suspected and asymptomatic cases to outline a percentile of active symptoms that were seen in healthy individuals and those bearing a similarity to the pre-existing disease. 80.9% contagiousness were mild (e.g., flu-like signs) and could recuperate without any medication, 13.8% were severe, causing pneumonia and breath shortness, 4.7% were serious and included respiratory failure, multiorgan failure, and septic shock. On an average, 2% of the reported cases showed fatality of the virus. Elderly patients having illness similar to the cardiovascular disease, chronic respiratory disease, hypertension, and diabetes are susceptible and at higher risk. The joint Mission of WHO-China published a report on 28th

February in which 55,000 cases were observed to have mild symptoms appearing during the second week of their infection and critical symptoms started appearing by the third and sixth weeks, respectively (Worldometers). At present highest mortalities are observed in USA followed by India and Brazil. Majority of the cases started with travelers flying in from infected regions and the virus spread by community gathering. Reinfection in treated patients was observed, especially in China, causing a concern over the dose efficacy and treatment pattern.

The main aim of this article is to uphold commonly used treatment procedures along with the possibility of curing side effects and other diseases and symptoms that might occur during COVID-19 infection with herbal remedies and phytochemicals. A basic understanding of the viral taxonomy, mechanism of infection, and identification methods are also provided for detailed identification of the causative agent.

11.2 STRUCTURE AND TAXONOMY

Coronaviruses (CoVs) are positive-stranded RNAs (Mr 6×10^6) with nucleoproteins that bear an envelope (Coutard et al., 2020; Tyrrell and Myint, 1996). They belong to the order Nidovirales, subfamily Orthocoronavirinae in the Coronaviridae family. They are classified as four genera such as alpha, beta, gamma, and delta coronaviruses (CoVs) which are further divided into lineages. Common human CoVs are HCoV-OC43 and HCoV-HKU1, belonging to beta CoV of A-lineage. HCoV-229E and HCoV-NL63 belong to alpha CoV. Other human CoVs are SARS-CoV, SARS-CoV-2 and MERS-CoV, which belongs to beta CoVs of the B and C-lineages (Cascella et al., 2020). According to an antiviral research held in China, the coronavirus possesses a furin-like protease pattern of recognition present in the juxtaposition of a maturation site of S-protein. There is a difference in the sequence amino acids of the S-protein of 2019-nCov that was not found in previously isolated coronavirus strains (Coutard et al., 2020). The virus being zoonotic in nature has undergone structural changes making it a dreaded human pathogen.

11.3 INFECTION AND PATHOGENICITY

The receptors identified for the binding of coronavirus are Aminopeptidase-N and a sialic acid-containing binder, which bind to ACE2 receptor. This virus gets entry to the host cells and un-coats the genome and positive-sense genomic RNA is exposed which is then immediately translated into viral replicase complex. This complex with the aid of host proteins (e.g., hnRNPA1) transcribes a set of positive-sense sub-genomic mRNAs (~7). The 3′ ends are common in all mRNAs but 5′ ends are unique and are translated by host ribosome into structural (E, S, M, N) and accessory proteins. The nucleoprotein is coded by the shortest mRNA and the other direct synthesis of the genome. N protein helps in packaging the genome into ribonucleocapsid and the virus particle undergoes maturation in Golgi complex and releases the host via exocytosis or budding. From the study in human volunteers' organ cultures, it was shown that the coronaviruses are fastidious in nature; hence, they grow only in differentiated epithelial cells respiratory system. The infected cells become vacuolated, show damaged cilia, and form syncytia. This damage induces inflammatory response and swelling which in turn obstructs the airways, stimulates sneezing, and raises the mucosal temperature leading to shortness of breath (Tyrrell and Myint, 1996; Zhong et al., 2012).

11.4 MOLECULAR IDENTIFICATION

Clinical samples need to be isolated and RNA extracted with a reliable kit like MagNA Pure 96 system (Roche, Penzberg, Germany). By the supernatant of cell culture, viral RNA can be extracted by mini kit (QIAGEN, Hilden, Germany). A 25 μL reaction mixture is to be prepared possessing 5 μL RNA, 12.5 μL 2 × reaction buffer provided with the Superscript-III by one step RT-PCR along with Platinum Taq polymerase, 0.4 μL of 50 mM magnesium sulfate solution, 1 μL reverse transcriptase/Taq mixture, and one μg bovine serum albumin (nonacetylated). The primer and probe sequences need to be added at an optimized concentration. This is to be followed by thermal cycling (55°C, 10 min) for reverse transcription, and then shifted to 95°C (3 min). Further, 45 cycles are to be performed at 95°C (15s) and 58°C (30 s). The results have to be compared with partial (>400 nt) and complete SARS-related virus genome sequence available in GenBank and aligned for confirmation (Corman et al., 2020). SHERLOCK COVID-19 test based on CRISPR technology (High Sensitivity Enzymatic Reporter UnLOCKing) is another way for diagnosis although the protocol has not been standardized for clinical samples (Kellner et al., 2019).

11.5 IMMUNOLOGICAL ASSAY

Serological testing like analysis of plasma and serum in blood has been expanded to testing the presence of antibodies immunoglobulin G (IgG) and immunoglobulin M (IgM) in sputum, saliva, and other biological fluids. These antibodies are not exclusively specific for the nucleocapsid protein and spike glycoprotein. A few days after the infection IgM becomes detectable in the serum followed by IgG, which can be detectable in the next couple of weeks. Detection of IgM suggests early stage of infection and IgG suggests presence of postinfection immunity. Several methods are available for testing including Enzyme-Linked Immunosorbent Assay (ELISA), neutralization bioassay, specific chemo sensors, and immune chromatographic lateral flow assay from which only ELISA-based assay is described in short.

It is a microtiter-well, plate-based ELISA technique is employed for detecting as well as for quantifying (proteins, peptides, antibodies, and hormones). It takes about 1–5 h for the results. In the case of SARS-CoV-2, a viral protein is coated in the plate well. Patient sample will bind specifically if antiviral antibody is present, followed by detection with tracer antibody to produce fluorescent-based or colorimetric exposition (Carter et al., 2020).

11.6 TREATMENT PROTOCOLS

Several drugs have been identified based on individual symptoms which might throw a light toward standardized treatment protocols. Commonly used procedure includes the use of Vero cell lines and rabbit sera. As per a recent article published in Cell Research, a study was conducted to analyze antiviral efficacy of 5 FAD-approved drugs (chloroquine, Nafamostat, Nitazoxanide, Penciclovir, and Ribavirin) and two broad-spectrum antiviral drugs (Remdesivir-GS-5734 and Favipiravir -T-705) against the clinical isolate 2019-nCoV in vitro in Vero E6 cells (ATCC-1586) (cytotoxicity was detected by CCK8 assay). The drugs chloroquine and Remdesivir were known to effectively inhibit viral infection in low concentrations. Viral load in cells was measured by qRT-PCR and viral nucleoprotein expression analysis is done by the Western Blot method (Wang et al., 2020).

11.6.1 REMDESIVIR

The broad-spectrum drug Remdesivir (GS-5734) is designed for the treatment of *Ebola* virus. It is a nucleoside analogue and one of the oldest classes of antiviral drug present. It blocks the RNA polymerase that coronaviruses need to replicate their genomes and multiply in the host body. As per the latest reports, it is also found to be active against the COVID-19 infection. This drug was successfully used to block the replication machinery of SARS and MERS coronavirus. The drug is also found to work against COVID-19 infection in isolated cells (Goodwin, 2020; National Institute of Health, 2020a; Olena, 2020).

11.6.2 LOPINAVIR/RITONAVIR

They are used for the treatment of HIV infection. This combination of drugs is also known as Kaletra. Lopinavir and ritonavir (LPV/R) are protease inhibitors. According to an article published in New England Journal, a trial of LPV/r was conducted among 199 COVID-19-positive cases and it was not found to be much effective against this infection. On the contrary, in South Korea, a 54-year-old female COVID-19-positive patient was effectively treated (Cao et al., 2020; Goodwin, 2020).

11.6.3 CHLOROQUINE

Chloroquine is a drug used to treat malaria-infected patients. It is also used in cases of autoimmune disorders. Various studies show this drug to be effective against Human-CoV. Chloroquine obstructs the virus replication ability. This drug enters the endosomes within our cell membrane. The endosomes are mildly acidic in nature; however, the drug's chemical structure increases the pH of the endosome compartments. Several viruses including SARS-CoV also cause acidification of endosomes to gain entry inside the cell membrane, let off their DNA or RNA, and start the replication process but the chloroquine interrupts this dangerous phase. This drug also stops the virus from attaching itself to the receptor known as angiotensin-converting enzyme 2 (ACE2) on some mammalian cells. On attachment of virus spike protein into the ACE2 receptor, a chemical reaction is triggered which interferes with the conformation of the receptor by allowing the virus to infect. The acceptable dosage of chloroquine seems to interfere with this process and also viral replication in general. It is assumed that whatever is applicable for SAR-CoV-1 might also be applicable to SARS-CoV-2. According to recent article published in Nature, a combined drug treatment comprising of Remdesivir and chloroquine was found to successfully inhibit the SARS-CoV2 from infecting in-vitro (A less toxic version of chloroquine and hydroxychloroquine can also be used) (Wang et al., 2020).

11.6.4 COMBINED TREATMENT

This combined drug treatment has also shown significant results in COVID-19-positive patients. As per a study published in *International Journal of Antimicrobial Agents*, it was found that the impact of hydroxychloroquine treatment along as well as in combination of hydroxychloroquine with azithromycin, the percentage of patients gave negative PCR results in the samples of nasopharynx varied among the groups (Table 11.1). On day 6 of post inclusion, 100% patients treated by hydroxychloroquine along with azithromycin combinations virologically cured than 57.1% of patients treated only with hydroxychloroquine, while only 12.5% in the control group (Figure 11.1) (Gautret et al., 2020).

11.6.5 APN01

The APN01 is a recombinant human Angiotensin Converting Enzyme 2 (rhACE2) to medicate the acute lung injury (ALI), the acute respiratory distress syndrome (ARDS), and the pulmonary arterial hypertension (PAH) developed by APEIRON. The ACE2 receptor expresses itself in epithelia of human airway and parenchyma of lungs, which was initially recognized as the gateway that the SARS virus to infect the cells. The ACE2 receptor is utilized by the new virus (e.g., 2019-nCoV) to go into the human cells. Hence, treatment with recombinant ACE2 can be employed not only to check the virus but also to protect the lung injury (PipelineReview, 2020).

11.6.6 FAVILAVIR

This drug was designed for the treatment of inflammation in the nose and throat. It has been approved in China to treat COVID-19 infection and is found to have been very effective in a clinical trial. It is a very potent

TABLE 11.1 Treatment Using Drug Regimens and Efficacy of Cure in Patients. The Proportion of Patients Virologically Cured (Negative Nasopharynx PCR) by Day, in COVID-19 Patients Treated with Hydroxyl Chloroquine Only, in COVID-19 Patients Treated in Combination of Hydroxyl Chloroquine Along with Azithromycin, and in Control COVID-19 Patients.

	Day 3 post inclusion			**Day 4 post inclusion**			**Day 5 post inclusion**			**Day 6 post inclusion**		
	A*	**B***	**C***	**A***	**B***	**C***	**A***	**B***	**C***	**A***	**B***	**C***
Control	1/16	6.3	0.002	4/16	25.0	0.05	3/16	18.8	0.002	2/16	12.5	<0.001
Only hydroxychloroquine treatment	5/14	35.7		7/14	50.0		7/14	50.0		8/14	57.1	
Combined treatment by hydroxychloroquine and azithromycin	5/6	83.3		5/6	83.3		6/6	100		6/6	100	

Source: Gautret et al. (2020).

A, number of negative results patients/total number of patients treated.*

B, % patients recovered, C*, p-value.*

drug used against RNA-based viral infections since it is known to inhibit the RNA-dependent RNA polymerase (RdRp). It has also been found to be advantageous in the treatment of influenza in Japan as well as China. The drug is not currently approved by FDA. This drug was produced on a mass scale in China to treat COVID-19 patients (The Science Times, 2020).

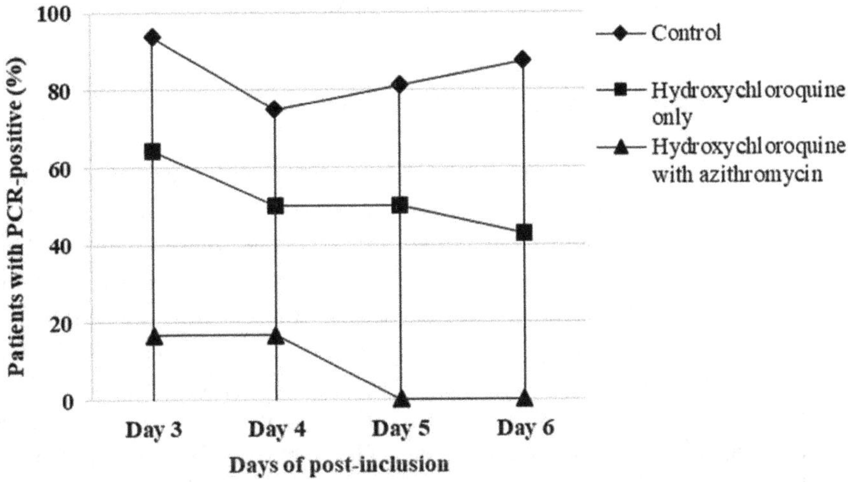

FIGURE 11.1 Percent patients with PCR-positive nasopharynx samples with 6-day trial including hydroxychloroquine and combination of hydroxychloroquine and azithromycin combination, respectively (Gautret et al., 2020).

11.6.7 FAVIPIRAVIR

The broad-spectrum antiviral drug differentially inhibits the RNA-dependent RNA polymerase, which is generally known to be effective against influenza viruses and also effective against viruses which are resistant to other antiviral drugs (Furuta et al., 2017). The Favipiravir is also used to treat COVID-19 patients.

11.6.8 mRNA-1273 TREATMENT

This experimental vaccine was developed by the National Institute of Allergy and Infectious Disease in collaboration with Moderna Inc., Cambridge (NIAID). This vaccine was developed utilizing the genetic platform of mRNA. It instructs the body's cells to express the viral protein which evokes a vigorous immune response. The vaccine mRNA-1273 showed a promising effect in animal models. The VRC as well as Moderna scientists are working on an experimental MERS vaccine targeting the spike protein. Once the genetic sequence of SAR–CoV2 was available, sequence was targeted to express stabilized spike protein of viruses in the already existing mRNA platform (National Institute of Health, 2020b).

11.6.9 CONVALESCENT BLOOD PLASMA TREATMENT

This can be a potential therapy for COVID-19 infection. Many studies have shown a shorter hospital stay as well as lower rate of mortality in patients treated with convalescent plasma compared to the untreated patients. This method of treatment has the approval of W.H.O since 2014, during the *Ebola* outbreak. The process is to basically acquire antiviral antibodies from previously infected patients who are now cured. These antibodies usually stay for months in the blood stream of patients. Researchers believe that incorporating these antibodies could possibly boost the immune response of the patient against the virus. This method of treatment also has its risks. There is danger of transfusing a patient with the wrong type of blood or accidently pushing other pathogens in the process of transfusion, but safety advancements in medical science have made these negative features rare. Japanese drug maker Takeda Pharmaceutical Co. claims that they are developing a new drug from the blood plasma of people who have already recovered from the infection (Chen et al., 2020; Hixenbaugh, 2020; Krishna, 2020).

Other than these medicines, many pharmaceutical companies and research groups are envisaged to develop vaccination methods to fight COVID-19. Recently, ChAdOx1 nCoV-19 vaccine developed by University of Oxford is under Human clinical trials. The vaccine is based on nonreplicating Chimpanzee adenovirus vector, ChAdOx1, modified to encode the SARS-CoV-2 spike protein. Entos Pharmaceuticals is also working to produce a vaccine for COVID-19 infection based on the Fusogenix drug delivery system, which is a Proteo-lipid vehicle programme to introduce genetic payload consisting several protein epitopes (from SARS-CoV-2) directly to the cells which will prompt the immune response to avoid the infection of COVID-19 in the body (Duddu, 2020). Covaxin is an indigenously formulated COVID-19 vaccine developed by India-based

Biotechnology Company called the Bharat Biotech with a partnership of the Indian Council of Medical Research (ICMR) and the National Institute of Virology (NIV). This vaccine utilizes an inactivated virus. The vaccine recently got its approval for the human trails (Raghavan, 2020). Along with traditional medicines researches are also trying to use Ayurvedic treatment methods to fight COVID-19 though strong evidences on the effectiveness of Ayurvedic treatment are yet to be established.

11.7 POTENTIAL HERBAL CONCOCTIONS

Various studies showed that plant-based phytochemicals can be an excellent alternative for several pulmonary and respiratory diseases. Owing to the well-known health-benefitting bioactive ingredients, the patients well received the plant-based medicines and they often preferred plant-based medications over chemically produced therapeutics. Many phytochemicals are currently in use for therapeutic as well as prophylactic treatment against cancer and inflammatory disorders because of their antimicrobial, antiviral, and anticancer attributes. The pharmaceutical industries are identifying and exploiting plant-based compounds from the rainforests and Himalayas are increasing swiftly in tropical and subtropical countries (Rezk et al., 2015; Masoodi et al., 2020; Ozturk et al., 2021a, b).

According to the study of Sengupta et al. (2020) the phytochemical analysis of the leaves of Rose tree (*Rhododendron* spp.), Vasaka (*Justicia Adhatoda*), Holy basil (*Ocimum tenuiflorum*), Kalmegh (*Andrographis paniculata*), Thankuni (*Centella asiatica*), and Lata (*Mikania micrantha*) possesses many bioactive compounds as well as antioxidants (Table 11.2). *Rhododendron* leaves and twigs possess the phenolic acids, those are known to possess anti-inflammatory, anti-HIV, and anti-nociceptive potential. In addition, the leaves and flowers *Rhododendron* are used to treat headache, diabetes, and rheumatism. The aqueous extracts of leaves of *M. micrantha* showed high zone of Inhibition (up to 24±0.7 mm) against pathogenic *Salmonella* spp. The extracts of *A. paniculata* also proved to contain high amounts of saponin as well as flavonoids. High amount of saponin and terpenoids were also found in the leaves of *O. tenuiflorum*, *C. asiatica*, and *M. micrantha*. The aqueous as well as ethanolic extracts of these plants also showed antimicrobial potential. Thus, extracts of these leaves could be used as prophylaxis as well as treatment toward respiratory tract infections and related problems (Sengupta et al., 2020).

TABLE 11.2 The Leaf Extract Phytochemical Analysis of *Andrographis paniculata*, *Centella asiatica*, *Mikania micrantha*, *Ocimum tenuiflorum* and *Rhododendron* spp.

Sample	Test for phytochemicals	Type of extracts			
		Ethanol	Methanol	Aqueous	Benzene
Andrographis paniculata	Saponins	+	+	+	N/A
	Flavonoids	–	+	+	N/A
	Steroids	+	+	+	N/A
	Terpenoids	+	+	+	N/A
Centella asiatica	Saponins	-	+	+	N/A
	Flavonoids	-	+	+	N/A
	Steroids	+	+	-	N/A
	Terpenoids	+	+	-	N/A
Mikania micrantha	Saponins	+	+	+	N/A
	Flavonoids	–	+	+	N/A
	Steroids	+	+	+	N/A
	Terpenoids	+	+	+	N/A
Ocimum tenuiflorum	Saponins	–	+	+	N/A
	Flavonoids	–	+	+	N/A
	Steroids	+	–	–	N/A
	Terpenoids	+	-	+	N/A
Rhododendron sp.	Saponins	+	+	+	–
	Flavonoids	+	+	+	–
	Steroids	+	+	+	+
	Terpenoids	+	+	+	+

Source: Adapted from Sengupta et al. (2020).
N/A: not available.

11.8 POSSIBLE PLANT-BASED ANTIASTHMATIC REMEDIES

COVID-19 is known to cause adverse effects in patients with underlying medical conditions like Asthma and also show symptoms like cough and fever which can be treated using herbal medicines. Current treatment regimens lack satisfactory success and are known to cause adverse effects. Alternative plant-based formulations can be an effective way in dealing with the problem (Taur and Patil, 2011). Some common Indian plants used for symptomatic treatment of asthma are as under.

11.8.1 AERVA LANATA

In a study conducted by Kumar et al. (2009), ethanol extract obtained from the aerial parts of *Aerva lanata* showed anti-asthmatic effects at 30 mg/kg and 60 mg/kg oral dosage in clonidine-induced catalepsy in the isolated goat tracheal chain preparation model as well as the mast cell degranulation in mice.

11.8.2 EUPHORBIA HIRTA

Euphorbia hirta is also known as asthma weed. In a study conducted by Youssouf et al. (2007), ethanolic extracts of aerial part at 100–1000 mg/kg have shown antihistaminic as well as antiallergic activity via the inhibition of the passive cutaneous anaphylaxis as well as paw anaphylaxis reaction. It also protects the mast cell from degranulation too.

11.8.3 FICUS BENGHALENSIS

Taur and Patil (2011) conducted a study using bark extracts (aqueous, ethanol, and ethyl acetate) including isolated fractions from the aqueous extract of *Ficus benghalensis* showing antihistamine activity via inhibition of clonidine-induced catalepsy in mice (dose, 50 mg/kg).

11.9 VACCINATION FOR COVID-19

Several case studies were carried out to determine the efficacy of the current vaccines.

11.9.1 CHADOX1 NCOV-19

It is also known as AstraZeneca/Oxford Vaccine. The findings of 4 randomized trial conducted in the Brazil, South Africa, and United Kingdom (during April 23 to Nov 4, 2020), participants enrolled were 23,848, while 11,636 participants (7548 in UK and 4088 in Brazil) were inducted in the analysis of interim primary efficacy. In those who received 2 vaccine doses, the efficacy was 62.1%, while in those participants who received a low dose followed by a standard dose, the efficacy was 90%. As a whole, the vaccine efficacy among both groups was found to be 70·4% (95·8% CI 54·8–80·6; 30 [0·5%] of 5807 vs. 101 [1·7%] of 5829) (Voysey et al., 2020).

11.9.2 BNT162B2 MRNA COVID-19 VACCINE

It is also known as Pfizer-BioNTech Vaccine. In a randomized study conducted in a group of 43,548 participants, 43,448 obtained injections (21,720 with BNT162b2 and up to 21,728 with placebo). The BNT162b2 mRNA vaccine was found to be 95% effective in preventing COVID-19 infection (Polack et al., 2020).

11.10 COMBATING IMMUNODEFICIENCIES

Improving diet is the first choice for immunity boosting. Consuming low-carbohydrate and protein-rich diet helps in improving the immunity. Some natural most used ingredients in Indian foods which have shown to boost immunity are Ginger and Turmeric. Vegetables and fruits rich in Beta carotene, ascorbic acid, and other vitamins are good for immunity (Narayana Health, 2020). Beta-carotene or carotenoids have pro-vitamin A activity that stimulated the production of various cytokines, enhanced the lymphocyte blastogenesis, increased the population of lymphocyte subsets, and also increased the lymphocyte cytotoxic activity (Chew, 1993). The vitamin C is a common constituent in pepper, cauliflower and tomato has pleiotropic functions to contribute electrons. It also acts as antioxidant as well as a cofactor of many gene regulatory enzymes. The vitamin C promotes oxidant-scavenging activity in the skin owing to accumulation in phagocytic cells (e.g., neutrophils) and helps in the production of reactive oxygen species (ROS), which kills the microbes. Vitamin C is also shown to promote the proliferation of B-cells as well as T-cells due to its gene regulatory activity (Carr and Maggini, 2017). It is also recommended by Narayana Health (2020) to consume foodstuffs rich in ω-3 fatty acids. The ω-3 fatty acids have been shown to regulate the proliferation of immune cells and regulate the production of cytokines. It gets incorporated into the phospholipids of neutrophils and then gets metabolized to prostaglandins, leukotrienes, and protectins, which modulate the function of neutrophils, phagocytic capacity, as well as production of ROS and cytokines (Gutiérrez et al., 2019).

A good sleep will give good brain function and proper body function. Lack of sleep prevents the body from resting and impairs body function that will ultimately impact immune system. Staying hydrated throughout the day will wash out toxins from the body. Also exercising daily, even light exercise is also effective, distressing the mind by practicing Yoga and Meditation are also needed to boost the immunity (Narayana Health, 2020).

Ministry of Ayush (2020), Government of India, also suggested some measures to boost the immunity by having spices: Turmeric, Cumin, Coriander, and Garlic in foodstuffs. Turmeric in milk ("Golden Milk") is another recommendation to boost the immunity (Ministry of Ayush, 2020).

11.11 CONCLUSIONS AND OUTLOOK

The world is facing a severe threat today with the death toll rising and numerous people getting infected, some being asymptomatic. The healthcare system around the world is struggling to cope up with this sudden outbreak of infection. In majority of the countries, the situation started with an immigrant from an infected country, which was followed by community spread, where there was a gathering or exchange of items. Frontline healthcare professionals and researchers worldwide are working throughout to combat the increasing mortalities and hospitalized cases. It was reported that the food habits like eating of bats were initially the trigger, since it was never till date a deadly human pathogen. The coronavirus family was first reported in 1958 but till December 2019, it has not caused vital respiratory tract infection in humans. Proper personal hygiene and sanitation play a major role in controlling this pandemic along with social distancing. Lockdown is being maintained in majority of the countries to combat viral infections. The infection is found to be at its peak in the third and fourth week post-introduction. It is very important to maintain proper health, sanitation and improve the immunity. Most of the infected people are in the age groups of 60 and above with intermittent infection in younger people, who were in direct contact. Lowering the temperature increases the pathogenicity is yet to be proved. A detailed study on the mode of infection, pattern, and prognosis is required. A cocktail of drugs used for HIV and malaria are being found to be most effective. Several newly found vaccines are under trial in various countries in a run to save the world from this disaster. Several vaccine candidates are being administrated to people in some countries. But, the availability of vaccines to a larger section of people will still take some time and demand prompt action. Underlying medical conditions like asthma, renal disorders, allergies, and rhinitis worsen the effects of COVID-19 infection in patients. Plant-based medicines can be used as a symptomatic remedy in patients affected by COVID-19 to minimize the suffering as well as morbidity. Risk of associated side effects of traditional medicines, antibiotics, and steroids can also be minimized by using phytoconstituents. Pharmaceutical companies are coming up with a promise for mass production of drugs using potential bioactive compounds. A positive side of the pandemic is that the environment is now booming with life and revitalized. Ozone holes have vanished, water is cleaner along with air. Pollution levels have dropped down due to lesser anthropogenic activities due to nationwide lockdown. The world is now breathing and recovering from the negative impacts of human civilization. Mortality rates have reached a plateau in a few countries, but the peak is decreasing with fewer cases of reinfection. Boosting immunity seems to be the need of the hour till the vaccines switch to their functions. Herd immunity if developed can also be a saviour in third world countries.

ACKNOWLEDGMENT

We thank our Honourable Vice Chancellor of West Bengal State University and DSTBT Government of West Bengal for logistic support.

KEYWORDS

- **2019-nCoV**
- **ChAdOx1**
- **hydroxychloroquine**
- **pandemic**
- **phytochemicals**

REFERENCES

Aljazeera. Coronavirus: All You Need to Know About Symptoms and Risks, 2020. https://www.aljazeera.com/news/2020/01/coronavirus-symptoms-vaccines-risks-200122194509687.html (accessed on Feb 11, 2021).

Cao, B.; Wang, Y.; Wen, D.; Liu, W.; Wang, J. et al. Trial of Lopinavir-Ritonavir in Adults Hospitalized with Severe COVID-19. *New Engl. J. Med.* **2020,** *382* (19), 1787–1799.

Carr, A. C.; Maggini, S. Vitamin C and Immune Function. *Nutrients* **2017,** *9* (11), 1211.

Carter, L. J.; Garner, L. V.; Smoot, J. W.; Li, Y.; Zhou, Q. et al. Assay Techniques and Test Development for COVID-19 Diagnosis. *ACS Cent. Sci.* **2020,** *6* (5), 591–605.

Cascella, M.; Rajnik, M.; Cuomo, A.; Dulebohn, S. C.; Di Napoli, R. Features, Evaluation and Treatment Coronavirus (COVID-19). In *StatPearls* **2020**.

Chen, L.; Xiong, J.; Bao, L.; Shi, Y. Convalescent Plasma as a Potential Therapy for COVID-19. *Lancet. Infect. Dis.* **2020,** *20,* 398–400.

Chew, B. P. Role of Carotenoids in the Immune Response. *J. Dairy. Sci.* **1993,** *76,* 2804–2811.

Corman, V. M.; Landt, O.; Kaiser, M.; Molenkamp, R.; Meijer, A. et al. Detection of 2019 Novel Coronavirus (2019-nCoV) by Real-Time RT-PCR. *Euro. Surveill.* **2020,** *25* (3), 2000045.

Coutard, B.; Valle, C.; de Lamballerie, X.; Canard, B.; Seidah, N. G.; Decroly, E. The Spike Glycoprotein of the New Coronavirus 2019-nCoV Contains a Furin-Like Cleavage Site Absent in CoV of the Same Clade. *Antiviral Res.* **2020,** *176*, 104742.

Covid19India. Coronavirus Outbreak in India. https://www.covid19india.org/ (accessed on Feb 11, 2021).

Duddu, P. Coronavirus treatment: Vaccines/Drugs in the Pipeline for COVID19, 2020. https://www.clinicaltrialsarena.com/analysis/coronavirus-mers-cov-drugs/(accessed on Feb 11, 2021).

Furuta, Y.; Komeno, T.; Nakamura, T. Favipiravir (T-705), A Broad Spectrum Inhibitor of Viral RNA Polymerase. *Proc. Jpn. Acad. Ser. B. Phys. Biol. Sci.* **2017,** *93* (7), 449–463.

Gautret, P.; Lagier, J C.; Parola, P.; Hoang, V. T.; Meddeb, L. et al. Hydroxychloroquine and Azithromycin as a Treatment of COVID-19: Results of an Open-Label Non-Randomized Clinical Trial. *Int. J. Antimicrob.* **2020,** 105949.

Goodwin, M. Treatment for Coronavirus Disease (COVID-19), 2020. https://www.healthline.com/health/coronavirus-treatment (accessed on February 11, 2021).

Gutiérrez, S.; Svahn, S. L.; Johansson, M. E. Effects of Omega-3 Fatty Acids on Immune Cells. *Int. J. Mol. Sci.* **2019,** *20* (20), 5028.

Hixenbaugh, M. FDA Is Working on a Treatment for Coronavirus with Blood from Recovered Patients, 2020. https://www.nbcnews.com/health/health-news/fda-working-treatment-coronavirus-blood-recovered-patients-n1165231 (accessed on Feb 11, 2021).

Kellner, M. J.; Koob, J. G.; Gootenberg, J. S.; Abudayyeh, O. O.; Zhang, F. Sherlock: Nucleic Acid Detection with CRISPR Nucleases. *Nat. Protoc.* **2019,** *14*, 2986–3012.

Krishna, A. S. Is There a Cure for Coronavirus? 2020. https://gulfnews.com/world/is-there-a-cure-for-coronavirus-1.1584539901471 (accessed on Feb 11, 2021).

Kumar, D.; Prasad, D. N.; Parkash, J.; Bhatnagar, S. P.; Kumar, D. Antiasthmatic Activity of Ethanolic Extract of *Aerva lanata* Linn. *Pharmacologyonline* **2009,** *2*, 1075–1081.

Lun, Z. R.; Qu, L. H. Animal to Human SARS-Associated Coronavirus Transmission. *Emerg. Infect. Disease.* **2004,** *10* (5), 959.

Masoodi, K. Z.; Amin, I.; Mansoor, S. et al. Botanicals from the Himalayas with Anticancer Potential—An Emphasis on Kashmir Himalayas. In: *Biodiversity and Biomedicine—Our Future*; Ozturk, M., Egamberdieva, D., Pešić, M., Eds., Chapter 11; Academic Press, 2020; pp 189–234.

Ministry of Ayush. Ayurveda's Immunity Boosting Measures for Self Care During COVID-19 Crisis, 2020. https://www.mohfw.gov.in/pdf/ImmunityBoostingAYUSHAdvisory.pdf (accessed on Feb 11, 2021).

Narayana Health. Boosting your Immune System Against Coronavirus: How to Minimize the Risk of Infection? 2020. https://www.narayanahealth.org/ (accessed on Feb 11, 2021).

National Institute of Health. NIH Clinical Trial of Remdesivir to Treat COVID-19 Begins, 2020a. https://www.nih.gov/news-events/news-releases/nih-clinical-trial-remdesivir-treat-COVID-19-begins (accessed on Feb 11, 2021).

National Institutes of Health. *NIH Clinical Trial of Investigation Vaccine for COVID-19 Begins*, 2020b. https://www.nih.gov/news-events/news-releases/nih-clinical-trial-investigational-vaccine-COVID-19-begins

Olena, A. Remdesivir Works Against Coronaviruses in the Lab, 2020. https://www.the-scientist.com/news-opinion/remdesivir-works-great-against-coronaviruses-in-the-lab- 67298 (accessed on Feb 11, 2021).

Ozturk, M.; Altay, V.; Efe, R. *Biodiversity, Conservation and Sustainability in Asia: Volume I: Prospects and Challenges in West Asia and Caucasus*; Springer Nature Switzerland AG, **2021a**. DOI: 10.1007/978-3-030-59928-7

Ozturk, M.; Khan, S. M.; Altay, V.; Efe, R.; Egamberdieva, D.; Khassanov, F. *Biodiversity, Conservation and Sustainability in Asia: Volume II: Prospects and Challenges in South and Middle Asia*; Springer Nature Switzerland AG, 2021b. DOI: 10.1007/978-3-030-73943-0

PipelineReview. APEIRON's Respiratory Drug Product to Start Pilot Clinical Trial to Treat Coronavirus Disease COVID-19 in China, 2020. https://pipelinereview.com/index.php/2020022673884/Proteins-and-Peptides/APEIRONs-respiratory-drug-product-to-start-pilot-clinical-trial-to-treat-coronavirus-disease-COVID-19-in-China.html (accessed on Feb 11, 2021).

Polack, F. P.; Thomas, S. J.; Kitchin, N.; Absalon, J.; Gurtman, A. et al. Safety and Efficacy of the BNT162b2 mRNA COVID-19 Vaccine. *N Engl J Med.* **2020,** *383* (27), 2603–2615.

Raghavan, P. Explained: What Is Covaxin, India's COVID-19 Vaccine Candidate; How Long Before Approval? 2020. https://indianexpress.com/article/explained/explained-what-is-covaxin-indias-COVID-19-vaccine-candidate-how-long-before-approval-6483553/ (accessed on Feb 11, 2021).

Rezk, A.; Al-Hashimi, A.; John, W.; Schepker, H.; Ullrich, MS.; Brix, K. Assessment of Cytotoxicity Exerted by Leaf Extracts from Plants of the Genus Rhododendron Towards Epidermal Keratinocytes and Intestine Epithelial Cells. *BMC. Compl. Alternative. Med.* **2015,** *15* (1), 364.

Sengupta, T.; Biswas, S.; Nath, S.; Mukherjee, I.; Das, P. Bioceutical and Antimicrobial Efficacy of Some Medicinal Plants of India. In *Natural Resources and their Ecosystem Services*, Mitra, A., Ed.; HSRA Publications: Bangalore, India, 2020; pp 126−139.

Taur, D. J.; Patil, R. Y. Some Medicinal Plants with Antiasthmatic Potential: A Current Status. *Asian. Pac. J Trop. Biomed.* **2011,** *1* (5), 413–418.

The Science Times. 'Favilavir': First Approved Drug to Possibly Treat Coronavirus, 2020. https://www.sciencetimes.com/articles/25053/20200317/favilavir-first-approve-drug-treat-coronavirus.htm (accessed on Feb 11, 2021).

Tyrrell, D. A. J.; Myint, S. H. Coronaviruses. In *Medical Microbiology*; Baron, S., Ed., 4th ed.; The University of Texas Medical Branch at Galveston, 1996. https://www.ncbi.nlm.nih.gov/books/NBK7782/

Voysey, M.; Clemens, S.; Madhi, S. A.; Weckx, L. Y.; Folegatti, P. M. et al. Safety and Efficacy of the ChAdOx1 nCoV-19 Vaccine (AZD1222) Against SARS-CoV-2: An Interim Analysis of Four Randomised Controlled Trials in Brazil, South Africa, and the UK. *Lancet.* **2020,** *397* (10269), 99–111.

Wang, M.; Cao, R.; Zhang, L.; Yang, X.; Liu, J. et al. Remdesivir and Chloroquine Effectively Inhibit the Recently Emerged Novel Coronavirus (2019-nCoV) In Vitro. *Cell. Res.* **2020,** *30*, 269–271.

Worldometers. Coronavirus symptoms (COVID-19), 2021. https://www.worldometers.info/coronavirus/coronavirus-symptoms/ (accessed on Feb 11, 2021).

Youssouf, M. S.; Kaiser, P.; Tahir, M.; Singh, G. D.; Singh, S. et al. Anti-Anaphylactic Effect of *Euphorbia hirta Fitoterapia* **2007,** *78* (7–8), 535–539.

Zhong, Y.; Tan, Y. W.; Liu, D. X. Recent Progress in Studies of Arterivirus- and Coronavirus-Host Interactions. *Viruses* **2012,** *4* (6), 980–1010.

PART V

Ethnomedicine and Lifestyle Diseases

CHAPTER 12

Ayurveda and Lifestyle Diseases

PURVI SAXENA and MARYAM SARWAT

Amity Institute of Pharmacy, Amity University, Noida, Uttar Pradesh, India

ABSTRACT

As lifestyle diseases continue to pose a threat to health across the world and have been a major cause of increased mortality rate, experts from all around the world have acknowledged the potency of herbal drugs in the treatment and prevention of lifestyle diseases like diabetes, hypertension, coronary artery disease, stress, obesity, etc. It has been reported that many modern-day medicines are carcinogenic and can lead to serious liver damage. There has been an increased global interest in traditional medicine. The most ancient therapy is Ayurveda. It is also called as the "science of longevity" as it offers a comprehensive system to live a long healthy life. In Western countries, about 40% population is consuming herbal medicines for the treatment of various diseases. Ayurveda provides a better solution in the form of a proper dietary management, "panchakarma" like detoxification and bio-purification procedures, medicaments, and rejuvenation therapies. The principle of Ayurveda is based on the complete physical, psychological, and spiritual well-being of an individual making it best suited for the treatment of lifestyle disorders. The alternative medicines use herbs, organic matter, and minerals while the preparation of herbal drugs includes the use of medicinal plants only. Some of the ayurvedic preparations have proven therapeutic efficacy against lifestyle diseases, for example, Udvartanam (powder

Ethnic Knowledge and Perspectives of Medicinal Plants, Volume 1: Curative Properties and Treatment Strategies. Munir Ozturk, Kandikere R. Sridhar, Maryam Sarwat, Volkan Altay, & Francisco Martín Huerta-Martínez (Eds.)

massage), Varunadi kashayam, Triphala churnam are used for the treatment of obesity. Sarpagandha churnam, Arjunarishtam, and Brahmi vati are used for hypertension and cardiovascular diseases. For dyslipidemia, Guggulu, Lasuna, Vrikshmla, and Kulatha are used. Ashwagandha, Jatamanji, somalatha, and sarpagandha are used to manage stress and sleep disorders. For uterine disorders, nonhormonal drugs like Asoka, Lodhra, Kumari, and Tila are used. Nimba, Guduchi, Haridra, and Sathavari are used for autoimmune diseases. With rapid economic developments and Western industrialization, it is evident that the lifestyle has been changed drastically in the past few decades. The prevalence of lifestyle diseases has reached alarming proportions in the world in recent years. Now, Ayurvedic and herbal drugs are considered the first choice of treatment because of increased side effects of modern medicines and high mortality rate due to lifestyle diseases. Globally, efforts have been made to enhance the development, production, and utilization of herbal drugs, hence increasing the growth of herbal drug industry. The main target is to promote health, prevent and manage lifestyle diseases for a healthy and happy life in the modern era.

12.1 INTRODUCTION

Individuals in developing countries fight mainly against infectious and communicable diseases. On the other hand, developed countries continue to struggle against lifestyle diseases (Ozturk and Hakeem, 2018, 2019a, b; Ozturk et al., 2014, 2016, 2018, 2020, 2021a, b). While there has been progress in treatment facilities, the human pathology continues to increase. Although life expectancy has been increased for many diseases, still a greater number of people suffer from lifestyle diseases. The increase in mortality rate is primarily due to lifestyle diseases. The major concern for the modern world is rapidly changing lifestyles and poor health practices. Professional burnout, stress, and sleep deprivation continue to affect our health in a toxic way contributing to morbidity, disability, and mortality due to lifestyle diseases (Rippe, 2018).

With the rapid development and industrialization, it is critical to assess the parameters leading toward these diseases and recognize the methods to tackle them. One of the methods to prevent lifestyle diseases is a balanced diet and proper physical exercise (Sharma and Majumdar, 2009). The basic requirement in nutrition must be fulfilled for us to stay healthy. Another approach is maintaining good lifestyle practices through Ayurveda which includes consumption of medicinal herbs, lifestyle management, and detoxification of the body (Gokani, 2014).

12.2 LIFESTYLE DISEASES

Lifestyle diseases are ailments that are based on the daily routine of people. The daily habits that push them toward a lazy routine and unhealthy diet result in chronic noncommunicable diseases (NCDs) which can be life-threatening. Around 40 million deaths reported globally are due to NCDs, which is 70% of total deaths around the globe (Tabish, 2017). In 2017, the mortality rate in India due to lifestyle diseases was 61.8% (Figure 12.1).

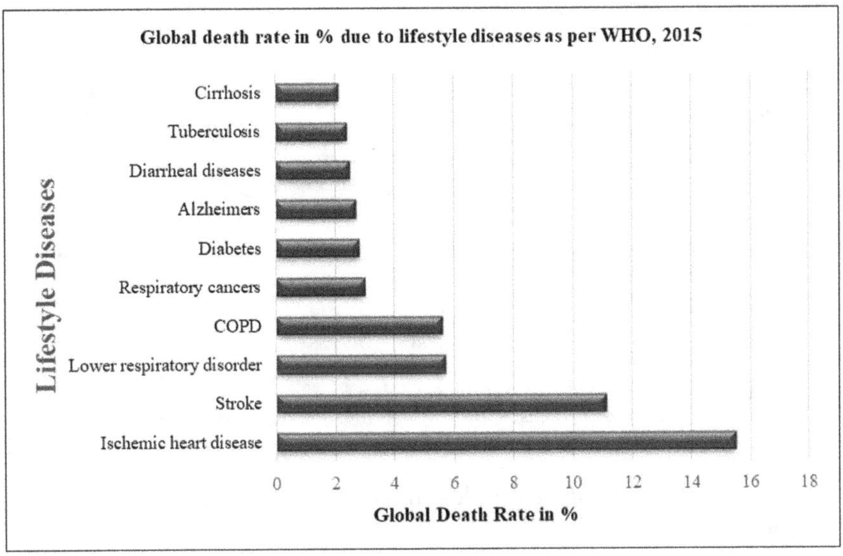

FIGURE 12.1 The annual death rate around the world due to various lifestyle diseases.
Source: WHO (2015).

Although, these diseases cannot be transmitted from person to person (hence termed noncommunicable diseases), but, the health risk, they possess, is very high due to which they come under the category of chronic diseases (Figure 12.2).

The causes include unhealthy lifestyle practices and poor diet. The most common factors are genetics, environment, and physiology. The main NCDs are cardiovascular diseases, respiratory diseases, and cancer (Tabish, 2017). The major reasons for cancer in many cases are poor physical activity, an unbalanced diet, smoking, tobacco use, and drinking alcohol (Manton, 1988).

They contribute to economic loss to a larger extent as poor families and middle-income countries are exclusively exposed to behavioral risk factors leading them toward poverty. In 2015, India faced an economic loss of 236$ million on account of lifestyle diseases only. The global impact of these diseases is responsible for high morbidity and mortality rates irrespective of age groups. The cases are aggressively increasing year by year and to tackle them correctly is the need of the hour.

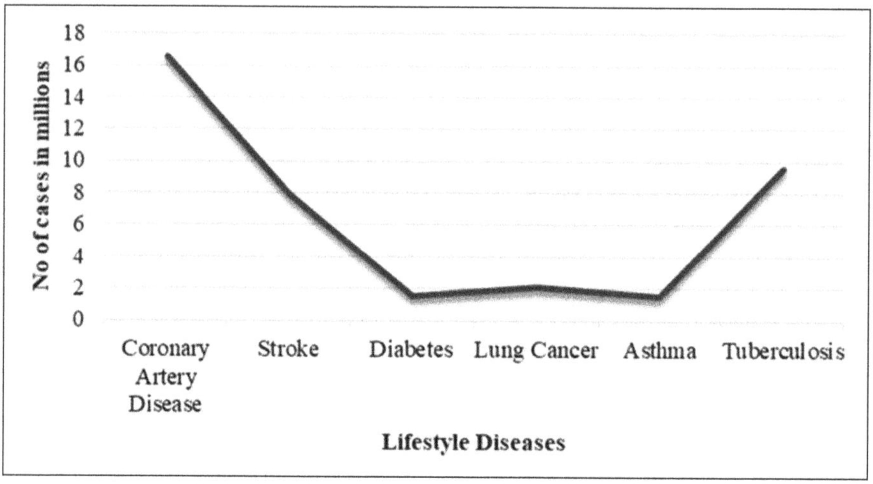

FIGURE 12.2 The number of cases for different lifestyle diseases as per WHO (2018).

Major risk factors can be divided into three major categories (Table 12.1) (Tabish, 2017):

1. Modifiable risk factors—diet changes, smoking, alcohol consumption, poor physical maintenance, etc.
2. Nonmodifiable risk factors—gender, genetics, age, race, etc.
3. Metabolic factors—hyperglycemia, hyperlipidemia, obesity, hypertension, etc.

12.3 AYURVEDA: THE ANCIENT SOLUTION TO MODERN PROBLEMS

Ayurveda provides a holistic approach for modern-day problems, one of them being lifestyle diseases. Since it is an age-old tried and tested healing system, it provides a better alternative for treating such diseases. It is mainly based on a mind–body–soul approach and restores the balance in the body. According to Ayurvedic principles, all chronic diseases are a result of an imbalance of the body–mind–soul. It not only focuses on treating the diseases, but also promotes the concept of a well-balanced life (Parasuraman et al., 2014). It focuses on rejuvenation and detoxification therapies that not only help to eradicate the health issues but also bring harmony in all aspects of life. It is truly "mother of all healing". It also includes various plants as resources for herbal medications; thus, it is more natural and comparatively better than modern-day medicines (Sreedevi and Tripathy, 2017).

TABLE 12.1 Various Risk Factors of Some Common Lifestyle Diseases.

Diseases	Risk factors
Cardiovascular Diseases	High blood pressure, tobacco use, physical inactivity, diabetes, heavy alcohol use, obesity, high salt in diet, genetics age, family history, race, ethnicity, abnormal blood coagulation, excess homocystine in blood.
Diabetes	Overweight /obesity, hypertension, low physical activity, heavy alcohol use, family history, age, distribution of fat in body, absence of beta cells in pancreas, presence of autoantibodies
Cancer	Smoking, heavy alcohol use, exposure of radiation, low physical activity, unhealthy diet, bad food habits, low intake fiber, immune deficiencies, family history, genetics, race, diabetes
Respiratory illness	Smoking, air pollution, tobacco use, dust and chemicals, genetics

Unlike allopathic medicines that are designed chemicals for specific receptors to provide symptomatic relief, Ayurveda is based on eliminating the root cause of the disease and prevents its reoccurrence. It offers different regimens like *dinacharya* (lifestyle), *ritucharya* (season), *panchakarma* (detoxification), and *rasayana* (rejuvenation) (Chandola, 2012). It is safe, efficacious, and cost-effective than most of the modern medicines. No reported side effect of ayurvedic drugs and excipients suggests that they are the better solution available for humanity (Alam et al., 2014). They promote longevity and vitality thereby offering a chance of a healthy, happy, and long life.

Some of the popular ayurvedic medicines include **Boswelia,** known as Indian frankincence or olibanum obtained from the resins of *Boswelia serrata* tree. The efficacy of this drug has been proved to be similar to nonsteroidal anti-inflammatory drugs (NSAIDs), but it is safer as compared to NSAIDs. It has been reported that it also increases the breathing capacity in patients with chronic respiratory diseases (Table 12.2).

Brahmi is another ayurvedic drug used with strong anti-inflammatory activity and improves the ability of the body to deal with stress and anxiety. It is a staple herb obtained from *Bacopa monieri*. **Curcumin** is an active constituent of *Curcuma longa*, commonly known as **turmeric.** Although it is used in food for flavor and color, it is a major ayurvedic remedy for various heart diseases as it increases the blood flow more effectively than certain pharmaceutical drugs. It is said to be more effective than Prozac in the treatment of depression.

Licorice root or **mulathi** is a wonderful drug that holds the central position in Ayurveda. The biological source is *Glycyrrhiza glabra*, containing the active constituent Glycyrrihizin (Altay et al., 2016; Ozturk et al., 2017; Pleskanovskaya et al., 2019). It is most effective in throat infections and digestive problems.

Bitter Melon produces antidiabetic effects by promoting the secretion of insulin. The biological source of bitter melon is *Mormodica charantia.*

Arjuna is the most potent cardiotonic agent available to date. It is widely used for chronic heart disease as it strengthens the cardiac muscle fibers to reduce the risk of heart failure. The biological source of arjuna is *Terminalia arjuna* and arjunolic acid is one of the major constituents responsible for hypotensive effect via diuresis (Parasuraman et al., 2014). **Ashoka** is another potent herb that is used for its diuretic effects due to the presence of leucoanthocyanidin and leucopelargonidin. The biological source is *Saraca indica*. **Pterocarpus** or **Kino tree** is *Pterocapus marsupium* which is used in diabetes as it exerts a hypoglycemic effect. The chemical constituent responsible for its activity is kinoin or kinotannic acid. **Gotu Kola** is known as **"the herb of longevity"** and is obtained from *Centella asiatica.* It is known to improve memory and reduce anxiety, depression, and stress (Parasuraman et al., 2014). **Ashwagandha** is a very popular ayurvedic remedy. It is a potent immunity booster, enhances muscle growth, lowers blood sugar level, and improves sleep in people with anxiety and sleep disorders. It is obtained from the small woody plant *Withania somnifera*.

Most cardiovascular problems arise as a result of many factors like age, gender, physical inactivity, blood cholesterol, etc. Ayurveda aims to control the risk factors by providing a balanced lifestyle to people with the help of natural therapies, meditation, and diet control. Stress and mental health issues can be prevented by internal medicines (Mathur and Mascarenhas, 2019). To have sound health one needs to keep his mind, body, and soul aligned together. With the help of ayurvedic practices, this alignment can be maintained and restored. Social life, work-life, and personal life create chaos internally leading to disturbances that precipitate several noncommunicable diseases. Traditional practices aim to provide peace to the individual and create harmony in an individual's life (Sreedevi and Tripathy, 2017).

Migraine is a condition where the patient experiences severe headache which interferes with the day to day life of the patient. The etiology of migraine is still unknown. Also, there is no cure in modern medicine for migraines yet. But a study was conducted where ayurvedic medicine was used to better understand the disease to provide a solution for the prevention of future attacks in chronic conditions. Ayurvedic models were utilized to offer additional therapy to give relief to the patients. Thus, we can say that thousands of years old system of medicine could be the solution to all our health problems specifically lifestyle-related issues.

TABLE 12.2 Some Important Drugs Used in Ayurveda Along with Their Active Constituents Responsible for Their Activity, Biological Source and Also the Part of the Plant Which Is Used in Ayurvedic Preparations.

Drugs	Biological source	Part used	Active constituent responsible for activity
Arjun	*Terminalia arjuna*	Bark	Arjunolic Acid
Turmeric	*Curcuma longa*	Rhizome	Curcumin
Boswellia	*Boswellia serrate*	Resin	Boswellic Acid
Ashwagandha	*Withania somnifera*	Roots	Withaferin-A
Pterocarpus	*Pterocarpus marsupium*	Heartwood	Kinoin or kinotannic acid
Brahmi	*Centella asiatica*	Leaves	Bacoside A
Liqorice	*Glycerrhiza glabra*	Roots	Glycyrrhizin
Bitter Melon	*Momordica charantia*	Fruits and seeds	Charantin
Ashoka	*Saraca indica*	Leaves	Leucoanthocyanidin and Leupelargonidin
Clove	*Eugenia caryophyllus*	Flower bud	Eugenol
Gudhuchi	*Tinospora cordifolia*	Stem	Tinosporin
Myrobalan	*Terminalia chebula*	Dried fruit	Anthraquinone
Cumin	*Cuminum cyminum*	Seeds	Cuminaldehyde
Gotu Kola	*Centella asiatica*	Dried aerial parts	Asiatic acid
Digitalis	*Digitalis purpurea*	Aerial Parts	Digoxin

12.4 MAJOR LIFESTYLE DISEASES AND AYURVEDIC DRUGS USED FOR THEIR TREATMENT

Some of the major lifestyle diseases that have become life-threatening for people today are discussed in the following section.

12.4.1 CARDIOVASCULAR DISEASES

The mortality rate is highest in patients with CVDs. It is responsible for more than 17 million deaths per year globally. It has been estimated that it will increase to 23 million per year by the year 2030 (Shaito et al., 2020). Cardiovascular disease (CVD) is the disease of heart or blood vessels. Major pathology is vascular impairment but it can be prevented. A healthy vascular endothelium performs many actions like vasodilation, antithrombotic, anti-inflammatory, and anti-atherogenic. But various risk factors contribute to endothelium dysfunction causing pathogenesis of atherosclerosis, coronary artery disease, and myocardial ischemia. The levels of high-density lipoprotein (HDL) and low-density lipoprotein (LDL) play a key role in keeping the endothelium healthy. High amount of LDL leads to plaque accumulation in arteries leading to blockage. This plaque causes the artery to become thinner and due to blood pressure, it ruptures. It attracts the platelets leading to thrombosis and causes complete blockage of coronary arteries. Thus leading to myocardial ischemia as blood flows toward heart is insufficient, which increases the heart beat to meet the oxygen demand, causing myocardial infarction. When this vicious cycle continues for a long time it causes myocardial remodeling which a major reason for congestive heart failure (CHF).

12.4.1.1 AYURVEDIC DRUGS FOR THE TREATMENT OF CVDS

There are various ayurvedic which are being used for the treatment of CVDs, namely (Shaito et al., 2020):

- *Digitalis purpurea* (chemical constituent obtained—Digoxin) is known to be an ionotropic drug which increases the cardiac contractility and is used in CHF.
- *Rauwolfia serpentine* (chemical constituent obtained—Reserpine) is used in hypertension.
- *Monascus purpureus* (chemical constituent obtained—Lovastatin) is used as an anti-hyperlipidemic drug.
- *Papaver somniferum* (chemical constituent obtained—Papaverine) is used as base for the synthesis of antihypertensive drugs.
- *Panax ginseng* (chemical constituent obtained—Ginsenosides) is used as an anti-hyperlipidemic and antihypertensive drug.
- *Allium sativum* (Garlic) is used for systolic hypertension.

- *Ginko biloba* also called as maidenhair tree and "living fossil" (chemical constituent obtained-Ginkolides) is used as an anti-inflammatory and antioxidant agent.
- *Ganoderma lucidum* consists of triterpeniods, nucleosides, polysaccharides which possess properties like antihypertensive, hepatoprotective, immunomodulation, hypocholesterolemic, and antioxidant.
- *Gynostemma pentaphyllum* is used for its antilipidemic, antioxidant, and antihypertensive actions.
- *Salvia miltiorrhiza* is used in angina pectoris (chest pain due to imbalance between oxygen demand and oxygen supply to the heart).

12.4.2 DIABETES

The second lifestyle disease leading to most deaths is diabetes mellitus. There are four types of diabetes: type 1, type 2, gestational, and prediabetes. 90% of the total cases are of type 2 Diabetes. Diabetes mellitus is a type of metabolic disorder where there is decrease in the level of insulin in body causing rise in blood glucose levels, that is, hyperglycemia. Insulin depletion in body can occur due to many pathways including development of insulin resistance in body, decrease in insulin secretion, downregulation of insulin receptors, destruction of beta cells in Islets of Langerhans in pancreas, and excess formation of glucose (high level of glucagon in body).

It is prevalent in children and can be of two types-

- Type 1A—Autoimmune type, where beta cells are completely destroyed leading to complete absence of insulin in the body.
- Type 1B—Idiopathic type, the reason is unknown.

Not much treatment options are available for type 1 diabetes.

Type 2 diabetes is known as insulin dependent is caused due to many reasons mentioned above. It is prevalent in 90% population in India and usually occurs in people with age above 40 years. More treatment options are available for type 2 diabetes including some herbal drugs.

12.4.2.1 AYURVEDIC DRUGS USED FOR TYPE 2 DIABETES (PANG ET AL., 2019)

- *Memecylon umbellatum* acts as an anti-inflammatory agent reducing the production of TNFα, interleukin-1β, and interleukin-6 as they destroy the beta cells in pancreas.

- Lycii Radicis Cortex in the root bark of *Lycium barbarum* inhibits NF-κB thereby inhibiting inflammatory response.
- *Momordica charantia* called as bitter melon inhibits the activation of NF- κB thus inhibiting inflammation.
- *Tinospora cordifolia* increases the superoxide dismutase (SOD) and catalase (CAT) enzymes which help in destroying the free radicals. By exerting its antioxidant property, it helps in preventing oxidative stress in patients.
- *Amomum cadamomum* helps to reduce plasma free fatty acids as lipotoxicity is also a major factor that contributes in the development of insulin resistance and beta cell dysfunction.
- *Acer pycnanthum* inhibits α-glucosidase and reduces blood glucose levels.
- *Lodhrasavam* contains 19 herbal ingredients which shows antidiabetic effects.
- *Ephedra sinica* changes gut microbiota and reduces fasting blood glucose levels.
- Gingerol exerts its antidiabetic action by increasing insulin secretion through glucagon like peptide-1 (GLP-1).
- *Psidium guajava* inhibits α-glucosidase and dipeptidyl peptidase-4 (DPP-4).

12.4.3 CANCER

Thirty percent of total cancer cases are due to the poor lifestyle and health management. Almost 7 million people die due to cancer each year. Cancer is considered a group of diseases where some body cells divide uncontrollably and spread to other parts of the body. Normally human cells divide and multiply whenever there is need but in case of cancer the division is not regulated (Masoodi et al., 2020). It results in the formation of tumor (mass of tissues). The cell growth in blood cancer does not form a solid tumor while other cancers form solid tumors. The abnormal cell division is genetic and may result due to mutation in genes. Therefore, cancer can be inherited from parents. Three main types of genes altered in cancer are proto-oncogenes, DNA repair genes, and tumor suppressor genes.

Proto-oncogenes take part in normal cell division but if altered in certain ways can lead to the development of cancers. Tumor suppressor genes control cell division and growth but mutation can cause cells to divide uncontrollably. DNA repair genes are important as they take part in repair of damaged DNA but changes in these can also lead to cancer.

The spread of tumor (primary tumor) to different part of the body (different from its origin) is called metastasis. Cancer cells travel via blood to other organs and form a secondary tumor. Also the cancer cells require more nutrition as they keep on dividing so they develop their own new blood vessels which is known as angiogenesis. Although there is no cure for cancer found till date but there are certain treatment options available. One option is the use of phytochemicals and ayurvedic drugs to treat cancer and provide relief to the patients.

12.4.3.1 AYURVEDIC DRUGS FOR CANCER

Some natural drugs used for the treatment of cancer are (Yin et al., 2013):

- *Scutellaria baicalensis*—is used in prostate cancer and contains baicalin, a flavone glycoside. Mechanism of action includes the inhibition of enzymatic synthesis of eicosanoids which are essential mediators of inflammation and tumor cell proliferation in prostate gland.
- *Platycodon grandiflorum*—is used in lung cancer, mainly for the reduction of therapy-associated toxicity. It is also beneficial for management of symptoms of cancer. It can also be used as an adjuvant to enhance the anticancer action of other drugs.
- *Veratrum californicum*—used to treat pancreatic cancer. Its mechanism of action includes inhibition of SHH signaling through direct binding to seven-helix bundle of SMO protein. Main chemical constituent is a steroidal alkaloid known as Cyclopamine. It also inhibits the conversion of bone marrow precursor cells into cancer cells.
- *Catheranthus roseus*—Vincristine and vinblastine prevent the polymerization of mitotic spindle and arrest the cell division in metaphase. They are used to treat many types of cancers like Hodgkin and Non-Hodgkin Lymphomas.
- *Taxus baccata* and *Taxus brevifolia*—Paclitaxel and docetaxel are two most common drugs that are used in ovarian and breast cancers. These act by promoting the polymerization of mitotic spindle thereby stabilizing the mitotic spindles.
- *Camptotheca accuminata*—Camptothecin obtained from this plant is used for colorectal cancer and ovarian cancer. It is a topoisomerase-I targeting agent.
- There are some supplements that can be used in the treatment of cancer as adjuvants:

- For lung cancer—Sheng-mai injection, Gu-gin granule, Feiji Recipe etc can be used.
- For hepatocellular carcinoma—Kava, Grapeseed, Echinacea, and *Hypericum perforatum* can be used.
- For bone tumor—Guliu capsule (GLC) is used.

12.4.4 CHRONIC RESPIRATORY DISEASES

It includes COPD and asthma which constitute 90% of deaths occurring in low-income countries. These are the most under-diagnosed conditions that eventually lead to the death of the patients. COPD is comprised of chronic bronchitis, chronic asthma, and emphysema. They all come under lung inflammatory diseases. The major pathophysiological pathway includes the role of inflammatory mediators like cytokines including interleukins (IL-1 AND IL-6), and TNF-α. They are released by different cells like neutrophils, T lymphocytes, and macrophages. Oxidative stress and smoking are two major reasons for the development of these chronic conditions. Transforming growth factor-β (TGF-β) is responsible for airway fibrosis leading to airway destruction. Ecosanoids like LTB_4 and PGE_2 are also involved in the inflammatory pathway.

12.4.4.1 AYURVEDIC DRUGS USED TO CURE RESPIRATORY DISORDERS

Various ayurvedic drugs are used to treat asthma and COPD include (Alamgeer et al., 2018; Rachana et al., 2016):

- *Curcuma longa*—Turmeric is known to be an anti-inflammatory agent. The active constituent of this plant is curcumin and is used to provide relief in asthmatic patients.
- *Zingiber officinale*—is a powerful expectorant used in chronic bronchitis. It also possesses anti-inflammatory, antiemetic, and antiviral properties.
- *Glycyrrhiza glabra*—also known as Yashti-Madhu is having antioxidant, expectorant, and anti-pyretic properties. The antioxidant action helps to reduce the oxidative stress and provides relief in asthma and COPD.
- *Ocimum sanctum*—treats bronchitis, influenza, cough, and cold by showing its mucolytic action.

- *Cuminum cyminum*—is known to be a powerful bronchodilator and has antimicrobial properties. Therefore, it cures common cold and cough as it prevents the formation of cough in the respiratory tract.
- *Adhatoda vasica*—is used in allergic conditions and bronchial asthma. The major active compound Vasicine has bronchodilatory action. It has been reported that intravenous administration of this drug clears the airway by decreasing mucus production and dilates the bronchi. It is a potent antioxidant as it increases glutathione levels.

All the above diseases are very much preventable if one decides to follow a balanced diet, maintain proper weight, include physical activities in daily routine, indulge in detoxification, and consume various natural components and drugs like tulsi, neem, garlic, clove, ginger, turmeric, cardamom, cinnamon, amla, etc. These methods not only boost immunity but also help in improving lifestyle and prevent a lot of chronic diseases that are caused mainly due to lifestyle changes.

12.5 PREVENTION OF LIFESTYLE DISEASES WITH AYURVEDA

Ayurveda has two major objectives—prevention of health and treatment of diseases in people. Due to the poor lifestyle and unhealthy eating habits, people are more prone to develop diseases. Ayurveda aims at complete well-being of an individual. It provides a better solution for overall restoration of health and happiness of the individual. Nowadays, people are shifting more toward ancient system of medicine for better results. *Shodhana, Shamana, Rasayana* therapy are used along with *dinacharya, ritucharya* which not only promotes health but also helps to enhance the quality of life and prolongs lifespan. It keeps a balance between *dosha, datu*, and *mala* (Chaudhary et al., 2017). The four components of daily life include *Ahara* (food), *Achara* (conduct), *Vichara* (thoughts), and *Vihara* (behavior). These components greatly affect a person and determine whether a particular individual is predisposed to noncommunicable diseases or not. According to the concept in Ayurveda if one of these components is disturbed, it leads to disturbances in *tridosha*, resulting in manifestation of diseases. The dietary requirements are extremely important for maintaining good health. In Ayurveda, every prescription requires a proper diet regime. It also suggests different combinations in diet that must be avoided at any cost or else they will cause dietary incompatibility. Also the *prakriti* of a person is considered before the dietary regime is designed. Ayurveda includes dietary supplements called

Rasayana which has rejuvenating and nourishing effect by enhancing *Agni Bala* (digestive power). It increases the nutritional status of an individual leading to improved quality of *dhatu* (tissue) (Sreedevi and Tripathy, 2017). All these methods help to strengthen the four components and create a balance between them improving the overall health of an individual.

12.6 CONCLUSIONS

Modern medicine may provide faster relief, but overall health benefits are obtained from Ayurveda, the ancient science of healing. With more advancements in therapies and treatments, people are realizing the importance of Ayurveda as it does not have any serious side effects. Moreover, the introduction of personalized medication and increase in cost of treatment leaves us with one, better and economical option. As we move toward complicated and targeted therapies that require extreme precision and expertise, the chances of failure increase a lot. Therefore, the best and simplest way to achieve better health and prolong one's lifespan is the combination of Ayurveda with technology, it may provide us good quality of health care. Since Ayurveda is a *prakriti*-based treatment, its combination with technology may help us achieve the impossible. The management of lifestyle diseases is of critical importance as it is like a pandemic which is claiming far more lives than other diseases altogether.

KEYWORDS

- **Ayurveda**
- **herbal drug**
- **herbal drug industry**
- **modern medicine**
- **traditional medicine**

REFERENCES

Alam, Md. T.; Parvez, N.; Sharma, P. K. FDA-Approved Natural Polymers for Fast Dissolving Tablets. *J. Pharma.* **2014,** 952970. DOI: 10.1155/2014/952970.

Alamgeer; Younis, W.; Asif, H.; Sharif, A.; Riaz, H.; Bukhari, I. A.; Assiri, A. M. Traditional Medicinal Plants Used for Respiratory Disorders in Pakistan: A Review of the Ethno-Medicinal and Pharmacological Evidence. *Chin Med.* **2018,** *13*, 48.

Altay, V.; Karahan, F.; Ozturk, M. et al. Molecular and Ecological İnvestigations on the Wild Populations of *Glycyrrhiza* L. Taxa Distributed in the East Mediterranean Area of Turkey. *J. Plant Res.* **2016,** *129* (6), 1021–1032.

Chandola, H. M. Lifestyle Disorders- Ayurveda with Lots of Potential for Prevention. *Ayu* 2012, *33*, 327.

Chaudhary, S.; Pramod, M.; Brahmanand, S.; Anamika, S. Preventive and Curative Aspects of Ayurveda in Lifestyle Diseases. *Int. J. Ayurveda Pharma Res.* 2017, *5*, 51–53.

Gokani, T. Ayurveda-the Science of Healing. *Headache* **2014,** *54*, 1101–1106.

Manton, K. G. The Global Impact of Non-Communicable Diseases: Estimates and Projections. *World Health Stat. Quart.* **1988,** *41*, 251–266.

Masoodi, K. Z.; Amin, I.; Mansoor, S. et al. Botanicals from the Himalayas with Anticancer Potential—An Emphasis on Kashmir Himalayas. In *Biodiversity and Biomedicine—Our Future*; Ozturk, M., Egamberdieva, D., Pešić, M., Eds., Chapter 11; Academic Press, 2020; pp 181–234.

Mathur, P.; Mascarenhas, L. Lifestyle Diseases: Keeping Fit for a Better Tomorrow. *Ind. J. Med. Res.* **2019,** *149* (Suppl). DOI: 10.4103/0971–5916.251669

Ozturk, M.; Hakeem, K. R. *Plant and Human Health—Vol. 1—Ethnobotay and Physiology*; Springer Science + Business Media: New York, 2018.

Ozturk, M.; Hakeem, K. R. *Plant and Human Health—Vol. 2—Phytochemistry and Molecular Aspects*; Springer Science + Business Media: New York, 2019a.

Ozturk, M.; Hakeem, K. R. *Plant and Human Health—Vol. 3—Phytochemistry and Therapeutic Uses*. Springer Science + Business Media, NY, **2019b**.

Ozturk, M.; Altay, V.; Gucel, S.; Guvensen, A. Halophytes in the East Mediterranean-Their Medicinal and Other Economical Values. In *Sabkha Ecosystems: Volume IV: Cash Crop Halophyte and Biodiversity Conservation Tasks for Vegetation Science*, Vol. 47; Springer: Netherlands; 2014; pp 241–272.

Ozturk, M.; Altay, V.; Altundağ, E.; Gucel, S. Halophytic Plant Diversity of Unique Habitats in Turkey: Salt Mine Caves of Çankırı and Iğdır. In *Halophytes for Food Security in Dry Lands*; Khan, M. A., Ozturk, M., Gul, B., Ahmed, M. Z., Eds., Chapter 18; Elsevier, 2016, http://dx.doi.org/10.1016/B971–0-11–801851–5.00011–2

Ozturk, M.; Altay, V.; Hakeem, K. R.; Akçiçek, E. *Liquorice from Botany to Phytochemistry*; SpringerBriefs in Plant Science, 2017. https://doi.org/10.1007/971–3-311–74241–3.

Ozturk, M.; Altay, V.; Latiff, A. et al. A Comparative Analysis of the Medicinal Plants Used for Diabetes Mellitus in the Traditional Medicine in Turkey, Pakistan, and Malaysia. In: *Plant and Human Health*; Ozturk, M., Hakeem, K. R., Eds., Vol. 1; Springer: Cham, Chapter 11; Springer International Publishing AG, 2018; pp 401–461.

Ozturk, M.; Egamberdieva, D.; Milica, P. *Biodiversity and Biomedicine-Our Future*; Academic Press, Elsevier Inc.: UK, USA, 2020.

Ozturk, M.; Altay, V.; Efe, R. *Biodiversity, Conservation and Sustainability in Asia: Volume I: Prospects and Challenges in West Asia and Caucasus*; Springer Nature: Switzerland AG, 2021a, DOI: 10.1007/971–3-031–59921–7

Ozturk, M.; Khan, S. M.; Altay, V.; Efe, R.; Egamberdieva, D.; Khassanov, F. *Biodiversity, Conservation and Sustainability in Asia: Volume II: Prospects and Challenges in South and Middle Asia*'; Springer Nature: Switzerland AG, 2021b. DOI: 10.1007/971–3-031–73941–0

Pang, G. M.; Li, F. X.; Yan, Y.; Zhang, Y.; Kong, L. L.; Zhu, P.; Wang, K. F.; Zhang, F.; Liu, B.; Lu, C. Herbal Medicine in the Treatment of Patients with Type 2 Diabetes Mellitus. *Chin. Med. J.* **2019,** *132*, 71–85.

Parasuraman, S.; Thing, G. S.; Dhanaraj, S. A. Polyherbal Formulation: Concept of Ayurveda. *Pharmacogn. Rev.* **2014,** *8*, 71–80.

Pleskanovskaya, S. A.; Mamedova, M. A.; Ashıralıyeva, M. A. et al. *Glycyrrhiza glabra* (Liquorice) in Turkmenistan—Medicinal and Biological Aspects. In *Plant and Human Health,—Pharmacology and Therapeutic Uses*; Ozturk, M., Hakeem, K. R., Eds., Vol. 3, Chapter 2; Springer Nature: Switzerland, 2019; pp 21–35.

Rachana, R.; Pant, M.; Basu, S.; Jain, A.; Goel, N.; Wadi, I. A Review on Herbal Therapy for Respiratory Ailments. *Int. J. Life Sci. Pharma Res.* **2016,** *6*, 11–12.

Rippe J. M. Lifestyle Medicine: The Health Promoting Power of Daily Habits and Practices. *Am. J. Lifestyle Med.* **2018,** *12*, 491–512.

Shaito, A.; Thuan, D. T. B.; Phu, H. T.; Nguyen, T. H. D.; Hasan, H.; Halabi, S.; Abdelhady, S.; Nasrallah, G. K.; Eid, A. H.; Pintus, G. Herbal Medicine for Cardiovascular Diseases: Efficacy, Mechanisms, and Safety. *Front Pharmacol.* **2020,** *11*, 422.

Sharma, M.; Majumdar, P. K. Occupational Lifestyle Diseases: An Emerging Issue. *Indian J. Occup. Environ. Med.* **2009,** *13*, 101–112.

Sreedevi, S.; Tripathy, R. N. Lifetsyle Disease and Ayurveda: An Overview and Prospective. *Int. J. Res. Ayurveda Pharm* 2017, *8*, 21–25.

Tabish, S. A. Lifestyle Diseases: Consequences, Characterstics, Causes and Control. *J. Cardiol. Curr. Res* **2017,** *9* (3), 00326.

WHO. The Annual Death Rate Around the World Due to Various Lifestyle Diseases, 2015.

WHO. The Number of Cases for Different Lifestyle Diseases, 2018.

Yin, S. Y.; Wei, W. C.; Jian, F. Y.; Yang, N. S. Therapeutic Applications of Herbal Medicines for Cancer Patients. *Evid. Based Compl. Altern. Med. eCAM* **2013,** Article ID 302426. DOI: 10.1155/2013/302426.

CHAPTER 13

The Multi-Targeting Efficacy and Therapeutic Effects of Ayurveda and Chinese Medicine: An Integrated Approach for Cancer Treatment and Management

MOHAMMAD AFSAR KHAN and HIFZUR R. SIDDIQUE

Molecular Cancer Genetics & Translational Research Lab, Section of Genetics, Department of Zoology, Aligarh Muslim University, Aligarh, India

ABSTRACT

Herbal-based traditional medicines have a long history of therapeutic application throughout the world. Ayurveda and Chinese herbs have been traditionally used as indigenous complementary and alternative medicine to treat various types of diseases since ancient times effectively. These medicines demonstrated fewer toxic effects, prolonged survival rates, and enhanced quality of life. Further, the use of Ayurvedic and Chinese medicine in combination with chemotherapy and radiotherapy enhances these therapies' efficacy. Cancer is a complex disease and the leading cause of death worldwide. The existing anticancer therapies do not address the challenges arising from tumor heterogeneity, such as developing drug resistance and the side effects of these therapies. In this context, different preclinical and clinical experiments show different modes of actions of Ayurveda and Chinese herbs in various

Ethnic Knowledge and Perspectives of Medicinal Plants, Volume 1: Curative Properties and Treatment Strategies. Munir Ozturk, Kandikere R. Sridhar, Maryam Sarwat, Volkan Altay, & Francisco Martín Huerta-Martínez (Eds.)

cancers, such as induction of apoptosis, modulation of tumor suppressor genes and oncogenes, interaction with the tumor microenvironment, inhibition of metastasis, and cancer stem cells proliferation. Interestingly, these medicines have less or no toxic effect on normal cells. This chapter will illustrate the efficacy of Ayurvedic and Chinese herbal medicine in combating different cancers, either alone or in combination with other therapies.

13.1 INTRODUCTION

Cancer is one of the deadly diseases contributed by genetic, epigenetic, and environmental factors. It has been estimated that one of the three people in the world develops cancer during their life span (https://www.who.int/news-room/fact-sheets/detail/cancer; Bray et al., 2018). The various factors responsible for cancer development involve mutations such as gain of function mutation in proto-oncogenes and loss of function mutation in tumor suppressor genes (TSG), gene amplifications, deletions, and translocations, as well as defects in the process of chromosomal segregation (Fouad and Aanei, 2017; Singh et al., 2020). The epigenetic basis of cancer involves changes like DNA methylation as well as histone and chromatin modification. Studies have shown that genetic and epigenetic changes exert a synergistic effect on the process of malignant transformation (Baylin and Jones, 2016; Fatma et al., 2020). According to a recent study, environmental factors in the malignant transformation are around 80–90%, resulting from smoking, alcohol consumption, diet, and reproductive behavior (Lewandowska et al., 2019). It has been reported that hepatitis B virus (HBV), hepatitis C virus (HCV), and human papillomavirus (HPV) infection is also responsible for 25% of cancer in low- and middle-income countries. The cumulative death due to these factors estimates around 9.6 million deaths in 2018, that is, out of every six deaths, one is due to cancer (https://www.who.int/news-room/fact-sheets/detail/cancer).

The transformation of normal cells to malignant cells results due to various abnormalities like the dysregulation of the cell signaling pathways, which influence the cell metabolism and cell survival and dysregulation of the proliferative sustainability of cells, evading the growth suppressor genes (p53, pRB), which negatively regulates cell proliferation (Singh et al., 2019, 2020). Tumor cells resist cell death by evolving a variety of strategies such as loss of function mutations in p53, activation of oncogenic signaling, downregulation of pro-apoptotic proteins (BIM, PUMA, BID), or increasing the expression of anti-apoptotic proteins (BCL-2, BCL-XL) to limit the process of programmed cell death (Hanahan and Weinberg, 2011; Parray et al., 2012). Furthermore, cancer cells also achieve replicative immortality by extending the telomeres' length via enhancing the telomerase activity, which results in developing resistance against senescence or apoptosis. Tumor cells also undergo angiogenic switching and form new blood vessels to acquire nutrients, oxygen supply and to evacuate metabolic wastes by upregulating angiogenic inducers (VEFG, FGF, MMP-9) and downregulating angiogenic inhibitors (TSP-1) (Fouad and Aanei, 2017; Hanahan and Weinberg, 2011). In addition to these characteristics, tumor cells also undergo invasion and metastasis through an alteration in the extracellular matrix (ECM), mainly by downregulating E-cadherin (Peinado et al., 2011). Extensive studies on the in-depth understanding of the various mechanisms involved in cancer progression are still exploring the complex phenomenon of cancer progression to design a precise and efficient therapeutic approach against cancer. Different advanced technologies and combinational therapies are currently under evaluation both in vitro and in vivo to combat this deadly disease (Khan et al. 2019). Currently, nanomedicine, targeted therapy, thermal ablation, and magnetic hyperthermia are the potential therapies that provide precise treatment options against cancer and reduce the limitations such as side effects arising from the various therapies used for treatment (Pucci et al., 2019). Combinational therapies like nanomedicine and targeted therapy improve the efficacy (Pucci et al., 2019) and therapeutic potential of the already tested anticancer agents whereas novel strategies like siRNA delivery, gene therapy, and immunotherapy provide effective and precise treatment against cancer (Singh et al. 2020; Pucci et al., 2019). Traditional Chinese Medicine (TCM) and Ayurveda are the two ancient herbal medicines used to prevent and treat various diseases and act as an antiviral, antibacterial, immune enhancer and in the treatment of neurological disorders (Figure 13.1). In this chapter, we review the role of Traditional Chinese Medicine (TCM) and Ayurveda (an Indian Traditional medicine) to treat various diseases, especially inflammatory conditions, and cancer. Furthermore, we will review the literature for the mechanism of action of these medicines and their potential therapeutic efficacy alone or in combination with chemotherapeutic drugs.

13.2 HISTORY OF TRADITIONAL CHINESE MEDICINE AND AYURVEDA

Herbs or herbal plants are used for decades, especially in ancient civilizations like China, Egypt, India, etc. Such herbal medicine has a wide range of therapeutic potential in diseases like skin problems, cardiovascular, viral, bacterial diseases, metabolism disorders like diabetes, inflammatory diseases, infectious diseases, and cancer. Herbal medicine constitutes either whole plant or plant parts, bioactive compounds extracted from the plants, or microscopic plants like fungi. Among the traditional medicine practiced from ancient to the modern world, TCM and Ayurveda have a considerable contribution in treating various diseases.

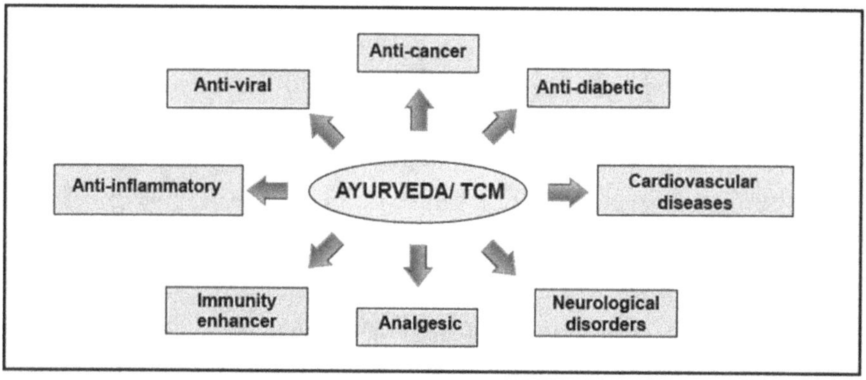

FIGURE 13.1 An illustration of the various medicinal properties of Ayurveda/traditional Chinese medicine.

13.2.1 TRADITIONAL CHINESE MEDICINE (TCM)

TCM was used over thousands of years to fight against different diseases. Since the founding of the People's Republic of China (1949), TCM and Western medicine have been used to improve public health. Bian Que, during the Warring States Period (770-221 BC), first put forward the four methods of diagnosis, which includes (i) Inspection (i.e., visual inspection to observe abnormalities in the patients like body secretions, complexion, tongue, etc.), (ii) Auscultation and Olfaction (to detect sound abnormalities in the patients like respiration sound and detecting odor emitted by the patient like breath, recreation or excretion, etc.), (iii) Inquiring (to enquire about the observable symptoms and relevant medical history of the patients), and (iv) Palpation (including pathological changes and functions of organs, predicting through the pulse and also by pressing the relevant body parts (Wang et al., 2008). Zhang Zhongjing during Han Dynasty (25–200 BC) collected and combined the rules and principles to measure the various illness patterns by the internal ailments in "*The Shang Han Za Bing Fun*" (Treatise on Febrile Diseases and Miscellaneous Illness). It includes the prevention, pathology, symptoms, therapy, and treatments of the diseases (Lu et al., 2004). The "*Shen Nong Ben Cao Jing*" (Shennong's Classic of Materia Medica, 200-250CE) is another collection that outlines the theory of compatibility of the medicinal ingredients explaining the property of drugs as "four natures" and "five flavors." It led to the formation of the foundation of TCM pharmaceutical theory development foundation. Li Shizhen was the first to scientifically categorize medicinal herbs during the Ming Dynasty (1368–1644AD). Western medicine and TCM were practiced, especially during the Mid-Qing Dynasty (1912–1949AD) (Lu et al., 2004). Presently, TCM is based on five characteristics which include (i) mind and body mean the interaction between mental and physical factors has coordination in the conditions of health and development of illness; (ii) dynamic balance is the most vital for body functions and thus restoring chaotic body functions to cure the disease; (iii) emphasis on individuality, that is, providing treatment based on syndrome differentiation by analyzing specific symptoms and physical signs; (iv) attention on preventive treatment, that is, emphasis on prevention before the disease appears by improving health through a balanced diet, balanced labor and rest, regular life and emotional adjustment; (v) simplicity, that is, without complex equipment, diagnose the patients. For example, the small splints used in osteopathy.

TCM provides enlightenment to society and helps to transform the world, but it also comes up with a systematic and holistic approach to explaining health and disease. TCM has a great contribution to Chinese history, which has faced various natural disasters, wars, and plaque and other neighboring countries. TCM has a globalization approach in the modern world, and around 183 countries and regions are more or less practicing the essence of TCM (Lu et al., 2004). According to World Health Organization (https://www.who.int/news-room/fact-sheets/detail/cancer), more than 100 countries have been approved to practice acupuncture and moxibustion, and some forms of TCM have also been registered in other countries like Russia, Cuba, Singapore, Vietnam, etc.

13.2.2 AYURVEDA—AN INDIAN TRADITIONAL MEDICINE

Ayurveda is based on traditional Indian medicine parallel to TCM, which is practiced in their respective geographical region. The foundation of Ayurveda has been laid by the ancient schools named "*Vaisheshika*" and "*Nyaya*" (school of logic). The *Vaisheshika* school propagates and inferences the pathological conditions for the treatment, whereas *Nyaya* school teaching is based on the patient's condition and the condition of disease before treatments begin (Jaiswal and Williams, 2017). The origin of Ayurveda is considered to be from *Brahma* (Hindu God), which is translated to ordinary people by different writings and oral narrations. The healing and holistic knowledge of Ayurveda is composed in the form of poetry called "*Shloka*" in Sanskrit. Among the four collections of religious texts called "*Vedas*" Sanskriti literature and the oldest scripture of Hinduism (*Yajur-*, *Rig-*, *Sam-*, and *Atharva Vedas*), the Rig Veda describes 67 plants as the healing cure (Jaiswal and Williams, 2017). "*Charaka Samhita*" is a compiled knowledge of *Vedas,* written by Agnivesha and edited by Charaka (Kumar et al., 2017). Other compilations that various scholars compile are Nighantu Granthas, Bhava Prakasha, and Madhava Nidana (Jaiswal and Williams, 2017). According to Ayurveda, the whole universe is made up of five elements called "*Pancha Mahaboota*," which includes *Vayu* (Air), *Aakash* (Space), *Jala* (Water), *Prithvi* (Earth), and *Teja* (Fire). By varying the conditions, these *Pancha Mahaboota* forms three basic humors, referred to as "Tridoshas" the three fundamental energies and principles, that is, (i) Vata Dosha, which maintains cellular transport, homeostatic balance, and the elimination of waste products. *Vata Dosha* is responsible for catabolism in the body. (ii) *Pita Dosha* regulates body temperature, hunger, and thrust management and maintains optic nerves' coordination. *Pita Dosha* is responsible for the metabolism of the body. (iii) *Kapha Dosha*, which governs all the lubrications in the body, including joints, lungs, and brain, is responsible for forming all the seven tissues called *Sapta dhatus* (i.e., plasma, blood, muscles, fat, bone, bone marrow, and reproductive fluid). The anabolism of the body is governed by the *Kapha Dosha* (Heinrich et al., 2004). An imbalance between these *Dosha* is responsible for all the illnesses and diseases.

*Tri Malas (*three major excreta*)* and *Trayo Dosa Agni (*the digestive fire inside the body*)* are the two factors that are considered important along with the *Doshas* and the *Dhatus* in the doctrine of Ayurveda. Among them, *trimalas* include the three types of waste products produced by the body due to the metabolic and digestive processes. These include the "M*utra"* (i.e., urine), "*Purisa"* (i.e., fecal matter), and "*Sveda"* (i.e., sweat). Ayurveda also describes how any imbalance between the *Tridoshas* leads to disturbance in the effective elimination of the waste products, thereby resulting in several metabolic diseases such as diarrhea, constipation, asthma, rheumatoid arthritis, and many more. The failure to eliminate the *Mutra Mala* from the body leads to infection of the urinary tract, cystitis, and gastric pain.

Similarly, if the *Sveda Mala* is not cleared from the body, it results in skin-related problems such as irritation and improper body fluid balance. In the doctrine of Ayurveda, the biological fire required for the functioning of all the metabolic processes is called "*Agni*." The human body includes three categories of *Agni*. Among them, the most important one is *Jatharagni which* is responsible for the digestive fire. *Jatharagni* is closely related to the body's *Pitta'* (fire) and ultimately to the "*Vatta*" (air). Any increase in the body's digestive fire due to an increase in the acidic conditions leads to an elevation in the *Pitta* levels, and its respective symptoms are also observed. The digestive fire is also involved in controlling the normal microflora, the digestive system's proper function, and the provision of energy to the whole body. Any interference in its balance leads to discomfort in the body's gastrointestinal tract and results in various pathological problems like ulcers, diarrhea, and constipation.

13.3 ROLE OF TCM AND AYURVEDA IN INFLAMMATORY DISEASES

Inflammation is an immune response triggered by various factors, including harmful pathogens, damaged cells, irradiation, or toxic chemicals or compounds. The characteristic features of inflammation at the tissue level comprise swelling, heat, or pain, as well as the loss of tissue function (Chen et al., 2018). During inflammation, the microcirculatory events involve changes such as a change in vascular permeability, recruitment of leucocytes, and also the release of inflammatory mediators like pro-inflammatory cytokines (Ferrero-Miliani et al., 2007). The common pathogenesis of inflammation led to various chronic diseases such as cardiovascular and bowel disease, arthritis, diabetes, and cancer. The various mechanisms of the generation of pro-inflammatory response involve (i) cell surface pathogen recognition pattern (PRRs) that includes toll-like receptors (TLRs), retinoic acid-inducible gene (RIG)-I-like receptors (RLRs), C-type lectin receptors (CLRs), as well as NOD-like receptors (NLRs) (Amarante-Mendes et al., 2018); (ii) activation of inflammatory pathways triggered by the microbial product and cytokines such as MAPK, JAK-STAT, and NF-κβ pathways (Chen et al., 2018; Henríquez-Olguín et al., 2015); (iii) release of inflammatory markers produced by activated inflammatory cells (i.e., macrophages and adipocytes). The inflammatory markers include inflammatory cytokines (IL-1, IL-6, IL-12, TNFs, IFNs, CSF, etc.), inflammatory proteins (e.g., CRP, serum amyloid A, haptoglobin, fibrinogen, etc.), and other inflammatory markers (i.e., ROS,

8-OHdG) (Chen et al., 2018); (iv) recruitment of inflammatory cells such as neutrophils followed by monocytes, NK-cells, T-cells, and B-cells (Robb et al., 2016). Various natural herbs from TCM have been proven to inhibit pro-inflammatory pathways and suppress the related inflammatory disease. For instance, Evodiamine, which is extracted from the plant *Evodiae fructus,* inhibits the production of COX-2-mediated PGE2 and inhibits the expression of iNOS through the inhibition of PI3K/AKT/p70S6K pathways. Moreover, it also inhibits hypoxia-inducible factor-1alpha (HIF-1) (Liu et al., 2009). Phylligenin, Naringenin, 6-Gingerol, Schicantherin bioactive substances have been shown to inhibit the production of pro-inflammatory cytokines and decrease the expression of lipopolysaccharides (LPS). Moreover, these substances also interfere and downregulate the MAPK, NF-κβ, and Activator Protein-1 (AP-1) (Pan et al., 2011). Cholalic acid and hyodeoxycholalic acid are well documented and prevent cerebral ischemia by inhibiting the inflammatory cytokines (IL-1ß, IL-6, and TNF-α) and are also found to be effective in the treatment of Alzheimer's disease (Pan et al., 2011; Hua et al., 2009). Curcumin, a strong anti-inflammatory agent, has been reported to be used to treat myocarditis (an inflammation of the heart muscles). Curcumin exerts its effects by inhibiting cytokines (IL-1I, TNF-α, GATA) and NF-κβ expression (Pan et al., 2011). Ginkgolide B, Glycyrrhetinic acid, and Monacolin K are effective in treating atherosclerotic disease. The basal mechanism of attenuation is by decreasing the generation of ROS, MMP-2, and pro-inflammatory cytokines. Further, it also enhances the expression of macrophage migration inhibitory factor (MIF) (Xie and Du, 2011). *Bi-Qi* capsule, a TCM formulation, reduces the CIA-induced inflammation, cartilage destruction, and synovial hyperplasia. *Bi-Qi* is widely used for the treatment and prevention of arthritis. *Bi-Qi* results in a reduction in the level of TNF-α, IL-18 cytokines in a dose-dependent manner (Wang et al., 2018). *Kudiezi* extracted from *Ixeris sonachifolia,* which is a whole herbal injection, is used to treat acute cerebral infraction by increasing the production of anti-inflammatory cytokines (eg-IL-10), decreasing pro-inflammatory cytokines (IL-6), and MMP-9 (Liu et al., 2018). *Ilex pubescens* herb, found mostly in the south of China, is used to treat cardiovascular disorders where it downregulates the production of NO and decreases the production of pro-inflammatory cytokines (IL-1ß, TNF-α). Moreover, it also enhances the Ca^{+2} dependent ATP enzyme activation (Peng et al., 2019). Herbs "*Qing Re Yao*" TCM medicine which is translated as the "medicine which removes heat," consists of 54 herbs that have anti-inflammatory activities or innate immune-modulating activity. The "*Qing Re Yao*" is effective against various types of inflammation related to the different organs, but it needs further investigation. This mixture of medicine acts on more than one inflammatory pathway. For instance, *Scutellaria baicalensis* has a role in the inhibition of iNOS, COX2, NF-κβ, and inflammatory cytokines (IL-1ß, IL-6, IL-12, and TNF-α). The combination therapy of "*Qing Re Yao*" showed a synergetic effect on inflammation-related diseases (Guan et al., 2018). *Wang-Bi* (WB) capsule, which consists of 17 herbal medicines including *Angelica pubescens, Climatis chinesis, Rehmannia glutinosa Libosch*, etc., therapeutic efficacy against Collagen-Induced Arthritis (CIA) in a mice model. The treatment of *Wang-Bi* shows that it decreases the inflammation of joints and prevents the destruction of bone marrow. Mechanism of action of *Wang-Bi* includes the inhibition of IL-1ß, IL-6, TNF-α, and NF-κβ (Cui et al., 2020). *Xiaoqinglong decoction* (XQLD) is a famous TCM formulation widely used in Asia with herbs like Pinellia Ternata, Liquorice root, and Chinese Magnolcavin Fruit, dried Ginger, White Paeony root, etc. are used for the treatment of chronic obstructive pulmonary disease (COPD). The oral administration of XQLD has several molecular and therapeutic effects like reduction in IL-4 and IL-5, promoting apoptosis, and downregulating p62 level (Zhen et al., 2018).

The role of Ayurveda in inflammation is also well documented. "*Divya Pidantaka Taila*" has a mixture of herbs, including the main ingredient Himalayan wildflower Roscoea alpine and other ingredients like *Aegle marmelos, R. cordifolia, B. aristata, P. zeylanica*, etc. are used for the treatment of inflammations, edema, and joint pain (Aggarwal et al., 2011). "*Daruharidra*" scientifically known as *Barberis aristata is well known for its anti-inflammatory activity and is* traditionally used by the tribes at Indian State Sikkim. It inhibits COX-2 and NF-κβ. Moreover, it also has anticancer activity, such as the inhibition of proliferation and invasion (Pandey et al., 2008). In Ayurvedic medicine, garlic extract (*Allium sativum*) is traditionally used for the cure of inflammation. A study reported that the extract of garlic could cure inflammation (e.g., bowel inflammation). The underlying mechanism of action involves inhibition of T-cell-mediated TH-1 cells and pro-inflammatory cytokines (IL-2, IL-6, IL-8, TNF-α), also upregulation of the anti-inflammatory cytokines, that is, IL-10 (Hodge et al., 2002). The Ayurvedic formulation "*Dashanga Ghana*" having ingredients of drugs like *Tagara, Sukshmaila, Haridra, Yashtimadhu, Kushta, Daruharidra, Shirisha,* and *Jatamamsi* has been reported to inhibit carrageenan-induced inflammation and formalin-induced inflammation in a rat model. Also, it has shown analgesic activity by modulating the opioid receptor or possibly by releasing endogenous analgesic factors (like endorphin), etc. (Ruknuddin et al., 2013). *Arjuna Ksheera Paka* (AKP), an Ayurvedic formulation composed of *Terminalia Arjuna,* has several therapeutic effects like cardioprotective and antioxidant activity. AKP shows dose-dependent anti-inflammatory activity in carrageenan-induced Paw edema. The stem bark of *T. arjuna* has several phytochemicals like terpenoids, tennis, flavonoids, saponin, etc. Also, AKP has milk protein, casein which enhances the bioavailability of AKP in vivo (Dube et al., 2016). *Divya Amvatari Ras* (DAR), traditional herbo-mineral medicine with more than six herbs, includes *Terminalia chebula, Terminalia bellirica, Plumbago zeylenica, Emblica officinalis, Ricinus communis*, and *Vachellia nilotica.* It also includes a herbal processed Sulphur and Mercury. It has also been reported to exhibit anti-arthritic and anti-inflammatory activity in collagen antibody-induced arthritis (CAIA). DAR treatments also downregulate pro-inflammatory cytokines (IL-6, TNF-α, COX-2, and NF-κβ in monocytes (THP-1)). Therefore, DAR with no adverse side effects could be used as a potential or alternative RA treatment (Balakrishna et al., 2019). Another polyherbal formulation *Guggulutiktaka ghritam* (GTG) is used as an Ayurvedic medicine to treat several chronic inflammations. GTG has several action mechanisms such as the suppression of pro-inflammatory cytokines (TNF-α, IL-1ß), lipoxygenase activity in controlling inflammation. Lupeol (*C. paniculatus*), piperine (*P. longum* and *P. nigrum*), rutin (*A. indica*), stigmasterol (*C. longa*), gallic acid (*A. indica*), piperlongumin (*P. longa*), and ferulic acid (*C. mukul*) is the bioactive molecules present in GTG (Mohan et al., 2019). Lupeol acts as a multi-target agent that exerts its anti-inflammatory, anti-arthritis, and anticancer effects by targeting molecular pathways like NF-κβ, PI3K/AKT Wnt/ß-catenin (Siddique et al., 2011). Piperine is an active alkaloid that shows prominent anti-inflammatory, anticancer, and immune-modulatory effects (Figures 13.2 and 13.3). Lutin and Stigmasterol can inhibit the proliferation, progression, and angiogenesis of cancer (Siddique et al., 2012). Phenolic acid-like galic acid and ferulic acid display great potential as cytotoxic anticancer agents, promoting apoptosis, targeting cell progression like angiogenesis and metastasis. It also displays epigenetic modulator properties (Abotaleb et al., 2020). *Ashwagandha* (*Withania somnifera*) is most commonly used in Ayurvedic medicine as an adaptogen known as "Indian *Ginseng*." The root of *Ashwagandha* consists of various alkaloids, flavonoids, and more than 40 withanolides. A recent study shows that *Ashwagandha* is used as an antioxidant and used to improve the body defense system and improve cell-mediated immunity. It also protects the cellular damage against free radicals and inhibits the pro-inflammatory cytokines. The antioxidant activity of *Ashwagandha* is due to the enhanced transport of Nrf2 to the nucleus, where it upregulates the expression of antioxidant enzymes (Farooqui et al., 2018). Ayurvedic medicine *Brahmi Gharita* which consist of the formulation of herbs like *Brahmi* (*Bacopa monnieri*), *Vaca* (*Acorus calamus*), old ghee (*Purana Gharita*), *Shankhphuphi* (*Convolvulus pluricaulis*), and *Kustha* (*Saussurea lappa*), have been used for various disorders like insomnia, remittent fever, as an anti-inflammatory and to enhance the memory. *Brahmi* found throughout the Indian subcontinent has a wide potential as a medicinal plant that acts as an analgesic, nootropic, and memory enhancer. The anti-inflammatory effect of "*Brahmi Gharita*" is due to Cynaropicrin (a sesquiterpene lactone) from *Saussurea lappa.* Cynaropicrin inhibits the production of inflammatory mediators like IL-2 and the proliferation of lymphocytes (Cho et al., 2000).

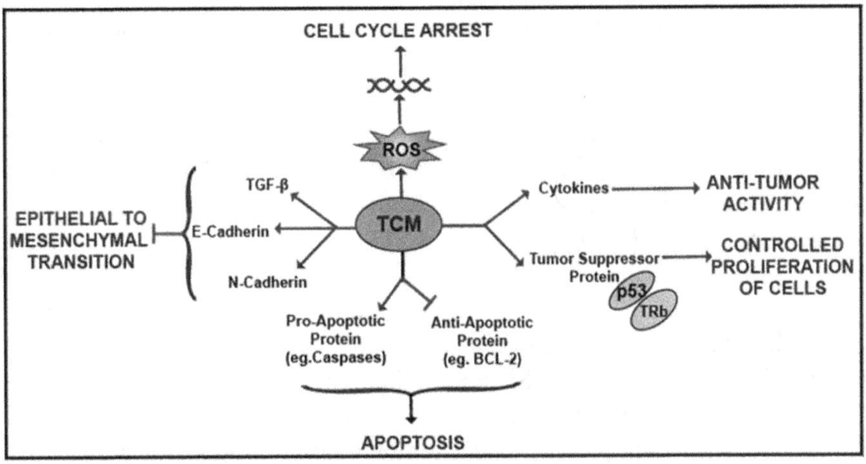

FIGURE 13.2 An illustration of the mechanism of anti-inflammatory action of TCM performed via attenuating or suppressing cell signaling and effector proteins.

13.4 ANTICANCER EFFECTS OF AYURVEDA/TCM AND NOVEL FORMULATIONS

The diagnosis and treatment have been discussed in the literature of ancient Chinese medicines like "The Yellow Emperor's Inner Canon" at cancer more than 2000 years ago. TCM has been shown to inhibit various cancer stages and has multiple molecular targets (Table 13.1). Hence, it improves the patient's life quality, health and also prevents recurrence and metastasis

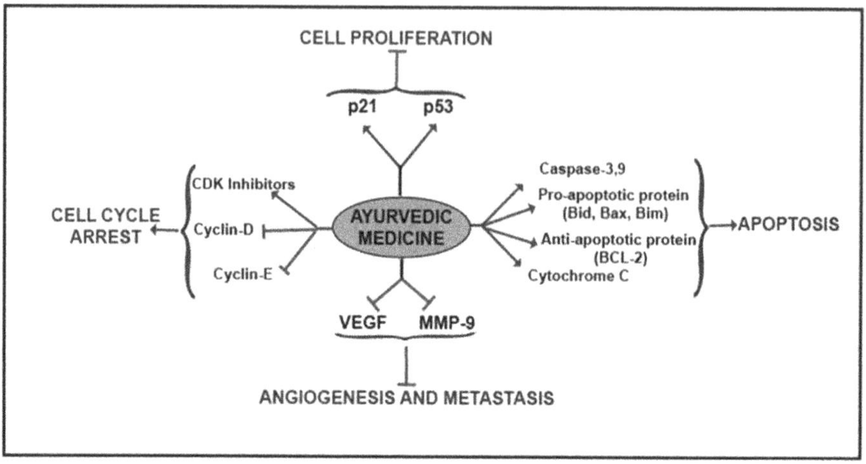

FIGURE 13.3 An illustration of the mechanism of the anticancer mechanism of action of Ayurvedic medicine.

(Liu et al., 2015). Moreover, TCM combined therapies have been shown to reduce the toxicity of chemotherapeutic drugs and enhance the potential of radiotherapy and chemotherapy. Treatment of cancer with TCM is either single herb-based (*Huang Qi, Ginseng, Chan Su,* etc.) or includes extracting various herbs. *Huang Qi* (*Radix astragali*), an ancient Chinese herb, has an immunomodulatory role. It activates immune cells like lymphocytes, NK-cells, macrophages, and their secretions like IL-6 and tumor necrosis factor (TNF). *Ginseng* (Ren Shen), another single herbal Chinese medicine, shows the modulation of the immune system and reduces the toxicity when combined with radiotherapy and chemotherapy. *Ginseng,* meaning "*man herb,*" comes from the Chinese word "*Jen Sheng,*" which has many species, namely *P. ginseng* and *P. quinquefolius* (American *Ginseng*). *Ginseng* is very effective against various types of cancers like liver, gastric, colon, and pancreatic cancer (Kao et al., 2001). *Ginseng* has various molecular targets, including activation of tumor suppressor proteins (p53, p21), retinoblastoma tumor suppressor protein dephosphorylation and activation, and pro-apoptotic proteins (Hofseth and Wargovich, 2007). *Ban Mao* (Mylabris), a single plant herb medicine, displays antitumor activity and inhibits cancerous cells' growth. The anticancer effect of Mylabris is due to various bioactive chemicals present in the herb, specially cantharidin which is extracted from the species *Mylabris phalerata* or *M. cichorii* (Liu and Chen, 2009). The Chinese herbal formulation *Shenqi Fuzheng* injection consisting of *Huang Qi* (*Radix Astragali*) and *Dang Shen* (*Codonopsis pilosula*) have been reported to show

TABLE 13.1 Anticancer Properties of Single/Mixed TCM Formulation and Related Herbs.

No	TCM	Cancer type	Herbs	Effects	Source
1	*Ginseng* (single)	Gastric cancer	*Panax ginseng* or *P. quinquefolius*	It inhibits cell growth and induces apoptosis	Hofseth and Wargovich (2007)
2	*Ban Mao* (single)	Hepatoma Oesophageal cancer	*Mylabris phalerata* or *M. cichorii*	Antitumor activity	Liu and Chen (2009)
3	*Shenqi Fuzheng*	Breast cancer	*Radix Astragali Codonopsis pilosula*	Antitumor activity, reduced toxicity induced by chemotherapy	Hoffman et al. (2020)
4	*Yangyinjiedu* (YYJD)	Lung cancer	*Radix Ophiopogonis* Five leaf *Gynostemma Astragalus, Paris polyphylla, glossy privet* fruit	The antiproliferative and pro-senescence effect, ROS-induced DNA damage	Zheng et al. (2017)
5	*Bu-Zhong-Yi-Qi-Tang* (BZYQT)	Hepatocarcinoma	*Radix Astragali Membranaceus, R. Ginseng, R. Angelicae, R. Bulpeuri, R. Glycyrrhizae, Rhizoma Zingiberis, Rhizoma Astractylodis, Rhizoma Astractylodis Macrocephalae, Pericarpium citripoonensis*	It inhibits cell growth and induces apoptosis	Kao et al. (2001)
6	*Realgar-Indigo-naturalis*	Promyelocytic leukemia	*Indigo naturalis* *Radix psudostellariae* *Salvia miltiorrhiza*	Induces cell cycle arrest, shows synergistic effect with ATI	Wang et al. (2008)
7	*Yanggan Jiedu Sanjie (YGJDSJ)*	Hepatocarcinoma	*Ligustrum lucidum, D. indica, S. nigrum, S. barbata, Euphorbia helioscopia, Ranunculus ternatus, C. wenyujin, Polygonum cuspidate*	Inhibits cancer progression, induces mesenchymal to epithelial morphology	Hu et al. (2019)
8	*Mio-Yi-Ai-Tang*	Lung cancer	*Solanum iyratum, Salviae chinensis, Hedyotis diffusa, Scutellaria barbata, Cephalotaxus fortunei, Fructus akebiae*	Anticancer activity, inhibits cell proliferation, synergistic effect with cisplatin	Li et al. (2020)

TABLE 13.1 *(Continued)*

No	TCM	Cancer type	Herbs	Effects	Source
9	*Fuzheng Qinggjie* granules (FZQJ)	Hepatocellular carcinoma	*Astragalus membranaceus, Ganoderma lucidum, Ligustrum lucidum, Rhizoma dioscoreae, Hedyotis diffusa, Prunella vulgaris*	Acts as adjuvant in chemotherapy, Enhances anticancer activity of CTX	Chen et al. (2017)
10	Herbal formulation	Breast cancer	*Camellia sinesis, Hedyotis diffusa, Andrographis paniculata, Acanthopanax senticosus*	Inhibits tumor progression and metastasis Prevents osteolysis	Yue et al. (2018)

promising anticancer effects, improved tumor response, and reduction in the toxicity induced by chemotherapy. It enhances immune cells like T-lymphocytes and NK-cells (Hoffman et al., 2020). *Bu-Zhong-Yi-Qi-Tang* (BZYQT) is another Chinese formulation composed mainly of glycyrrhizin, astragaloside IV, and ginsenosides RB1 and Rg1, and saikosaponin a and c. BZYQT has multiple molecular targets that exhibit cell cycle arrest (G0/G1), DNA fragmentation, and apoptosis in hepatocarcinoma cells HepG2, Hep3B, and HA22T cells (Kao et al., 2001). Chinese formulation *Realgar-Indigo naturalis,* which principally consists of *Indigo naturalis, Radix psudostellariae, Salvia miltiorrhiza,* and ATI (tetraarsenic tetrasulfide, tanshione, Indirubin), shows therapeutic efficacy against promyelocytic leukemia, a disease characterized by immature promyelocytes accumulation in the bone marrow and chromosomal translocation. ATI shows a synergistic effect and induces cell cycle arrest at G_0/G_1 phase in APL cells and led to the hypo-phosphorylation of Rb (Wang et al., 2008). Another TCM is *Yangyinjiedu* (YYJD), which has optimized five herbal ingredients, namely *Radix ophiopogonis, Fiveleaf gynostemma, Astragalus, Paris polyphylla,* and Glossy Privet Fruit, which shows antiproliferative and pro-senescence effect in lung cancer cells. YYJD exerts its effect by inducing ROS generation, DNA damage, cell cycle arrest at the G2/M phase, and colony formation of lung cancer cells (Zheng et al., 2017). Yue et al. (2018) formulated an innovative herbal formulation to investigate anti-metastatic, anti-angiogenic, and immune-modulatory effects against breast cancer in a mouse model. The herbal formula consists of four herbs, that is, *Camellia sinensis, Hedyotis diffusa, Andrographis paniculata,* and *Acanthopanax senticosus*. The formulation exhibits a reduction in breast tumor size and metastasis and has bone protective effects, that is, osteolysis. It has also been reported to modulate immune CD^{+8} T-cells, Treg-cells, and MDSC (myeloid-derived suppressor cell) population in the immune-competent model upregulates the antitumor cytokine IL-12 (Yue et al., 2018). *Yanggan Jiedu Sanjie* (YGJDSJ) has demonstrated its inhibitory effects on epithelial-mesenchymal transition and inhibition of cancer progression in human hepatocarcinoma (Bcl-7402) cells. The herbal formulation reportedly reversed the TGF-ß1 induced morphology, that is, mesenchymal to epithelial morphology, by upregulating the E-cadherin and inhibiting the N-cadherin. The SMAD3 phosphorylation and snail expression have also been inhibited by YGJDSJ (Hu et al., 2019). *Mio-Yi-Ai-Tang*, a Chinese herbal formulation consisting of six herbs, that is, *Solanum iyratum, Herba salviae chinensis, Hedyotis diffusa, Scutellaria barbata, Cephalotaxus fortunei,* and *Fructus akebiae* has been shown to inhibit cell proliferation and induce apoptosis in case of lung cancer. It has synergistic effects with the therapeutic drug cisplatin when given in combination. The treatment of both drugs showed an enhancement in the percentage of cells in the S and G2 phase of the cell cycle, suggesting their similar action mechanisms. Miao and cisplatin synergistically inhibit ß-catenin and AXIN, which further inhibits transcription of C-MYC (Li et al., 2020). TCM practitioners often used Fuzheng Guben herbs like Ganodorma, Fructus lycii, Ginseng species, and A. membranaceous, strengthening the immune system via the activation of B-cells T-cells, NK-cell, macrophages, and enhancement in the production of cytokines and it also prevents the cyclophosphamide-induced bone marrow damage. Whereas the *Qingre Jiedu* herbs like *Hedyotis diffusa*, *Lobelia chinensis* Lour, *Prunella vulgaris,* etc., have a role in the inhibition of cell proliferation angiogenesis. *Fuzheng Qinggjie* granules (FZQJ), a combination of two traditional herbs, that is, *Fuzheng Guben* and *Qingre Jiedu,* has been reported to enhance the anticancer activity of cyclophosphamide and also alleviates the cyclophosphamide-induced decrease of WBC and platelets. Further, it also increases CD^{3+} and CD^{4+} T-lymphocytes. Hence, FZQJ serves as a potential adjuvant during radiotherapy or chemotherapy (Chen et al., 2017).

Ayurvedic medicines in cancer treatment are widely studied as conventional and alternative medicine. The studies demonstrated that Ayurvedic medicine has a great potential to treat cancer and reduce chemotherapeutic drugs' side effects (Table 13.2). Herbo-mineral and metallic Ayurvedic formulation *Mauktikyukta Kamdudha* (MKD) having immunity booster properties; "*Mauktikyukta Praval Panchamruta*" (MPP) and *Suvarnabhasmdi* (SBD), which are known to reduce stress-induced depression, improve digestion and immunity, etc. These medicines were reported to show reduced toxicity and improved cancer patient lifespan treated with chemotherapeutic drugs. Thus, the combination of Ayurvedic medicine has no adverse effect on a chemotherapeutic drug's anticancer activity (Deshmukh et al., 2014). Garlic extract (*Allium sativum*) has been shown to inhibit cancer progression. In vitro studies on leukemia cells have shown the antiproliferative effect of garlic compound, Ajoene. Ajoene induces mitochondria-dependent apoptosis, leading to the activation of a cascade of Caspases and enhancing their activity like enhancement in the activity of Caspases-3, the release of Cytochrome c, and downregulation in the anti-apoptotic proteins like BCL-2 (Dirsch et al., 1998). *Arkeshwara Rasa* (AR), which contains a mixture of plant herbs including *Terminalia belerica*, *T. chebula*, *Phyllanthus emblica*, *Plumbago zeylanica*, and *Calotropis procera,* etc. and Mercuric Sulphide (HgS), shows an anticancer activity against pancreatic cancer

TABLE 13.2 Therapeutic Effects of Some Ayurvedic Herbs/Medicine in Various Cancer Types.

Ayurvedic medicine	Cancer type	Mechanism of action	Source
Arkeshwara Rasa	Pancreatic cancer	Inhibits cell growth, enhances lactate dehydrogenase (LDH) enzyme	Nafiujjaman et al. (2015)
Tulsi (Vrinda)	Lung cancer	Induces mitochondrial-dependent apoptosis, activation of caspases 3, 9 and cytochrome c release, downregulates anti-apoptotic protein Bcl-2	Magesh et al. (2009)
Triphala	Breast cancer Gynecological cancer	Reduces cell growth and induces apoptosis, Induction of ROS and DNA damage, antiproliferative activity Downregulation of PI3K/Akt/mTOR- NF-κβ /p53 pathway	Sandhya et al. (2006), Zhao et al. (2018)
Garlic extract	Leukemia	Antiproliferative effect and induces mitochondrial-dependent apoptosis, Enhancement of caspase 3, release of cytochrome c, downregulation of Bcl-2	Dirsch et al. (1998)
Amla	Ovarian cancer	Induces autophagy independent of apoptosis Inhibits NF-κβ signaling	Zhao et al. (2015)
Ashwagandha	Lung cancer Prostate cancer Breast cancer	Reduces cell growth and Induces apoptosis Upregulates the p53 expression Downregulation of anti-apoptotic protein Bcl-2	Palliyaguru et al. (2016)
Turmeric	Lung cancer	Induces apoptosis and inhibits angiogenesis and metastasis Upregulates pro-apoptotic protein Downregulates MMP-9 and VEGF	Wilken et al. (2011)
Licorice root	NSCLC	Induces apoptosis Enhances expression of caspase and cleavage of PARP. Attenuated the expression of Cyclin D1 and cyclin E	Kangsamaksin et al. (2017)

cells (MIA-PaCa-2) (Nafiujjaman et al., 2015). *Tulsi* (*Ocimum sanctum*), also called *Vrinda,* "Mother medicine of nature," also has lots of medicinal properties. Various bioactive molecules are present in *Ocimum sanctum* like flavonoids, eugenol, and Linolenic acid, which have antiproliferative and anticancer activities. Apigenin, one of the flavonoids present in the Tulsi plant, has wide anti-cancerous effects and inhibits various key cell signaling pathways in abnormal proliferative cells (Singh et al. 2019). The DMBA-induced skin papillomas in mice treated with *Ocimum sanctum* inhibit chemical-induced carcinogenesis and their metabolic activation (Prashar et al., 1998). Ethanol-extract of *Ocimum sanctum* (EEOS) shows anticancer activity in lung carcinoma A549 cells. The underlying basis of cytotoxicity involves cleavage of poly (ADP-ribose) polymerase (PARP), mitochondria-dependent apoptosis by activating Caspase-9 and Caspase-3, the release of Cytochrome c, and an increase in the ratio of pro-apoptotic protein (BAX) to anti-apoptotic proteins (BCL-2). Moreover, EEOS inhibits the AKT and ERK pathways (Magesh et al., 2009). *Brahma Rasayana* (BRM) and *Chyavanaprash* (CHM) also show protective effects against doxorubicin-induced cardiotoxicity. The combinational treatment prevents the release of lactate dehydrogenase (LDH), creatine-kinase-MB (CK-MB), and glutamic oxaloacetic transaminase (GOT) from mitochondria which arises after the doxorubicin treatment. It thus prevents the free radical induced-dox damage, thereby improving the chemotherapeutic drug's efficacy (Suhailbani et al. 2016). *Triphala* is an Ayurvedic formulation constituting dried fruit powder of three plants: *Terminalis chebula* (chebulic myrobalan), *Emblica officinalis* also known as Indian gooseberry *Terminalia belerica (*Bedda nut tree*)*. This herbal *Terminalis chebula* has many bioactive compounds like chebulin, gallic acid, terflavin, luteolin, tannic acid, and other flavonoids and alkaloids, whereas *P. emblica* is having compounds like quercetin (well known for its anticancer activity), tannins, gallic acid, other flavonoids and vitamin C (Prasad and Srivastava, 2020). *Triphala*, also known as "*Bras Bu gSum Thang*" in Tibetan medicine, has a diverse composition and includes polyphenols, flavonoids, glycosides, phenolic acid, sterols, amino acid, and fatty acids, etc.

Triphala's role is well studied in promoting health and immunity enhancement; however, recent studies demonstrated its potential toward anti-inflammatory, anti-mutagenic, and anticancer effects. *Triphala* has also shown its therapeutic efficacy in various cancer types, including breast, pancreas, prostate, cervical cancer, etc. (Prasad and Srivastava, 2020). The selective cytotoxicity of *Triphala* has been demonstrated by Sandhya et al. (2006), where a similar concentration of *Triphala* reduces cell growth and induces apoptosis underlying enhanced ROS generation and DNA damage in MCF-7 and barcl-95 cell lines. In contrast, it does not cause any cytotoxicity in normal breast epithelial cells (Sandhya et al., 2006). In another study, *Triphala* showed antiproliferative and anticancer activity by elevating BAX/BCL-2, downregulating c-MYC, and cyclin D1 expression (Vadde et al., 2015). The antiproliferative activity of *Triphala* against female reproductive cancer involves the dysregulation of some important mitogenic pathways like P13K/Akt/mTOR, MAPK/ERK, and NF-κβ /p53 pathways (Zhao et al., 2018).

Amla (Indian Gooseberry) is originally native to India and is widely used to make pickles and dishes as a vegetable. *Amla,* scientifically known as *Phyllanthus emblica*, has been used for the treatment of cancer. The fruit of *Phyllanthus emblica* contains various polyphenols, tannin derived compounds, and it shows antiproliferative and anticancer activity by inducing autophagy-related pathways independent of the apoptotic pathways in ovarian cancer cells and also by inhibiting NF-κβ (Zhao et al., 2015). Ashwagandha (*Withania somnifera*) is an ancient medicine used as an adaptogen, that is, it helps fight body stress and has also demonstrated anticancer properties. Out of 23 species of *Withania*, only two species, namely *W. somnifera* and *W. coagulan*, have medicinal properties. Leaf extract of Aswagandha exerts anticancer effects by upregulating the tumor suppressor p53 or enhancing the expression of anti-apoptotic protein BCL-2 (Palliyaguru et al., 2016). Turmeric (*Curcuma longa)* has long been used as Ayurvedic medicine for centuries and has diverse physiological effects, including antioxidant, anti-inflammatory, antiseptic, and anticancer. Curcumin, which is a main bioactive compound, is responsible for these effects. Curcumin has been proven to have anticancer activities like arresting cell cycle by enhancing the expression of CDK inhibitors, Cyclin D, Cyclin E expression or inducing apoptosis by upregulating pro-apoptotic protein (BAX, BAD, and BIM) or inhibiting angiogenesis and metastasis by inhibiting the expression of VEGF, MMP-9 protein (Wilken et al., 2011; Kangsamaksin et al., 2017).

Licorice (*Glycyrrhiza glabra)* is the oldest herbal plant used to treat various diseases like allergic reactions, antioxidant, anti-inflammatory conditions. The root extract of Licorice shows potential cytotoxic effects in various cancers due to various bioactive compounds, including glycyrrhetic acid (GA), phenolic acid, and various flavones. Various mechanisms like induction of apoptosis exert the therapeutic potential by arresting the cell cycle at the G1 phase and attenuating the expression of cyclin D1, cyclin

E, enhancing the caspase activity and cleavage of poly (ADP-ribosyl) polymerase (PARP) in the case of NSCLC cells (Song et al., 2014).

Neem (*Azadirachta indica*) is one of the traditional herbs used to treat various diseases. This Ayurvedic herb consists of many biologically active compounds like nimbolide, limnoids, and azadirachtin, which shows marked anticancer activities by inhibiting cell proliferation and induction of apoptosis, inhibiting angiogenesis, and metastasis, scavenging free radicals and suppressing various oncogenic signaling pathways (Moga et al., 2018). The mechanism of apoptosis by Neem extract involves the enhancement of pro-apoptotic proteins (BIM, BAD) and PTEN expression. Moreover, it inhibits angiogenesis by inhibiting angiopoietin and vascular endothelial growth factor-A (VEGF-A) (Arumugam et al., 2014). Azadirachtin has been shown to arrest the cell cycle by downregulating Cyclin B, Cyclin D1 and enhances the expression of p21 in HeLa cells, whereas nimbolide enhances the expression of caspases and inhibits anti-apoptotic protein survivin (Hao et al., 2014).

13.5 AYURVEDA AND TCM IN OTHER DISEASES

A number of plant species (approximately 12,000) with numerous medicinal properties have been categorized into Ayurveda. The benefits and importance of these plants have been mentioned in more than 200 books including, 57 *Nighantus*, 140 *Vyakhyas*, and 6 *Samhitas*, and codified into the morphological description (*Rupa gnana*), pharmacy (*Bhaishajya kalpana*), and pharmacology (*Dravya guna shastra*) (Thomas et al., 2020). It has been observed that Ayurveda has great implications in malnutrition-related problems and various other disorders. "*Swarna bindu prashana*" (SBP), a metallic preparation of medicines, is widely used in Ayurveda. The main components of SBP are "*Swarna prashan*" (gold nanoparticle), "*Madhu*" (honey), "*Gou ghrita*" (cow ghee), and other "*Medhya dravyas*" (memory booster). SBP can be used in vaccine development and immunotherapies because of its shape, size, surface, functionality, and charges. Furthermore, the role of SBP has been identified in dendritic cell maturation and T-cell activation (Nelaturi et al., 2020). Ayurveda is used in tissue nutrition, which is a continuous process after conception and persists till death. Tissue nutrition is different in all phases of life (Agrawal et al., 2020). Recently, the ministry of AYUSH (Government of India) recommended "*Ayush Kwath*" having basil, cinnamon, ginger, and black pepper to improve innate immunity for combating the infection COVID-19, a pandemic disease spread in December 2019 due to the virus SARS-CoV-2.

Marich, *Tulsi*, Sunthi, and *Dalchini* are easily available and commonly used as drugs at home. *Ayush Kwath,* with these ingredients, has antiviral, immune-modulatory, antioxidant, anti-platelet, anti-inflammatory, anti-atherosclerotic, reno-protective, and hepato-protective properties (Gautam et al., 2020). Further, this polyherbal formulation's preclinical and clinical trials need to be done to evaluate its efficacy and safety. The role of *Withania somnifera* (Ashwagandha) is explained in *Susruta Samhita, Charaka Samhita,* and other ancient texts as "*Balya*" (increases strength), "*Vajikari*" (spermatogenic), "*Brusya*" (sexual performance enhancer), "*Kamarupini*" (libido-enhancing), "*Pustida*" (nourishing). Later, the role of *Ashwagandha* is also reported in the treatment of anxiety and some other central nervous system (CNS) disorders (Mukherjee et al., 2020). *Aucklandia costus Falc.* is a native of the Himalayan region and has been recommended to treat leukoderma, kidney, liver, blood disorders, Qi stagnation, and *tridosha.* The oral intake of root and powder of *A. costus* with warm water can cure gastric diseases. Further, the powder of *A. costus* has been reported to have a significant effect against blisters, skin to cure boils, and leprosy (Nadda et al., 2020). Ayurveda medicines significantly affect acetylcholinesterase expression, oxidation products, β-amyloid senile plaques, inflammatory pathways, specific brain receptors involved in Alzheimer's disease (AD) (Calfio et al., 2020).

The main goal of TCM was to get balanced nutrition providing all the nutrients to achieve balance and harmony within the body (Zhao et al., 2020). "Scoparone," an ingredient of *Artemisia capillaris Thunb*, is useful in treating cholestasis, hepatic dysfunction, and jaundice for over 1000 years. Recently, it has been found that Scoparone also has antioxidant, anti-inflammatory, anti-apoptotic, hypolipidemic, and anti-fibrotic properties. Scoparone has a potential against various liver diseases like acute liver injury, alcohol-induced hepatotoxicity, fulminant hepatitis, non-alcoholic fatty liver disease, and fibrosis (Hui et al., 2020). Recently, it has been observed that TCM also plays an important role in Addison's disease (AD) through altering the gut microbiota (GM) (Sun et al., 2020). Further, TCM has been found to play an important role in many allergic diseases. *Glycyrrhizae Radix et Rhizoma* is known as one of the popular herbal drugs in China and has a potential for various medicinal purposes due to its water-soluble side-chain nonpolar saponins. *Aurantii Fructus* (AF) and *Aurantii Fructus Immaturus* (AFI), used as herbal medicines in China, are widely employed in treating various liver diseases with high morbidity and mortality rates. Various ingredients have been isolated from AFI and AF, including flavonoids, alkaloids, volatile oils, and coumarins (Wu et al., 2020). *Rhubarb,* also known as "*Rhei* or *Dahuang,*" one of the most primitive and important medicinal plants in China, belongs to the Polygonaceae family, from 270 BC in "*Shen Nong Ben Cao Jing.*" *Rhubarb* has a potential against bacterial, inflammatory, cancer, anti-fibrotic diseases. To enhance the effects of TCM, the use of micro/nanomaterials, which are capable of adsorption and sensing due to their chemical and physical properties, has been encouraged (Xiang et al., 2020). They are classified based on micro/nano-adsorbents, matrix materials into the following categories: porous materials, metal-based micro/nanomaterials, carbon-based materials, hybrid micro/nanomaterials, and graphene/graphite-liked micro/nanomaterials (Qian and Kai, 2020). *Xuebijing* (XBJ) injection, which is a Chinese injection consisting of *Carthamus tinctorius* L. (*Carthami Flos, hong hua, Asteraceae*), *Ligusticum chuanxiong* Hort. (*Chuanxiong Rhizoma, Chuan xiong, Umbelliferae*), *Angelica sinensis* (Oliv.) Diels (*Angelicae sinensis Radix, dang gui, Umbelliferae*), *Paeonia lactiflora* Pall. (*Paeoniae radix rubra, chi shao, Ranunculaceae*) *Salvia miltiorrhiza* Bge. (*Salviae miltiorrhizae Radix Et Rhizoma, Dan shen, Labiatae*) have been widely used for the treatment of sepsis in China with few side effects (Li et al., 2020).

Interestingly, Ayurveda and Chinese medicines are non or less toxic on a normal cell. It has been shown that taking these medicines along with other medicines or western drugs shows synergistic effects. *Curculigo orchiodies* significantly normalize the hyperglycemia-induced oxidative stress, lipid profile and normalize the renal functions (Singla and Singh, 2020). In another report, it has been shown that Ayurveda, combined with drugs, improves the quality and quantity of semen and reduces anxiety. In a clinical trial, it has been observed that TCM along with Ultrasound subgingival scaling shows synergetic effects in chronic periodontitis of elderly patients. Dexamethasone and Carnosine were found to show synergetic effects compared to when given alone and minimize seawater inhalation in a rat model's lung. *Progynova* combined with *Dingkun Dan* was also found to improve endometrial receptivity via the upregulation of VEGF mRNA, β-catenin, and downregulation of MMP-9 mRNA the injured rats (Vasudevan et al., 2020).

It has also been found that these medicines can be taken with nanoformulations, which is more effective. *Triphala,* which is an Ayurvedic medicine, is widely used for different microbial infections. The hydrogel containing nanoemulsion and a cream formulation has been prepared using Ayurvedic drugs to assess the antimicrobial activity (Omran et al., 2020). A number of injections have been made to boost the effects and directly inject the medicines into the body's blood. In a study conducted on Oesophageal cancer (OC), it has been found that Kang-ai injection and conventional treatment were helpful in patients. *Ciwujia* injection has been reported to act on anticoagulation, concurrent diseases, strengthening the mind's body, and regulation (Sun et al., 2020). Intraperitoneal injection of *Fengbaisan* combined with EX527 was effective against chronic obstructive pulmonary diseases (COPD) by altering the SIRT1 expression and inhibition of exoplasmic reticulum stress. In the future, studies and researches on TCM and Ayurveda may expand due to various studies; some of them have been mentioned above.

13.6 CONCLUSIONS AND FUTURE PERSPECTIVES

Preclinical and clinical trials show that TCM and Ayurveda may help to treat cancer and inflammatory diseases. Various promising results have been shown in clinical studies, but solid conclusions are yet to be drawn from them. Various useful effects have already been documented about TCM and Ayurveda, and many effects are ready to be sent to clinical trials. Studies are governing Ayurveda and TCM's role in altering the signaling pathways involved in the pathogenesis of cancer initiation, progression, and metastasis. TCM and Ayurveda may be promising therapeutic agents taking via. Nano-formulation, and along with drugs/phytochemicals to combat different cancer types. These approaches enhance the bioavailability of Ayurveda and Chinese medicines to the cells and exert synergistic effects. There are many traditional medicines present around us, and we still don't know about their role in cancer or any other diseases. Many researchers worldwide are focusing on TCM and Ayurveda and observing their role against various diseases. In the future, it may be possible that the use of TCM and Ayurveda along with a drug or other agent will be an excellent agent to fight against the different types of cancer.

ACKNOWLEDGMENTS

The authors are thankful to the Department of Zoology, AMU, Aligarh for providing necessary laboratory facilities. MAK expresses their sincere gratitude to CSIR, India, for Fellowships. HRS is thankful to the UGC [Grant No. F.30-377/2017(BSR)] and DST-SERB (Grant No. EMR/2017/001758), New Delhi, for providing financial help.

KEYWORDS

- **Ayurveda**
- **cancer**
- **chemotherapy**
- **Chinese herbs**
- **targeting pathways**

REFERENCES

Abotaleb, M.; Liskova, A.; Kubatka, P.; Büsselberg, D. Therapeutic Potential of Plant Phenolic Acids in the Treatment of Cancer. *Biomolecules* **2020,** *10*, 221.

Aggarwal, B. B.; Prasad, S.; Reuter, S.; Kannappan, R.; Yadav, V.; Park, B.; Kim, J.; Gupta, S. C.; Phromnoi, K.; Sundaran, C.; Prasad, S.; Chaturvedi, M. M.; Sung, B. Identification of Novel Anti-Inflammatory Agents from Ayurvedic Medicine for Prevention of Chronic Diseases: "Reverse Pharmacology" and "Bedside to Bench" Approach. *Curr. Drug Targets* **2011,** *12*, 1595–1653.

Agrawal, S.; Verma, V.; Gehlot, S. Explication on Tissue Nutrition in Prenatal and Postnatal Life: An Ayurveda Perspective. *J. Ayurveda Integr. Med.* **2020.**

Amarante-Mendes, G. P.; Adjemian, S.; Branco, L. M.; Zanetti, L. C.; Weinlich, R.; Bortoluci, K. R.; Pattern Recognition Receptors and the Host Cell Death Molecular Machinery. *Front. Immunol.* **2018,** *9*, 2379.

Arumugam, A.; Agullo, P.; Boopalan, T.; Nandy, S.; Lopez, R.; Gutierrez, C.; Narayan, M.; Rajkumar, L. Neem Leaf Extract Inhibits Mammary Carcinogenesis by Altering Cell Proliferation, Apoptosis, and Angiogenesis. *Cancer. Biol. Ther.* **2014,** *15*, 26–34.

Balakrishna, A.; Varshney, A.; Paudel, S.; Joshi, K.; Sakat, S.; Joshi, D.; Joshi, K.; Ranjan, R.; Gupta, A.; Bhattacharya, K.; Varshney, A. Anti-Inflammatory and Anti-Arthritic Efficacies of an Indian Traditional Herbo-Mineral Medicine 'Divya Amvatari Ras' in Collagen Antibody-Induced Arthritis (CAIA) Mouse Model Through Modulation of IL-6/IL-1β/TNF-α/NFκB Signaling. *Front. Pharmacol.* **2019,** *10*, 659.

Baylin, S. B.; Jones, P. A. Epigenetic Determinants of Cancer. *Cold Spring Harb. Perspect. Biol.* **2016,** *8*, a019505.

Bray, F.; Ferlay, J.; Soerjomataram, I.; Siegel, R. L.; Torre, L. A.; Jemal, A. Global Cancer Statistics 2018: GLOBOCAN Estimates of Incidence and Mortality Worldwide for 36 Cancers in 185 Countries. *CA Cancer J. Clin.* **2018,** *68*, 394–424.

Calfio, C.; Gonzalez, A.; Singh, S. K.; Rojo, L. E.; Maccioni, R. B. The Emerging Role of Nutraceuticals and Phytochemicals in the Prevention and Treatment of Alzheimer's Disease. *J. Alzheimers Dis*. **2020,** *10*, 3233.

Chen, L.; Deng, H.; Cui, H.; Fang, J.; Zuo, Z.; Deng, J.; Li, Y.; Wang, X.; Zhao, L. Inflammatory Responses and Inflammation-Associated Diseases in Organs. *Oncotarget* **2018,** *9*, 7204.

Chen, X. Z.; Cao, Z. Y.; Zhang, Y. Q.; Li, J. N.; Liao, L. M.; Du, J. Fuzheng Qingjie Granules Potentiate the Anti-Cancer Effect of Cyclophosphamide by Regulating Cellular Immune Function and Inducing Apoptosis in Hepatoma 22 Tumor-Bearing Mice. *Oncol. Lett.* **2017,** *13*, 3261–3268.

Cho, J. Y.; Baik, K. U.; Jung, J. H.; Park, M. H. In Vitro Anti-Inflammatory Effects of Cynaropicrin, a Sesquiterpene Lactone, from Saussurea lappa. *Eur. J. Pharmacol.* **2000,** *398*, 399–407.

Cui, H.; Shu, H.; Fan, D.; Wang, X.; Zhao, N.; Lu, C.; Lu, A.; He, X. Wang-Bi Capsule Alleviates the Joint Inflammation and Bone Destruction in Mice with Collagen-Induced Arthritis. *Evid. Based Complement. Altern. Med.* **2020,** 1015083.

Deshmukh, V.; Kulkarni, A.; Bhargava, S.; Patil, T.; Ramdasi, V.; Gangal, S.; Gatar, S.; Godse, V.; Datar, S.; Gujar, S.; Sardeshmukh, S. Effectiveness of Combinations of Ayurvedic Drugs in Alleviating Drug Toxicity and Improving Quality of Life of Cancer Patients Treated with Chemotherapy. *Supportive Care Cancer* **2014,** *22*, 3007–3015.

Dirsch, V. M.; Gerbes, A. L.; Vollmar, A. M. Ajoene, a Compound of Garlic, Induces Apoptosis in Human Promyeloleukemic Cells, Accompanied by Generation of Reactive Oxygen Species and Activation of Nuclear Factor kappaB. *Mol. Pharmacol.* **1998,** *53*, 402–407.

Dube, N.; Nimgulkar, C.; Bharatraj, D. K. Validation of Therapeutic Anti-Inflammatory Potential of Arjuna Ksheera Paka—A Traditional Ayurvedic Formulation of Terminalia Arjuna. *J. Tradit. Complement Med.* **2016,** *7*, 414–420.

Farooqui, A. A.; Farooqui, T.; Madan, A.; Ong, J. H.; Ong, W. Y. Ayurvedic Medicine for the Treatment of Dementia: Mechanistic Aspects. *Evid. Based Complement. Alternat. Med.* **2018,** 2481076.

Fatma, H.; Santosh, S.; Siddique, H. R. Epigenetic Modifications of c-MYC: Role in Cancer Cell Reprogramming, Progression and Chemoresistance. *Semin. Cancer Biol.* **2020**.

Ferrero-Miliani, L.; Nielsen, O. H.; Andersen, P. S.; Girardin, S. E. Chronic Inflammation: Importance of NOD2 and NALP3 in Interleukin-1beta Generation. *Clin. Exp. Immunol.* **2007,** *147*, 227–235.

Fouad, Y. A.; Aanei, C. Revisiting the Hallmarks of Cancer. *Am J. Cancer Res.* **2017,** *7*, 1016–1036.

Gautam, S.; Gautam, A.; Chhetri, S.; Bhattarai, U. Immunity Against COVID-19: Potential Role of Ayush Kwath [Published Online Ahead of Print, 2020 Aug 17]. *J. Ayurveda Integr. Med.* **2020**.

Guan, F.; Lam, W.; Hu, R.; Kim, Y. K.; Han, H.; Cheng, Y. C. Majority of Chinese Medicine Herb Category "Qing Re Yao" Have Multiple Mechanisms of Anti-Inflammatory Activity. *Sci. Rep.* **2018,** *8*, 1–1.

Hanahan, D.; Weinberg, R. A. Hallmarks of Cancer: The Next Generation. *Cell* **2011,** *144*, 646–674.

Hao, F.; Kumar, S.; Yadav, N.; Chandra, D. Neem components as Potential Agents for Cancer Prevention and Treatment. *Biochimica et Biophysica Acta* **2014,** *1846*, 247–257.

Heinrich, M.; Barnes, J.; Gibbons, S.; Williamson, E. *Fundamentals of Pharmacognosy and Phytopharmacy*, 2004.

Henríquez-Olguín, C.; Altamirano, F.; Valladares, D.; López, J. R.; Allen, P. D.; Jaimovich, E. Altered ROS Production, NF-κB Activation and Interleukin-6 Gene Expression Induced by Electrical Stimulation in Dystrophic MDX Skeletal Muscle Cells. *Biochim Biophys Acta* **2015,** *185*, 1410–1419.

Hodge, G.; Hodge, S.; Han, P. *Allium sativum* (Garlic) Suppresses Leukocyte Inflammatory Cytokine Production In Vitro: Potential Therapeutic Use in the Treatment of Inflammatory Bowel Disease. *Cytometry* **2002,** *48*, 209–215.

Hoffman, R. D.; Li, C. Y.; He, K.; Wu, X.; He, B. C.; He, T. C.; Gao, J. L. Chinese Herbal Medicine and Its Regulatory Effects on Tumor Related T-Cells. *Front. Pharmacol.* **2020,** *11*, 492.

Hofseth, L. J.; Wargovich, M. J. Inflammation, Cancer, and Targets of Ginseng. *J. Nutr.* **2007,** *137*, 183S–185S. https://www.who.int/news-room/fact-sheets/detail/cancer

Hu, B.; An, H. M.; Yan, X.; Zheng, J. L.; Huang, X. W.; Li, M. Traditional Chinese Medicine Formulation Yanggan Jiedu Sanjie inhibits TGF-β1-Induced Epithelial-Mesenchymal Transition and Metastatic Potential in Human Hepatocarcinoma Bel-7402 Cells. *BMC Complement. Altern. Med.* **2019,** *19*, 67.

Hua, Q.; Zhu, X. L.; Li, P. T.; Liu, Y.; Zhang, N.; Xu, Y.; Jia, X. The Inhibitory Effects of Cholalic Acid and Hyodeoxycholalic Acid on the Expression of TNFα and IL-1β After Cerebral Ischemia in Rats. *Arch. Pharma. Res.* **2009,** *32*, 65–73.

Hui, Y.; Wang, X.; Yu, Z.; Fan, X.; Cui, B.; Zhao, T.; Mao, L.; Feng, H.; Lin, L.; Yu, Q.; Zhang, J.; Wang, B.; Chen, X.; Zhao, X.; Sun, C. Scoparone as a Therapeutic Drug in Liver Diseases: Pharmacology, Pharmacokinetics and Molecular Mechanisms of Action. *Pharmacol. Res.* **2020,** *160*, 105170.

Jaiswal, Y. S.; Williams, L. L. A Glimpse of Ayurveda—The Forgotten History and Principles of Indian Traditional Medicine. *J. Tradit. Complement Med.* **2017,** *7*, 50–53.

Kangsamaksin, T.; Chaithongyot, S.; Wootthichairangsan, C.; Hanchaina, R.; Tangshewinsirikul, C.; Svasti, J.; Lupeol and Stigmasterol Suppress Tumor Angiogenesis and Inhibit Cholangiocarcinoma Growth in Mice Via Downregulation of Tumor Necrosis Factor-α. *PLoS One* **2017,** *12*, e0189628.

Kao, S. T.; Yeh, C. C.; Hsieh, C. C.; Yang, M. D.; Lee, M. R.; Liu, H. S.; Lin, J. G. The Chinese Medicine Bu-Zhong-Yi-Qi-Tang Inhibited Proliferation of Hepatoma Cell Lines by Inducing Apoptosis via G0/G1 Arrest. *Life Sci.* **2001,** *69*, 1485–1496.

Khan, M. A.; Singh, D.; Siddique, H. R. Animal Models in Cancer Chemoprevention. *Int. J. Zoo. Anim.* **2019,** *2*, 000171.

Kumar, S.; Dobos, G. J.; Rampp, T.; The Significance of Ayurvedic Medicinal Plants. *J. Evid. Based Complem. Altern. Med.* **2017,** *22*, 494–501.

Lewandowska, A. M.; Rudzki, M.; Rudzki, S.; Lewandowski, T.; Laskowska, B. Environmental Risk Factors for Cancer—Review Paper. *Ann. Agric. Environ. Med.* **2019,** *26*, 1–7.

Li, B.; Zhang, W.; Tan, T.; Liu, W.; Luo, X.; Zhang, J.; Yang, Y.; Li, R.; Ge, Z. Chinese Herbal Formulas Miao-Yi-Ai-Tang Inhibits the Proliferation and Migration of Lung Cancer Cells Through Targeting β-Catenin/AXIN and Presents Synergistic Effect with Cisplatin Suppressing Lung Cancer. *Bio. Med. Res. Int.* **2020,** 2761850.

Liu, D.; Chen, Z.; The Effects of Cantharidin and Cantharidin Derivates on Tumour Cells. *Anti-Cancer Agents Med. Chem.* **2009,** *9*, 392.

Liu, J.; Wang, S.; Zhang, Y.; Fan, H. T.; Lin, H. S. Traditional Chinese Medicine and Cancer: History, Present Situation, and Development. *Thorac. Cancer* **2015,** *6*, 561–569.

Liu, X.; Jin, X.; Chen, B.; Liu, X.; Liang, X.; Fang, X.; Wu, H.; Fu, X.; Zheng, H.; Ding, X.; Duan, N.; Zhang, Y. Effects of Kudiezi Injection on Serum Inflammatory Biomarkers in Patients with Acute Cerebral Infarction. *Dis. Markers* **2018,** 7936736.

Liu, Y. N.; Pan, S. L.; Liao, C. H.; Huang, D. Y.; Guh, J. H.; Peng, C. Y.; Chang, Y. L.; Teng, C. M. Evodiamine Represses Hypoxia-Induced Inflammatory Proteins Expression and Hypoxia-Inducible Factor 1α Accumulation in RAW264.7. *Shock* **2009,** *32*, 263–269.

Lu, A. P.; Jia, H. W.; Xiao, C.; Lu, Q. P. Theory of Traditional Chinese Medicine and Therapeutic Method of Diseases. *World J. Gastroenterol.* **2004,** *10*, 1854–1856.

Magesh, V.; Lee, J. C.; Ahn, K. S.; Lee, H. J.; Lee, H. J.; Lee, E. O.; Shim, S. H.; Jung, H. J.; Kim, J. S.; Kim, D. K.; Choi, S. H.; Ahn, K. S.; Kim, S. H. *Ocimum sanctum* Induces Apoptosis in A549 Lung Cancer Cells and Suppresses the In Vivo Growth of Lewis Lung Carcinoma Cells. *Phytother. Res.* **2009,** *23*, 1385–91.

Moga, M. A.; Bălan, A.; Anastasiu, C. V.; Dimienescu, O. G.; Neculoiu, C. D.; Gavriş, C. An Overview on the Anticancer Activity of *Azadirachta indica* (Neem) in Gynecological Cancers. *Int. J. Mol. Sci.* **2018,** *19*, 3898.

Mohan, M. C.; Abhimannue, A. P.; Kumar, B. P. Modulation of Pro-Inflammatory Cytokines and Enzymes by Polyherbal Formulation Guggulutiktaka Ghritam. *J. Ayurveda Integr. Med. Med.* **2019,** S0975–9476.

Mukherjee, P. K.; Banerjee, S.; Biswas, S.; Das, B.; Kar, A.; Katiyar, C. K. *Withania somnifera* (L.) Dunal—Modern Perspectives of an Ancient Rasayana from Ayurveda. *J. Ethnopharmacol.* **2020,** *264*, 113157.

Nadda, R. K.; Ali, A.; Goyal, R. C.; Khosla, P. K.; Goyal, R. *Aucklandia costus* (Syn. *Saussurea costus*): Ethnopharmacology of an Endangered Medicinal Plant of the Himalayan Region. *J. Ethnopharmacol.* **2020,** *263*, 113199.

Nafiujjaman, M.; Nurunnabi, M.; Saha, S. K.; Jahan, R.; Lee, Y. K.; Rahmatullah, M. Anti-Cancer Activity of Arkeshwara Rasa—A Herbo-Metallic Preparation. *AYU* **2015,** *36*, 346–350.

Nelaturi, P.; Nagarajan, P.; Sabapathy, S. K.; Sambandam, R. Swarna Bindu Prashana—An Ancient Approach to Improve the Infant's Immunity. *Biol. Trace Element Res.* **2020,** *27*, 1–4.

Omran, Z.; Bader, A.; Porta, A.; Vandamme, T.; Anton, N.; Alehaideb, Z.; El-Said, H.; Faidah, H.; Essa, A.; Vassallo, A.; Halwani, M. Evaluation of Antimicrobial Activity of Triphala Constituents and Nanoformulation. *Evid. Based Complement. Alternat. Med.* **2020,** 6976973.

Palliyaguru, D. L.; Singh, S. V.; Kensler, T. W.; *Withania somnifera*: From Prevention to Treatment of Cancer. *Mol. Nutr. Food Res.* **2016,** *60*, 1342–1353.

Pan, M. H.; Chiou, Y. S.; Tsai, M. L.; Ho, C. T.; Anti-Inflammatory Activity of Traditional Chinese Medicinal Herbs. *J. Tradit. Complement. Med.* **2011,** *1*, 8–24.

Pandey, M. K.; Sung, B.; Kunnumakkara, A. B.; Sethi, G.; Chaturvedi, M. M.; Aggarwal, B. B. Berberine Modifies Cysteine 179 of IkappaBalpha Kinase, Suppresses Nuclear Factor-kappaB-Regulated Anti-Apoptotic Gene Products, and Potentiates Apoptosis. *Cancer Res.* **2008,** *68*, 5370–5379.

Parray, A.; Siddique, H. R.; Nanda, S.; Konety, B. R.; Saleem, M. Castration-Resistant Prostate Cancer: Potential Targets and Therapies. *Biol. Targets Therap.* **2012,** *6*, 267–276.

Peinado, H.; Lavotshkin, S.; Lyden, D. The Secreted Factors Responsible for Pre-Metastatic Niche Formation: Old Sayings and New Thoughts. *Semin. Cancer Biol.* **2011,** *21*, 139–146.

Peng, T.; Jiang, Y.; Farhan, M.; Lazarovici, P.; Chen, L.; Zheng, W. Anti-Inflammatory Effects of Traditional Chinese Medicines on Preclinical In Vivo Models of Brain Ischemia-Reperfusion-Injury: Prospects for Neuroprotective Drug Discovery and Therapy. *Front Pharmacol.* **2019,** *10*, 204.

Prasad, S.; Srivastava, S. K.; Oxidative Stress and Cancer: Chemopreventive and Therapeutic Role of Triphala. *Anti-oxidants (Basel).* **2020,** *9*, 72.

Prashar, R.; Kumar, A.; Hewer, A.; Cole, K. J.; Davis, W.; Phillips, D. H. Inhibition by an Extract of *Ocimum sanctum* of DNA-Binding Activity of 7,12-dimethylbenz[a]Anthracene in Rat Hepatocytes In Vitro. *Cancer Lett.* **1998,** *128*, 155–60.

Pucci, C.; Martinelli, C.; Ciofani, G. Innovative Approaches for Cancer Treatment: Current Perspectives and New Challenges. *E-Cancer Med. Sci.* **2019,** *13*, 961.

Qian, J.; Kai, G. Application of Micro/Nanomaterials in Adsorption and Sensing of Active Ingredients in Traditional Chinese Medicine. *J. Pharm. Biomed. Anal.* **2020,** *190*, 113548.

Robb, C. T.; Regan, K. H.; Dorward, D. A.; Rossi, A. G. Key Mechanisms Governing Resolution of Lung Inflammation. *Semin. Immunopathol.* **2016,** *38*, 425–448.

Ruknuddin, G.; Biswajyoti, P.; Kumar, P. P.; Krishnaiah, A. B.; Basavaiah, R. Anti-Inflammatory and Analgesic Activities of Dashanga Ghana: An Ayurvedic Compound Formulation. *Int. J. Nutr. Pharmacol. Neurol. Dis.* **2013,** *3*, 303–308.

Sandhya, T.; Lathika, K. M.; Pandey, B. N.; Mishra, K. P. Potential of Traditional Ayurvedic Formulation, Triphala, as a Novel Anti-Cancer Drug. *Cancer Lett.* **2006,** *23*, 206–214.

Siddique, H. R.; Liao, D. J.; Mishra, S. K.; Schuster, T.; Wang. L.; Matter, B.; Campbell, P. M.; Villalta, P.; Nanda, S.; Deng, Y.; Saleem, M. Epicatechin-Rich Cocoa Polyphenol Inhibits Kras-Activated Pancreatic Ductal Carcinoma Cell Growth In Vitro and in a Mouse Model. *Int. J. Cancer* **2012,** *131*, 1720–31.

Siddique, H. R.; Mishra, S. K.; Karnes, R. J.; Saleem, M. Lupeol, a Novel Androgen Receptor Inhibitor: Implications in Prostate Cancer Therapy. *Clin. Cancer Res.* **2011,** *17*, 5379–91.

Singh, D.; Khan, M. A.; Siddique, H. R.; Apigenin, A. Plant Flavone Playing Noble Roles in Cancer Prevention Via Modulation of Key Cell Signaling Networks. *Recent Pat. Anticancer Drug Discov.* **2019,** *14*, 298–311.

Singh, D.; Khan, M. A.; Siddique, H. R. Emerging Role of Long Non-Coding RNAs in Cancer Chemoresistance: Unravelling the Multifaceted Role and Prospective Therapeutic Targeting. *Mol. Biol. Rep.* **2020,** *47*, 5569–5585.

Singla, K.; Singh, R. Nephroprotective Effect of Curculigo Orchiodies in Streptozotocin-Nicotinamide Induced Diabetic Nephropathy in Wistar Rats. *J. Ayurveda Integr. Med.* **2020,** S0975–9476.

Song, J.; Ko, H. S.; Sohn, E. J.; Kim, B.; Kim, J. H.; Kim, H. J.; Kim, C.; Kim, J. E.; Kim, S. H. Inhibition of Protein Kinase C α/βII and Activation of c-Jun NH2-Terminal Kinase Mediate Glycyrrhetinic Acid Induced Apoptosis in Non-Small Cell Lung Cancer NCI-H460 Cells. *Bioorg. Med. Chem. Lett.* **2014,** *24*, 1188–1191

Suhailbani, E.; Menon, A.; Nair, C. K. Protective Effect of Ayurvedic Formulations Against Doxorubicin-Induced Cardiotoxicity: Preliminary Studies on Brahma Rasayana and Chyavanaprash. *J. Cancer Res. Ther.* **2016,** *12*, 561–564.

Sun, Y. X.; Jiang, X. J.; Lu, B.; Gao, Q.; Chen, Y. F.; Wu, D. B.; Zheng, W. Y.; Yang, L.; Li, H.; Yu, B. Roles of Gut Microbiota in Pathogenesis of Alzheimer's Disease and Therapeutic Effects of Chinese Medicine. *Chin. J. Integr. Med.* **2020**.

Thomas, V.; Nair, S. N. V.; Ved, D. K.; Shankar, D. Controversial Identities of Medicinal Plants in Classical Literature of Ayurveda. *J. Ayurveda Integr. Med.* **2020,** 30374–30377.

Vadde, R.; Radhakrishnan, S.; Reddivari, L.; Vanamala, J. K. Triphala Extract Suppresses Proliferation and Induces Apoptosis in Human Colon Cancer Stem Cells Via Suppressing c-Myc/Cyclin D1 and Elevation of Bax/Bcl-2 Ratio. *Biomed. Res. Int.* **2015,** 649263.

Vasudevan, V. K.; Unnikrishnan, P.; Muraleedharan, A.; Krishnarajabhatt, H. S. A Comprehensive Ayurvedic Treatment Along with Counseling in Oligoasthenozoospermia with Previous Intrauterine Insemination Failure—A Case Report. *J. Ayurveda Integr. Med.* **2020,** S0975–9476.

Wang, C.; de Pablo, P.; Chen, X.; Schmid, C.; McAlindon, T. Acupuncture for Pain Relief in Patients with Rheumatoid Arthritis: A Systematic Review. *Arthritis Rheum.* **2008,** *59*, 1249–1256.

Wang, K.; Zhang, D.; Liu, Y.; Wang, X.; Zhao, J.; Sun, T.; Jin, T.; Li, B.; Pathal, J. L. Traditional Chinese Medicine Formula Bi-Qi Capsule Alleviates Rheumatoid Arthritis-Induced Inflammation, Synovial Hyperplasia, and Cartilage Destruction in Rats. *Arthritis Res. Therap.* **2018,** *20*, 43.

Wilken, R.; Veena, M. S.; Wang, M. B.; Srivatsan, E. S. Curcumin: A Review of Anti-Cancer Properties and Therapeutic Activity in Head and Neck Squamous Cell Carcinoma. *Mol. Cancer* **2011,** *10*, 12.

Wu, J.; Huang, G.; Li, Y.; Li, X. Flavonoids from Aurantii Fructus Immaturus and Aurantii Fructus: Promising Phytomedicines for the Treatment of Liver Diseases. *Chin. Med.* **2020,** *15*, 89.

Xiang, H.; Zuo, J.; Guo, F.; Dong, D. What We Already Know About Rhubarb: A Comprehensive Review. *Chin. Med.* **2020,** *15*, 88.

Xie, W.; Du, L. Diabetes Is an Inflammatory Disease: Evidence from Traditional Chinese Medicines. *Diab. Obes. Metab.* **2011,** *13*, 289–301.

Yue, G. G.; Lee, J. K.; Chan, B. C.; Kwok, H. F.; Hoi, S. W.; Sze, D. M.; Fung, K. P.; Leung, P. C.; Lau, C. B. An Innovative Anti-Cancer Chinese Herbal Formula Exhibited Multi-Targeted Efficacies in Metastatic Breast Cancer Mouse Model. *Chin. Med.* **2018,** *13*, 64.

Zhao, T.; Sun, Q.; Marques, M.; Witcher. Anticancer Properties of *Phyllanthus emblica* (Indian Gooseberry). *Oxid. Med. Cell Longev.* **2015,** 950890.

Zhao, X.; Tan, X.; Shi, H.; Xia, D. Nutrition and Traditional Chinese Medicine (TCM): A System's Theoretical Perspective. *Eur. J. Clin. Nutr.* **2020.**

Zhao, Y.; Wang, M.; Tsering, J.; Li, H.; Li, S.; Li, Y.; Liu, Y.; Hu, X. An Integrated Study on the Anti-Tumor Effect and Mechanism of Triphala Against Gynecological Cancers Based on Network Pharmacological Prediction and In Vitro Experimental Validation. *Integr. Cancer Therap.* **2018,** *17*, 894–901.

Zhen, G.; Jing, J.; Fengsen, L. Traditional Chinese Medicine Classic Herbal Formula Xiaoqinglong Decoction for Acute Exacerbation of Chronic Obstructive Pulmonary Disease: A Systematic Review Protocol. *Medicine (Baltimore)* **2018,** *97*, e13761.

Zheng, T.; Que, Z.; Jiao, L.; Kang, Y.; Gong, Y.; Yao, J.; Ma, C.; Bi, L.; Dong, Q.; Zhao, X.; Xu, L. Herbal Formula YYJD Inhibits Tumor Growth by Inducing Cell Cycle Arrest and Senescence in Lung Cancer. *Sci. Rep.* **2017,** *7*, 1–9.

CHAPTER 14

Immunomodulatory Compounds Derived from Medicinal Plants as Promising Therapeutics for Cancer

SAJIDA and ASHWINI PRABHU

Yenepoya Research Centre, Yenepoya (Deemed to be University), Mangalore, Karnataka, India

ABSTRACT

Imbalance in the immune system functions is associated with several diseases, including inflammatory diseases, autoimmune diseases, and cancer. Several synthetic drugs that can target the immune system have been designed and in use. However, these drugs do have certain limitations and may pose adverse reactions. Hence, the search for newer immunotherapeutics is gaining attention in the recent past. Immunomodulators are the substances that regulate the efficiency of the immune responses. A variety of immunomodulators derived from traditionally used plant sources have been developed that can specifically inhibit or enhance the functions of different immune cells such as cytotoxic T lymphocytes, lymphocytes, macrophages, natural killer (NK) cells, and neutrophils. The immunomodulators are particularly beneficial in designing immune therapies against various disorders. Several metabolites such as polysaccharides, flavonoids, alkaloids, and terpenoids derived from plants have been used to treat immune disorders and infections due to their immune stimulatory activity. Certain studies have demonstrated the efficacy of phytocompounds like capsaicin, colchicine, capsaicin, curcumin, epigallocatechol-3-gallate, genistein,

Ethnic Knowledge and Perspectives of Medicinal Plants, Volume 1: Curative Properties and Treatment Strategies. Munir Ozturk, Kandikere R. Sridhar, Maryam Sarwat, Volkan Altay, &
Francisco Martín Huerta-Martínez (Eds.)

quercetin, resveratrol, and andrographolide as immunostimulators in cancer. This chapter discusses the various immunomodulatory plant metabolites that could be developed into cancer immunotherapeutics based on their potential preclinical and clinical leads. The key signaling pathways that are targeted by these immunomodulatory compounds are also elaborated.

14.1 INTRODUCTION

The immune system is one of the complex organizations of cells and molecules with special property to protect the cells from any infection. These cells recognize infection or abnormality in the cell system and invade by the release of certain biomolecules to destroy the infection. There are two kinds of invading system: innate and adaptive. Innate immune system or natural immune system encompasses physical, chemical, and cellular responses, which involves the action of macrophages, dendritic cells, endothelial cells, granulocytes, natural killer cells, epithelial cells, and platelets. These cells act on infectious agents by phagocytosis and chemotactic action/inflammation and release the specific proteins to the site of infection to invade them. Adaptive immunity is contributed by the cellular and humoral responses. Adaptive immunity is antigen-specific and antigens are engulfed by the antigen-presenting cells (APCs). The APCs present the antigens to naïve T or B cells in MHC I/II molecule and activate lymphocytes. Active T lymphocytes produce Cytotoxic T lymphocytes (CTLs), Treg cells, and NK cells that release the pro-inflammatory and inflammatory cytokines/interleukins like IFN-γ, IL-6, TNF-α, etc. Active B lymphocytes release antigen-specific monoclonal antibodies and block the activity of the foreign molecule or abnormal cells (Luster, 2002; Hudspeth et al., 2013).

The immune system maintains normal tissue homeostasis. Thymus remains an important organ in the production, development, and homeostasis of T cells. The T cells differentiate between self and foreign antigens. These migrating T cells are predetermined by the T-cell receptors (TCRs) and TCRs recognize MHC molecules and produce invading molecules against the malignancy or infection. As tumor cells originate from the normal cells, the regulation of immune function remains the same in malignant and nonmalignant cells.

Globally, cancer is regarded as one of the major causes of death (Masoodi et al., 2020). It is a complex system with neoplastic cells, tainted extracellular matrix microenvironment, and supporting mesenchymal, endothelial cells with the infiltration of inflammatory immune cells. This cancer architecture contributes to the genomic instability, epigenetic modifications, uncontrolled proliferation, regulation of anti-apoptotic pathways, and activation of aggressive angiogenesis for invasion and metastasis (Hanahan and Weinberg, 2011) (Figure 14.1). At the early stage of tumor, natural killer cells (NK cells) and CD8+ cells recognize and eradicate the tumor cells. Cancer immunosuppression involves the escape of neoplastic or tumorigenic cells from the primary site to secondary lymphoid organs and peripheral vessels from the immunogenic detection and elimination by the immune cells. Neoplastic cells escape from the immunogenic detection and elimination, thereby helping other tumorigenic cells to escape from the recognition of the immune cell and cause immunosuppression. This immunosuppressive mechanism creates the tumor microenvironment (TME) by the survived cells and macrophages get converted into M1 phenotype. The TME enhances the secretion of molecular suppressors of immune response such as VEGF, TGF-β, IL-10, and prostaglandin E2. It also activates T-cell suppressors as well as inhibits the checkpoint activators such as PD-1, PD-L1, and CTLA-4. In metastatic stages, immune tolerance is associated with the release of pro-tumoral macrophages, regulatory T and B cells, immature dendritic cells (DCs), and pre-metastatic neutrophils. Tumorigenesis is a complex process consisting of initiation, progression, and metastasis. Major factors involved in the tumorigenesis are extracellular matrix (ECM), stromal cells, and TME. Adipose tissue establishes the hypoxic condition and releases proinflammatory cytokines and chemokines for enabling tumor initiation. Adipose tissue accumulates periadipocytes which increases the activity of macrophages and monocytes and helps cancer growth locally (Goodwin and Stambolic, 2015). Blood and lymphatic cells play a different and complex role in various stages of tumorigenesis. Under hypoxic condition, the tumor cells migrate into the blood stream and activate endothelial cells to stimulate HIF-1α secretion and dimerization of HIF-1α and HIF-1β. This dimer helps in the secretion of growth factors such as VEGF, FGF, PDGF, and angiogenin prerequisite for cancer cell growth and angiogenesis (Whiteside, 2008; Wang et al., 2017). Figure 14.1 depicts the mechanistic insights into the checkpoints of cancer progression.

Natural products are well known for their wide use in the therapeutic approach for various diseases (Ozturk et al., 2020, 2021a, b). Phytochemicals are well known for their pharmacological effects on cancer progression by modulating the multiple pathways that are involved in cancer cell growth. Certain medicinal plants such as *Curcuma longa, Curcuma amada, Allium*

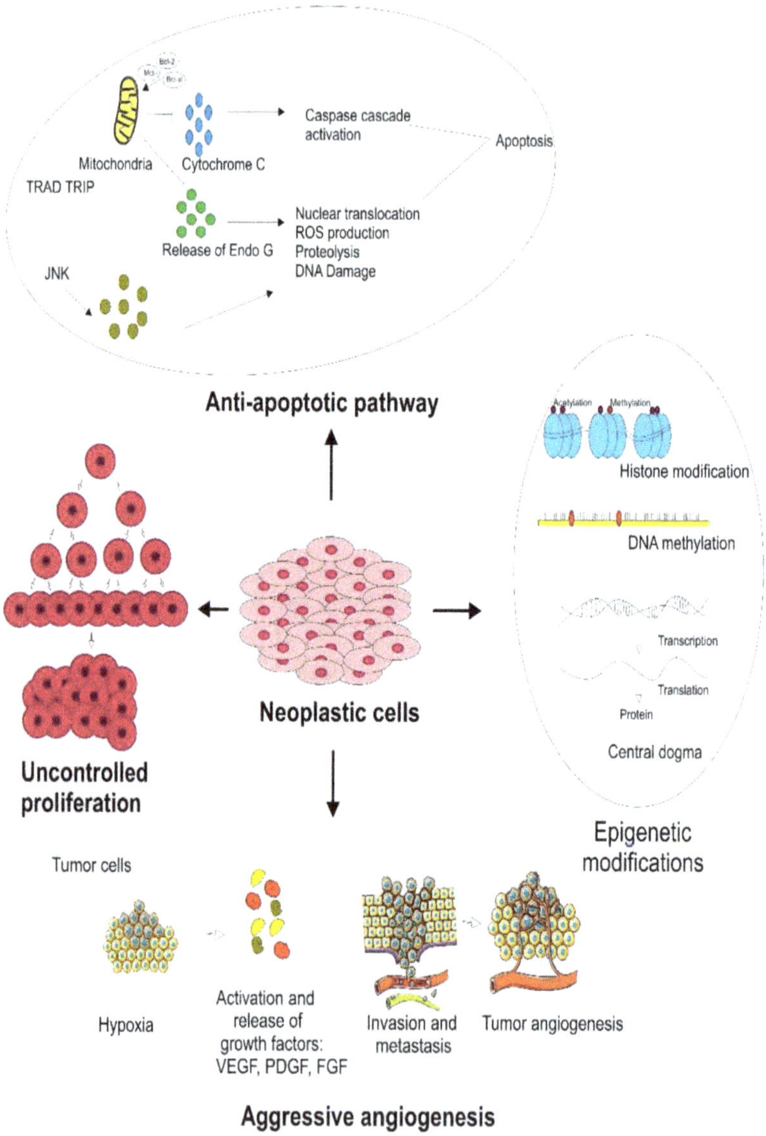

FIGURE 14.1 Architecture of cancer cells: Neoplastic cells undergo series of modifications in cellular as well as in genetic level. Cancer cells undergo uncontrolled growth without cell death causing the abnormal proliferation and metastasis. Overgrown cell mass results in the phenomenon of oxygen tension called hypoxia, which stimulates series of signaling pathways. These pathways play a role cancer cell progression, invasion, metastasis, and aggressive neo-vascularization. Cellular stress inhibits the normal functioning of cells and inhibits the pro-apoptotic and apoptotic signaling molecules. Also, altered epigenetic modifications such as histone modifications and DNA methylation and acetylation are encountered.

sativum, Cathranthus roseus, Zingiber officinale, Morinda citrifolia, Vitis vinifera, etc. are used to treat various diseases such as arthritis, jaundice, fever, inflammation, and other infectious diseases traditionally. These plants contain antioxidant-rich secondary metabolites including curcumin, allicin, resveratrol, Epigallocatechin gallate (EGCG), vinblastine, S-allyl-cysteine (SAC), E/Z-ajoene, diallyltrisulfide (DATS), gingerol, and others that serve as promising chemopreventive agents. Several bioactive compounds derived from plants showed anti-proliferative and anti-metastatic effects on various cancers via the modulation of signaling pathway effectors. Phytocompounds induce antioxidant enzymes like GSH, GST, GPxn and help in the activation of apoptotic pathways including Caspase-3, 7, 8, 9, 10, 12, and p53. Anti-neoplastic effect is mediated by inducing the expressions of cycloxygenase (COX), MAPK/ERK, TNK, Akt, PI3K, Bax, Bak, Bcl-2, cytokines, and matrix metalloproteinases and also by the modulation of DNA repair damage. Further, cancer cell death is triggered by the G2/M phase cell cycle arrest with the inhibition of Cdc2, CDK2, and CDK4 kinases (Iqbal et al., 2017). These CDK and Cdcs provide key support for the expansion, differentiation, and balancing of immune cells in the system. CDKs regulate the monocytes to secrete the cytokine IFN-β; meanwhile, CDK suppresses the overexpression of IL-1β and $p16^{INK4A}$ that is required to suppress IL-6. $p27^{KIP1}$ has a role in the macrophage mesenchymal migration, which promotes tumor infiltration. CDKs balance the expression of $p27^{KIP1}$and NFκB activity (Laphanuwat and Jirawatnotai, 2019). This review addresses traditionally used plant materials that have potential to combat cancer or cancer-related ailments. Table 14.1 gives an account of oncology clinical trials in various phases carried out using certain phytocompounds.

14.2 ROLE OF NATURAL COMPOUNDS IN CANCER PREVENTION

14.2.1 VINBLASTINE

Vinblastine (VBL) is a plant alkaloid, produced by the periwinkle plant *Catharanthus roseus*. The VBL enhances the immune system against cancer and also causes apoptosis in cancer cells. Dendritic cells (DCs) are essential in eliciting the immune response against cancer cells. Immature DCs get deactivated by the immunosuppressive action of TME. VBL activates the immature DCs and turns them into mature DCs and presents the tumor antigen to CD8 T cells and, in turn, activates the host immune system to

TABLE 14.1 Clinical Trials on Natural Compounds: Effect of Natural Compounds on Various Cancer Patients.

Active compound	Dose/Duration	Type of cancer	Phase	Outcome	Adverse effect	References
Vinblastin	0.1 mg/kg every 3 weeks with IFNα2a was administered subcutaneously at 3 million units three times a week	Advanced renal cell cancer	Phase I	Patients achieved disease stabilization 10% of patients experienced partial remission	Fatigue, fever, and flu-like symptoms	Pyrhonen et al. (1999)
	Dacarbazine (250 mg/ m^2)+vinblastine (6 mg/m^2 per day+ bleomycin (15 units/ m^2) was administered by 24-h infusion from day 1 to day 5, and cisplatin (50 mg/m^2) To limit bleomycin, vinblastin, and cisplatin administered. Courses were repeated on a cycle of four weeks	Metastatic melanoma	Phase III	10% of patients showed partial remission	Dose-limiting objective gastrointestinal and hematologic toxicity	Luikart et al. (1984)
	Vinblastine (3 mg/m^2) + cyclophosphamide (50 mg)+rofecoxib (25 mg) orally daily for 850 weeks	Advanced solid tumors	Phase II	Extremely tolerated Median time to tumor progression was 103 days for all patients and 289 days for patients experiencing clinical benefit Median overall survival rate was 253 days and 375 days for patients experiencing clinical benefit	Neutropenia in 25% of patients grade 1 alopecia in single patient no grade 3/4 adverse events	Young et al. (2006)
	Nilotinib orally twice daily (BID) in combination with once-weekly vinblastine injections for a maximum of 12 cycles of 28 days	Recurrent low-grade glioma	Phase I	disease control rate was 85.3% 12-month progression-free survival was 37.1%	Neutropenia Reversible adverse non hematologicala adverse effects	Vairy et al. (2020)

TABLE 14.1 *(Continued)*

Active compound	Dose/Duration	Type of cancer	Phase	Outcome	Adverse effect	References
Curcumin	8 g/d orally for 8 weeks	Advanced pancreatic cancer	Phase II	Low oral bioavailability of drug 73% tumor regression and increase in the serum cytokine levels Modulation of peripheral blood mononuclear cells	No adverse effect reported	Dhillon et al. (2008)
	2 g and 4g daily for 30 days	Colorectal neoplasia	Phase IIA	Decrease number of aberrant crypt foci (ACF) No change in PGE_2 concentration Anticarcarcinogenesis activity by curcumoid complex in the serum	59% had grade 1 and 2 toxicity No grade 3/4 toxicity	Carroll et al. (2011)
Taxol	80 mg/m^2 paclitaxel (P) intravenously (IV) on days 1, 8, and 15 and 90 mg/m^2 epirubicin (E) IV on day 1 with a dosing interval of 21 days for four cycles	Advanced HER 2-negative breast cancer	Phase II	Did not show any improved response rate Would show response in the HER2-positive breast cancer	Neutropenia leukopenia	Jiang et al. (2020)
EGCG	800 mg EGCG, 1200 mg EGCG, or placebo orally once daily for 14–28 days	Bladder Cancer	Phase II	94% completed study Reduction in proliferating cell nuclear antigen (PCNA) and clusterin with chemopreventive action	Mild to severe grade 1–3 adverse effects	Gee et al. (2017)
	440 µM EGCG after final radiotherapy	Esophagus Cancer	Phase II	EGCG tolerated most patients Clinical response is 86.3%	Mild heart burn and nausea Allergic reaction observed	Li et al. (2019)

conflict cancer cells. Apart from DC maturation, VBL also enhances the apoptosis in melanoma cells and CTL infiltration into tumor site (Tanaka et al., 2009). The VBL is known for its chemotherapeutic potential against cancer by inhibiting the tumor cell proliferation via mitotic arrest and induction of apoptotic cell death. It induces the phosphorylation of c-Jun protein and activates the JNK pathway (Kolomeichuk et al., 2008).

Several studies have demonstrated the combination of VBL with different chemotherapeutic agents for enhancing the therapeutic outcome. Antitumor activity is mediated by VBL in the human epidermoid carcinoma cell line, wherein VBL promotes apoptosis by modulating the expressions of JNK, ERK, and p53 signaling molecules. Since VBL inhibits the expression of the ERK signaling pathway, cell death is promoted. Based on the promising results obtained from in vivo and in vitro approaches pertaining to the immunomodulatory and antineoplastic effects on tumor cells, several clinical studies on VBL and its analogues alone or in combination with other conventional therapies have been carried out. Furthermore, VBL (at dosages of 3, 4, 5, and 6 mg/m^2 per week) was combined with nilotinib (115, 230, and 350 mg/m^2) in recurrent low-grade glioma patients. Around 40% of the patients completed the treatment without severe side effects. Among 35 patients, two patients experienced febrile neutropenia and six patients experienced severe adverse effects such as neutropenia, hypertension, seizure, respiratory infection, vomiting, and others (Vairy et al., 2020). Interferon alfa-2a (IFNα-2a) helps in balancing the erythrocyte sedimentation rate (ESR) without inducing weight loss in cancer patients. IFNα-2a was combined with VBL (median dose of 2.3 mg/wk and a cumulative dose 62 mg). VBL treatment median dose was 2.4 mg/wk with a cumulative dose 36 mg for 12 months. Survival rate increased up to 67.6 weeks with some adverse effects (Pyrhonen et al., 1999). Cyclooxygenase (COX) inhibitor acts as a chemotherapeutic agent against bladder cancer by inducing apoptosis and activating the immunomodulatory mechanisms. Further, this phenomenon leads to the inhibition of cancer growth via inhibition of angiogenesis and antiproliferative effects on cancer stem cells. A total of 51 dogs were recruited and introvenosouly administered with vinblastin (2 or 2.5 mg/m^2) based on body weight $\geq$ 15 kg or < 15 kg for every two weeks along with proxicam dosage of 0.3 mg/kg. Administration proxicam enhances VBL to prevent COX release and increased the survival rate with grade 1 and 2 toxicities in the dogs with bladder cancer (Knapp et al., 2016). The effects of VBL on alleviating the cancer cell survival, growth, accretion, and metastasis are indicated in Figure 14.2.

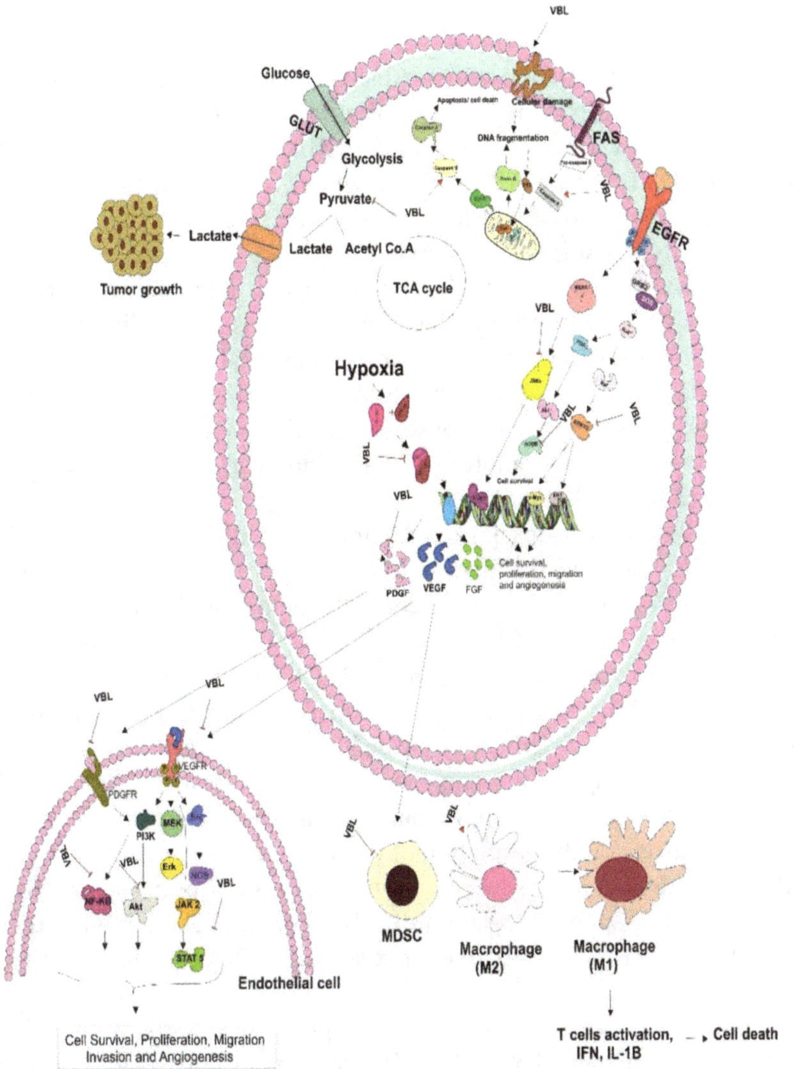

FIGURE 14.2 Anticancer effect of vinblastin (VBL) by regulating the various signaling pathways and immunogenic response. The VBL causes the cellular damage, DNA damage, and releases ROS. ROS generated by stress and Caspase 8 activates Bax and Bcl 2, followed by the activation of caspase cascades to destroy the cells. Cell survival, proliferation, invasion, angiogenesis, and metastasis is regulated by the EGFR pathway, VBL suppresses the expression of mTOR, ERK1/2, and JNKs. Meanwhile, hypoxic condition regulates the production of growth factors such as VEGF, PDGF, FGFs and treatment with VBL inhibits the expression of these growth factors and aggressive angiogenesis. It also inhibits the regulation of MDSCs to tumor site, thereby activating the macrophages to act against tumor cells via T-cell activation, IFN, and IL-1β expression.

14.2.2 ALLICIN

Garlic is a spice used in the culinary dishes (Ozturk et al., 2012). Garlic is well known for its antioxidant and anti-inflammatory activities, which is due to the presence of various active compounds like diallyl sulfide (DAS), diallyl disulfide (DADS), diallyltrisulfide (DATS), diallylthiosulfonate (allicin), S-allyl-cysteinesulfoxide (alliin). E/Z-ajoene, S-allyl-cysteine (SAC), and Allicin/diallylthiosulfonate is a major bioactive organosulfur compound of *Allium sativum* (garlic). Allicin also acts as an immunomodulatory agent to recover the cell injury by changing the levels of alkaline phosphatase, alanine aminotransferase, aspartate aminotransferase, glutathione, and superoxide dismutase (Suddek, 2014). Dendritic cells are responsible for eliciting the primary response to infection or injury via activation of lymphocytes. Allicin promotes DC maturation with an increased expression of CD40 (Feng et al., 2012).

Garlic extract contains high concentrations of allicin, which can inhibit the cancer cell growth and proliferation. Oomen et al. (2004) found the antitumor effects of allicin on different cancer cells including HeLa (human cervical cancer), L-929 (mouse fibrosarcoma), SiHa (cell line of human cervical cancer), and SW480 (human colon cancer), wherein this compound induced significant growth arrest and caspase-induced apoptosis. Furthermore, allicin has the potential to fragment DNA. Allicin acts on gastric adenocarcinoma cells by restraining proliferation via cell cycle arrest in S-phase and also had no deleterious effects on normal intestinal cells (Mansingh et al., 2018). Allicin also acts on the formation of ulcerative colitis by the deactivation of AP-1/NF-κB/signal transducer inhibition of transcription factor (STAT-1), inhibition of p38phosphorylation of JNK and extracellular signal-regulated kinase 1/2 (ERK1/2)-regulated peroxisome proliferators-activated receptor (PPAR)-γ (Shi et al., 2017).

Further, to investigate the selective proliferative effects of allicin on cancer cells, Zhang and Yang (2017) carried out a study wherein the results revealed that allicin inhibits the invasion and metastasis of cancer cells. In case of cervical cancer, the nuclear factor such as erythroid 2-related factor 2 (NRF2) is accountable for the invasion and metastasis. Treatment with allicin suppressed the expression of NRF2 and hemeoxygenase 1 by the inactivation of phosphoinositide 3-kinase/protein kinase B (PI3K/AKT) signaling. Blockade of NRF2 expression obstructs the growth, invasion, and metastasis in cervical cancer cells.

14.2.3 CURCUMIN

Phytopolyohenol curcumin belongs to the class of curcuminoid, the active compound from the Indian spice *Curcuma longa*, with a wide range of therapeutic properties. Traditionally, Indians and Chinese have been using curcumin to treat several diseases like jaundice, anorexia, diabetic wounds, rheumatism, etc. Based on these evidence, several scientists across the world studied the effect of curcumin using preclinical and clinical models and revealed that the therapeutic property of curcumin is due to its anti-inflammatory and antioxidant activity. Curcumin also can modulate the expression of transcription factors and cause cell cycle arrest. Curcumin showed antiproliferative effects on several cancer cells via the induction of apoptosis, p53 stabilization, mTOR, Wnt, Notch, PI3K, signaling inhibition, AMPK activation, cell cycle inhibition, inhibition of oncogenes, inactivation of NF-kB, metastasis inhibition, angiogenesis inhibition, miRNA regulation, DNA damage, and repair. Metabolic activity plays a key role in cancer progression and metastasis and therefore by altering the metabolic activity, cancer cell growth could be controlled. As lactate release is increased, glucose uptake in the presence of oxygen is enhanced, which is considered a hallmark for the tumor progression. Curcumin helps in inhibiting the uptake of oxygen and release of lactate in various cancers through the silencing of pyruvate kinase M2 (PKM2) and also inhibits mTOR and HIF1α expression (Siddiqui et al., 2018). Secreted frizzled-related protein (SFRP) family is inactivated by promoter methylation to convert into oncogenes, mainly involved in Wnt/β-catenin signaling pathway. FDA approved anti-DNA methylation agent called 5-aza2′-deoxycytidine (DAC), which is administered in combination with curcumin to enhance the therapeutic efficacy against tumor growth. Inhibition of ovarian cancer growth via the downregulation of SFRP5 protein and demethylation of the promoter gene was reported (Yen et al., 2019) by the release of tumor suppressor proteins. Curcumin also helps in inhibiting the colony forming and migratory potential of cells through epithelial–mesenchymal transition (EMT) process. In case of neuroblastoma, curcumin downregulates ERK1/2 and activates intrinsic apoptotic pathways. This apoptosis depends on the expression of brain expressed X-linked (Bex) genes, a pro-apoptotic gene. Curcumin induced apoptosis in neuroblastoma cells in a dose-dependent way with an increase in the expressions of procaspases-3, 9 and phosphorylated ERK1/2 expression as well as dose-dependent induction of Bex gene (Sidhar and Giri, 2017).

Further, curcumin also enhanced the sensitivity of chemo or radiotherapy to various cancers. Pancreatic cancer is a highly aggressive and resistant tumor. Curcumin induced cell death in pancreatic cancer in adjunction with radiotherapy by enhancing the cell cycle arrest at G2/M phase (Schwarz et al., 2020).

Cancer cell growth is regulated by mTORC1/2 and can be inhibited by PP242, which belongs to the class of small-molecule protein kinase inhibitor which has the potential to suppress leukemia cells by targeting adenosine triphosphate (ATP) binding site of mTOR to subdue PI3K/AKT/mTOR signaling in Ph^+ B-cell acute lymphoblastic leukemia and T-cell lymphoma. Cancer cells with activated mTOR pathway show resistance to PP242 and defer to undergo apoptosis. To enhance the apoptotic efficacy, curcumin was combined with PP242 and results revealed a significant increase in apoptosis via the inhibition of mTOR1/2 expression. Further, this combination also increased cytosolic Ca^{2+} release from endoplasmic reticulum followed by the lysosomal damage (Seo et al., 2018).

14.2.4 TAXOL

Taxol or paclitaxel, present in the bark and leaf of the plants *Corylus avellana, Taxus baccata*, and *T. canadensis,* is extensively used to treat various organ cancers (ovarian, breast, and lung). Paclitaxel promotes the arrest of mitotic phase of cell cycle of neoplastic cells via binding to the β-tubulin of microtubule (Xie and Zhou, 2017). Further, its apoptotic effect on cancer cells through different signaling pathways, caspase-3 activation, increased expression of Bax, cytochrome-c expression, and chromatin condensation was elucidated. Besides, paclitaxel can cause a significant increase in the ROS and malondialdehyde (MDA) expression which enhances the immune response against cancer cells. Also, various signaling pathway molecules including AKT/MAPK were inhibited along with phosphorylated p38 and p90 ribosomal protein S6 kinase protein (Ren et al., 2018). Paclitaxel can also inhibit the invasion as well as migration of cancer cells through inhibiting PI3K protein. Cell survival depends on the expression of protein P-GSK3B. Phosphorylation of GSK3B protein induces apoptosis as well as inhibits the cell migration and invasion by downregulation of PI3K/Akt signaling molecules (Ma et al., 2018).

Paclitaxel not only destroys the cancer cells but also activates immune system against cancer via the regulation of dendritic cells (DCs), macrophages, Natural killer cells (NKs), and specific T cells (Vassileva et al., 2008).

These phagocytic cells release the tumor antigens and activated cells release pro-inflammatory cytokines, and inhibit Treg cells. Hence, to enhance the effect of paclitaxel, it can be combined with adoptive immune cells or other conventional therapies. Combination therapy of paclitaxel, carboplatin, and bevacizumab has been used to treat NSCLC, breast cancer, ovarian cancer, and various other tumor types (Spigel et al., 2015). After the therapeutic success of paclitaxel, several analogues have been synthesized and showed promising results in the in vitro/in vivo studies. The mechanism was further investigated to evaluate the safety of the analogues for different cancers (breast, lung, pancreatic, and urethral bladder) (Ojima et al., 2016).

14.2.5 GINGEROL

Gingerol is a bioactive compound from ginger rhizomes (*Zingiber officinale* Roscoe). It is used in the traditional systems of medicine because of its antimicrobial, anticancer, antioxidant, anti-inflammatory, and antiallergic properties. Gingerol exerted anticancer activity on various cancers including cervical, breast, blood, liver, prostate, colorectal, ovarian, and lung cancer. Cytotoxic activity of ginger is credited mainly to the activation of NAG1 and caspase 3 leading to apoptosis. It also enhances cell cycle arrest at the G1 phase, inhibits MAPK/AP-1 signaling pathway, and downregulates cyclin D1 molecules (Mahmoodally et al., 2019). Anti-tumorigenic and pro-apoptotic activity of gingerol on colon cancer by the inhibition of leukotriene A(4) hydrolase expression as well as induction of G2/M arrest is reported (Lin et al., 2012). Gingerol also induces Bax and caspase activation (Brantley-Finley et al., 2003). Based on the preclinical reports, clinical trials were performed. The results revealed that there was a dose-dependent toxicity at higher concentrations (2000 mg) and mild toxicity signs such as fatigue, headache, GI symptoms, etc were observed (Zick et al., 2009).

14.2.6 EPIGALLOCATECHIN-3-GALLATE

The epigallocatechin-3-gallate (EGCG) is an active catechin part and parcel of green tea (*Camellia sinensis*), well known for its antioxidant as well as anti-inflammatory activity. This compound induced apoptosis and inhibited tumor progression by altering different signaling pathways. In lung cancer cells, EGCG exhibited anti-proliferative effect by inhibiting colony formation, cell migration, MMP independent invasion, and phosphorylation of

AMPK and mTOR signaling pathways (Chen et al., 2020). EGCG inhibited the progression of hepatocellular carcinoma via the induction of apoptosis and different molecular pathways such as downregulation of NF-κB, p53, EGFR, modulation of PI3K–Akt–mTOR; FGF, and VEGF pathways (Bimonte et al., 2019).

Nano complex of EGCG with lanthanide metal ions enhanced noteworthy antitumor effects on in vitro and in vivo models of melanoma. Melanoma cell migration was inhibited by the complex, and also enhanced apoptosis through increased expression of caspase 7/cleaved PARP expression and downregulation of procaspase 3. In mice model, EGCG treatment showed a significant decrease in the lung melanoma (Li et al., 2019a).

14.2.7 RESVERATROL

Resveratrol (RSV) is a polyphenol found in grape skin, peanuts, hops and abundantly present in the roots of *Polygonum cuspidatum* commonly known as Japanese knotweed. Several studies have shown that RSV can restrain COX-1 and 2 inflammatory molecules and sirtuin-dependent apoptosis. RSV promotes apoptosis and also enhances the release of proinflammatory molecules (Vervandier-Fasseur and Latruffe, 2019). The nutrient deprivation autophagy factor-1 (NAF-1) is involved in calcium metabolism and it is antiapoptotic and antiautophagic in nature. RSV regulated the cellular reactive oxygen species (ROS) and Nrf2 activation in drug-resistant pancreatic cancer and suppressed the activity of NAF-1. Modulation of these proteins induced apoptosis and cancer cell death (Cheng et al., 2018).

The RSV is known for its inhibitory effects on cancer cells by apoptosis and cell cycle arrest via modulating the VEGF and angiogenin expression to inhibit the cancer growth. Along with that, RSV can modulate immune cells to fight against cancer and other infectious diseases. Likewise, Falchetti et al., (2001) demonstrated how RSV enhanced the immune response to the infection. RSV stimulates the release of CD 8+ and CD 3+ T cells which produce cytokines such as IL-2, IL-4, and IFN-α. Further, it enhances the proliferation of CD 3+ & CD28+ T cells along with the enhanced activity of Cytotoxic T lymphocytes (CTL) at a lower concentration of RSV (2.5 μg/ml) (Falchetti et al., 2001). A new study demonstrated tumor rejection release of NK cells and macrophages into the tumor microenvironment in xenograft model human papillomavirus tumor and also releases inflammatory cytokine IL-2 and enhances the apoptosis (Mukherjee et al., 2018). Tumor microenvironment inhibits T-cell proliferation in the presence of PD-L1 protein and also PD-L1 expression is enhanced by the histone acetylation/deacetylation. Treatment with RSV decreased PD-L1 levels with the upregulation of T-cell proliferation and also modulates expression of NFκB in colorectal and breast cancer cells (Lucas et al., 2018).

Tumor cells are recognized by the immune cells in the presence of major histocompatibility complex of class I chain-related proteins A as well as B (MICA and MICB). But antibodies against NK group 2 member D (NKG2D) and miR-17-92 block the expression of MICA and MICB with the enhancement of breast cancer (MCF-7, Hs 578T, BCap37, and MDA-MB-231 cells) cell survival. In breast cancer cells, RSV upregulates MICA as well as MICB expression by downregulating the c-Myc expression which inhibits the miR-17-92 transcription and blocks NKG2D antibodies. Further, RSV regulates antitumor effect by the release of NK cells to the tumor site and osmotic lysis of cells (Pan et al., 2017). RSV showed a significant effect on cancer inhibition in preclinical studies and based on these results, the pharmacological effect of RSV was evaluated on healthy volunteers. Healthy individuals administered with repeated doses of RSV 1000 mg/day for 28 days showed an increase in the circulating immune cells. It was also found that administered dose was safe and tolerable with the increased circulation of $\gamma\delta$ T cells and regulatory T cells. Intake of RSV significantly increased plasma antioxidant with a slight decrease in proinflammatory cytokines TNF-α and MCP-1 (Espinoza et al., 2017). Patients with colorectal cancer ingested doses of 0.5 and 1.0 g RSV daily for 29 days and found these doses were tolerable with no adverse effects. After 29 days, resection biopsy of colorectal cancer showed a 5% decrease in the proliferation and also daily doses ameliorated anticancer effects (Patel et al., 2010).

14.2.8 PROCYANIDIN

Grape (*Vitis vinifera*) seed and the peel is rich in procyanidin, a chemopreventive and chemotherapeutic agent. Procyanidin is a phenolic compound with the pharmacological property to improve cardiovascular health, hypertension, hyperlipidemia, and atherosclerosis. Procyanidin-rich grape extract showed the anticancer effect on the breast cancer cells via the downregulation of CDK4, MAPK/ERK1/2, and MAPK/p38 and also induced CDKI Cip1/p21 in MDAMB cells. Further, it inhibits the cell growth as well as induces cell cycle arrest at G1 phase (Agarwal et al., 2000). PGI_2 (PGI) is an effective vasodilator and inhibitor of platelet activation and aggregation. In non-small cell lung cancer (NSCLC), expression of PGI_2 is downregulated.

Presence of procyanidin in grape enhances 6-keto PGF1α. 6-keto PGF1α is a metabolite of PGI_2, along with the reduced expression of COX-2 and caspase-3, induced apoptosis (Mao et al., 2016).

14.2.9 DAMNACANTHAL

Damnacanthal is an active compound of *Morinda citrifolia* L. (family, Rubiaceae), commonly named as Noni. Noni is well known for its medicinal properties against various diseases. From Noni, over 150 bioactive compounds have been identified, the major compound is Damnacanthal (3-hydroxy-1-methoxy-anthraquinone-2-aldehyde). Investigation of Damnacanthal (Noni's active anthraquinone compound) on colorectal tumorigenesis showed a promising outcome. The antitumor effect was exhibited by the compound due to cell cycle arrest and caspase-dependent apoptosis. It also induced NAG1 [(nonsteroidal anti-inflammatory drug (NSAID)-activated gene-1)] activation involved in transforming cell growth by the release of pro-apoptotic and anti-tumorigenic activity. Induced NAG-1 protein inhibited the colony formation and cellular migration with an increased expression of p53 (Nualsanit et al., 2012). It has been observed that in cervical cancer, growth is inhibited by upregulated apoptotic proteins such as p53 and Bax affecting the intrinsic pathway of mitochondria via the modulation of caspase-9 and caspase-3 expression. It also helps in reducing the expression of anti-apoptotic proteins such as Bcl-X_L Bcl-2 and survivin (Gupta et al., 2013). This alteration in the gene/protein could help in inhibiting the cancer cell growth or invasion. Hepatocellular growth factor (HGF)/c-Met signaling pathway plays a crucial role in the growth, proliferation, and progression of cancer cells. Hence, targeting HGF/c-Met pathway in hepatocellular carcinoma would be better to therapeutic approach. Garcia-Vilas et al., (2015) showed a chemopreventive effect of Damnacanthal on hepatocellular carcinoma cells by inhibiting the HGF/c-Met pathway. Damnacanthal inhibits the cell growth by inducing c-Met phosphorylation as well as arrest cell cycle.

14.2.10 CROCETIN

Carotenoid crocetin is a major component derived from the flower stigma of spice saffron (*Crocus sativus* L), widely used as a food additive (Kafi et al., 2018). Saffron showed chemopreventive and chemoprotective activity against various cancers. Saffron induced dose-dependent caspase-induced apoptosis in non-small cell lung cancer cells (Samarghandian et al., 2013). Crocetin inhibits lipid peroxidation and stimulates the activity of catalase, GSH-Px, GST, and superoxide dismutase (SOD) to prevent the oxidative damage and enhance the immunostimulatory environment. Further, crocetin downregulates aryl hydrocarbon-hydroxylase (AHH), gamma-glutamyltransferase (GGT), and lactate dehydrogenase (LDH) induced by reactive oxygen species (ROS) and scavenges free radicals to prevent cancer progression. Several regulatory proteins such as Cdc-2, Cdc-25c, and cyclin B1 that activate cell cycle are inhibited by crocetin and this compound also arrests cell cycle at G2/M phase (Gutheil et al., 2012). Treatment of breast cancer cells with crocetin showed cell cycle arrest by microtubule depolymerization. Crocetin binds to tubulin and inhibits the assembly of microtubule-associated protein (MAP) rich tubulin to block the proliferation of cancer cells (Hire et al., 2017).

Moreover, saffron carotenoid crocetin enhances NK-cell activity specific to the cancer cells. Crocetin also showed the anti-inflammatory effect on methylcholanthrene induced tumor in a rodent model and responsible for inhibition of cervical cancer via the declined release of IL-1β, TNF-α, and polymorphonuclear cells (PMN) and COX2 production (Bolhassani et al., 2014; Chen et al., 2015). These studies have shown crocetin would be a better therapeutic agent to treat cancer by immunomodulation as well as by directly acting on the cancer cells.

14.3 CONCLUSIONS

Immune response activation is an important major function of the human body toward the antigen invasion. There is an increasing evidence that natural compounds derived from ethnic knowledge can act as potential anticancer agents by regulating the immunomulation and also by acting on the various pathways involved in cancer cell growth, proliferation, and migration. Anticancer effects of certain ethnic phytochemicals are mainly exerted by the activation of immune cells and release of cytokines to the tumor microenvironment, thereby suppressing the tumor development and metastasis. Although many of these compounds are used globally, their efficacies and target signaling cascades have been studied sporadically with the limited completed clinical trials. Highlights are given on the cellular and molecular mechanisms regulated by the phytochemicals in immune cells and downstream effector pathways. Such compounds or derivatives thereof can be developed into complementary therapeutics after appropriate preclinical and clinical validations.

KEYWORDS

- **cancer**
- **immunomodulation**
- **phytochemicals**
- **signaling pathways**
- **therapy**

REFERENCES

Agarwal, C.; Sharma, Y.; Zhao, J.; Agarwal, R. A Polyphenolic Fraction from Grape Seeds Causes Irreversible Growth Inhibition of Breast Carcinoma MDA-MB468 Cells by Inhibiting Mitogen- Activated Protein Kinases Activation and Inducing G1 Arrest and Differentiation. *Clin. Cancer Res.* **2000,** *6*, 2921–2930.

Bimonte, S.; Albino, V.; Piccirillo, M.; Nasto, A.; Molino, C.; Palaia, R.; Cascella, M. Epigallocatechin-3-Gallate in the Prevention and Treatment of Hepatocellular Carcinoma: Experimental Findings and Translational Perspectives. *Drug Design Dev. Ther.* **2019,** *13*, 611–621.

Bolhassani, A.; Khavari, A.; Bathaie, S. Z. Saffron and Natural Carotenoids: Biochemical Activities and Anti-Tumor Effects. *Biochim. Biophys. Acta.* **2014,** *1845*, 20–30.

Brantley-Finley, C.; Lyle, C. S.; Du, L.; Goodwin, M. E.; Hall, T.; Szwedo, D.; Kaushal, G. P.; Chambers, T. P. The JNK, ERK and p53 Pathways Play Distinct Roles in Apoptosis Mediated by the Antitumor Agents Vinblastine, Doxorubicin, and Etoposide. *Biochem. Pharmacol.* **2003,** *66*, 459–469.

Carroll, A. E.; Benya, R. V.; Turgeon, D. K.; Vareed, S.; Neuman, M. Phase IIA Clinical Trial of Curcumin for the Prevention of Colorectal Neoplasia. *Cancer Prev. Res.* **2011,** *4*, 354–364.

Chen, B. H.; Hsieh, C. H.; Tsai, S. Y.; Wang, C. Y.; Wang, C. C. Anticancer Effects of Epigallocatechin-3-Gallte Nanoemulsion on Lung Cancer Cells Through the Activation of AMP-Activated Protein Kinase Signaling Pathway. *Sci. Rep.* **2020,** *10*, 5163.

Chen, B.; Hou, Z. H.; Dong, Z.; Li, C. D. Crocetin Downregulates the Proinflammatory Cytokines in Methylcholanthrene Induced Rodent Tumor Model and Inhibits COX-2 Expression in Cervical Cancer Cells. *BioMed Res. Int.* **2015,** *2015*, 829513.

Cheng, L.; Yan, B.; Jiang, Z.; Zhou, C.; Cao, J.; Qian, W.; Li, J.; Sun, L.; Ma, J.; Ma, Q.; Sha, H. Resveratrol-Induced Downregulation of NAF-1 Enhances the Sensitivity of Pancreatic Cancer Cells to Gemcitabine via ROS/Nrf2 Signaling Pathways. *Oxid. Med. Cellular Longev.* **2018,** 9882018.

Dhillon, N.; Aggarwal, B. B.; Newman, R. A.; Wolff, R. A.; Kunnumakkara, A. B.; Abbruzzese, J. L.; Ng, C. S.; Badmaev, V.; Kurzrock, R. Phase II Trial of Curcumin in Patients with Advanced Pancreatic Cancer. *Clin. Cancer Res.* **2008,** *14*, 4491–4499.

Espinoza, J. L.; Trung, L. Q.; Inaoka, P. T.; Yamada, K.; An, D. T.; Mizuno, S.; Nakao, S.; Takami, A. The Repeated Administration of Resveratrol Has Measurable Effects on Circulating T-Cell Subsets in Humans. *Oxid. Med. Cell Longev.* **2017,** ***2017***, 6781872.

Falchetti, R.; Fuggetta, M. P.; Lanzilli, G.; Tricarico, M.; Ravagnan, G. Effects of Resveratrol on Human Immune Cell Function. *Life Sci.* **2001,** *70*, 81–96.

Feng, Y.; Zhu, X.; Wang, Q. Allicin Enhances Host Proinflammatory Immune Responses and Protects Against Acute Murine Malaria Infection. *Malaria J.* **2012,** *11*, 268.

Garcia-Vilas, J. A.; Quesada, A. R.; Medina, M. A. Damnacanthal, a Noni Anthraquinone, Inhibits C-Met and Is a Potent Antitumor Compound Against Hep G2 Human Hepatocellular Carcinoma Cells. *Sci. Rep.* **2015,** *5*, 8021.

Gee, J. R.; Saltzstein, D. R.; Kim, K.; Kolesar, J.; Huang, W. A Phase II Randomized, Double-Blind, Presurgical Trial of Polyphenon E in Bladder Cancer Patients to Evaluate Pharmacodynamics and Bladder Tissue Biomarkers. *Cancer Prev. Res.* **2017,** *10*, 1–10.

Goodwin, P. J.; Stambolic, V. Impact of the Obesity Epidemic on Cancer. *Ann. Rev. Med.* **2015,** *66*, 281–296.

Gupta, R. K.; Banerjee, A.; Pathak, S.; Sharma, C.; Singh, N. Induction of Mitochondrial-Mediated Apoptosis by *MorindaCitrifolia* (Noni) in Human Cervical Cancer Cells. *Asian Pac. J. Cancer Prev.* **2013,** *14*, 237–242.

Gutheil, W. G.; Reed, G.; Ray, A.; Dhar, A. Crocetin: An Agent Derived from Saffron for Prevention and Therapy for Cancer. *Curr. Pharm. Biotechnol.* **2012,** *13*, 173–179.

Hanahan, D.; Weinberg, R.A. Hallmarks of Cancer: The Next Generation. *Cell.* **2011,** *144*, 646–674.

Hire, R. R.; Srivastava, S.; Davis, M. B.; Konreddy, A. K.; Panda, D. Antiproliferative Activity of Crocin Involves Targeting of Microtubules in Breast Cancer Cells. *Sci. Rep.* **2017,** *7*, 44984.

Hudspeth, K.; Silva-Santos, B.; Mavilio, D. Natural Cytotoxicity Receptors: Broader Expression Patterns and Functions in Innate and Adaptive Immune Cells. *Front. Immunol.* **2013,** *4*, 69.

Iqbal, J.; Abbasi, B. A.; Mahmood, T.; Kanwal, S.; Ali, B.; Shah, S.A.; Khalil, A. T. Plant-Derived Anticancer Agents: A Green Anticancer Approach. *Asian Pac. J. Trop. Biomed.* **2017,** *7*, 1129–1150.

Jiang, Y. Z.; Ge, L. P.; Jin, X.; He, M.; Liu, Y.; Chen, L.; Zhuo, W.J.; Wu, J.; Liu, G.Y. et al. Randomized Phase II Clinical Trial and Biomarker Analysis of Paclitaxel Plus Epirubicin Versus Vinorelbine Plus Epirubicin as Neoadjuvant Chemotherapy in Locally Advanced HER2-Negative Breast Cancer with TEKT4 Variations. *Breast Cancer Res. Treatment.* **2020.** https://doi.org/10.1007/s10549–020–05940–8.

Kafi, M.; Kamili, A. N.; Husaini, A. M. et al. An Expensive Spice—Saffron (Crocus sativus L.)—Case Study from Kashmir, Iran and Turkey. In: Global Perspectives on Underutilized Crops; Ozturk. M. et al., Eds., Chapter 4; Springer International Publishing AG, part of Springer Nature, 2018; pp 109–149.

Knapp, D. W.; Ruple-Czerniak, W.; Ramos-Vara, J. A.; Naughton, J. F.; Fulkerson, C. M.; Honkisz, S. I. A Nonselective Cyclooxygenase Inhibitor Enhances the Activity of Vinblastine in a Naturally-Occurring Canine Model of Invasive Urothelial Carcinoma. *Bladder Cancer.* **2016,** *2*, 241–250.

Kolomeichuk, S. N.; Terrano, D. T.; Lyle, C. S.; Sabapathy, K.; Chambers, T. C. Distinct Signaling Pathways of Microtubule Inhibitors-Vinblastine and Taxol Induce JNK-Dependent Cell Death But Through AP-1 Dependent and AP-1 Independent Mechanisms Respectively. *FEBS J.* **2008,** *275*, 1889–1899.

Laphanuwat, P.; Jirawatnotai, S. Immunomodulatory Roles of Cell Cycle Regulators. *Front. Cell Dev. Biol.* **2019,** *7*, 23.

Li, K.; Xiao, G.; Richardson, J. J.; Tardy, B. L.; Ejima, H.; Huang, W.; Guo, J.; Liao, X.; Shi, B. Targeted Therapy Against Metastatic Melanoma Based on Self-Assembled Metal-Phenolic Nanocomplexes Comprised of Green Tea Catechin. *Adv. Sci.* **2019a**, *6*, 1801688.

Li, X.; Xing, L.; Zhang, Y.; Xie, P.; Zhu, W.; Meng, X.; Wang, Y.; Kong, L.; Zhao, H.; Yu, J. Phase II Trial of Epigallocatechin-3-Gallate in Acute Radiation-Induced Esophagitis for Esophagus Cancer. *J. Med. Food.* **2019,** 1–7.

Lin, C. B.; Lin, C. C.; Gregory, J. T. 6-Gingerol Inhibits Growth of Colon Cancer Cell LoVo via Induction of G2/M Arrest. *Evid. Based Compl. Altern. Med.* **2012,** *2012*, 326096.

Lucas, J.; Hsieh, T. C.; Halicka, H. D.; Darzynkiewicz, Z.; Wu, J. M. Upregulation of PD-L1 Expression by Resveratrol and Piceatannol in Breast and Colorectal Cancer Cells Occurs via HDAC3/p300-Mediated NF-κB Signaling. *Int. J. Oncol.* **2018,** *53*, 1469–1480.

Luikart, S. D.; Kennealey, G. T.; Kirkwood, J. M. Randomized Phase III Trial of Vinblastine, Bleomycin, and Cis-Dichlorodiammine-Platinum Versus Dacarbazine in Malignant Melanoma. *J. Clin. Oncol.* **1984,** *2*, 164–168.

Luster, A. D. The Role of Chemokines in Linking Innate and Adaptive Immunity. *Curr. Opin. Immunol.* **2002,** *14*, 129–135.

Ma, D.; Li, S.; Cui, Y.; Li, L.; Liu, H.; Chen, Y.; Zhou, X. Paclitaxel Increases the Sensitivity of Lung Cancer Cells to Lobaplatin via PI3K/Akt Pathway. *Oncol. Lett.* **2018,** *15*, 6211–6216.

Mahmoodally, M. F.; Aumeeruddy, M. Z.; Rengasamy, K. R. R.; Roshan, S.; Hammad, S.; Pandhee, J.; Hu, X.; Zengin, G. Ginger and Its Active Compounds in Cancer Therapy: From Folk Uses to Nanotherapeutic Applications. *Semin. Cancer Biol.* **2019,** 1044–579X.

Mansingh, D. P.; Dalpati, N.; Sali, V.K.; Vasanthi, A. H. R. Alliin the Precursor of Allicin in Garlic Extract Mitigates Proliferation of Gastric Adenocarcinoma Cells by Modulating Apoptosis. *Pharmacogn. Mag.* **2018,** *14*, S84–S91.

Mao, J. T.; Smoake, J.; Park, H. K.; Lu, Q.Y.; Xue, B. Grape Seed Procyanidin Extract Mediates Antineoplastic Effects against Lung Cancer via Modulations of Prostacyclin and 15-HETE Eicosanoid Pathways. *Cancer Prev. Res.* **2016,** *9*, 925–932.

Masoodi, K. Z.; Amin, I.; Mansoor, S. et al. Botanicals from the Himalayas with Anticancer Potential—An Emphasis on Kashmir Himalayas. In *Biodiversity and Biomedicine—Our Future*; Ozturk, M., Egamberdieva, D., Pešić, M., Eds., Chapter 11; Academic Press, 2020; pp 189–234.

Mukherjee, S.; Hussaini, R.; White, R.; Atwi, D.; Fried, A.; Sampat, S. TriCurin, a Synergistic Formulation of Curcumin, Resveratrol, and Epicatechingallate, Repolarizes Tumor-Associated Macrophages and Triggersan Immune Response to Cause Suppression of HPV+ Tumors. *Cancer Immunol. Immunother.* **2018,** *67*, 761–774.

Nualsanit, T.; Rojanapanthu, P.; Gritsanapan, W.; Lee, S. H.; Lawson, D.; Baek, S. J. Damnacanthal, a Noni Component, Exhibits Anti-Tumorigenic Activity in Human Colorectal Cancer Cells. *J. Nutr. Biochem.* **2012,** *23*, 915–923.

Ojima, I.; Lichtenthal, B.; Lee, S.; Wang, C.; Wang, X. Taxane Anticancer Agents: A Patent Perspective. *Exp. Opin. Ther. Pat.* **2016,** *26*, 1–20.

Oomen, S.; Anto, R. J.; Srinivas, G.; Karunagarn, D. Allicin (from Garlic) Induces Caspase-Mediated Apoptosis in Cancer Cells. *Eur. J. Pharmacol.* **2004,** *485*, 97–103.

Ozturk, M.; Altay, V.; Efe, R. *Biodiversity, Conservation and Sustainability in Asia: Volume I: Prospects and Challenges in West Asia and Caucasus*; Springer Nature: Switzerland AG, 2021a. DOI: 10.1007/978–3-030–59928–7

Ozturk, M.; Egamberdieva, D.; Milica, P. *Biodiversity and Biomedicine-Our Future*; Academic Press, Elsevier Inc.: UK, USA, 2020.

Ozturk, M.; Gucel, S.; Altay, V.; Altundağ, E. Alliums, an Underutilized Genetic Resource in the East Mediterranean. Proc. 6th IS on Edible Alliaceae. *Acta Hort.* **2012,** *969* (ISHS 2012), 303–309.

Ozturk, M.; Khan, S. M.; Altay, V.; Efe, R.; Egamberdieva, D.; Khassanov, F. *Biodiversity, Conservation and Sustainability in Asia: Volume II: Prospects and Challenges in South and Middle Asia*; Springer Nature: Switzerland AG, 2021b. DOI: 10.1007/978-3-030-73943-0

Pan, J.; Shen, J.; Si, W.; Du, C.; Chen, D.; Xu, L.; Yao, M.; Fu, P.; Fan, W. Resveratrol Promotes MICA/B Expression and Natural Killer Cell Lysis of Breast Cancer Cells by Suppressing c-Myc/miR-17 Pathway. *Oncotarget.* **2017,** *8*, 65743–65758.

Patel, K. R.; Brown, V.A.; Jones, D. J. L.; Britton, R.G.; Hemnigway, D.; Miller, A.S.; West, K. P.; Booth, T. D.; Perloff, M.; Crowell, J. A.; Brenner, D. E.; Steward, W. P.; Gescher, A. J.; Brown, K. Clinical Pharmacology of Resveratrol and Its Metabolites in Colorectal Cancer Patients. *Cancer Res.* **2010,** *70*, 7392–7399.

Pyrhonen, B. S.; Salminen, E.; Ruutu, M.; Lehtonen, T.; Nurmi, M.; Tammela, T.; Juusela, H. Prospective Randomized Trial of Interferon Alfa-2a Plus Vinblastine Versus Vinblastine Alone in Patients With Advanced Renal Cell Cancer. *J. Clin. Oncol.* **1999,** *17*, 2859–2867.

Ren, X.; Zhao, B.; Chang, H.; Xiao, M.; Wu, Y.; Liu, Y. Paclitaxel Suppresses Proliferation and Induces Apoptosis Through Regulation of ROS and the AKT/MAPK Signaling Pathway in Canine Mammary Gland Tumor Cells. *Mol. Med. Rep.* **2018,** *17*, 8289–8299.

Samarghandian, S.; Borji, A.; Farahmad, S. K.; Afshari, R.; Davoodi, S. *Crocus sativus* L. (Saffron) Stigma Aqueous Extract Induces Apoptosis in Alveolar Human Lung Cancer Cells through Caspase-Dependent Pathways Activation. *BioMed Res. Int.* **2013,** 417928.

Schwarz, K.; Dobiasch, S.; Nguyen, L.; Schilling, D.; Combs, S.E. Modification of Radio-sensitivity by Curcumin in Human Pancreatic Cancer Cell Lines. *Sci. Rep.* **2020,** *10*, 3815.

Seo, S. U.; Woo, S. M.; Lee, H. S.; Kim, S. H.; Min, K. J.; Kwon, T. K. mTORC1/2 Inhibitor and Curcumin Induce Apoptosis Through Lysosomal Membrane Permeabilization-Mediated Autophagy. *Oncogene*. **2018,** *37*, 5205–5220.

Shi, L. M.; Lin, Q. L.; Li, X. H.; Nie, Y.; Sun, S. G.; Deng, X. Y.; Wang, L.; Lu, J.; Tang, Y.P.; Luo, F. J. Alliin, a Garlic Organosulfur Compound, Ameliorates Gut Inflammation Through MAPK-NF-κB/AP-1/STAT-1 Inactivation and PPAR-7 Activation. *Mol. Nutr. Food Res.* **2017,** *61*, 1601013.

Siddiqui, F. A.; Prakasam, G.; Chattopadhyay, S.; Rehman, A. U.; Padder, R. A.; Ansari, M. A. Curcumin Decreases Warburg Effect in Cancer Cells by Down-Regulating Pyruvatekinase M2 via mTORHIF1α inhibition. *Sci. Rep.* **2018,** *8*, 8323.

Sidhar, H.; Giri, R. K. Induction of Bex Genes by Curcumin Is Associated with Apoptosis and Activation of p53 in N2a Neuroblastoma Cells. *Sci. Rep.* **2017,** *7*, 41420.

Spigel, D. R.; Patel, J. D.; Reynolds, C. H.; Garon, E. B.; Hermann, R. C.; Govindan, R. Quality of Life Analysis from the Randomized Open-Label, Phase III Point Break Study of Pemetrexed-Carboplatin-Bevacizumab Followed by Maintenance Pemetrexed-Bevacizumab Versus Paclitaxel-Carboplatin-Bevacizumab Followed by Maintenance Bevacizumab in Patients. *J. Thorac. Oncol.* **2015,** *10*, 353–359.

Suddek, G. M. Allicin Enhances Chemotherapeutic Response and Ameliorates Tamoxifen-Induced Liver Injury in Experimental Animals. *Pharm. Biol.* **2014,** *52*, 1009–1014.

Tanaka, H.; Matsushima, H.; Nishibu, A.; Clausen, B. E.; Takashima, A. Dual Therapeutic Efficacy of Vinblastine as a Unique Chemotherapeutic Agent Capable of Inducing Dendritic Cell Maturation. *Cancer Res.* **2009,** *69*, 6987–6994.

Vairy, S.; Teuff, G. L.; Bautista, F.; Carli, E. D. Phase I Study of Vinblastine in Combination with Nilotinib in Children, Adolescents, and Young Adults with Refractory or Recurrent Low-Grade Glioma. *Neuro-Oncol. Adv.* **2020,** *2*, 1–12.

Vassileva, V.; Allen, C. J.; Piquette-Miller, M. Effects of Sustained and Intermittent Paclitaxel Therapy on Tumor Repopulation in Ovarian Cancer. *Mol. Cancer. Ther.* **2008,** *7*, 630–637.

Vervandier-Fasseur, D.; Latruffe, N. The Potential Use of Resveratrol for Cancer Prevention. *Molecules.* **2019,** *24*, 4506.

Wang, M.; Zhao, J.; Zhang, L.; Wei, F.; Lian, Y.; Wu, Y.; Gong, Z.; Zhang, S.; Zhou, J.; Cao, K.; Li, X.; Xiong, W.; Li, G.; Zeng, Z.; Guo, C. Role of Tumor Microenvironment in Tumorigenesis. *J Cancer*. **2017,** *8*, 761–773.

Whiteside, T. L. The Tumor Microenvironment and Its Role in Promoting Tumor Growth. *Oncogene*. **2008,** *27*, 5904–5910.

Xie, S.; Zhou, J. Harnessing Plant Biodiversity for the Discovery of Novel Anticancer Drugs Targeting Microtubules. *Front. Plant Sci.* **2017,** *8*, 720.

Yen, H. Y.; Tsao, C.W.; Lin, Y. W.; Kuo, C. C.; Tsao, C.H.; Liu, C.Y. Regulation of Carcinogenesis and Modulation Through Wnt/β-Catenin Signaling by Curcumin in an Ovarian Cancer Cell Line. *Sci. Rep.* **2019,** *9*, 17267.

Young, S. D.; Whissell, M.; Noble, J. C. S.; Cano, P. O.; Lopez, P. G.; Germond, C. J. Phase II Clinical Trial Results InvolvingTreatment with Low-Dose Daily Oral Cyclophosphamide, Weekly Vinblastine, and Rofecoxib in Patients with Advanced Solid Tumors. *Clin. Cancer Res.* **2006,** *12*, 3092–3098.

Zhang, Q.; Yang, D. Allicin Suppresses the Migration and Invasion in Cervical Cancer Cells Mainly by Inhibiting NRF2. *Exp. Ther. Med.* **2017,** *17*, 1523–1528.

Zick, S. M.; Djuric, Z.; Ruffin, M. T.; Litzinger, A. J.; Normolle, D. P.; Feng, M. R.; Brenner, D. E. Pharmacokinetics of 6-, 8-, 10-Gingerols and 6-Shogaol and Conjugate Metabolites in Healthy Human Subjects. *Cancer Epidemiol. Biomarkers Prev.* **2009,** *17*, 1930–1936.

CHAPTER 15

Contribution of Indian Traditional Medicine in Cancer Treatment: An Update

NEHA KATHURIA and SHAZIA RASHID

Amity Institute of Biotechnology, Amity University Uttar Pradesh, Noida, India

ABSTRACT

According to the World Health Organization, cancer is the second most common cause of death worldwide. Conventional cancer treatment includes surgery, radiation therapy, and chemotherapy, which often kills healthy cells and results in many side effects to patients. Therefore, there is a need for new methods to treat cancer with minimum side effects and this has led to research on natural compounds for cancer treatment. As Indian terrain is very diverse and home to a huge wealth of medicinal plants, researchers are working extensively on many natural plants and medicinal compounds from Indian subcontinent. Indian traditional medicine that largely comprises two important branches, Ayurveda and Unani system of medicines has been used for hundreds of years for the treatment of various diseases. Besides their use in traditional medicine, plants have always been a good source of pharmacologically active molecules, known as Phyto-compounds. In this chapter, Indian traditional system of medicines will be explored for their role in the treatment and management of cancer and highlight current research

Ethnic Knowledge and Perspectives of Medicinal Plants, Volume 1: Curative Properties and Treatment Strategies. Munir Ozturk, Kandikere R. Sridhar, Maryam Sarwat, Volkan Altay, & Francisco Martín Huerta-Martínez (Eds.)

that is focused on understanding their molecular mechanisms to impart wider acceptability for their use in treatment.

15.1 INTRODUCTION

Without a doubt, cancer has become the deadliest disease accounting for one in sixth deaths in 2018 according to the World Health Organization (Masoodi et al., 2020). Conventional cancer treatment incorporates for the most part medicines which however besides treating cancer, begin to influence the normal cells in the human body causing side effects. This has led to research into alternate, safer methods of cancer treatment. India has been known for restorative plants and medications and its greatness in traditional medicines has been celebrated all over the world (Ozturk et al., 2021a, b). The cancer treatment with Ayurveda goes back to the seventh century BC when Atreya and Dhanwanthari used herbal medicines for treating the early stages of cancer (Poornima and Efferth, 2016). In India, traditional medicine was mostly used by people who live in inaccessible rural areas with limited access to allopathic medicines (Borins, 1987). Due to lack of scientific evidence on the mechanism of action and working, the Indian Traditional Medicine did not get recognition among the Western world researchers until WHO gave importance and consideration to the Indian system of Traditional Medicine (Jangid and Dixit, 2019). Since various improvements have been made in modern medicine, the mechanisms of the Indian traditional medicinal system have earned pace and have reached a level of worldwide acceptance (Chauhan et al., 2015; Krishna et al., 2020). Several traditional pharma sectors like Dabur, Himalaya, Zandu, Hamdard, and modern pharma companies like Ranbaxy, Lupin, and Allembic are utilizing India's herbal formulations in their medications (Kamboj, 2000). Traditional Indian methods of treatment broadly incorporate six branches, Ayurveda, Siddha, Unani, Yoga, Naturopathy, and Homeopathy (Poornima and Efferth, 2016).

15.2 INDIAN SYSTEMS OF MEDICINE

15.2.1 AYURVEDA

The term Ayurveda comes from the Sanskrit language which is made up of two words: ayus (meaning life) and veda (meaning knowledge). The main motive of Ayurveda is providing healthy living while maintaining the balance of the body (the teaching of Indian traditional medicine). Ayurveda is also known as Astanga Ayurveda, which means made up of eight parts. The eight major divisions of Ayurveda are as follows (Ravishankar and Shukla, 2007):

1. Kayachikitsa (Internal Medicine): deals with various physical as well as psychological diseases like diabetes, kidney problems, liver diseases, etc.
2. Kaumar Bhritya (Pediatrics): deals with child care and children-related problems.
3. Bhootavidya (Psychiatry): deals with psychiatric problems and diseases and is believed to be caused by supernatural forces.
4. Shalakya (Otorhinolaryngology and Ophthalmology): deals with diseases of eyes, nose, ears, tongue, dental problems, head, neck, throat, that is, diseases above the clavicle.
5. Shaly (Surgery): it is a surgical branch of Ayurveda which means the removal of unwanted, irritating elements from the body with the help of surgery. For example hemorrhoids.
6. Agada Tantra (Toxicology): it is also known as the branch of toxicology which deals with the treatment of toxins released from food poisoning, snake bites, insect and animal bites, etc.
7. Rasayana (Geriatrics): Rasayana is a Sanskrit word which means restoration of youthful vigor by promoting health at both macro and microcellular levels.
8. Vajikarana (Aphrodisiacs and Eugenics): deals with the treatment of sexual dysfunctions.

Ayurveda considers wellbeing as the balance of the three natural humous (doshas), the seven body tissues (dhatus), legitimate assimilation furthermore, a condition of happiness or joy of the spirit, sense, and brain (Ravishankar and Shukla, 2007). Consequently, remembering all the parts of Ayurveda, treatment includes the rebuilding of the parity of upset doshas through managing diet, rectifying life-routine and conduct, organization of medications, and falling back on preventive nonsedate treatments known as Panchkarma (five procedures) and Rasayana (restoration) treatment (Poornima and Efferth, 2016). A recent case study reported a 60-year-old female suffering from uncontrolled type-2 diabetes mellitus and chronic kidney disease (stage 4) was prescribed hemodialysis. She was treated with shamanaaushdhi, Mustadiyapana Basti, and with specific pathyaahara. After 9 days, her tests reflected a change in her waste production capacity and aligned her doshas. Therefore, with the help of proper assessment, Ayurveda can be used to align all the doshas, dushya, and vyadhi avasti (Rachana et al.,

2019). Along with the natural treatment, Ayurveda provides a cost-effective treatment as well.

15.2.2 SIDDHA

On the other hand, Siddha's culture of medication is an accepted achievement and image of Tamil culture which started in Southern parts of India. Siddha medication is developed from Dravidian culture and grew in the hour of Indus valley human progress. Chinese alchemy, Taoism, and Taoist Pathology are considered a principal source of inspiration for Siddha's speculative chemistry. It is accepted that in obsolescent time, the core of the treatment with Siddha was created by 18 siddhar (a class of Tamil sages). Even though Siddha's arrangement of medication resembles Ayurveda in numerous perspectives, it has its way of thinking and idea, holistic approach, and way of life situated measures (Sen and Chakraborty, 2014; Subbarayappa, 2001). Siddha's concept of treatment is based on three major cosmic forces namely—"Vaatha" (the creative/anabolic forces), "Kapha" (the destructive/catabolic forces), "Pitha" (the protective force). The ayurvedic five elements and these forces of Siddha go hand in hand and are believed that they interconnected with each other. So, therefore, it was believed that aligning these three forces together would help to treat a large number of diseases (Borins, 1987).

15.2.3 UNANI

Unani medicine is considered to be the medicine that was converted into art with the help of scientific inputs given by the great Hippocrates, an ancient Greek physician (460 B.C.) and further down the road by Galen, Roman physician, surgeon, and philosopher. Unani medicine is based on the approach where the body has four major humors namely blood, phlegm, yellow bile, and black bile (Borins, 1987). Unani arrangement of medication is the combination of the contemporary traditional therapeutic framework in Egypt, Syria, Iran, Iraq, China, India, and several other east nations. It began in Greece and later developed in Arab. Bedouin and Persian pioneers in the 11th century presented Unani medication in India, the framework got recognition and advancement during Mughal rule during the 16th–18th century (Lone et al., 2012). Unani medicine is based on three types of therapies—Regimental therapy, Dietotherapy, Pharmacotherapy (Borins,

1987). Regimental therapy includes special treatment methods where the body's capacity to produce waste materials like sweat, urine, and excreta is increased which in turn helps to improve immunity, strengthens defence mechanisms, and provides better health. On the other hand, Dietotherapy includes treatment that focuses primarily on the diet by improving the quality and quantity of the food. This approach is also called "natural healers." And the third approach of Pharmacotherapy includes treatment by the usage of natural drugs obtained from plants, animal parts, and certain minerals.

15.2.4 YOGA AND NATUROPATHY

Naturopathy and Yoga are the drugless, noninvasive, and proof-based arrangement of medications that confers normal treatments, based on the hypothesis of imperativeness, toxemia, one mending limit of the human body, and the standards of sound living. This methodology to health care stresses instruction, self-duty, and therapies to bolster and animate a person's self-recuperating limit. The principles of naturopathy were first utilized by the Hippocratic School of Medicine in around 400 BC. Yoga and naturopathy go hand in hand (Shrivastava et al., 2015). Where naturopathy is a form of treatment where the effectiveness is proven over a while and is also referred to as time-tested principles. However, naturopathy has a little different and unique way of treatment. The body has treated all things considered. These methods of treatment are designed in a way that there is no specific cause for the disease rather a tedious check is performed on the whole day and factors like daily lifestyle, sleeping time, eating habits, etc. are all taken into consideration for the treatment (Rastogi, 2012). Yoga, on the other hand, is known as the conscious union of mind with supreme consciousness. This includes the eight limbs of Yoga (the eight-fold paths) with various stages like yama, niyama, asana, pranayama, pratyahara, dharana, dhyana, and samadhi. Each of these limbs has varied meanings and effects in the therapy of Yoga.

- Yama is a practice of self-control, sobriety, and self-monitoring
- Niyama is awareness, practices, and self-learning and training
- Asana is a posture for meditation
- Pranayama is breathing control and regulation practices
- Pratyahara is dealing with internal realization and retreatment of senses
- Dharana means concentration
- Dhyana is meditation

- Samadhi is the final stage of an eight-fold path which is a stage of enlightenment that is a connection with divine order (Taneja, 2014).

15.2.5 HOMEOPATHY

Homeopathic medications are made from a combination of substances (for example, plants, minerals, or chemicals). In request to reduce toxicity, the restorative substances are diluted progressively and shaken energetically between every dilution. Hahnemann created homeopathy by giving therapeutic substances to volunteers and contemplating the side effects which they endured (a procedure is known as a "demonstrating" or a Homeopathic Pathogenesis Trial). Hahnemann then applied the therapeutic substances during sickness that had comparable side effects (Relton et al., 2017). It is a branch of AYUSH and is based on the idea that the body has the capability of healing itself. It is commonly known as "like cures like" which is based on the principle of vital response: is an automatic healing response present in all human beings. This principle states that the body is aware of how to fight any unusual event within by producing symptoms that are a part of curing the illness. The medicine is provided according to the symptoms produced which further acts as a stimulus to the vital response and boosts the body's natural healing capacity (Kaur et al., 2019; D'Huyvetter and Cohrssen, 2002).

15.3 INDIA: THE LAND OF MEDICINAL PLANTS

Of the world's 297000 flora species, 8000 species of flora are found in the Indian Himalayan region (Schippmann et al., 2002; Ozturk et al., 2021a, b). Out of which, 22% of flora species found are medicinal plants. The continuous developing acknowledgment of restorative plants is because of a few reasons, incorporating heightening confidence in homegrown medication (Kala et al., 2006). Ayurveda, the oldest medical system in the Indian subcontinent, has alone reported approximately 2000 medicinal plant species, followed by 1121 reported in Siddha and 751 in Unani (Kala et al., 2006). Around 81 types of Himalayan restorative plants are known to be utilized for the extraction of oil. Of the all-out 675 types of Himalayan wild edibles, 171 are utilized for the treatment of sicknesses (Rawal and Dhar, 2001). The bioactive compounds found in medicinal plants are commonly known as phyto-chemicals. These compounds have been used against many diseases since time immemorial; hence, the demand for medicinal plant products has increased tremendously in recent years. The dependence on medicinal plants is also because of social inclinations. In certain local cultures of north India, medicinal plants have been worshipped as divine beings, goddesses, and minor gods (Kala et al., 2006).

Some of the commonly found medicinal plants in India are (Pandey et al., 2013):

- *Asparagus racemosus* (Shatavari): Shatavari is commonly found in Rajasthan. The major parts of the plant with medicinal properties are roots and leaves. It is used in the treatment of hysterectomies and also improves immunity. Also it helps to purify the blood and is a supplement of female hormones (Kamboj, 2000).
- *Commiphora mukul* (Guggul): Guggul is generally found in the Northern areas of India. The gum extracted from the bark for these plants possesses medicinal properties. It is used in joint treatment and immune-care. It helps to maintain lower levels of cholesterol and can be used in the treatment of cold (Mukherjee et al., 2001).
- *Cyperus scariosus* (Nagarmusta): Nagarmusta is generally found in Chhattisgarh, UP, and Bihar. The rhizomes of the plant keep the genitourinary system and liver healthy (Pandey et al., 2013).
- *Garcinia cambogia* (Garcinia): Garcinia is mostly found in Kerala and Karnataka. The fruits of these plants are used for heart disorder treatment and are a rich source of vitamin C (Pandey et al., 2013).
- *Glycyrrhiza glabra* (Yashtimadhu, Licorice): Yashtimadhu is commonly used in Northeast India. The bark and flower of these plants relieve muscle spasms, used for the gastrointestinal tract. It is an antioxidant and is known to prevent cancer (Isbrucker et al., 2006, Mukherjee et al., 2001; Ozturk et al., 2017a).
- *Gymnema sylvestre* (Gurmarar): Gurmarar is used in western and southern India. The stem of this plant is used as a medicinal plant as it increases insulin production and regulates sugar metabolism (Kamboj, 2000).
- *Melia azadirachta* (Nimba, Neem): Nimba is used in most parts of India. It possesses detoxifying properties, promotes healing, and is beneficial for the digestive, circulatory, and respiratory systems (Pandey et al., 2013).
- *Nardostachys jatamansi* (Jatamansi, Musk root): Jatamansi is found in Eastern Himalayas. The leaves, roots, and fruit of this plant are used for menopause-related problems (like late menopause or heavy menstruation) and it is also effective for treating mental disorders. It

is generally known as a relaxing plant and used in Ayurvedic formulations (Kamboj, 2000).

- *Piper longum* (Pippali, Indian Long Pepper): Pippali is commonly found in the households of Northern India. The fruit of the plant improves digestion and the respiratory system. It also keeps the lungs healthy and enhances metabolism (Kamboj, 2000).
- *Terminalia chebula* (Haritaki): Haritaki is found in North India. The fruit, bark, and roots act as a detoxifying agent and a rich source of vitamin C. It is also known to be antimutagenic (Mukherjee et al., 2010). In Ayurveda, it one of the components of "Triphala" which is a combination of three fruit extracts.
- *Tinospora cordifolia* (Guduchi): The tropical region of India is rich in the vegetation of Guduchi. The leaves are a rich source of vitamin C and boost immunity. It helps to strengthen and increase the production of immune cells (Kamboj, 2000).
- *Zingiber officinale* (Sunthi, Ginger): Sunthi is found in most parts of India. The stem of the plant helps in improving digestion, enhances bowel movement, and prevents nausea (Umadevi et al., 2013).

15.4 ANTICANCER PLANTS FROM INDIA

Plants are known to be the most natural and important component of traditional medicine (Altay and Çelik, 2011; Altay and Karahan, 2012; Altay et al., 2015a, b; Ozturk et al., 2017b, c, 2018a, b, c, d, e, f, g, 2020, 2021a, b). India being the land of rich diversity for flora and fauna has now attracted the attention of scientists and researchers worldwide to explore the rich traditional Indian system of medicine. One of the recent studies showed that people consuming natural herbal products have a lesser chance to develop cancer (Shaikh et al., 2016). For example, soyabean (a species of native legume) is known as a rich source of anticancer agents, saponins. Thus, there is a demand for detailed study and screening of plant extracts for anticancer compounds and agents. Some of the common anticancer herbal compounds found in India are listed below (Figure 15.1). However, the consumption of these herbs should be under the strict observation of doctors (Umadevi et al., 2013).

- *Aloe barbadensis* (Aloe Vera): Commonly known as Aloe Vera, the plant possesses a variety of medicinal properties apart from very effective anticancer properties. Bioactive compounds isolated from

Aloe Vera show effective action toward cancer cells. It is also known to contain "super carbohydrates" that have shown protection against some cancers like liver cancer. When used in combination with chemotherapy and radiation, it helps to reduce the side effects because of its tremendous antioxidant profile. It is an immunity enhancer and helps in skincare as well. A lot of bioactive compounds from this plant are under research for their anticancer properties (Kim et al., 1999).

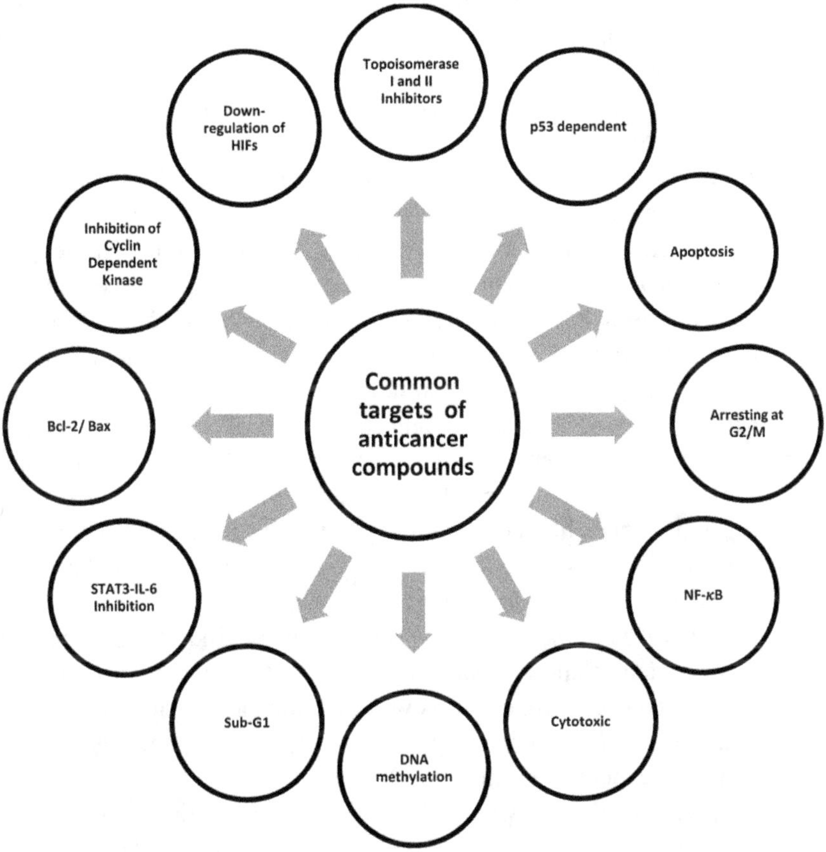

FIGURE 15.1 Common targets of anticancer compounds.

[The above figure illustrates common targets of anticancer compounds involved in the process of carcinogenesis. There is a main circle in the middle with the caption "Some Common Anti-carcinogenic mechanisms," other circles are made from the main circle with arrows. The other circles are 12 in number. The various mechanisms specified in the 12 circles are "Topoisomerase I and II Inhibitors," "p53 dependent," "Apoptosis," "Arresting at G2/M," "NF-κB," "Cytotoxic," "DNA methylation," "Sub-G1," "STAT3-IL-6 Inhibition," "Bcl-2/ Bax," "Inhibition of Cyclin-Dependent Kinase," "Down-regulation of HIFs"].

- *Alpinia galanga* (Galangal): Bioactive compounds like Acetoxy-chavicol-acetate (ACA), Pinocembrin, and flavonoid like Galangin are isolated from the Galangal plant which possesses anticancer activities. They are proven to be effective against breast, colon, lung, prostate, etc. cancer cells (Samarghandian et al., 2014; Umadevi et al 2013).
- *Andrographis paniculate* (Kalmegh): Kalmegh possesses various medicinal properties against diabetes, skin diseases, high blood pressure, ulcers, and influenza besides showing anticancer properties. Bioactive compounds found in this plant induce apoptosis by arresting G0/G1 phase of the cell cycle. It is also antioxidant and anti-HIV. It also helps to reduce chemotherapy and radiation side effects (Nyeem et al., 2017).
- *Berberis vulgaris* (Daruharidra): Daruharidra shows anticancer activity by arresting the cell cycle at G1 stage and then induces apoptosis, arresting cancer cell growth. It is also used in Homeopathic medicine and helps to provide treatment against cold, fever, heart and lung diseases, kidney problems, etc (Abd El-Wahab et al., 2013).
- *Curcuma longa* (Turmeric/Haldi): Turmeric/Haldi is one of the most important spices in the Indian household which possesses anticancer activity along with enhancing the taste of food. The bioactive compounds isolated from the plant are found to cause apoptosis at every step of the cell cycle. It shows anticancer activity against various types of cancer like colon, oral, breast, skin, prostate, liver, and lung cancers. It is also anti-inflammatory, antioxidant, and enhances the immune system (Johnson and Mukhtar, 2007).
- *Emblica officinalis* (Amla): Also known as "Indian gooseberry," it an important plant used since times ancient in Ayurveda. It possesses many medicinal properties as well as anticancer properties. It is also antioxidant and effective against breast, uterus, pancreas, stomach, and liver cancer (Sairam et al., 2002).
- *Glycyrrhiza glabra* (Mukethi): Mukethi is one of the most used herbs in Ayurveda, commonly referred to as "sweet root" as it tastes sweeter than sugar. It is antioxidant, antimicrobial, analgesic, and shows anticancer properties against cancers of breast, lung, stomach, colon, liver, and kidney cancer (Kaur et al., 2019).
- *Glycine max* (Soya/Soyabean): The bioactive compounds like Isoflavones and saponins which stops the growth and spread of cancer cell in a variety of cancers like breast, stomach, colon, ovary, and liver cancer (Ahmad et al., 2014).

- *Nigella sativa* (Kalonji): Kalonji is another important plant that is used in the Indian traditional system of medicine of Ayurveda, Siddha, and Unani. The seeds and oil of this plant are of great importance for a long time ago. It possesses a very strong anticancer activity against malignant ascites, malignant lymphoma, malignant melanoma, and leukemia (Tembhurne et al., 2014).
- *Ocimum sanctum* (Tulsi): Along with medicinal properties, Tulsi is worshipped as a sacred plant in the Northern Parts of India. It is also an important plant used in Ayurveda. Bioactive compounds like eugenol, orientin, and vicenin are effective against breast cancer, liver cancer, and fibrosarcoma as well. When used along with chemotherapy and radiation, it helps to reduce the harmful side effects as well. It is antioxidant in nature (Dharmani et al., 2004, Baliga et al., 2013).
- *Tinospora cordifolia* (Giloya): Giloya is known for its antistress, anti-inflammatory, and anticancer properties. It is effective against cancers of the lung, cervix, throat, and malignant ascites (Bala et al., 2015).
- *Withania somnifera* (Ashwagandha): Ashwagandha is extracted from the plant which is known for its anticancer properties against cancers of the breast, lung, and colon. It has several other bioactive compounds that possess anticancer properties and also are antiproliferative and antiangiogenic as well as consisting of medicinal properties like antioxidant, antistress, immunomodulatory, anti-inflammatory, and antiaging. It too helps to reduce the side effect of chemotherapy and radiation (Singh et al., 2011).

15.5 ANTICANCER COMPOUNDS FOUND IN INDIA AND THEIR SCIENTIFIC EVIDENCE

On performing extensive studies, various mechanisms of anticancer agents have been discovered which are proved helpful against carcinogenesis. Phytochemicals exhibit anti-carcinogenic activities that restrict the cancer initiation and growth by interfering with cell growth through mechanisms like cellular proliferation, differentiation, apoptosis, angiogenesis, and metastasis (Pratheeshkumar et al., 2012). Common mechanisms like necrosis and apoptosis are usually found in most of the phytochemicals which suppress the proliferative drive of tumors and are mainly related to cell death or arrest the cell during its growth phases in the cell cycle (Mukherjee et al., 2014). Also, the Nrf2, NFκB, and AP-1 signaling pathways mediated by phytochemicals prevent multi-step processes by exerting anti-inflammatory and antioxidative stress effects. It should also be noted that several drugs that are derived from phytochemicals are based on redox-active compounds that serve as antitumor activities. For example, studies show that phytochemicals like 4HPR, resveratrol, curcumin, xanthohumol, the isothiocyanate PEITC, and CDDO triterpenoids produce a prooxidant state inside tumor cells which is possible by promoting either reactive oxygen species (ROS) generation by mitochondria or NADPH oxidases, induction of redox imbalance through glutathione depletion, or impairment of glutathione biosynthesis while they, on the other hand, act as an antioxidant and activate the superoxide dismutase (SOD) activity in the tumor cells (Tosetti et al., 2009).

Looking for affirmative medicine for cancer has always been the need of the hour. With so many discoveries being carried out around the world in Western medicine, India sets its foot into the alternative medicine system because of its rich diversity and fruitful results in curing cancer through natural medicine. When different varieties of plants, microorganisms, and aquatic organisms were studied closely, the report showed over 25 years 63% of anticancer drugs were obtained from these natural sources (Das and Satyalakshmi, 2012). The major disadvantage of synthetic drugs lies with their side effects and their harm to the normal and sound cells of the body thus deteriorating it. With the advancement in technology, several important anticancer compounds have been found in Indian medical plants which are listed below:

β-hydroxyecdysterone, Cordioside, Columbin: These compounds are isolated from the plant *Tinospora cordifolia* (Hindi name: Giloya). The plant is found abundant in the Northern parts of India. This extract has shown a prominent anticancer effect in the skin cancer model of mice (Reddy and Rajasekhar, 2015). However, anticancer properties of more compounds from these plant sources are under investigation. The compounds are used for treating diabetes and possess antitoxic, antioxidant activities, antimicrobial activities, antidiabetic activities, and cytotoxic effects (REF). Also they are used for treating arthritis, chronic fever, vomiting, and piles (Reddy and Rajasekhar, 2015; Umadevi et al., 2013; Desai et al., 2008).

Curcumin: It is a type of polyphenol which is isolated from *Curcuma longa* (Hindi name: Haldi) which is one of the most commonly used Indian spice found in southwest India. Curcumin is believed to show an anticancer potential and causes inhibition in cell proliferation and apoptosis via certain degenerating expressions of NF-kappa B, Activator protein 1 (AP-1), Epidermal growth receptors (EGR-1). Aggarwal et al. (2003) performed preclinical studies about curcumin consumption and its toxic effect on human cells and found that clinically used curcumin extract is safer for daily use and did not depict any toxic effect. It is one of the most commonly used household Indian spices. It exhibits the property of anticancer as well as anti-inflammatory and has been showing promising results to cure cancers by the proliferation of breast tumor cells, inhibits proliferation of cancer of colon and kidney (Umadevi et al., 2013; Desai et al., 2008; Aggarwal et al., 2003).

Colchicine: It is an alkaloid isolated from a poisonous plant *Colchicum autumnale* (Hindi name: Hirantutiya) found in the southern region of Karnataka State in South India. It disrupts a dynamic equilibrium between tubulin and its polymeric form, the microtubule, causing inhibition of the tumor. Because of the high toxicity of the plant, it is not used in clinical trials, but it is believed that this plant exerts antiproliferative effects through the inhibition of microtubule formation by blocking the cell cycle at the G2/M phase and triggering apoptosis. It is however useful in treating gout and familial Mediterranean fever (Mukherjee et al., 2014; Prakash et al., 2013; Kumar, 2000).

Epigallocatechin-3-Gallate: It is one of the main bioactive elements of green tea *Camellia sinensis*. It accounts for 50–80% of catechins. It is found in Darjeeling, Assam, Nilgiri in India. The compound inhibits NF-κB activity, MAPK pathway, AP-1 activity, and EGFR-mediated downstream signaling pathways. It has been reported to consist of anti-inflammatory, antioxidant, anti-infective, anticancer, anti-angiogenetic, and chemopreventive properties (Prakash et al., 2013; Pratheeshkumar et al., 2012; Singh et al., 2011).

Betulinic Acid: It is a pentacyclic triterpenoid isolated from *Ziziphus nummularia* (Hindi name: Jhar Beri) found throughout the arid and semiarid tracts of India, Pakistan Afghanistan, Egypt, Iran, Iraq, and Israel. Betulinic acid helps in the inhibition of microtubule assembly, interacts with DNA topoisomerase II, inhibits cell proliferation via the activation of reactive oxygen species (ROS); it also causes apoptosis by a p53- and CD95-independent mechanism. It has been reported to cause cytotoxicity against a brain tumor and neuroectodermal cells (Prakash et al., 2013; Desai et al., 2008).

Lignans, Flavanoids, and Tannins: It is isolated from *Phylanthus amarus* (Hindi Name: Amla) found in tropical, subtropical, and warmer parts of India. It one of the most commonly used plants in Ayurveda. The *P. amarus* extract possess antitumor activities, can induce apoptosis, and cause interference in DNA repair mechanisms (Prakash et al., 2013; Desai et al., 2008).

Bullatacin: It is isolated from the fruit of *Annona atemoya* (Hindi name: Sharifa). The parts of the plant like roots, leaves, and fruit are used generally for medicinal purposes and drug development. The extract shows anticancer properties by inducing process of chromatin margination and tumor cell condensation and hence pursued by apoptosis (Prakash et al., 2013; Desai et al., 2008).

Campothecin: It was first isolated from *Mappia foetida / Nothapodytes foetida* (Hindi name: Amruta) found in South India. A recent study also revealed that the endophytic fungus growing on the plant also produced and released campothecin. It helps to inhibit poly nucleic acid biosynthesis and causing the fermentation of DNA in vitro; it is also an effective inhibitor of nucleic acid synthesis in HeLa cells. It has an antitumor activity which showed efficacy in ovarian and small cell lung cancer (Prakash et al., 2013; Mukherjee et al., 2010; Desai et al., 2008).

Withaferin A: It was originally isolated from *Withania somnifera* (Hindi Name: Ashwagandha); the plant is of great commercial value and used in Ayurveda for its significant medicinal values. It is found in Karnataka, UP, Punjab, Himachal Pradesh, MP, Gujarat, Rajasthan, Maharashtra, Haryana, and Orissa. When used against cancer cell lines it produces an apoptosis response by activation of ROS species and also sometimes by activation of RNOS generation. It is antiaging, anti-peroxidative, anti-inflammatory, antitumor, antistress, antioxidant, immuno-modulatory, and comprises rejuvenating properties (Desai et al., 2008).

Andrographolide: It is a colorless, crystalline ring-like structure extracted from *Andrographis paniculate* (Hindi name: Kalmegh). This compound is found in the highest quantity in the seeds of the plant. The plant is commonly found in India and Sri Lanka. It is known to be the lead component in cancer drug development as it shows cytotoxic effects against a variety of tumors. It is found to be effective against human epidermoid cancer cells, lymphocytic leukemia cells, breast cancer cells, and colon cancer cells. The plant is found to be effective in the treatment of jaundice, cholestasis, and hepatotoxins. It also shows anti-HIV activity (Desai et al., 2008).

15.6 CANCER TREATMENT WITH INDIAN TRADITIONAL MEDICINE

Treating cancer has always been one of the major challenges for researchers as well as a clinician since most of the existing treatments are not effective enough to provide full protection from this disease and also are associated with severe side effects in many instances. Thus, there is an urgent need to identify efficient treatment strategies with minimum side effects. India has a huge wealth of natural resources (flora and fauna) and practices that are used as the treatment strategies for a variety of diseases, including cancer. This knowledge has culminated in ancient written texts and practiçes followed by local healers and medical practitioners. The treatment strategies are grouped into categories: Ayurveda, Siddha, Unani, Yoga & Homeopathy, and Naturopathy. Each category concerning cancer treatment has been discussed below.

15.6.1 CANCER TREATMENT WITH AYURVEDA SYSTEM OF MEDICINE

Treatment of cancer under this branch of medicine is based on plant drug systems and natural substances for healing. The drug preparation in Ayurveda is believed to be similar to that of allopathy (conventional treatment using chemical drugs) as it is based on targeting specific tissues and organs. Generally, these preparations have proven to be more successful when used as a cotherapy along with radiation and chemotherapy. The preparations are known to be the mixtures of extracts from potent anticancer plants, for example, "Triphala" is known to be the combination of three plant extracts which is widely known for its anticancer properties (Pilmeijer, 2017). Furthermore, extensive research and clinical trial tests over some specific phytochemicals are still being conducted to produce the basis for evidence-based medicine (EVB) (Ganguly, 2014). Some recommended methods in classical texts of the Ayurvedic system of medicine include—internal purification, applying of paste (from the herb-based extracts) for external treatment of cancer, fomentation (the method of applying external heat and warmth to wounds), and lysis of cancer through the process of bloodletting (the method of surgically removing blood for therapeutic purposes) (Manohar, 2014). Prakash et al. in 2020 reported a study where a patient suffering from Acute Promyelocytic Leukaemia (APML), which is a form of blood cancer, was treated with oral Ayurvedic medications along with a planned diet, prescribed by an Ayurvedic practitioner. It was observed, after 340 days of treatment, the patient had significantly improved and no harmful side effects were observed and the patient resumed his normal life.

15.6.2 CANCER TREATMENT WITH UNANI SYSTEM OF MEDICINE

In the Unani system of medicine, cancer is commonly referred to as Sartan ("crab" in Arabic) which means cancer sticks to the organism like a crab does to its prey. Only a few physicians in Unani like Galen (129-199AD), Rhazes (854-925), Abulcasis (936-1013), and Avicenna (980-1037) studied cancer in detail and were able to develop few formulations for the treatment of cancer. Unani medicines are used as chemotherapeutic agents and also as adjuvants. While the chemotherapeutic agents are still under clinical developments and trials, adjuvants are proven to be reliable (Standard Unani Medical Terminology, 2012). Adjuvant therapy promotes the prevention of cancer and old Unani texts have laid down six basic principles of therapy for cancer treatment. These are Air (Hawa), Food and Drink (Makool o Mashroob), Bodily Movement and Repose (Harkat o Sukoon Badani), Psychic Movement and Repose (Harkat o Sukoon Nafsani), Sleep and Wakefulness (Naum o Yaqza), Retention and Evacuation (Ihtibas o Istifragh) (Naaz and Ahmed, 2017). Some of the guidelines to follow these principles are available in Training Manual, Integration of Unani Medicine in NPCDCS 2016 and include:

- Breathing fresh and pollution-free air.
- Avoiding the use of tobacco chewing and smoking.
- Avoiding junk and preserved foods, alcohol, carbonated drinks, etc.
- Nonvegetarian diet should be avoided.
- Naturally, nutritional-rich food like turmeric, tomatoes, garlic, flaxseed, spinach, broccoli, pomegranates, walnuts, etc should be consumed daily if possible.
- Exercising for 30–45 min at least five days every week.
- Emotions like, for example, anger, fear, sadness should be avoided in extreme.
- Practicing spiritual peaceful life.
- Sleeping for 6–8 h regularly.
- Proper urination, perspiration, and menstruation should be ensured.

Regimental therapy is another form of therapy that focuses on the improvement of life for cancer patients. The various regimens of Regimental therapy are Dalak (Massage therapy), Hammam (Balneotherapy), and Shamum (Aromatherapy). All the three regimens have their principles and theories which are proven successful in the area of cancer (Naaz and Ahmed, 2017).

15.6.3 CANCER TREATMENT WITH SIDDHA SYSTEM OF MEDICINE

Another component of Indian Traditional medicine is Siddha. It is based on interventions by medicinal herbs and plants for the treatment of cancer. Siddha's ancient medical texts have specified some of the important medicines that are capable of treating cancer like Rasa Ganthi Meluku, Nanthimai,

Rasaparpam, Vangaparpam, Senkoddai ghee, Sengoddai illagam which are all made from natural sources (Sujeethasai and Soruban, 2019). In 2005, Sowmyalakshmi et al. reported an intervention using Semecarpus Lehyam (SL), a Siddha medicine for the treatment of breast cancer. SL is a herbal medicine obtained from serial extraction using four organic solvents and has shown potent anticancer properties. SL was shown to be more effective against MDA 231 cells. Hence, this herbal amalgamation is used against the hormone ER-negative breast cancers. Another study by Ganapathy et al. in 2019 reported a comparative evaluation of the two organic-based Siddha medicines, MahaVallathy Leghiyam (MVL) and Neeradi Muthu Vallathy Leghiyam (NMVL), for anticancer potential against oral cancer cell lines in vitro. The study concluded that NVML showed better anticancer potential and was able to inhibit the proliferation of cancer cells by the mechanism of apoptosis. This study promoted the use of NVML which is considered for long-term use for the adjuvant therapy in Siddha medicine.

15.6.4 CANCER TREATMENT WITH YOGA AND NATUROPATHY SYSTEM OF MEDICINE

In comparison to allopathic medicine, Yoga is a nonpersuasive, cost-effective, and nontoxic, and spiritual enhancing treatment remedy for most diseases (Pirri, 2011). According to some already proven theories, Yoga helps to avoid tumor growth as well. Cancer is a disease where the body's immune system plays an important role in developing abnormal cells, Yoga is a practice that can help strengthen the body's immune system and promote immune cell development, and increases its production. Yoga also helps to reduce depression, stress, and anxiety and keep the body functioning in homeostasis. Several cases reported from Meares showed regression in tumor growth in patients who performed Yoga regularly (Agarwal et al., 2018). It was noted in a survey that Americans have spent more than 10 billion dollars annually on Yoga (Field, 2011; Field, 2016; Jeter et al., 2014) which is being practiced for its health and fitness benefits. However, more studies need to be carried out to determine the role of Yoga and its healing benefits for cancer. Naturopathy is a treatment based on the natural ability of the body to heal itself once the body is surrounded by a healthy environment. There is not much scientific evidence available to support Naturopath as a mode of treatment for cancer. However, in some cases, naturopathy is used only as an additional treatment with other known cancer cures (Cassileth and Deng, 2004).

15.6.5 CANCER TREATMENT WITH HOMEOPATHY SYSTEM OF MEDICINE

The status of Homeopathy for cancer treatment has not gained pace worldwide as the evidence for working of this medicine for cancer treatment still lacks. Thus, the efficacy of Homeopathic drugs is used only as an additional therapy (Singh et al., 2019). However, Saha et al. (2015) reported the use of homeopathic treatment in an in-vitro experiment used a homeopathic remedy, which resulted in apoptosis in non-small cell lung carcinoma. Various studies have shown that homeopathic medicine can be useful for increasing the quality of life of cancer patients. However, more concrete scientific evidence needs to be available to support this mode of treatment and for the time being Homeopathy is used as an additional therapy (Ahlawat, 2018).

15.7 ACCEPTABILITY OF INDIAN TRADITIONAL MEDICINE WORLDWIDE

The phytochemicals extracted from traditional herbal medicine, especially under Ayurveda, have started to gain worldwide attention which would help to make Indian Traditional system of medicine a part of the modern system of medicine (Sen and Samanta, 2014). Ayurveda with its worldwide acceptance has now been recognized all over the world and is gaining pace day by day. India has well-established government institutes for research on synthetic drugs and natural products like the Central Drug Research Institute (CDRI), Council of Scientific and Industrial Research (CSIR), Central Institute of Medicinal and Aromatic Plants, National Botanical Research Institute, Regional Research Laboratories, and National Chemical laboratories which play a key role in the advancement of Ayurveda (Sen and Samanta, 2014). The Department of Ayurveda, Yoga & Naturopathy, Unani, Siddha & Homeopathy (AYUSH) of the Ministry of Health & Family Welfare (AYUSH) are involved in promoting advances and developments in the area of natural medicine. The department of AYUSH along with its two partners ICMR and CSIR work together to achieve safety, efficacy and ensure effective production of Ayurvedic drugs against some life-threatening diseases. The collaborative effort of these institutes focuses on important objectives such as quality control, drug assessment, maintaining pharmacopeial standards (these are the standards that ensure the quality and safety of medicines by appropriate testing), overseeing the working of the Pharmacopeial Laboratory of Indian

Medicines (PLIM), partnership with the Quality Council of India (QCI), and overseeing the functioning of Indian Medicine Pharmaceutical Company Limited (IMPCL). AYUSH also ensures Good Manufacturing Practices (GMP) and Drug Quality Control (Singh et al., 2011).

All the drug developments and formulations by these Indian facilities are further guided by the WHO (World Health Organisation). According to the guidelines of the WHO, herbal medicines are classified into four major categories of (Chaudhary et al., 2011):

Category 1: Indigenous herbal medicines
Category 2: Herbal medicines in systems
Category 3: Modified herbal medicines
Category 4: Imported products with a herbal medicine base.

WHO has played an important part in the global acceptance of Ayurveda. WHO has assigned AYUSH with several Appraisal Project Work (APW) and Direct Financial Cooperation (DFC) projects that have helped the Indian traditional medicine to gain pace on the world stage (Shah, 2019). The safety of all Ayurvedic medicines is assessed by clinical trials, as well as ensured by the data presented in other research papers. AYUSH and WHO work in hand and hand to ensure the efficacy of Ayurvedic medicines where WHO conjoins as an academic associate and provides logical support (Chaudhary et al., 2011).

Ayurveda is also included in the health care system of several countries like the United Kingdom (U.K.), the United Arab Emirates, Sweden, Indonesia, and the USA besides 30 other countries that are also accepting and relying on the natural medicine system (Sen and Chakarborty, 2014). Ayurvedic system of medicine is being researched, studied, and practiced for the last four decades in the Society of Ayurveda established in 1969 by the Osaka Medical School, Japan (Sen and Chakraborty, 2017). The popularity of the Ayurvedic system of medicine is also reported in Buenos Aires, Argentina where it has been introduced as a "lifestyle" medicine and a rapid increase in the popularity has been observed among the middle and upper cases of the country (Freidin and Ballesteros, 2015). Moreover, in Italy, Ayurveda is recognized as a complete healthcare system (Morandi et al., 2010). However, in the 17th century, both Yoga and Ayurveda were accepted all over Britain post-war (Newcombe, 2008). A survey conducted in 2007 reported that over 200,000 Americans used Ayurvedic medicines in the U.S.A. (Sen and Chakraborty, 2017). The trend is further on the rise due to rigorous scientific research into this system of medicine.

15.8 TOWARD A BRIGHTER FUTURE

India has a wealth of natural resources and flora is one of the most important resources contributing to a wide variety of applications. Out of 17,000–18,000 flowering species of plants, 6000–7000 species are in medicinal usage for Ayurveda and hold tremendous potential in the future as drugs (Katoch et al., 2017) Ayurvedic system has now been recognized in countries like Nepal, Sri Lanka, Bangladesh, UK, and USA and around 75% of 100 million subcontinental population is appreciating the benefits of Ayurvedic system (Sen and Chakraborty, 2017). The demand for Indian traditional natural medicines has increased all over the world and with more advancement in technology in scientific research, there is a growing interest in exploring the mechanism of action and targeted use and delivery of the traditional medicines in different diseases and particularly for cancer. Since the Indian traditional medicine system has shown fewer or no side effects and is effective against many diseases, the need for Indian medicine has increased over the years and is proved advantageous for the economic growth of India (Sen and Chakraborty, 2014). The benefit and demand of the Ayurvedic system of medicine have promoted India as one of the medical tourist destinations for people from countries like the UK, USA, Canada, China, Bangladesh, and Sri Lanka which has resulted in almost 1.27 million medical tourists visiting India in search of better treatment through natural medicine (Sen and Chakraborty, 2017). Indian traditional medicine can provide a holistic, safer, and effective treatment for many diseases due to which it has drawn worldwide attention. The preference of patients toward traditional medicines due to limited or no side effects increased safety, low cost compared to modern/allopathic medicine and inclination toward self-medication is the reason for increased interest in herbal medicines worldwide (Sharma et al., 2011). Apart from medical organizations and pharmaceutical industries, the education system and education statutory bodies have been successful in establishing Ayurvedic Medical Colleges which provide an updated and more extensive education on the Ayurvedic system of medication under the guidance of UGC (University Grants Commission). Currently, India has over 500 teaching hospitals, 70,000 vaidyas, and thousands of government-funded dispensaries associated with the Ayurvedic system of medicine and its related areas under the Indian traditional medicine system (Shah, 2019).

However, Indian traditional medicine still faces huge challenges due to the lack of comparable evidence-based studies and proof of mechanisms to enhance the confidence of the Western population. Besides, the medicinal plants and compounds are not properly catalogued and organized in the database resulting in limited accessibility for research. But with the development of government-funded research laboratories and research targeted to study the Indian traditional system of medicine has encouraged clinical trials to be conducted for generating evidence and form a basis for evidence-based medicine (EBM). Supporting this, ICMR has developed the Clinical Trial Registry of India (CTRI), a platform that provides a detailed catalogue of the on-going clinical trials and the organizations conducting these trials which have made EBM more powerful. For instance, searching for the keyword "Ayurveda" on the official website of CTRI displayed a list of on-going clinical trials in an organized manner. This has helped organize and collate the data and provide strong support for EBM research (Rao et al., 2018). Thus, it helps in promoting the research and development and generates support for the global acceptability of Indian Traditional medicines which might eventually replace modern medicines in the future.

The Indian traditional medicine system is largely based on the body's healing power and self-defence mechanisms which make it more efficient and safer compared to conventional allopathic drugs. However, this system of medicine has to overcome some major challenges such as lack of extensive evidence-based research and systematic clinical trials against diseases due to which trust and confidence are absent in this system in the Western world. To sum up, the Indian traditional system of medicine has the potential to revolutionize the disease management and well-being of people and offer advantages like nontoxicity, safety, cost-effective method, healthy lifestyle, and personalized treatment which may become a way of life in the future.

KEYWORDS

- **Ayurveda**
- **anticancer compounds**
- **Indian traditional medicine**
- **Phyto-compounds**
- **Unani**

REFERENCES

Abd El-Wahab, A. E.; Ghareeb, D. A.; Sarhan, E. E.; Abu-Serie, M. M.; El Demellawy, M. A. In Vitro Biological Assessment of *Berberis vulgaris* and Its Active Constituent, Berberine: Antioxidants, Anti-Acetylcholinesterase, Anti-Diabetic and Anticancer Effects. *BMC Complem. Altern. Med.* **2013**, *13*, 218.

Agarwal, R. P.; Afek, A. M. Yoga into Cancer Care: A Review of the Evidence-Based Research. *Int. J. Yoga* **2018**, *11* (1), 3–29.

Aggarwal, B. B.; Kumar, A.; Bharti, A. C. Anticancer Potential of Curcumin: Preclinical and Clinical Studies. *Anticancer Res.* **2003**, *23* (1A), 363–398.

Ahlawat, A. Role of Homeopathic Drugs as Anti-Cancer Agents. *Int. J. Hom. Sci.* **2018,** *2* (1), 21–23.

Ahmad, A.; Hayat, I.; Arif, S.; Masud, T.; Khalid, N.; Ahmed, A. Mechanisms Involved in the Therapeutic Effects of Soybean (*Glycine max*). *Int. J. Food Prop.* **2014**, *17* (6), 1332–1354.

Altay, V.; Çelik, O. Antakya semt pazarlarındaki bazı doğal bitkilerin etnobotanik yönden araştırılması. *Biyoloji Bilimleri Araştırma Dergisi* **2011**, *4* (2), 131–139.

Altay, V.; Karahan, F. Tayfur Sökmen Kampüsü (Antakya-Hatay) ve çevresinde bulunan bitkiler üzerine etnobotanik bir araştırma. *Karadeniz Fen Bilimleri Dergisi* **2012**, *2* (7), 11–28.

Altay, V.; Karahan, F.; Sarcan, Y. B.; Ilçım, A. An Ethnobotanical Research on Wild Plants Sold in Kırıkhan District (Hatay/Turkey) Herbalists and Local Markets. *Biol. Divers. Conserv.* **2015b**, *8* (2), 81–91.

Altay, V.; Keskin, M.; Karahan, F. An assessment of the Plant Biodiversity of Mustafa Kemal University Tayfur Sokmen Campus (Hatay-Turkey) for the View of Human Health. *Int. J. Sci. Technol. Res.* **2015a**, *1* (2), 81–103.

Bala, M.; Pratap, K.; Verma, P. K.; Singh, B.; Padwad, Y. Validation of Ethnomedicinal Potential of Tinospora Cordifolia for Anticancer and Immunomodulatory Activities and Quantification of Bioactive Molecules by HPTLC. *J. Ethnopharmacol.* **2015**, *175*, 131–137.

Baliga, M. S.; Jimmy, R.; Thilakchand, K. R.; Sunitha, V.; Bhat, N. R.; Saldanha, E.; Rao, S.; Rao, P.; Arora, R.; Palatty, P. L. *Ocimum sanctum* L (Holy Basil or Tulsi) and Its Phytochemicals in the Prevention and Treatment of Cancer. *Nutr. Cancer* **2013**, *65* (1), 21–35.

Borins, M. Traditional Medicine in India. *Can. Fam. Phys.* **1987,** *33*, 1061.

Cassileth, B. R.; Deng, G. Complementary and Alternative Therapies for Cancer. *Oncologist.* **2004**, *9*, 81–89.

Chaudhary, A.; Singh, N. Contribution of World Health Organization in the Global Acceptance of Ayurveda. *J. Ayurveda Integr. Med.* **2011**, *2* (4), 179–186.

Chauhan, A.; Semwal, D. K.; Mishra, S. P.; Semwal, R. B. Ayurvedic Research and Methodology: Present Status and Future Strategies. *Ayu* **2015**, *36* (4), 361–369.

D'Huyvetter, K.; Cohrssen, A. Homeopathy. *Primary Care* **2002**, *29* (2), 1.

Das, B.; Satyalakshmi, G. Natural Products-Based Anticancer Agents. *Mini-Rev Org. Chem.* **2012**, *9*, 169–177.

Desai, A. G.; Qazi, G. N.; Ganju, R. K.; El-Tamer, M.; Singh, J.; Saxena, A. K.; Bedi, Y. S.; Taneja, S. C.; Bhat, H. K. Medicinal Plants and Cancer Chemoprevention. *Curr. Drug Metabol.* **2008**, *9* (7), 581–591.

Dharmani, P.; Kuchibhotla, V. K.; Maurya, R.; Srivastava, S.; Sharma, S.; Palit, G. Evaluation of Anti-Ulcerogenic and Ulcer-Healing Properties of *Ocimum sanctum* Linn. *J. Ethnopharmacol.* **2004**, *93* (1–3), 197–206.

Field, T. Yoga Clinical Research Review. *Complement. Ther. Clin. Pract.* **2011**, *17*, 1–8.

Field, T. Yoga Research Review. *Complement. Ther. Clin. Pract.* **2016**, *24*, 141–161.

Freidin, B.; Ballesteros, M. Choosing Ayurveda as a Healthcare Practice in Argentina. *Curr. Sociol.* **2015**, *63* (5), 661–684.

Ganapathy, P.; Elumalai, K.; Arumugam, M. K.; Amulya, C. S.; Manivel, R. Anticancer Potential of Siddha Formulations Against Oral Cancer Cell Line In Vitro. *Trends Med.* **2019**, *19*, 1–6.

Ganguly, S. Ayurveda for Cancer Therapy. *World J. Pharma. Res.* **2014**, *3* (9), 1471–1479.

Isbrucker, R. A.; Burdock, G. A. Risk and Safety Assessment on the Consumption of Licorice Root (*Glycyrrhiza* sp.), Its Extract and Powder as a Food Ingredient, with Emphasis on the Pharmacology and Toxicology of Glycyrrhizin. *Regul. Toxicol. Pharmacol.* **2006**, *46* (3), 161–192.

Jangid, D. K.; Dixit, D. Global Acceptance of Ayurveda—A Sincere Goal & Obstacles in Its Way. *Wjpmr* **2019**, *5* (4), 91–99.

Jeter, P. E.; Nkodo, A. F.; Moonaz, S. H.; Dagnelie, G. A Systematic Review of Yoga for Balance in a Healthy Population. *J. Altern. Complement. Med.* **2014**, *20*, 221–232.

Johnson, J. J.; Mukhtar, H. Curcumin for Chemoprevention of Colon Cancer. *Cancer Lett.* **2007**, *255* (2), 170–181.

Kala, C. P.; Dhyani, P. P.; Sajwan, B. S. Developing the Medicinal Plants Sector in Northern India: Challenges and Opportunities. *J. Ethnobiol. Ethnomed.* **2006**, *2*, 1.

Kamboj, V. P. Herbal Medicine. *Curr. Sci.* **2000**, *78* (1), 35–39.

Katoch, D.; Sharma, J. S.; Banerjee, S.; Biswas, R.; Das, B.; Goswami, D.; Harwansh, R. K.; Katiyar, C. K.; Mukherjee, P. K. Government Policies and Initiatives for Development of Ayurveda. *J. Ethnopharmacol.* **2017**, *197*, 25–31.

Kaur, H.; Chalia, D.; Manchanda, R. Homeopathy in Public Health in India. *Homeopathy* **2019**, *108* (02), 071–087.

Kim, H. S.; Kacew, S.; Lee, B. M. In Vitro Chemopreventive Effects of Plant Polysaccharides (*Aloe barbadensis, Lentinus edodes, Ganoderma lucidum* and *Coriolus versicolor*). *Carcinogenesis* **1999**, *20* (8), 1637–1640.

Krishna, S.; Dinesh, K. S.; Nazeema, P. K. Globalizing Ayurveda—Opportunities and Challenges. *Int. J. Health Sci. Res.* **2020**, *10* (3), 51–68.

Kumar, A. Traditional Indian Ayurvedic Medicines: Some Potential Plants for Bioenergy, Medicine from India. *Instit. Nat. Med. Toyama Med. Pharma. Univ. Jpn* **2000**, *27*, 1–15.

Lone, A. H.; Ahmad, T.; Anwar, M.; Sofi, G.; Imam, H.; Habib, S. Perception of Health Promotion in Unani Herbal Medicine. *J. Herb. Med.* **2012**, *2* (1), 1–5.

Manohar, P. R.; Descriptions and Classification of Cancer in the Classical Ayurvedic Texts. *Indian J. Hist. Sci.* **2014**, *50*, 181–195.

Masoodi, K. Z.; Amin, I.; Mansoor, S. et al. Botanicals from the Himalayas with Anticancer Potential—An Emphasis on Kashmir Himalayas. In *Biodiversity and Biomedicine—Our Future*; Ozturk, M., Egamberdieva, D., Pešić, M., Eds., Chapter 11; Academic Press, 2020; pp 181–234.

Morandi, A.; Tosto, C.; Sartori, G.; Roberti di Sarsina, P. Advent of a Link Between Ayurveda and Modern Health Science: The Proceedings of the First International Congress on Ayurveda, "Ayurveda: The Meaning of Life-Awareness, Environment, and Health". *Evid. Based Complement Altern. Med.* **2010**, *2011*.

Mukherjee, A.; Basu, S.; Sarkar, N.; Ghosh, A.; Advances in Cancer Therapy with Plant Based Natural Products. *Curr. Med. Chem.* **2001**, *8* (12), 1461–1486.

Mukherjee, P. K.; Bahadur, S.; Harwansh, R. K.; Chaudhary, S. K. Shifting Paradigm for Validation of Medicinal Plants in Indian Traditional Medicine. *Indian Drugs* **2014**, *51* (8), 5–14.

Mukherjee, P. K.; Venkatesh, P.; Ponnusankar, S. Ethnopharmacology and Integrative Medicine—Let the History Tell the Future. *J. Ayurv. Integr. Med.* **2010**, *1* (2), 100–109.
Naaz, F.; Ahmed, S. Integration of Unani Medicine in Cancer Management. *WJPR* **2017**, *6* (6), 451–461.
Newcombe, S. A Social History of Yoga and Ayurveda in Britain, 1950–1995, Ph.D. Thesis Submitted at the Faculty of History, University of Cambridge, 2008.
Nyeem, M. A.; Mannan, M. A.; Nuruzzaman, M.; Kamrujjaman, K. M.; Das, S. K. Indigenous King of Bitter (*Andrographis paniculata*): A Review. *Faslnamah-i Giyahan-i Daruyi* **2017**, *5* (2), 311–324.
Ozturk, M.; Altay, V.; Altundağ, E.; Ibadullayeva, S. J.; Aslanipour, B.; Gönenç, T. M. Herbals in Iğdır (Turkey), Nakhchivan (Azerbaijan), and Tabriz (Iran). In *Plant and Human Health*; Ozturk, M., Hakeem, K. R., Eds., Vol. 1, Springer: Cham, Chapter 6, **2018c**, pp 191–266.
Ozturk, M.; Altay, V.; Efe, R. *Biodiversity, Conservation and Sustainability in Asia: Volume I: Prospects and Challenges in West Asia and Caucasus*; Springer Nature Switzerland AG, 2021a. DOI: 10.1007/971-3-031-59921-7
Ozturk, M.; Altay, V.; Gonenç, T. M. Herbal from High Mountains in the East Mediterranean. In *Drug Discovery from Herbs-Approaches and Applications*; Bhojraj, S. et al., Eds.; NAM S & T Centre, DAYA Publishing House: New Delhi, India, Chapter 24, 2017b; pp 321–367.
Ozturk, M.; Altay, V.; Gucel, S.; Altundağ, E. Plant Diversity of the Drylands in Southeast Anatolia-Turkey: Role in Human Health and Food Security. In *Plant Biodiversity: Monitoring, Assessment and Conservation*; Ansari, A. A., Gill, S. S., Eds., Chapter 5; CABI UK, 2017c; pp 81–124.
Ozturk, M.; Altay, V.; Hakeem, K. R.; Akçiçek, E. *Liquorice from Botany to Phytochemistry*; SpringerBriefs in Plant Science, 2017a. https://doi.org/10.1007/971-3-311-74241-3
Ozturk, M.; Altay, V.; Latiff, A. et al. A Comparative Analysis of the Medicinal Pteridophytes in Turkey, Pakistan, and Malaysia. In *Plant and Human Health*; Ozturk, M., Hakeem, K. R., Eds., Vol. 1; Springer: Cham, Chapter 9, Springer International Publishing AG, 2018d; pp 341–390.
Ozturk, M.; Altay, V.; Latiff, A. et al. A Comparative Analysis of the Medicinal Plants Used for Diabetes Mellitus in the Traditional Medicine in Turkey, Pakistan, and Malaysia. In *Plant and Human Health*; Ozturk, M., Hakeem, K. R., Eds., Vol. 1; Springer: Cham, Chapter 11, Springer International Publishing AG, 2018e; pp 401–461.
Ozturk, M.; Altay, V.; Latiff, A. et al. Potential Medicinal Plants Used in the Hypertension in Turkey, Pakistan, and Malaysia. In *Plant and Human Health*; Ozturk, M., Hakeem, K. R., Eds., Vol. 1; Springer: Cham, Chapter 16, Springer International Publishing AG, 2018f; pp 591–618.
Ozturk, M.; Altay, V.; Orçen, N. et al. A Little Known and a Little Consumed Natural Resource: *Salicornia*. In *Global Perspectives on Underutilized Crops*; Ozturk, M. et al., Eds., Chapter 3; Springer International Publishing AG, 2018a; pp 81–108.
Ozturk, M.; Altundağ, E.; Ibadullayeva, S. J.; Altay, V.; Aslanıpour, B. A Comparative Analysis of Medicinal and Aromatic Plants Used in the Traditional Medicine of Iğdır (Turkey), Nakhchivan (Azerbaijan), and Tabriz (Iran). *Pak. J. Bot.* **2018b**, *50* (1), 331–343.
Ozturk, M.; Egamberdieva, D.; Milica, P. *Biodiversity and Biomedicine-Our Future*; Academic Press, Elsevier Inc.: UK, USA, 2020.
Ozturk, M.; Gökler, I.; Altay, V. Medicinal Bryophytes Distributed in Turkey. In *Plant and Human Health*; Ozturk, M., Hakeem, K. R., Eds., Vol. 1; Springer: Cham, Chapter 8, Springer International Publishing AG, 2018g; pp 321–348.

Ozturk, M.; Khan, S. M.; Altay, V.; Efe, R.; Egamberdieva, D.; Khassanov, F. *Biodiversity, Conservation and Sustainability in Asia: Volume II: Prospects and Challenges in South and Middle Asia*; Springer Nature Switzerland AG, 2021b. DOI: 10.1007/971–3-031–73941–0

Pandey, M. M.; Rastogi, S.; Rawat, A. K. S. Indian Traditional Ayurvedic System of Medicine and Nutritional Supplementation. *Evid. Based Complement. Altern. Med.* **2013**, *2013*, 1–12.

Pilmeijer, A. Cancer & Ayurveda as a Complementary Treatment. *Int. J. Complement Altern. Med.* **2017**, *6* (5), 1.

Pirri, C. Integrating Complementary and Conventional Medicine. *Cancer Forum* **2011**, *35*, 31–39.

Poornima, P.; Efferth, T. Ayurveda for Cancer Treatment. *Med. Aromat. Plants* 2016, *5* (5), 1.

Prakash, B.; Prakash, S.; Tiwari, S. Acute Promyelocytic Leukemia: 37 Years Long Ongoing Survival in a de novo Patient with Metal-Based Ayurvedic Treatment. *Asian J. Oncol.* **2020**, *1*, 1–2.

Prakash, O.; Kumar, A.; Kumar, P.; Ajeet, A. Anticancer Potential of Plants and Natural Products: A Review. *Am. J. Pharmacol. Sci.* **2013**, *1* (6), 101–115.

Pratheeshkumar, P.; Sreekala, C.; Zhang, Z.; Budhraja, A.; Ding, S.; Son, Y. Cancer Prevention with Promising Natural Products: Mechanisms of Action and Molecular Targets. *Anti-Cancer Agents Med. Chem.* **2012**, *12* (10), 1151–1184.

Rachana, M. S.; Totad, M.; Girish, K. J.; Vasantha, B.; Vibhu, P. Ayurvedic Management of Chronic Kidney Disease: A Case Report. *J. Ayurveda Integr. Med. Sci.* **2019**, *4*, 281–290.

Rao, V.; Maulik, M.; Gupta, J.; Panchal, Y.; Juneja, A.; Adhikari, T.; Pandey, A.; Clinical Trials Registry—India: An overview and new developments. *Indian Journal of Pharmacology*, **2018**, *50* (4), 208–211.

Rastogi, R. Naturopathy in India: Current Status and Future Challenges. *Ann. Ayurv. Med.* **2012**, *1*, 151–157.

Ravishankar, B.; Shukla, V. J. Indian Systems of Medicine: A Brief Profile. *Afr. J. Trad. Complement. Altern. Med. AJTCAM* **2007**, *4* (3), 319–337.

Rawal, R. S.; Dhar, U. Protected Area Network in Indian Himalayan Region: Need for Recognizing Values of Low Profile Protected Areas. *Curr. Sci.* **2001**, *81*, 175–183.

Reddy, N.; Rajasekhar, R. *Tinospora cordifolia* Chemical Constituents and Medicinal Properties: A Review. *Sch. Acad. J. Pharm.* **2015**, *3*, 64–369.

Relton, C.; Cooper, K.; Viksveen, P.; Fibert, P. Thomas, K.; Prevalence of Homeopathy Use by the General Population Worldwide: A Systematic Review. *Homeopathy* **2017**, *106* (2), 69–78.

Saha, S.; Bhattacharjee, P.; Guha, D.; Kajal, K.; Khan, P.; Chakraborty, S.; Mukherjee, S.; Paul, S.; Manchanda, R.; Khurana, A.; Nayak, D.; Chakrabarty, R.; Sa, G.; Das, T. Sulphur alters NFκB-p300 Cross-Talk in Favour of p53-p300 to Induce Apoptosis in Non-Small Cell Lung Carcinoma. *Int. J. Oncol.* **2015**, *47* (2), 573–582.

Sairam, K.; Rao, Ch. V.; Babu, M. D.; Kumar, K.; Agrawal, V. K.; Goel, R. K. Antiulcerogenic Effect of Methanolic Extract of *Emblica officinalis*: An Experimental Study. *J. Ethnopharmacol.* **2002**, *82* (1), 1–9.

Samarghandian, S.; Hadjzadeh, M. A.; Afshari, J. T.; Hosseini, M. Antiproliferative Activity and Induction of Apoptotic by Ethanolic Extract of Alpinia Galanga Rhizhome in Human Breast Carcinoma Cell Line. *BMC Complement. Altern. Med.* **2014**, *14*, 192.

Schippmann, U.; Leaman, D. J.; Cunningham, A. B. *Impact of Cultivation and Gathering of Medicinal Plants on Biodiversity: Global Trends and Issues*; Inter-Department Working Group on Biology Diversity for Food and Agriculture: Rome, FAO, 2002.

Sen, S.; Chakraborty, R. Revival, Modernization and Integration of Indian Traditional Herbal Medicine in Clinical Practice: Importance, Challenges and Future. *J. Trad. Complement. Med.* **2017**, *7* (2), 234–244.

Sen, S.; Chakraborty, R. Toward the Integration and Advancement of Herbal Medicine: A Focus on Traditional Indian Medicine. *Botan. Targets Therap.* **2014**, *2015* (5), 31–44.

Sen, T.; Samanta, S. K. Medicinal Plants, Human Health and Biodiversity: A Broad Review. *Biotechnol. App. Biodivers. Adv. Biochem. Eng./Biotechnol.* **2014**, *147*, 51–110.

Shah, S. Ayurveda: The Conventional Indian Medicine System and Its Global Practice. *Int. J. Innov. Sci. Technol.* **2019**, *4* (1), 11–33.

Shaikh, A.; Shrivastava, D.; Apte, D.; Navale, S. Medicinal Plants as Potential Source of Anticancer Agents: A Review. *J. Pharmacogn. Phytochem.* **2016**, *5* (2), 291–295.

Sharma, A. K.; Kumar, R.; Mishra, A.; Gupta, R. Problems Associated with Clinical Trials of Ayurvedic Medicines. *Rev. Brasil. Farmacog.* **2011**, *20*, 271–281.

Shrivastava, S. R.; Shrivastava, P. S.; Ramasamy, J. Mainstreaming of Ayurveda, Yoga, Naturopathy, Unani, Siddha, and Homeopathy with the Health Care Delivery System in India. *J. Trad. Complement. Med.* **2015**, *5* (11), 6–8.

Singh, C.; Bhinda, D.; Kumar, D.; Homeopathy in the Treatment of Cancer Patients: A Review. *Int. J. Homoeopath. Sci.* **2019,** *3* (1), 61–64.

Singh, N.; Verma, P.; Pandey, B. R.; Gilca, M. Role of withania somnifera in Prevention and Treatment of Cancer: An Overview. *Int. J. Pharma. Sci. Drug Res.* **2011**, *3* (4), 271–279.

Sowmyalakshmi, S.; Nur-E-Alam, M.; Akbarsha, M. A.; Thirugnanam, S.; Rohr, J.; Chendil, D.; Investigation on Semecarpus Lehyam—A Siddha Medicine for Breast Cancer. *Planta* **2005**, *220* (6), 910–918.

Standard Unani Medical Terminology. Central Council for Research in Unani Medicine, Ministry of AYUSH, Govt. of India: New Delhi, 2012.

Subbarayappa, B. V. The Roots of Ancient Medicine: An Historical Outline. *J. Biosci.* **2001**, *26* (2), 131–143.

Sujeethasai, K.; Soruban, T. A Study of Plants, Animals and Minerals which are Used "Puttru Noi" (Cancer) Treatment in the Authentic Siddha and Traditional Text Book. *J. Complement. Altern. Med. Res.* **2019**, *7* (3), 1–7.

Taneja, D. K. Yoga and Health. *Indian J. Community Med.* **2014,** *39* (2), 68.

Tembhurne, S. V.; Feroz, S.; Sakarkar, D. M. A Review on Therapeutic Potential of *Nigella sativa* (kalonji) Seeds. *J. Med. Plants Res.* **2014**, *8* (3), 166–167.

Tosetti, F.; Noonan, D. M.; Albini, A. Metabolic Regulation and Redox Activity as Mechanisms for Angioprevention by Dietary Phytochemicals. *Int. J. Cancer* **2009**, *125* (9), 1991–2003.

Training Manual, Integration of Unani Medicine in NPCDCS (National Programme for Prevention and Control of Cancer, Diabetes, Cardiovascular Diseases and Stroke). Published by Central Council for Research in Unani Medicine, Ministry of AYUSH, Government of India: New Delhi, 2016.

Umadevi, M.; Kumar, K. P.; Bhowmik, D.; Duraivel, S. Traditionally Used Anticancer Herbs in India. *J. Med. Plant Res.*, **2013**, *1*, 51–74.

CHAPTER 16

A Comprehensive Review on Medicinal Properties of Dawa-ul-Kurkum and Its Ingredients Against Liver Ailments in the Light of Ancient Wisdom and Modern Research

SAJIDA SUMAIYA[1,2], MEENAKSHI GUPTA[1], ARCHANA SHARMA[1], TANVEER NAVED[1], JAMAL AKHTAR[3], and MARYAM SARWAT[1]

[1]*Amity Institute of Pharmacy, Amity University, Noida, Uttar Pradesh, India*

[2]*School of Unani Medical Education and Research, Jamia Hamdard, New Delhi, India*

[3]*Central Council for Research in Unani Medicine, Janakpuri, New Delhi, India*

ABSTRACT

Unani system of medicine, originated in Greece and introduced in India by Arab and Persian settlers, has been recognized globally due to its easy accessibility and relatively safer effects. The formulations used in the Unani system are from plants, animals, or mineral origin. Among various formulations used for chronic ailments, Dawa-ul-Kurkum (DuK) is counted as one of the highly effective medicine for the ailments of the liver and spleen. The Unani literature

Ethnic Knowledge and Perspectives of Medicinal Plants, Volume 1: Curative Properties and Treatment Strategies. Munir Ozturk, Kandikere R. Sridhar, Maryam Sarwat, Volkan Altay, & Francisco Martín Huerta-Martínez (Eds.)

considers DuK as an anti-inflammatory (*muhallil*), sedative (*musakkin*), deobstruent (*mufatteh-e-sudad*), carminative (*kasir-e-riyah*) liver tonic (*muqawwijigar*), curative for diseases related to kidney (*muqawwigurda*), urinary bladder (*muqawwimasana*), stomach, and intestine (*medawaam'a*). Through databases, DuKs ingredients individually are proved to be anti-inflammatory, antioxidant, hepatoprotective, memory enhancer, neuroprotective (for Alzheimer's and Parkinson's disease), antitumor, and anticancer activities among various other specific effects. This chapter summarizes the information on the pharmacology and clinical research of individual ingredients of DuK as accessed through scientific journals and classical Unani literature. We have also tried to focus on the numerous possibilities for using DuK as an alternate therapy, alone, or in combination with other medications.

16.1 INTRODUCTION

The Unani medicine system is a broad medical system; it treats chronic diseases related to all organs of the human body. It deals precisely with many states of diseases and health; and offers promotive, protective, remedial, and rehabilitative healthcare (Naaz and Ahmed, 2017). In the Unani medical system, the human body is considered as a single unit made up of seven components: Elements *(arkaan)*, temperament (*mizaj*), humours *(akhlat)*, organs (*a'zaa*), spirits *(arwaah)*, faculties *(quwaa)*, functions *(afa'al)*, collectively known as *Umoor-e-Tabaiya* (Rahman, 2006). According to the Unani philosophy, the body is comprised of four elements: earth *(teen)*, air (*hawa*), water (*ma'a*), and fire *(naar)*], which have diverse temperaments, that is, cold, hot, wet, and dry respectively (Rahman et al., 2008). When these four elements intermix and interact with each other, a new compound comes into existence having a new temperament *(mizaj)*, that is, cold dry, hot wet, cold wet, and hot dry. The human body has simple (*mufrad*) as well as compound (*murakkab*) organs, which attain their nutrition through the four humors [yellow bile (*safra*), black bile *(sauda)*, phlegm *(balgham)*, and blood *(dam)*]. Every individual humor possesses its precise temperament, like yellow bile is hot and dry, black bile is cold and dry, phlegm is cold and moist, and blood is hot and moist (Rahman, 2006; Rahman et al., 2008). Human beings attain a temperament conferring to the majority of the humors in their body which then shows the person's state of health. A person's temperament may be phlegmatic, sanguine, melancholic, or choleric. Depending upon the temperament of a person, and the disease, a line of treatment is chosen.

Among various polyherbal formulations (murakkab) used for chronic ailments, DuK is considered to be one of the highly effective formulations for ailments of the liver and spleen (Figure 16.1). DuKs effects are credited due to its anti-inflammatory (muhallil) activity, analgesic & sedative (musakkin), deobstruent (mufatteh-e-sudad), carminative (kasir-e-riyah), and tonic for liver (muqawwijigar), kidney (muqawwigurda), urinary bladder (muqawwimasana), stomach, and intestine (medawaam'a) (Hafeez et al., 2018; Kabeeruddin, 2018). It is beneficial for reducing obesity (Jafri et al., 2015) and in the management of jaundice (Ansari et al., 2017). According to modern research, DuK has been shown to protect the liver against the damage induced by D-Galactosamine in rat models through the oxidant-antioxidant homeostatic balance (Gulati et al., 2019).

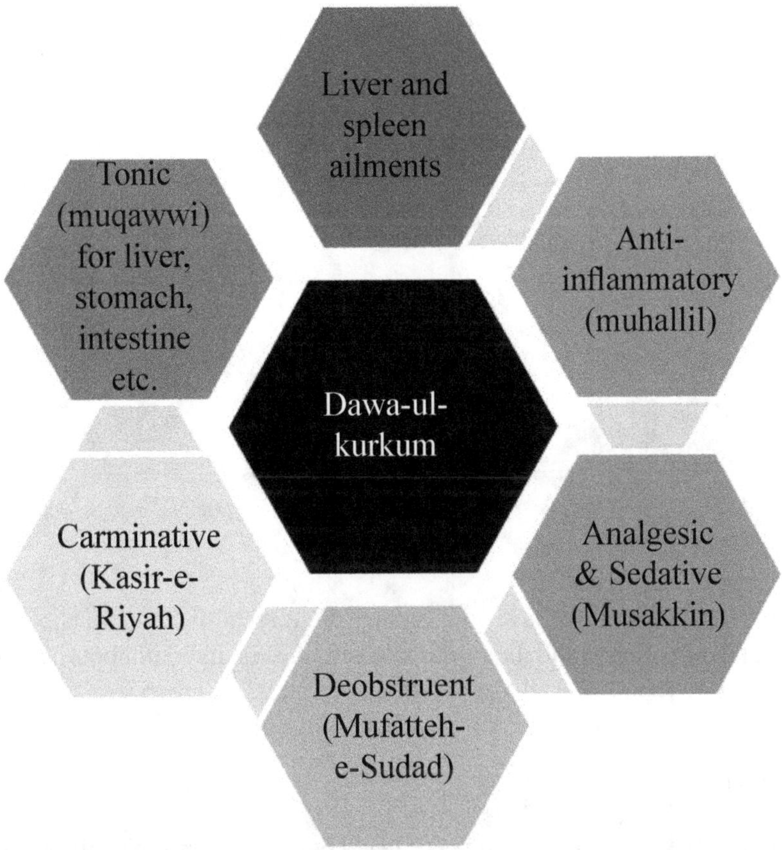

FIGURE 16.1 Diagrammatic representation showing the activities of Dawa-ul-Kurkum according to the classical texts of Unani medicine.

Based on the number of ingredients, DuK is categorized as Dawa-ul-Kurkum kabeer (higher number of ingredients) and Dawa-ul-Kurkum sagheer (lesser number of ingredients) in the National Formulary of Unani Medicine, part- I (NFUM-I) (Anonymous, 2006; Kabeeruddin, 2018). We have addressed Dawa-ul-Kurkum sagheer as DuK (constituents summarized in Table 16.1) here (Figure 16.2). The formulation's name is derived from its main ingredient Kurkum (a Persian word) denoting saffron (zaafran).

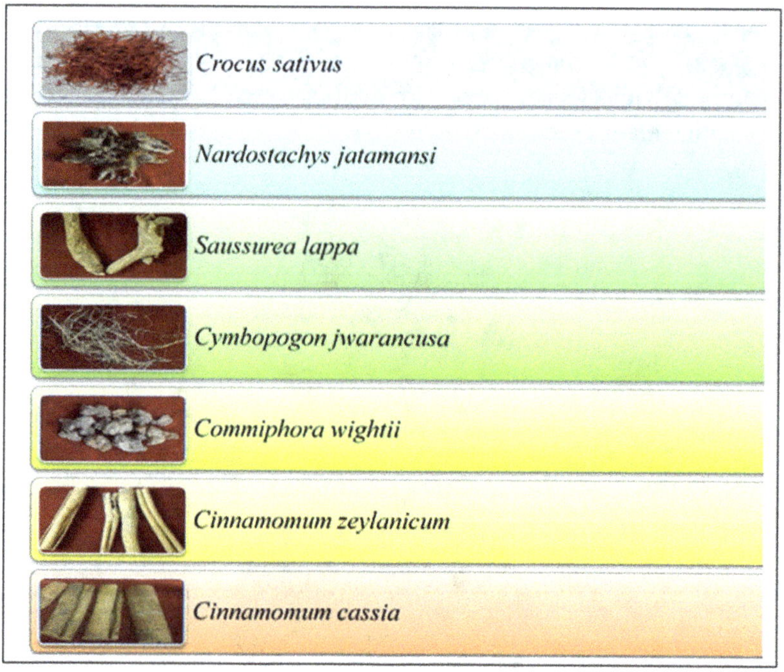

FIGURE 16.2 Constituents of Dawa-ul-Kurkum with its original images depicting its morphological features.

In this chapter, we have highlighted the effects of DuK on the human body, its ingredients, and their probable activities on liver ailments according to Unani literature as well as modern research and its prospects.

16.2 METHODS

An extensive literature search was carried out to explore the available information in Unani literature regarding DuK and its ingredients. The online search engines such as PubMed, Scopus, and Google Scholar were explored

TABLE 16.1 Medicinal Importance of the Ingredients of Dawa-ul-Kurkum*.

No	Botanical name of the Herb/ Common name	Medicinal properties as per Unani literature	Activities	Possible mechanism of Action	References
1	*Crocus sativus* (Zaafran)	Detergent (*jaali*), astringent (*qabiz*), anti-inflammatory (*muhallil*), aphrodisiac (*muqawwibaah*), tonic (*muqawwi*) for vital organs (heart, brain and liver)	Antiproliferative activity against hepatocellular carcinoma (HCC)	Arrests cell cycle at S and G2/M phases and downregulates inflammation; Inhibits telomerase and downregulateshTERT. Inhibition of STAT3 activation	Amin et al., 2011, 2016; Noureini and Wink, 2012; Kim and Park, 2018
			Protective effect on the liver tissues, attenuate oxidative stress in streptozotocin-induced diabetic rats	Expression of miRNA- 122 and downregulation of signaling pathway MAPK and MAPKAP	Altinoz et al., 2014; Samarghandhian et al., 2016; Yaribeygi et al., 2018; Hassani et al., 2017
2	*Nardostachysjatamansi* (Sumbuluttib)	Anti-inflammatory (muhallil), calorifacient (musakkhin), deobstruent (mufatteh), detergent (Jaali), chiefly used as a tonic (muqawwi) for liver and brain, and also as carminative (kasirriyah)	Reduces liver damage by decreasing serum transaminase and alkaline phosphatase against thioacetamide-induced hepatotoxicity and CCl_4 induced hepatotoxicity		Ali et al., 2000; Dandagi et al., 2008
			Protects liver tissues against radiation-induced damage		Gowda et al., 2011
			Antiproliferative and anticancer activity against HepG-2 cells		Bhagat et al., 2013; Chaudhary et al., 2015
3.	*Cinnamomum cassia* (Tajqalmi)	Carminative (kaasir e riyah) and astringent (qabiz), tonic (muqawwi) for stomach and liver	Anti-inflammatory, antihypertriglyceridemia, antidiabetic, hepatoprotective, antitumor, and anticancer		Mohammad and Dwettinck, 2017; Liao et al., 2012

TABLE 16.1 *(Continued)*

No	Botanical name of the Herb/ Common name	Medicinal properties as per Unani literature	Activities	Possible mechanism of Action	References
			In vitro antiproliferative and antiapoptotic activity on HepG2 cells	p53 induction and CD95 (APO-1) signaling pathways	Ng and Wu, 2011; Dutta and Chakraborty, 2018
4.	*Cymbopogonjwaran-cusa* (Izkhar)	Deobstruent (*mufatteh*), anti-inflammatory (*muhallil*), carminative (*kaasir e riyah*), tonic (*muqawwi*) for stomach and astringent (*qabiz*)	Antioxidant, antiallergic, antiparasitic, analgesic and antipyretic, hypolipidemic and hypoglycemic, hepatoprotective, and anticancer.		Prasad et al., 2013
			Flukicidal against buffalo's liver flukes, it paralyzes them leading to death.		Shafiq et al., 2015
			Reduction of body weight, lipid parameters, and blood glucose levels in rat models		Khan et al., 2018
5.	*Commiphorawightii* (Murmakki)	Antiseptic (*daaf'eta'ffun*), desiccative (*mujaffif*), detergent (*jaali*), carminative (*kasirriyah*), tonic (*muqawwi*), antihelminthic (*qaatilkirm e shikam*), anti-inflammatory (*muhallil*), deobstruent	Against diabetes, arthritis, asthma and other respiratory diseases, intestinal bowel disease, pancreatitis, cancer, Alzheimer's disease, and skin diseases		Shishodia et al., 2008; Kunnumakkara et al., 2018, Bhardwaj and Alia, 2019

TABLE 16.1 (Continued)

No	Botanical name of the Herb/ Common name	Medicinal properties as per Unani literature	Activities	Possible mechanism of Action	References
		(*mufatteh*), and calorifacient (*musakkhin*).	Anti-inflammatory activity on murine macrophages	Inhibits liposachharides-induced inflammatory cytokines in NF-κB signaling pathway	Zhang et al., 2016
			Alleviates hepatic hyperlipidemia and oxidative stress in streptozotocin-induced diabetic rats	Lowers hepatic glucose-6-phosphatase (G-6-Pase)	Bhardwaj et al., 2014
			Inhibition of cell proliferation in HepG2 cells	Activation of intrinsic mitochondrial pathways and cell cycle arrest and eventual apoptosis	Shi et al., 2015; Bhat et al., 2017
			Antiangiogenesis and antitumor effect and sensitizes hepatocellular carcinoma	Through nuclear factor-kB and STAT3 downregulation and upregulation of DR5 (death receptor) for TRAIL (tumor necrosis factor-related apoptosis inducing ligand)	Moon et al., 2011
6.	*Saussurealappa*(Qust)	Detergent (*jaali*), blood absorbent (*jazib e damm*), anti-inflammatory (*muhallil*), and desiccative (*mujaffif*). Tonic for vital organs (heart, liver, and brain) & nerves,	Anti-inflammatory, antioxidant, hepatoprotective, gastro-protective, antispasmodic, immunomodulatory, anticonvulsant, antidiabetic, and antihelminthic		Madhuri et al., 2012

TABLE 16.1 *(Continued)*

No	Botanical name of the Herb/ Common name	Medicinal properties as per Unani literature	Activities	Possible mechanism of Action	References
		carminative (*kasir e riyah*), and antihelminthic for stomach and intestine	Reverses and accelerates reversion of CCl_4 induced liver fibrosis in rats	Aantioxidant and anti-inflammatory activity through suppression of activated liver stellate cells and induction of apoptosis	El-sayed et al., 2015
			Alleviation of paracetamol induced liver damage in rabbits	Antioxidant and free radical scavenging activity	Kadhem et al., 2019
			Antitumor effects in HCC	Inhibition of epithelial growth factor receptor (EGFR) mediated pathway	Lin et al., 2016
			Cytotoxic activity in HepG2 cells	Arresting the cells in G_1 cell cycle phase via the intrinsic mitochondrial pathway	Shati et al., 2020
7.	*Cinnamomum-zeylanicum* (Darchini)	Tonic (*muqawwi*), carminative (*kasirriyah*). demulcent (*mulattif*) and dessicative (*mujaffif*)	Antioxidant, anti-inflammatory, hepatoprotective, hypoglycemic and hypolipidemic, antiulcerogenic, anesthetic, antiallergenic, antipyretic, and anticancer		Rao and Gan, 2014

TABLE 16.1 *(Continued)*

No	Botanical name of the Herb/ Common name	Medicinal properties as per Unani literature	Activities	Possible mechanism of Action	References
			Hypolipidemic effect	Ameliorates hepatic glycogen level by improving the liver's glycogenesis process	Hassan et al., 2012
			Hepatoprotective effect against paracetamol-induced hepatotoxicity	Antioxidant and radical scavenging activity	El-Hadary, 2015
			Anticancer effect on HepG2 cells		Varalakshmi et al., 2014; El-Nabi et al., 2016

**Information about Medicinal Properties as per Unani literature is procured from Hakeem (2011) and Khan (2012).*

for the modern pharmacological activities of individual ingredients and their role in various liver ailments.

16.3 DUK COMPOSITION

16.3.1 CROCUS SATIVUS (ZAFRAAN)

The perennial herb *C. sativus* L., family Iridaceae is grown in India, China, Azerbaijan, Greece, France, Iran, Spain, Italy, Morocco, Turkiye, Mexico, and Egypt (Kafi et al., 2018; Sumaiya et al., 2020). Saffron and its active metabolites (crocin, crocetin, picrocrocin, and safranal) are reported to cure various ailments of the eyes, brain, kidney, liver, etc. (Sarwat and Sumaiya 2020). Its bioactive compounds protect liver tissues and attenuate oxidative stress in streptozotocin-induced diabetic rats (Altinoz et al., 2014; Samarghandhian et al., 2016; Yaribeygi et al., 2018), and in acetaminophen &rifampicin induced hepatotoxicity (Moossavi et al. 2016). It exhibits a protective effect on hepatic tissues in BPA Bisphenol A) induced liver toxicity by inhibition of oxidative stress, expression of miRNA- 122, and downregulation of signaling pathway MAPK and MAPKAP (Hassani et al., 2017). The anti-inflammatory activity of saffron is attributed to its strong radical scavenging and antioxidant activity (Poma et al., 2012). The in vivo and in vitro studies suggested that saffron possesses antiproliferative activity against hepatocellular carcinoma (HCC) and induces apoptosis (Amin et al., 2011); in HepG2 cells, it arrests cell cycle at S and G2/M phases and downregulates inflammation (Amin et al., 2016), and inhibits telomerase and downregulateshTERT (Noureini and Wink, 2012). Saffron's carotenoids inhibit STAT3 activation and promote apoptosis in HepG2 and Hep3B cells (Kim and Park, 2018).

The Unani literature highlights saffron as the detergent (jaali), astringent (qabiz), anti-inflammatory (muhallil), aphrodisiac (muqawwibaah), tonic (muqawwi) for vital organs (heart, brain, and liver), and the whole body while its main activity mentioned as a tranquilizer, analgesic (musakkin), and catalytic. When it is added in formulation, it works as a catalyst. Saffron is used in the form of local application to reduce inflammation of the liver (Hakeem, 2011; Khan, 2012).

16.3.2 NARDOSTACHYS JATAMANSI (SUMBULUTTIB)

N. jatamansi (family Valerianaceae), a perennial herb of Alpine Himalayas, is used for a long time in various chronic diseases. The active components present in *N. jatamansi* (NS) exhibit antioxidant, anti-inflammatory, and hepatoprotective activities among others. NS extract reduces liver damage by decreasing serum transaminase and alkaline phosphatase against thioacetamide-induced hepatotoxicity (Ali et al., 2000). Radiotherapy used in cancer treatment leads to the production of reactive oxygen species. The extract of *N. jatamansi* protects the liver tissues against such radiation-induced damage (Gowda et al., 2011) and also shows antiproliferative and anticancer activity in Hep-2 cells (Bhagat et al., 2013; Chaudhary et al., 2015). NS is a component of F3 formulation that has shown hepatoprotective activity against CCl4-induced hepatic toxicity (Dandagi et al., 2008). It inhibits gluconeogenesis in the liver, improves insulin sensitivity, and hence alleviates hyperglycemia (You et al., 2018). The Unani text has established its basic activities as an anti-inflammatory (muhallil), calorifacient (musakkhin), deobstruent (mufatteh), and detergent (jaali). It is chiefly used as a tonic (muqawwi) for the liver and brain, and also as a carminative (kasir-e-riyah).

NS boosts the activities of the heart, liver, and brain; reduces flatulence, ascites, jaundice, and inflammation of the liver, stomach, uterus, and urinary bladder (Hakeem, 2011; Khan, 2012).

16.3.3 CINNAMOMUM CASSIA (TAJQALMI)

C. cassia (CC) bark, known as Chinese cassia or Chinese cinnamon, of family Lauraceae, is a bark of a tropical aromatic evergreen tree. Commonly used as a spice and additive agent globally, its appearance is thicker and shorter than *Cinnamomum zeylanicum* (Zhang et al., 2019). The significant benefits of CC have been reported on human health as an anti-inflammatory, antihypertriglyceridemia, antidiabetic, hepatoprotective, antitumor, and anticancer agent, mainly due to its phytochemical constituents (Muhammad and Dwettinck, 2017). The anti-inflammatory activity of active constituents of CC extract (cinnamic aldehyde, cinnamic alcohol, cinnamic acid, and coumarin) was established by Liao et al. in their in vivo and in vitro studies (Liao et al., 2012). In a study, CS extract showed that it can considerably alter liver antioxidant enzymes and the level of blood glucose in streptozotocin-induced animals (IM et al., 2014) and the type-2 diabetic animal model (Yan et al., 2015). Methanolic extract of CC extract recovers the antioxidant system and protects the liver tissues against long-term use of titanium dioxide nanoparticles- TiO2-NPs (Shakeel et al., 2018) and Nickel nanoparticles- Ni-NPs (Iqbal et al., 2020). Administration of an active ingredient of CC, which is 2-methoxycinnamaldehyde (2-MCA) in rat model protects against hepatic ischemia-reperfusion injury via anti-inflammatory and antiapoptotic properties (Golshahi et al., 2019). The constituents of CC show antiproliferative and antiapoptotic activity on HepG2 cells through p53 induction and CD95 (APO-1) signaling pathways (Ng and Wu, 2011; Dutta and Chakraborty, 2018).

The Unani texts mention CC has basic effects of energy enhancer on the body, and it also works as carminative (*kaasir-e-riyah*) and astringent (*qabiz*). It works chiefly as a tonic (*muqawwi*) for the stomach and liver. CC is mixed with other formulations that are a) beneficial for liver and stomach, and b) used as an astringent powder in diarrheal diseases (Hakeem, 2011; Khan, 2012).

16.3.4 CYMBOPOGON JWARANCUSA (IZKHAR)

C. jwarancusa (Jones.) of the family Poaceae, is counted as an aromatic perennial grass and used as condiment and medicine (Avoseh et al., 2015). Its name is derived from two Sanskrit words "jwar" and "ankusha," which means "fever and breaker," respectively. The plant shows many pharmacological activities like antioxidant, antiallergic, antiparasitic, analgesic and antipyretic, hypolipidemic and hypoglycemic, hepatoprotective, and anticancer (Prasad et al., 2013). Methanolic extract of *C. jwarancusa* (CJ) works as flukicidal against buffalo's liver flukes as it inhibits their motility, paralyzes them leading to their death (Shafiq et al., 2015). The ethanolic extract of CJ reduces body weight, lipid parameters, and blood glucose levels in rat models (Khan et al., 2018). CJ is one of the components of the Unani formulation *Majoondabeedulward*, which exhibits a hepatoprotective effect against the acetaminophen-induced liver damage in the animal model and restores the liver enzymes (Shakya and Shukla, 2011). The in vitro study of CJ oil shows cytotoxic and anticancer activity in Hep-2cells (Dar et al., 2011; Dutta et al., 2016).

The Unani literature mentioned its activities as deobstruent (*mufatteh*), anti-inflammatory (*muhallil*), carminative (*kaasir-e-riyah*), tonic (*muqawwi*) for stomach, and astringent (*qabiz*). The flower of CJ is considered of high efficacy as compared to the rest of the part. The main effect of CJ is seen in ascites and inflammation of the liver and spleen for which it is used in the compound formulation as decoction or alone. For firm swellings of the liver and stomach, CJ is used in the form of paste for local application (Hakeem, 2011; Khan, 2012).

16.3.5 COMMIPHORA WIGHTII (MURMAKKI)

C. wightii (guggul) tree of the Burseraceae family is found in parched regions of subcontinents of India mainly India, Bangladesh, and Pakistan. A single tree yields around 200–250 gm of dry resin in each collection season (Sarup et al., 2015). Studies have illustrated *C. wightii* (CW) to be intensely potent against various enduring illnesses like diabetes, arthritis, asthma and other respiratory diseases, otitis media, intestinal metaplasia, infectious diseases, intestinal bowel disease, pancreatitis, cancer, Alzheimer's disease, and skin diseases (Shishodia et al., 2008). It works as antioxidant, anti-inflammatory, hypolipidemic and cardioprotective, neuroprotective, hepatoprotective, anti-tumor, and anticancer agent (Kunnumakkara et al., 2018; Bhardwaj and Alia, 2019). The antioxidant activity of gum extract is evident as it inhibits the DPPH free radicals (Vani et al., 2016). Guggulsterone, an active component of guggul has shown anti-inflammatory activity on murine macrophages, and it inhibits liposachharides-induced inflammatory cytokines in the NF-κB signaling pathway (Zhang et al., 2016). A study by Bhardwaj and group suggests that CW extract alleviates hepatic hyperlipidemia and oxidative stress. It also lowers hepatic glucose-6-phosphatase (G-6-Pase) activity and thereby improves carbohydrate metabolism in streptozotocin-induced diabetic rats (Bhardwaj et al., 2014). Guggulsterone has antiangiogenesis and antitumor effects and sensitizes HCC by suppressing nuclear factor-kB and STAT3 activity and upregulating death receptor DR5 for TRAIL (tumor necrosis factor-related apoptosis-inducing ligand). This effect is associated with eIF2a and CHOP activation (Moon et al., 2011). It induces cell cycle arrest and eventual apoptosis and inhibits cell proliferation in HepG2 cells by activation of intrinsic mitochondrial pathways (Shi et al., 2015; Bhat et al., 2017). It also enhances doxorubicin's cytotoxic effect on PLC/PRF/5R cells via Cox-2/P-gp dependent pathway (Xu et al., 2017; Kunnumakkara et al., 2018). CW also reduces the harmful side effects of chemotherapy agents like cisplatin, cetuximab, and erlotinib, and works as a noteworthy agent for preventive and complementary therapy (Leeman-Neil et al., 2009).

The Unani text suggests CW of Mekkah as the best type among all its varieties. The basic activities mentioned in the literature include antiseptic (*daaf'eta'ffun*), dessicative (*mujaffif*), detergent (*jaali*), carminative (*kasir-e-riyah*), tonic (*muqawwi*), antihelminthic (*qaatil-e-kirm–e-shikam*), anti-inflammatory (*muhallil*), deobstruent (*mufatteh*), and calorifacient (*musakkhin*). CW has an antiseptic effect due to which it is used as a preventive cure in epidemics. Its strong anti-inflammatory effect mediates its use in gout, sciatica, and other joint disorders in the form of oral suspension or as a paste for local application (Hakeem, 2011).

16.3.6 SAUSSUREA LAPPA (QUST)

The perennial herb of *S. lappa* (SL) C.B. Clarke, family- Compositae, order- Asterales, is commonly known as Costus. With a long and stout root of 60cm, it has a characteristic peculiar odor (Pandey et al., 2007). Its pharmacological activities according to various studies include anti-inflammatory, anti-oxidant, hepatoprotective, gastro-protective, antispasmodic, immunomodulatory, anticonvulsant, antidiabetic, and antihelminthic (Madhuri et al., 2012). The aqueous methanolic extract of SL protects the liver and reduces hepatitis and hepatic damage induced by D-galactosamine and lipopolysaccharides in mice (Yaeesh et al., 2010). SL root extract reverses and accelerates the reversion of CCl_4-induced liver fibrosis in rats via its antioxidant and anti-inflammatory activity, and also through suppression of activated liver stellate cells and induction of apoptosis (El-sayed e al., 2015). Its aqueous extract exhibits a hepatoprotective effect and reduces hepatic damage produced by the intoxication of deltamethrin, by ameliorating the altered liver biomarkers and cellular structure (Alnahdi et al., 2016). The paracetamol-induced liver damage in rabbits is alleviated by the treatment of ethanolic extract of SL via its anti-oxidant and free radical scavenging activity (Kadhem et al., 2019). Active metabolites extracted from *S. lappa* root were studied for its anticancer effect. Compounds like costunolide and dehydrocostus lactone suppress hepatitis B virus surface antigen (HBsAg) gene expression in Hep3B and HepA2 cells at mainly mRNA level (Chen et al., 1995; Choi et al., 2013). Separately, dehydrocostuslactone inhibits cell proliferation and induces apoptosis coupled with the endoplasmic reticulum (ER) stress in hepatic carcinoma cells HepG2 and PLC/PRF/5 (Hsu et al., 2009; Zahara et al., 2014; Tian et al., 2017). The SL oil exerts antitumor effects in HCC via inhibition of the epithelial growth factor receptor mediated pathway (Lin et al., 2016). The secondary metabolite of SL extract shows cytotoxic and anticancer activity in HepG2 cells by arresting the cells in G_1 cell cycle phase via the intrinsic mitochondrial pathway (Shati et al., 2020).

The ancient Unani text highlights its activities on external use as the detergent (*jaali*), blood absorbent (*jazib-e-damm*), anti-inflammatory (*muhallil*), and desiccative (*mujaffif*). On internal use, it works as a tonic for vital organs (heart, liver, and brain) & nerves, carminative (*kasir-e-riyah*), and antihelminthic for the stomach and intestine. SL is also used in inflammation of the spleen, and ascites. Its main function is considered as a tonic for vital organs (Hakeem, 2011; Khan, 2012).

16.3.7 C. ZEYLANICUM (DARCHINI)

The inner bark of the tropical evergreen plant *C. zeylanicum* (CZ) from the genus *Cinnamomum*, has its own medicinal and culinary importance worldwide (Ranasinghe et al., 2013). It possesses properties like antioxidant, anti-inflammatory, hepatoprotective, hypoglycemic and hypolipidemic, antiulcerogenic, anesthetic, antiallergenic, antipyretic, and anticancer among many others (Rao and Gan, 2014). The CZ extract strongly exhibits a hypolipidemic effect and ameliorates the hepatic glycogen level by improving the liver's glycogenesis process (Hassan et al., 2012). The oil and ethanolic extract of CZ show hepatoprotective effect against paracetamol-induced hepatotoxicity due to its antioxidant and radical scavenging activity (El-Hadary, 2015; Abd El Fadil et al., 2020). CZ extract protects the liver tissues from damage caused due to the administration of CCl_4 (Eidi et al., 2012; Bellassoued et al., 2018), and acetaminophen (Hussain et al., 2019). The anticancer effect of CZ extract is reported in HepG2 cells as it induces growth inhibition and apoptosis (Varalakshmi et al., 2014; El-Nabi et al., 2016). Pretreatment with CZ shows a reduction in the cytotoxic effect of DEN (diethylnitrosamine) on liver tissues, with restoration in nuclear shape and slight regeneration of tubular structure (Sathya et al., 2014).

According to Unani literature, CZ works as a tonic (*muqawwi*), carminative (*kasir-e-riyah*), demulcent (*mulattif*) and dessicative (*mujaffif*). It provides energy to the stomach and liver and produces constipation in the intestine. CZ is used as a single drug as well as a component of any formulation. Its main function is considered to be tonic for vital organs (heart, liver, brain) (Hakeem, 2011; Khan, 2012).

16.4 CONCLUSIONS

The DuK formulation has been in use for ages as mentioned in multiple texts and literature of Unani medicine for the diseases of liver and spleen due to coldness, as a tonic for different organs of the body, and also as carminative. As we assessed the pharmacological activities of the ingredients of DuK individually, almost all of them have been used to treat the liver, its architecture, and biomarkers, in the form of anti-inflammatory, antioxidant, hepatoprotective, hypolipidemic, hypoglycemic, antitumor, and anticancer agents. It was seen that the Unani texts also highlighted their effectiveness as an anti-inflammatory (*muhallil*), analgesic (*musakkin*), desiccative (*mujaffif*), detergent (*jaali*), diuretic (*mudir e bol*), deobstruent (*mufatteh*), and tonic for vital organs (heart, liver, and brain) (*muqawwiaaza e raeesa*). These effects collectively enhance the efficacy of the formulation. The aforementioned activities (Modern + Unani) are suggestive of its use in liver diseases as an adjuvant to conventional therapy. DuK when combined with other conventional therapy may help to synergize the effects, reduce the side effects of the conventional drugs, improve the patients' quality of life, and also can be used in preventive cures.

KEYWORDS

- **Unani medicine**
- **alternative therapy**
- **dawa-ul-kurkum**
- **anti-inflammatory (*muhallil*)**
- **tonic (*muqawwi*)**

REFERENCES

Abd El Fadil, H.; Moustafa, A.; Khalifa, H.; Hossam, A.; Behairy, A. Cinnamon Extract Ameliorates Liver Damage and Oxidative Stress Induced By Paracetamol in Male Rats. *Damanhour J. Vet. Sci.* **2020,** *3*, 12–20.

Ali, S.; Ansari, K. A.; Jafry, M. A.; Kabeer, H.; Diwakar, G. Nardostachys Jatamansi Protects Against Liver Damage Induced by Thioacetamide in Rats. *J. Ethnopharmacol.* **2000,** *7*, 359–363.

Altinoz, E.; Oner, Z.; Elbe, H.; Turkoz, Y.; Cigremis, Y. Protective Effect of Saffron (Its Active Constituent, Crocin) on Oxidative Stress and Hepatic Injury in Streptozotocin Induced Diabetic Rats. *Gene Therap. Mol. Biol.* **2014,** *16*, 160–171.

Alnahdi, H. S.; Ayaz, N. O.; Elhalwagy, M. E. Prophylactic Effect of Cousts *Saussurea lappa* Against Liver Injury Induced by Deltamethrin Intoxication. *Int. J. Clin. Exp. Pathol.* **2016,** *9*, 387–394.

Amin, A.; Hamza, A. A.; Bajbouj, K.; Ashraf, S. S.; Daoud, S. Saffron: A Potential Candidate for a Novel Anticancer Drug Against Hepatocellular Carcinoma. *Hepatology* **2011,** *54*, 857–867.

Amin, A. A; Hamza, A.; Daoud, S.; Khazanehdari, K.; Al Hrout, A.; Baig, B.; Chaiboonchoe, A.; E Adrian, T.; Zaki, N.; Salehi-Ashtiani, K. Saffron-Based Crocin Prevents Early Lesions

Of Liver Cancer: In Vivo, In Vitro and Network Analyses. *Recent Patents Anti-Cancer Drug Discov.* **2016,** *11*, 121–133.

Anonymous. *National Formulary of Unani Medicne (NFUM), Part-I*; Ministry of Health and Family Welfare, Department of AYUSH: New Delhi, 2006; p 88.

Ansari, M. S.; Alam, M.; Ahmad, W. Commonly Used Unani Formulations in Jaundice Patients Attending Jarahiyat Section: A Case Series. *Int. J. Med. Res.* **2017,** *2*, 34–36.

Avoseh, O.; Oyedeji, O.; Rungqu, P.; Nkeh-Chungag, B.; Oyedeji, A. *Cymbopogon* Species; Ethnopharmacology, Phytochemistry and the Pharmacological Importance. *Molecules* **2015,** *20* 7438–7453.

Bellassoued, K.; Ghrab, F.; Hamed, H.; Kallel, R.; van Pelt, J.; Lahyani, A.; Makni Ayadi, F.; El Feki, A. Protective Effect of *Cinnamomum zeylanicum* L. Bark Essential Oil, on Hepatic and Renal Toxicity Induced by CCl4 in rats, 2018.

Bhardwaj, M.; Soni, A.; Mishra, S.; Tripathi, S. Protective Effect of *Commiphora wightii* in Metabolic Activity of Streptozotocin (STZ) Induced Diabetes in Rats. *J. Diab. Endocrinol.* **2014,** *5*, 19–28.

Bhardwaj, M.; Alia, A. *Commiphora wightii* (Arn.) Bhandari. Review of Its Botany, Medicinal Uses, Pharmacological Activities and Phytochemistry. *J. Drug Deliv. Therap.* **2019,** *9*, 613–621.

Bhagat, M.; Pandita, R. M.; Saxena, A. K. In Vitro and In Vivo Biological Activities of *Nardostachys jatamansi* Roots. *Med. Aromat. Plants* **2013,** *2*, 2167–0412.

Bhat, A. A.; Prabhu, K. S.; Kuttikrishnan, S.; Krishnankutty, R.; Babu, J.; Mohammad, R. M.; Uddin, S. Potential Therapeutic Targets of Guggulsterone in Cancer. *Nutr. Metabol.* **2017,** *14*, 1–11.

Chaudhary, S.; Chandrashekar, K. S.; Pai, K. S. R.; Setty, M. M.; Devkar, R. A.; Reddy, N. D.; Shoja, M. H. Evaluation of Antioxidant and Anticancer Activity of Extract and Fractions of *Nardostachys jatamansi* DC in Breast Carcinoma. *BMC Complement. Altern. Med.* **2015,** *15*, 1–13.

Chen, H. C.; Chou, C. K.; Lee, S. D.; Wang, J. C.; Yeh, S. F. Active Compounds from *Saussurea lappa* Clarks That Suppress Hepatitis B Virus Surface Antigen Gene Expression in Human Hepatoma Cells. *Antiviral Res.* **1995,** *27*, 99–109.

Choi, Y. K.; Cho, S. G.; Woo, S. M.; Yun, Y. J.; Jo, J.; Kim, W.; Shin, Y. C.; Ko, S. G.. *Saussurea lappa* Clarke-Derived Costunolide Prevents TNFα-Induced Breast Cancer Cell Migration and Invasion by Inhibiting NF-κB Activity. *Evid. Based Complement. Altern. Med.* **2013.**

Dandagi, P. M.; Patil, M. B.; Mastiholimath, V. S.; Gadad, A. P.; Dhumansure, R. H. Development and Evaluation of Hepatoprotective Polyherbal Formulation Containing Some Indigenous Medicinal Plants. *Indian J. Pharma. Sci.* **2008,** *70*, 265–268.

Dar, M. Y.; Shah, W. A.; Rather, M. A.; Qurishi, Y.; Hamid, A.; Qurishi, M. A. Chemical Composition, In Vitro Cytotoxic and Antioxidant Activities of the Essential Oil and Major Constituents of *Cymbopogon jawarancusa* (Kashmir). *Food Chem.* **2011,** *129*, 1606–1611.

Dutta, S.; Munda, S.; Lal, M.; Bhattacharyya, P. R. A Short Review on Chemical Composition Therapeutic Use and Enzyme Inhibition Activities of *Cymbopogon* Species. *Indian J. Sci. Technol.* **2016,** *9*, 1–9.

Dutta, A.; Chakraborty, A. Cinnamon in Anticancer Armamentarium: A Molecular Approach. *J. Toxicol.* ***2018.***

El-sayed, H. R. H.; Abd-Elmonem, M. M.; Gabr, O. M.; Badria, F. A. E. *Saussurea lappa* Root Extract Accelerates the Reversion of Liver Fibrosis Induced by Carbon Tetrachloride in Rats. *Benha Med. J.* **2015,** *32*, 116–125.

El-Hadary, A. E. A. Antioxidant and Hepatoprotective Effect Of *Cinnamomum zeylanicum* Oil Against Paracetamol Induced Hepatotoxicity In Male Rate. *J. Agric. Chem. Biotechnol* **2015,** *6*, 407–418.

Eidi, A.; Mortazavi, P.; Bazargan, M.; Zaringhalam, J. Hepatoprotective Activity of Cinnamon Ethanolic Extract Against CCI4-Induced Liver Injury in Rats. *Excli. J.* **2012,** *11*, 495–507.

El-Nabi, S. H.; El-Garawani, I.; El-Berry, A. The Apoptotic Properties of *Cinnamomum zeylanicum* and *Cymbopogon citratus* on Human Hepatocellular Carcinoma Cell Line (HepG2). *Eur. J. Pharma. Med. Res.* **2016,** *3*, 44–48.

Golshahi, H.; Araghi, A.; Baghban, F.; Farzad-Mohajeri, S. Protective Effects of 2-Methoxy-cinnamaldehyde an Active Ingredients of *Cinnamomum cassia* on Warm Hepatic Ischemia Reperfusion Injury in Rat Model. *Iran. J. Basic Med. Sci.* **2019,** *22*, 1400–1407.

Gowda, K. D.; Shetty, L.; Krishna, A. P.; Kumari, N. S.; Sanjeev, G.; Naveen, P. Protective Effect of *Nardostachys jatamansi* Root Extract Against Radiation Induced Damage on Liver and Kidney Functions in Albino Wistar Rats. *J. Pharm. Res.* **2011,** *4*, 2462–2465.

Gulati, K.; Reshi, M. R.; Rais-ur-Rahman; Akhtar, J.; Ray, A. Hepatoprotective Effects of Dawa-Ul-Kurkum, a Unani Polyherbal Preparation and the Possible Mechanisms in Experimental Model of D-Galactosamine Induced Liver Damage in Rats. *EC Pharmacol. Toxicol.* **2019,** *7*, 948–960.

Hafeez, A.; Siddiqui, M. A.; Khan, A. M.; Azeez, A. Evaluation of the Efficacy of Dawa-ul-Kurkum in Su-e-Mizaj Kabid Barid (Non-Alcoholic Fatty Liver Disease): A Randomized Single Blind Placebo Controlled Study. *J. Biol. Sci. Opin.* **2018,** *6*, 44–52.

Hakeem, H. M. A. *Bustanul Mufradat*; Aijaz Publishing House: Delhi, 2011.

Hassan, S. A.; Barthwal, R.; Nair, M. S., Haque, S. S. Aqueous Bark Extract of *Cinnamomum zeylanicum*: A Potential Therapeutic Agent for Streptozotocin-Induced Type 1 Diabetes Mellitus (T1DM) Rats. *Trop. J. Pharma. Res.* **2012,** *11*, 429–435.

Hassani, F. V.; Mehri, S.; Abnous, K.; Birner-Gruenberger, R.; Hosseinzadeh, H. Protective Effect of Crocin on BPA-Induced Liver Toxicity in Rats Through Inhibition of Oxidative Stress and Downregulation of MAPK and MAPKAP Signaling Pathway and miRNA-122 Expression. *Food Chem. Toxicol.* **2017,** *107*, 395–405.

Hsu, Y. L.; Wu, L. Y.; Kuo, P. L. Dehydrocostuslactonc, a Medicinal Plant-Derived Sesquiterpene Lactone, Induces Apoptosis Coupled to Endoplasmic Reticulum Stress in Liver Cancer Cells. *J. Pharmacol. Exp. Therap.* **2009,** *329*, 808–819.

Hussain, Z.; Khan, J. A.; Arshad, A.; Asif, P.; Rashid, H.; Arshad, M. I. Protective Effects of *Cinnamomum zeylanicum* L.(Darchini) in Acetaminophen-Induced Oxidative Stress, Hepatotoxicity and Nephrotoxicity in Mouse Model. *Biomed. Pharmacother.* **2019,** *109*, 2285–2292.

IM, K. K.; Issac, A.; Ninan, E.; Kuttan, R.; Maliakel, B. Enhanced Anti-Diabetic Activity of Polyphenol-Rich De-Coumarinated Extracts of *Cinnamomum cassia. J. Funct. Foods* **2014,** *10*, 54–64.

Iqbal, S.; Jabeen, F.; Peng, C.; Ijaz, M. U.; Chaudhry, A. S. *Cinnamomum cassia* Ameliorates Ni-NPs-Induced Liver and Kidney Damage in Male Sprague Dawley Rats. *Human Exp. Toxicol.* **2020,** *39*, 1565–1581.

Jafri, M. A.; Ansari, A. N.; Khalid, M.; Danishmand, A. T. Siman-e-Mufrit (Obesity)-A Modern Pandemic Controlled by Ancient Greeko-Arab Medicine. *Int. J. Health Sci. Res.* **2015,** *5*, 330–333.

Kabeeruddin, M. *Bayaz e Kabeer*, Vol II; Maktaba Al-Shifa, Kucha Chilan, Daryaganj: New Delhi, 2018; p 354.

Kadhem, M. Protective of Ethanolic Extract of *Saussurea lappa* Against Paracetamol-Induced Hepatic and Renal Damage in Male Rabbits. *Asian J. Pharma. Clin. Res.* **2019,** *12* (9), 68–73.

Kafi, M.; Kamili, A. N.; Husaini, A. M. et al. An Expensive Spice-Saffron (*Crocus sativus* L.) - Case Study from Kashmir, Iran and Turkey. In *Global Perspectives on Underutilized Crops*; Ozturk. M. et al., Eds., Chapter 4; Springer International Publishing AG, part of Springer Nature, 2018; pp 109–149.

Khan, H. M. A. *Muheet e Azam*, Vols. I, II and III; Central Council of Research in Unani Medicine: New Delhi, **2012.**

Khan, S. J.; Afroz, S.; Khan, R. A. Antihyperlipidemic and Anti-Hyperglycemic Effects of *Cymbopogon jwarancusa* in High-Fat High-Sugar Diet Model. *Pak. J. Pharma. Sci.* **2018,** *31*, 1341–1345.

Kim, B.; Park, B. Saffron Carotenoids Inhibit STAT3 Activation and Promote Apoptotic Progression in IL-6-Stimulated Liver Cancer Cells. *Oncol. Rep.* **2018,** *39* (4), 1883–1891.

Kunnumakkara, A. B.; Banik, K.; Bordoloi, D.; Harsha, C.; Sailo, B. L.; Padmavathi, G.; Roy, N. K.; Gupta, S. C.; Aggarwal, B. B. Googling the Guggul (*Commiphora* and *Boswellia*) for Prevention of Chronic Diseases. *Front. Pharmacol.* **2018,** *9*, 686.

Leeman-Neill, R. J.; Wheeler, S. E.; Singh, S. V.; Thomas, S. M.; Seethala, R. R.; Neill, D. B.; Panahandeh, M. C.; Hahm, E. R.; Joyce, S. C.; Sen, M.; Cai, Q. Guggulsterone Enhances Head and Neck Cancer Therapies Via Inhibition of Signal Transducer and Activator of Transcription-3. *Carcinogenesis* **2009,** *30*, 1848–1856.

Liao, J. C.; Deng, J. S.; Chiu, C. S.; Hou, W. C.; Huang, S. S.; Shie, P. H.; Huang, G. J. Anti-Inflammatory Activities of *Cinnamomum cassia* Constituents In Vitro and In Vivo. *Evid. Based Complement. Altern. Med.* **2012.**

Lin, X.; Peng, Z.; Fu, X.; Liu, C.; Xu, Y.; Ji, W.; Fan, J.; Chen, L.; Fang, L.; Huang, Y; Su, C. Volatile oil from *Saussurea lappa* Exerts Antitumor Efficacy by Inhibiting Epithelial Growth Factor Receptor Tyrosine Kinase-Mediated Signaling Pathway in Hepatocellular Carcinoma. *Oncotarget* **2016,** *7*, 79761–79773.

Madhuri, K.; Elango, K.; Ponnusankar, S. *Saussurea lappa* (Kuth Root): Review of Its Traditional Uses, Phytochemistry and Pharmacology. *Orient. Pharma. Exp. Med.* **2012,** *12*, 1–9.

Moon, D. O.; Park, S. Y.; Choi, Y. H.; Ahn, J. S.; Kim, G. Y. Guggulsterone Sensitizes Hepatoma Cells to TRAIL-Induced Apoptosis Through the Induction of CHOP-Dependent DR5: Involvement of ROS-Dependent ER-Stress. *Biochem. Pharmacol.* **2011,** *82*, 1641–1650.

Moossavi, M.; Hoshyar, R.; Hemmati, M.; Farahi, A.; Javdani, H. An In Vivo Study on the Hepato-Protective Effects of *Crocus sativus, Ziziphus jujuba* and *Berberis vulgar*is Against Acute Acetaminophen and Rifampicin-Induced Hepatotoxicity. *Clin. Phytosci.* **2016,** *2*, 16.

Muhammad, D. R. A.; Dewettinck, K. Cinnamon and Its Derivatives as Potential Ingredient in Functional Food—A Review. *Int. J. Food Prop.* **2017,** *20*, 2237–2263.

Naaz, F.; Ahmed, S. Integration of Unani Medicine in Cancer Management. *World J. Pharma. Res.* **2017,** *6*, 450–461.

Ng, L. T.; Wu, S. J. Antiproliferative Activity of *Cinnamomum cassia* Constituents and Effects of Pifithrin-Alpha on Their Apoptotic Signaling Pathways in Hep G2 Cells. *Evid. Based Complement. Altern. Med.* **2011.**

Noureini, S. K.; Wink, M. Antiproliferative Effects of Crocin in HepG2 Cells by Telomerase Inhibition and hTERT Down-Regulation. *Asian Pac. J. Cancer Prev.* **2012,** *13*, 2305–2309.

Pandey, M. M.; Rastogi, S.; Rawat, A. K. S. Saussurea Costus: Botanical, Chemical and Pharmacological Review of an Ayurvedic Medicinal Plant. *J. Ethnopharmacol.* **2007,** *110*, 379–390.

Poma, A.; Fontecchio, G.; Carlucci, G.; Chichiricco, G. Anti-Inflammatory Properties of Drugs from Saffron Crocus. *Anti-Inflammatory Anti-Allergy Agents Med. Chem.* **2012,** *11*, 37–51.

Prasad, C.; Singh, D.; Shukla, O. Antioxidant Activity and Trace Elements Profile of Extracts of *Cymbopogon jwarancusa* (Jones.) leaves. *J. Pharmacogn. Phytochem.* **2013,** *2*, 33–37.

Rahman, S. Z. Impact of Human Medicines on Environment–A New Emerging Problem. *Population Envis.* **2006,** *3*, 3–4.

Rahman, S. Z.; Khan, R. A.; Latif, A. Importance of Pharmacovigilance in Unani System of Medicine. *Indian J. Pharmacol.* **2008,** 40, S17- S20.

Ranasinghe, P.; Pigera, S.; Premakumara, G. S.; Galappaththy, P.; Constantine, G. R.; Katulanda, P. Medicinal properties of 'true'cinnamon (*Cinnamomum zeylanicum*): a systematic review. *BMC Complementary and Alternative Medicine* **2013,** *13*, 275.

Rao, P. V.; Gan, S. H. Cinnamon: A Multifaceted Medicinal Plant. *Evid. Based Complement. Altern. Med.* **2014**.

Samarghandian, S.; Asadi-Samani, M.; Farkhondeh, T.; Bahmani, M. Assessment the Effect of Saffron Ethanolic Extract (*Crocus sativus* L.) on Oxidative Damages in Aged Male Rat Liver. *Der Pharmacia Lettre* **2016,** *8*, 283–290.

Sarup, P.; Bala, S.; Kamboj, S. Pharmacology and Phytochemistry of Oleo-Gum Resin of Commiphora wightii (Guggulu). *Scientifica* **2015**.

Sarwat, M.; Sumaiya, S. *Saffron The Age-Old Panacea in a New Light*; Academia Press, 2020.

Sathya, M.; Rajeshwari, V.; Sakthishree, K. Influence of Aqueous Extract of *Cinnamomum zeylanicum* on the Progression of Cancer in Diethylnitrosamine Induced Rat Liver. *Eur. J. Exp. Biol.* **2014,** *4*, 190–195.

Shafiq, A.; Kanwal, R.; Ullah Qureshi, R.; Riaz Chaudhry, F. In Vitro Screening of *Cymbopogon jwarancusa* and *Conyza canadensis* Against Liver Flukes. *Trop. Biomed.* **2015,** *32*, 407–412.

Shakeel, M.; Jabeen, F.; Iqbal, R.; Chaudhry, A. S.; Zafar, S.; Ali, M.; Khan, M. S.; Khalid, A.; Shabbir, S; Asghar, M. S. Assessment of Titanium Dioxide Nanoparticles (TiO_2-NPs) Induced Hepatotoxicity and Ameliorative Effects of Cinnamomum Cassia in Sprague-Dawley Rats. *Biol. Trace Element Res.* **2018,** *182*, 57–69.

Shakya, A. K.; Shukla, S. Evaluation of Hepatoprotective Efficacy of Majoon-e-Dabeed-ul-Ward Against Acetaminophen-Induced Liver Damage: A Unani Herbal Formulation. *Drug Dev. Res.* **2011,** *72*, 346–352.

Shati, A. A.; Alkahtani, M. A.; Alfaifi, M. Y.; Elbehairi, S. E. I.; Elsaid, F. G.; Prasanna, R.; Mir, M. A. Secondary Metabolites of *Saussurea costus* Leaf Extract Induce Apoptosis in Breast, Liver, and Colon Cancer Cells by Caspase-3-Dependent Intrinsic Pathway. *BioMed. Res. Int.* 2020.

Shi, J. J.; Jia, X. L.; Li, M.; Yang, N.; Li, Y. P.; Zhang, X.; Gao, N.; Dang, S. S. Guggulsterone Induces Apoptosis of Human Hepatocellular Carcinoma Cells Through Intrinsic Mitochondrial Pathway. *World J. Gastroenterol.* **2015,** *21*, 13277–13287.

Shishodia, S.; Harikumar, K. B.; Dass, S.; Ramawat, K. G.; Aggarwal, B. B. The Guggul for Chronic Diseases: Ancient Medicine, Modern Targets. *Anticancer Res.* **2008,** *28*, 3647–3664.

Sumaiya, S.; Naved, T.; Sharma, A.; Sarwat, M. Amelioration of Liver Ailments by Saffron (*Crocus sativus*) and Its Secondary Metabolites. In *Saffron*; Academic Press, 2020; pp 1–20.

Tian, X.; Song, H. S.; Cho, Y. M.; Park, B.; Song, Y. J.; Jang, S.; Kang, S. C. Anticancer Effect of *Saussurea lappa* Extract Via Dual Control of Apoptosis and Autophagy in Prostate Cancer Cells. *Medicine* **2017,** *96*.

Vani, P.; Sreekanth, D.; Manjula, P.; Keerthi, B.; Kistamma, S.; Mohan, B.; Reddy, A. N; Mohan, C. H. Phytochemical Investigation, Antibacterial Activity and Antioxidant Activity of the Endangered Tree *Commiphora wightii* (Arn.) Bhandari. *J. Pharmacogn. Phytochem.* **2016,** *5*, 21–25.

Varalakshmi, B.; Anand, A. V.; Karpagam, T.; Bai, J. S.; Manikandan, R. In Vitro Antimicrobial and Anticancer Activity of *Cinnamomum zeylanicum* Linn Bark Extracts. *Int. J. Pharma. Pharma. Sci.* **2014,** *6*, 12–18.

Xu, H. B.; Fu, J.; Huang, F.; Yu, J. Guggulsterone Sensitized Drug-Resistant Human Hepatocarcinoma Cells to Doxorubicin Through a Cox-2/P-gp Dependent Pathway. *Eur. J. Pharmacol.* **2017,** *803*, 57–64.

Yaeesh, S.; Jamal, Q.; Shah, A. J.; Gilani, A. H. Antihepatotoxic Activity of *Saussurea lappa* Extract on D-Galactosamine and Lipopolysaccharide-Induced Hepatitis in Mice. *Phytother. Res.* **2010,** *24*, S229–S232.

Yan, Y. M.; Fang, P.; Yang, M. T.; Li, N.; Lu, Q.; Cheng, Y. X. Anti-Diabetic Nephropathy Compounds from *Cinnamomum cassia*. *J. Ethnopharmacol.* **2015,** *165*, 141–147.

Yaribeygi, H.; Mohammadi, M. T.; Sahebkar, A. Crocin Potentiates Antioxidant Defense System and Improves Oxidative Damage in Liver Tissue in Diabetic Rats. *Biomed. Pharmacother.* **2018,** *98*, 333–337.

You, H. N.; Park, M. H.; Hwang, S. Y.; Han, J. S. *Nardostachys jatamansi* DC Extract Alleviates Insulin Resistance and Regulates Glucose Metabolism in C57BL/KsJ-db/db Mice Through the AMP-Activated Protein Kinase Signaling Pathway. *J. Med. Food* **2018,** *21*, 324–331.

Zahara, K.; Tabassum, S.; Sabir, S.; Arshad, M.; Qureshi, R.; Amjad, M. S.; Chaudhari, S. K. A Review of Therapeutic Potential of *Saussurea lappa*-An Endangered Plant from Himalaya. *Asian Pac. J. Trop. Med.* **2014,** *7*, S60–S69.

Zhang, J. H.; Shangguan, Z. S.; Chen, C.; Zhang, H. J.; Lin, Y. Anti-Inflammatory Effects of Guggulsterone on Murine Macrophage by Inhibiting LPS-Induced Inflammatory Cytokines in NF-κB Signaling Pathway. *Drug Design Dev. Therap.* **2016,** *10*, 1829.

Zhang, C.; Fan, L.; Fan, S.; Wang, J.; Luo, T.; Tang, Y.; Chen, Z.; Yu, L. *Cinnamomum cassia* Presl: A Review of Its Traditional Uses, Phytochemistry, Pharmacology and Toxicology. *Molecules* **2019,** *24*, 3473.

CHAPTER 17

Herbal Medicines for the Treatment of Neurodegenerative Disorders

SHRUTI TYAGI[1], RAJENDRA AWASTHI[2], NEERUPMA DHIMAN[1], BHUPESH SHARMA[1], and GIRIRAJ T. KULKARNI[3]

[1]*Department of Pharmaceutics, Amity Institute of Pharmacy, Amity University Uttar Pradesh, Noida, Uttar Pradesh, India*

[2]*Department of Pharmaceutical Sciences, School of Health Sciences & Technology, University of Petroleum and Energy Studies (UPES), Dehradun, Uttarakhand, India*

[3]*Gokaraju Rangaraju College of Pharmacy, Hyderabad, Telangana, India*

ABSTRACT

Synthetic drugs prescribed to treat mental disorders can produce euphoric effects. These drugs also damage neurons due to the seizures, stroke, and direct toxic effects on brain cells. Repeated drug use may lead to the brain disorders due to the change in function of multiple brain circuits controlling decision-making power, impulse control, pleasures, memory, learning, and other activities. This makes harder for the individual with an addiction to experience the pleasure in response to natural phenomenon, such as, sex, positive social interactions, etc. Hence, over the past two to three decades, herbal therapeutics are encouraged over synthetic medicines. This article highlights various neurodegenerative disorders, current therapies, and their limitations. Special emphasis has been given to use of herbal medicines,

Ethnic Knowledge and Perspectives of Medicinal Plants, Volume 1: Curative Properties and Treatment Strategies. Munir Ozturk, Kandikere R. Sridhar, Maryam Sarwat, Volkan Altay, & Francisco Martín Huerta-Martínez (Eds.)

which can overcome the drawbacks associated with synthetic drugs, in the management of neurodegenerative disorders.

17.1 INTRODUCTION

Neurodegenerative disorders lead to progressive neurodegeneration and brain damage. Neurons are the building blocks of central nervous system (CNS), which has less or no tendency to regrow or renew. Hence, the damaged neurons show several CNS-related adverse effects. Neurodegenerative disorder is an umbrella term that includes Parkinson's disease (PD) and PD-related disorders, Alzheimer's disease (AD), and other dementias like, Attention deficit hyperactivity disorder (ADHD) and Huntington's disease. AD-related dementias are responsible for the greatest burden of neurodegenerative diseases, which is identified as a major crusade of morbidity worldwide.

Since 1992, every year October 10th has been observed as world mental health day to create global mental health awareness. WHO estimated depression as a second leading cause of morbidity worldwide by 2020, followed by cardiac diseases (Perry and Howes, 2011). India is, unfortunately, the leading country in adolescent and young age suicides due to the mental health issues caused by poor socio-economy, substance abuse, gender inequality, and poor health infrastructure. Unfortunately, India has less than four thousand psychiatrists for more than a billion population. A stigma of mental illness in the society is biggest barriers for mental treatment. Because of the stigma, people do not prefer going to a mental health professional for an early-stage evaluation (Perry and Howes, 2011).

17.2 COMMON BRAIN DISORDERS

Mental disorders not only include insanity, or depression, but it also includes emotional disorders. The human brain acts as a factory, which receives and generates chemical impulses known as messages. The nerve cells have special functions like learning, thinking, remembering, and hearing. Brain cells are also involved in the processing and storage of information to communicate with other cells. To continue this process, the brain requires a large amount of energy and oxygen. Deficiency of energy and oxygen may lead to the neurodegenerative disorders like AD, PD, HD, etc. In this section, a brief description has been appended to explore the basic information and understanding of common brain disorders (Hassan et al., 2014).

17.2.1 ALZHEIMER'S DISEASE (AD)

AD was originally defined as dementia. This implies an acquired mental disorder with loss of intellectual abilities to interfere with social or occupational functioning. It is associated with localized loss of neurons and shrinkage of basal forebrain and hippocampus. Beta-amyloid peptide is associated with the development of AD. Although there is no cure for AD with synthetic drugs, but to a certain level, it can be controlled with beta-amyloid peptide. It has been reported that the natural antioxidants, such as vitamin C, vitamin E, and β-carotene are useful in the cleaning of free radicals generated during the disease progression. The memory loss is resulted due to the shortage of acetylcholine. The level of this transmitter in the brain can be increased by inhibiting activity of acetyl cholinesterase enzyme (which split or break down the transmitter substance). Synthetic drugs which inhibit the breakdown of acetylcholine may delay the disease progression (Perry and Howes, 2011; Hassan et al., 2014; Yiannopoulou and Papageorgiou, 2013).

17.2.2 HUNTINGTON'S DISEASE

Huntington's disease was first explained in the 19th century by American physician George Huntington. It is caused by an inherited defect in a single gene. The onset of disease symptoms can begin at any age, however, mostly it starts from 34 to 45 years of age. Various causative factors of this disease have been described. However, the exact mechanism of disease is still need to be explored. There is no cure for HD, although the treatments to relieve some of the symptoms are available. The characteristic disease symptoms are random, jerky, and chorea. Rigidity and dystonia become apparent with the disease progression, which results in the dominant physical symptoms (Frank, 2014; Finkbeiner, 2011).

17.2.3 PARKINSON'S DISEASE (PD)

It is a progressive disorder of movement showing continuous shivering, mainly in older people. It is related to the dementia with common indications like tremor at rest usually starting in the hands. The muscle rigidity can be noticed as an increased resistance in passive limb movement and hypo kinesis suppression of voluntary muscles. In PD, the levels of dopamine, 5-hydroxyl tryptamine, acetylcholine, and norepinephrine tend to decrease in the substantia nigra and the carpus striatum of the brain. A short relief is possible with synthetic drugs, but complete cure is difficult (Jankovic and Aguilar, 2008; Rios et al., 2016).

17.2.4 *ATTENTION DEFICIT HYPERACTIVITY DISORDER (ADHD)*

ADHD is considered as a disorder of children. However, it is not limited to children only. In ADHD patients, the brain neurotransmitters controlling attention are less active. The cause of such chemical imbalance is not as yet well understood. However, it has been suggested that a gene may be responsible as the disorder often runs in families. It has been observed that the adults given stimulants have fewer ADHD symptoms and some of them may feel better concentration, but complete cure is often not realized (De Sousa and Kalra, 2012; Curatolo et al., 2010).

17.3 CURRENT THERAPIES TOWARD NEURODEGENERATIVE DISORDERS

Donepezil (Aricept) is approved to treat all stages of AD, rivastigmine (Exelon) is approved to treat mild to moderate AD, and galantamine (Razadyne) is approved to treat mild to moderate AD (Yiannopoulou and Papageorgiou, 2013). Other than the drugs, novel therapies such as targeting the excitotoxicity and misfolding protein aggregations, targeting the mitochondrial dysfunction and related pathways, targeting neuro-inflammation using drugs like minocycline and use of orally bioavailable compounds such as tetra peptide (PO21), etc. have also been reported (Van Bulck et al., 2019). Symptomatic as well as disease-modifying therapies have been also employed to treat AD (Cummings et al., 2019).

Drugs affecting brain dopaminergic system (antiparkinsons drugs) are levodopa (l-dopa), carbidopa, benserazide, bromocriptine, selegiline, rasagiline, entacapone, tolcapone, amantadine, etc. (Jankovic and Aguilar, 2008). Novel approaches used to treat PD are targeting α-synuclein aggregation, targeting mitochondrial dysfunction and oxidative stress, targeting autophagy, targeting intracellular calcium ions homeostasis alteration, targeting metal ions homeostasis alteration, etc. (Van Bulck et al., 2019). Stimulant medications commonly prescribed for attention deficit disorder include methylphenidate (Ritalin, Concerta, Metadate, Methylin) and certain amphetamines (Dexedrine, Dextrostat, Adderall) (De Sousa and Kalra, 2012).

Xenazine (tetrabenazine) is the first medication approved by the United States Food and Drug Administration (US FDA) for HD, risperidone, haloperidol, and chlorpromazine are often used off-label to treat HD due to their chorea suppression effect (Frank, 2014). A study suggests that A 1 R, A 2A R-containing heteromers can also consider as targets for HD-related drug development (Blum et al., 2018). Cell replacement therapies are also investigated based on the potential of replacing medium spiny striatal neurons that degenerate during diseased condition (Kieburtz et al., 2018).

17.4 SIDE EFFECTS OF THE ALLOPATHIC TREATMENT

Most common adverse events associated with PD treatment using synthetic therapeutics are nausea, dyskinesia, somnolence, compulsive behaviors, psychosis, peripheral edema, melanoma, and weight loss (Chou, 2008). Gastrointestinal manifestations, bradycardia, syncope, agitation, MRI abnormalities compatible with edema and microhemorrhages especially in ε-4 carriers, vasogenic edema, and arrhythmia association of drugs with non-melanoma skin cancer, altered levels of hepatic enzymes, and reduction of immunoglobulins have been also reported adverse effects associated with AD treatment using synthetic drugs. Cerebral microbleeds and vasogenic edema were other serious occurrences along with serious hepatotoxicity (Stella et al., 2015).

Adverse events associated with HD treatment are depression, drowsiness, tachycardia, hypotension, hypertension, extrapyramidal symptoms, withdrawal emergent neurological syndrome, tardive syndromes, insomnia, restlessness, anxiety, agitation, confusion, lactation, gynecomastia, impotence, dry mouth, blurred vision, urinary retention, parkinsonism, gastrointestinal distress, neuroleptic malignant syndrome, sedation, tardive dyskinesia, visual disturbances, tachycardia, elevated liver enzymes, and weight gain (Videnovic, 2013). The most common adverse effects of ADHD therapy are anorexia, nausea, abdominal pain, sleep disturbances, decreased appetite, weight loss, and irritability (De Sousa and Kalra, 2012).

17.5 TRADITIONAL APPROACHES FOR THE TREATMENT OF NEURODEGENERATIVE DISORDERS

Synthetic drugs currently used for the treatment of neurodegenerative disorders cause many side effects as well as adverse effects on human health.

To overcome these limitations, scientists are investigating new frontier to treat such disorders using traditional systems of medicine such as Ayurveda, Unani, and Siddha. The popularity of Chinese medicines is increasing day-by-day. Herbal remedies are considered to be safe and are routinely used worldwide since ancient times for the treatment of several disorders. Herbal treatment considers the whole human body as a single system. Unlike Allopathy system, traditional system aims for highest therapeutic responses with minimum or nil side effects. Ayurvedic medicines have quite complex formula with thirty or more ingredients, including a sizable number of ingredients that have undergone "alchemical processing," chosen to balance Vata, Pitta, or Kapha. Several disorders, such as convulsions, lockjaw, shaking palsy, paralysis, etc. due to the imbalance of Vata may cause neurodegenerative diseases. Vataraktha Chikitsa, a classical literature of Ayurveda, shows that the complex disorders affecting nervous system originate from an imbalance of Vata (Joy, 2016). Oxygen is the mediator of electron - transport mechanism. A dysfunction in the electron-transport mechanism can cause disrupted homeostatic regulation. A large number of experimental and clinical studies reported major disruption in homeostatic regulation in neurodegenerative conditions. Respiratory chain deficits, mitochondria dysfunction, exacerbated reactive oxygen species production, low hemoglobin levels, deficiency in the terminal complex of the mitochondrial electron transport chain-cytochrome C oxidase (COX), defects in oxidative phosphorylation (Oxphos) have been observed in the pathophysiology of neurodegenerative conditions (Joy, 2015).

17.5.1 HERBS DESCRIBED IN TRADITIONAL MEDICINE FOR NEURODEGENERATIVE DISORDERS

Use of hundreds of plants individually or in combination for the treatment of brain-related disorders is encouraged by the traditional system of medicine. Herbal therapeutics presents a new frontier for the successful treatment of neurodegenerative disorder. Most of the prescriptions include more than one plant part which supports the synergistic approach of Ayurvedic drugs. Herbal medicines have the potential to cure most of the mental diseases except genetically rooted brain disorders. Examples of the plants used for the treatment of neurodegenerative disorders are presented in Table 17.1.

TABLE 17.1 Plants Used for the Treatment of Neurodegenerative Disorders.

Common name	Biological name/ family	Part used	Active constituents	Therapeutic applications	References
Prickly chaff flower	*Achyranthes aspera*/ Amaranthaceae	Leaves, seeds, and whole plant juice	Oleanolic acid glycosides, amino acids, terpenoids, saponins, betains, and achyranthins	The seed powder of this plant provides relief from stiffness and headache, and can be used to treat the symptoms of AD	Fahey (2005)
Malabar nut	*Justicia adhatoda, Adhatoda vasica*/ Acanthaceae	Leaves and whole plant	Vasicine, vasicinone	The extract of this plant is used to treat loss of memory, tumors, and some of the symptoms of AD and PD	Claeson et al. (2000); Ali et al. (2013); Rasool et al. (2014)
Brahmi	*Bacopa monnier*/ Plantaginaceae	Costuss-peciosus root	Bacosides A, B, C	The extract is used to treat loss of memory, AD, PD, HD and ADHD	Hassan et al. (2014); Jansen et al. (2014); Rao et al. (2012); Jadiya et al. (2011); Choudhary et al. (2013); Ahn et al. (2016); Akram and Nawaz (2017); Singhal et al. (2012)
Bhang	*Cannabis sativa*/ Cannabinaceae	Leaves	Tetrahydro cannabinoids	The bhang extract is used to treat sleeplessness, AD, HD, PD, and ADHD	Aso and Ferrer (2016); Sagredo et al. (2012); Bassi et al. (2017); Kelly et al. (2017)
Shankh-pushpi	*Convolvulus microphyllus*/ Convolvulaceae	Acorus calamus roots	Convoline, convolamine	The root powder is recommended to improve the memory power and treat AD	Hassan et al. (2014); Rao et al. (2012)
Banyan tree	*Ficus benghalensis*/ Moraceae	Root bark, leaves	Bengalenosides, leuco pelargonidin glycoside	The root bark powder with sugar and cow's milk improves memory power and used to treat AD and PD	Panday and Rauniar (2016); Bhangale and Acharya (2016)

TABLE 17.1 *(Continued)*

Common name	Biological name/ family	Part used	Active constituents	Therapeutic applications	References
Kapikachhu	*Mucuna pruriens*/ Fabaceae	Seeds	L- Dopa, amines, alkaloids	The powder of the seeds of this plant tends to treat PD	Jansen et al. (2014); Vaidya and Devasagayam (2007); Lampariello et al. (2012)
Ginkgo-silver apricot (Chinese Medicines)	*Ginkgo biloba*/ Ginkoaceae	Leaves and seeds	Flavanoids, terpenic lactones, ginkgolides A, B, C, J, and M	Powdered extract is used to treat cognitive dysfunction, dementias, AD, HD, PD, and ADHD	Hassan et al. (2014); Rasool et al. (2014); Choudhary et al. (2013); Ahn et al. (2016); Akram and Nawaz (2017); Singhal et al. (2012); Janssen et al. (2010); Salehi et al. (2010); Tanaka et al. (2013)
Ginseng (Chinese medicines)	*Panax ginseng*/ Araliaceae	Aerial parts and roots	Ginsenosides (Rb1group and Rg1group)	It is widely used as an immunomodulator, memory enhancer and to treat stress, trauma, anxiety, PD, HD, and ADHD	Rasool et al. (2014); Choudhary et al. (2013); Ahn et al. (2016); Akram and Nawaz (2017); Singhal et al. (2012); Van Kampen et al. (2014); Cho (2012)
Drumstick tree	*Moringa oleifera*/ Moringaceae	Seed oil	Proteins, vitamin A, minerals, essential amino acids, antioxidants, flavonoids and isothiocyanates	The oil extract of this tree acts as anti-inflammatory, antioxidant, and neuro-protective agent. It is used to treat HD, PD, AD, and ADHD	Akram and Nawaz (2017); Kou et al. (2018); Vergara-Jimenez et al. (2017); Jaafaru et al. (2018); Sutalangka et al. (2013)
Ashwa-gandha	*Withania somnifera*/ Solanaceae	Long brown tuberous roots	Alkaloids, steroidal lactones, tropine, and cuscohygrine	Used to treat stress, anxiety, PD, HD, AD, and ADHD	Hassan et al. (2014); Jansen et al. (2014); Rao et al. (2012); Choudhary et al. (2013); Akram and Nawaz (2017); Singhal et al. (2012); Sehgal et al. (2012);

TABLE 17.1 *(Continued)*

Common name	Biological name/ family	Part used	Active constituents	Therapeutic applications	References
					Singhal et al. (2010); Ahmad et al. (2005); Kumar and Kumar (2009); Andrade (1996)
Pennywort	*Centella asiatica*/ Apiaceae	Roots and leaves	Asiaticosides, brahmosides, brahminosides and centellosides	Extracts of this plant are used to treat anxiety PD, AD, and HD	Hassan et al. (2014); Jansen et al. (2014); Rao et al. (2012); Choudhary et al. (2013); Singhal et al. (2012); Andrade (1996)
Country mallow	*Sida cordifolia*/ Malvaceae	Whole plant	Alkaloids- β-phenethylamine, ephedrine, pseudo-ephedrine, S-(+)-Nb-methyltryptophan methyl ester, hypaphorine, vasicinone, vasicinol, choline, and betaine	The whole plant extracts used to treat PD	Jansen et al. (2014); Khurana and Gajbhiye (2013)
Kava	*Piper methysticum*/ Piperaceae	Leaves and roots	Kavalactones - kavain, dihydrokavain, methysticin, dihydromethysticin, yangonin, and desmethoxyyangonin, flavokavain A, flavokavain B, and flavokavain C	Used to treat HD, AD, PD and ADHD	Sarris et al. (2011); Tzeng and Lee (2015); Tanaka et al. (2010)

TABLE 17.1 *(Continued)*

Common name	Biological name/ family	Part used	Active constituents	Therapeutic applications	References
Turmeric	*Curcuma longa*/ Zingiberaceae	Rhizome and root	Diarylheptanoids, curcuminoids such as curcumin, demethoxycurcumin and bisdemethoxycurcumin	Curcuminoids tend to inhibit the MAO type A receptor and is used for the treatment of AD, PD, HD	Hassan et al. (2014); Rao et al. (2012); Choudhary et al. (2013); Akram and Nawaz (2017); Singhal et al. (2012); Mythri and Bharath (2012)
Intellect tree	*Celastrus paniculatus*/ Celastraceae	Seeds	Steroid, terpenoid, carbohydrate, alkaloid, saponin, and phenolic compounds	Powdered seeds show cognition-enhancing and antioxidant properties and protects neuronal cells against glutamate-induced toxicity via modulating glutamate receptor function. It is used to treat AD, HD and PD.	Hassan et al. (2014); Rao et al. (2012); Andrade (1996); Godkar et al. (2003); Malik et al. (2017)
Spikenard	*Nardostachys jatamansi*/ Caprifoliaceae	Rhizome and roots	Acaciin, ursolie acid, octacosanol, kanshone A, nardosinonediol, nardosinone, aristolen-9beta-ol, oleanolic acid, beta-sitosterol, spirojatamol, nardostachysin, jatamols A and B, and calarenol	Treat dementia, loss of memory, AD and PD	Joy (2015); Andrade (1996); Ahmad et al. (2006)

TABLE 17.1 *(Continued)*

Common name	Biological name/ family	Part used	Active constituents	Therapeutic applications	References
Gugglu	*Commiphora mukul, C. molmol, C. whighitii*/ Burseraceae	Resins from barks	Commiphoric acids, commiphorinic acid, heerabomyrrhols, terpenes, sesquiterpenoids, cuminic aldehyde, eugenol, and the ketone steroids Z-and E-guggulsterone, and guggulsterols I, II, and III	Lowers serum LDL cholesterol and triglyceride levels. It shows antioxidant, antiacetylcholine esterase activity and is used in the treatment of AD	Hassan et al. (2014); Joy (2015); Akram and Nawaz (2017); Singhal et al. (2012)
Sweet flag	*Acorus calamus*/ Acoraceae	Leaves, stems, and roots, rhizome	Alpha-asarone, Beta-abalone, eugenol	The ethanolic and hydroethanolic extracts are used in the treatment of memory loss, AD, and PD	Hassan et al. (2014); Singhal et al. (2012); Andrade (1996)
Brazil nut	*Bertholletia excels*/ Lecythidaceae	Nut oil	Lecithin, choline	Enhance acethylcholine concentration in the brain, used to treat AD	Hassan et al. (2014); Singhal et al. (2012); Stockler-Pinto et al. (2014)
Blue pea	*Clitoria ternatea*/ Leguminosae	Rhizome	Triterpenoids, flavonol glycosides, anthocyanins, steroids, cliotides	Enhance acethylcholinein concentration in brain and act as nootropic, anxiolytic, antidepressant, anticonvulsant and antistress agent, used to treat AD and PD	Hassan et al. (2014); Margret et al. (2015); Talpate et al. (2014); Jain et al. (2003)

TABLE 17.1 *(Continued)*

Common name	Biological name/ family	Part used	Active constituents	Therapeutic applications	References
Saffron crocus	*Crocus sativus*/ Iridaceae	Pistils	Crocin	Crocin tends to inhibit fibrillogenesis and show antioxidant effect, used in the treatment of AD and PD	Hassan et al. (2014); Akram and Nawaz (2017); Khazdair et al. (2015); Pitsikas (2015)
Liquorice	*Glycyrrhiza glabra*/Fabaceae	Root	Glycyrrhizin, isoflavene glabrene, isoflavane - glabridin, anethole	Act as neuroprotective agent; protect apoptotic neuronal cell death induced by Aβ fragments and used to treat AD, HD and PD	Hassan et al. (2014); Akram and Nawaz (2017); Singhal et al. (2012); Chakravarthi and Avadhani (2013); Hwang and Chun (2012); Michel et al. (2013)
Snowdrop	*Galanthus nivalis*/ Amaryllidaceae	Bulb	Galanthamine	A specific inhibitor of the acetylcholinesterase enzyme and to potentiate cholinergic nicotinic neurotransmission, hence used in the treatment of AD	Hassan et al. (2014); Singhal et al. (2012); Pinho et al. (2013)
Toothed clubmoss	*Huperzia serrata*/ Lycopodiaceae	Whole plant	Lycopodium alkaloids, acetylcholinesterase inhibitor huperzine A	Toothed clubmoss act as a selective acetylcholinesterase inhibitor. Huperzine-A reduces the abnormally high radical activity, can be used in the treatment of AD	Hassan et al. (2014); Singhal et al. (2012)
St. John's wort	*Hypericum perforatum*/ Hypericaceae	Dried crude herb	Hyperforin, hypericin	Hyperforin is an arachidonate 5-lipoxygenase inhibitor and COX-1 inhibitor, it improves memory and learning, hence it can treat AD	Hassan et al. (2014)

TABLE 17.1 *(Continued)*

Common name	Biological name/ family	Part used	Active constituents	Therapeutic applications	References
Giloy	*Tinospora cordifolia*/ Menispermaceae	Whole plant	Columbin, tinosporaside, jatrorhizine, palmatine, berberine, tembeterine, tinocordifolioside, phenylpropene disaccharides, choline, tinosporic acid, tinosporal, and tinosporon	Immunostimulant and increases the synthesis of acetylcholine, enhance cognitive function, hence can be used to treat AD	Hassan et al. (2014); Akram and Nawaz (2017); Singhal et al. (2012)
Nettle leaf	*Urtica dioica*/ Clusiaceae	Leaves	Alpha-linolenic acid, omega-3 acid, carotenoids	Elevate the mood in some Alzheimer's patients	Hassan et al. (2014); Singhal et al. (2012)
Magnolia bark	*Magnolia officinalis*/ Magnoliaceae	Bark	Magnolol and honokiol	Offers reduction of memory impairment and inhibits the acetyl cholinesterase enzyme activity, hence used to treat AD	Hassan et al. (2014); Akram and Nawaz (2017); Singhal et al. (2012)
Maca	*Lipidium meyenii*/ Brassicaceae	Root	Glucotropaeolin, m-methoxyglucotropaeolin, benzyl glucosinolates, polyphenols, (1R,3S)-1-methyl-1,2,3,4-tetrahydro-β-carboline-3-carboxylic acid, and p-methoxybenzyl isothiocyanate	Offers reduction of memory impairment and inhibits the acetyl cholinesterase enzyme activity, hence used to treat AD	Hassan et al. (2014); Akram and Nawaz (2017); Singhal et al. (2012)

TABLE 17.1 *(Continued)*

Common name	Biological name/ family	Part used	Active constituents	Therapeutic applications	References
Passion flower	*Passiflora incarnate*/ Passifloraceae	Root and leaves	Beta-carboline harmala alkaloids, harman, harmaline, harmalol, harmine, and harmol	Improves the symptoms of ADHD	Ahn et al. (2016)
Valerian	*Valeriana officinalis*/ Caprifoliaceae	Root	Actinidine, chatinine, shyanthine, valerianin E, and valerine	Improve the symptoms of ADHD, enhance the cognition in various animal models, enhance dopamine postsynaptic receptor functioning etc., hence, to treat AD, ADHD and PD.	Ahn et al. (2016); Andrade (1996)
Common fig	*Ficus carica*/ Moraceae	Figs	Gallic acid, chlorogenic acid, syringic acid, (+)-catechin, (−)-epicatechin, and rutin	The figs of this plant at lower doses exhibit mild memory enhancing effect and at higher doses it evokes better learning ability and alter behavior, hence used to treat AD	Akram and Nawaz (2017)
Chinese parsley	*Coriandrum sativum*/Apiaceae	Fresh leaves and the dried seeds	Vitamin A, vitamin C, and vitamin K	The seeds and leaves of this plant offer memory enhancing effects. Due to its antioxidant, anti-inflammatory and cholesterol lowering activities, it can be used to treat AD and PD	Akram and Nawaz (2017)

TABLE 17.1 (*Continued*)

Common name	Biological name/ family	Part used	Active constituents	Therapeutic applications	References
Yerba mate	*Ilex paraguariensis*/ Aquifoliaceae	Leaves	It contains vitamin B12, B1 and C	The leaves of the plant improves short and long term memory and treat vascular dementia, which improves memory, hence can be used in the treatment of neurodegenerative disorders	Akram and Nawaz (2017)
Amla	*Emblica officinalis*/ Euphorbiaceae	Fruit	Ascorbic acid, emblicanin A, emblicanin B, punigluconin and pedunculagin	The whole fruit tends to decrease Oxidative stress and enhanced memory; hence it is used in the treatment of AD.	Akram and Nawaz (2017)
Ginger	*Zingiber officinale*/ Zingiberaccae	Rhizome	Zingerone, shogaols https://en.wikipedia.org/wiki/ Shogaoland gingerols	The rhizome of ginger being antioxidant and memory enhancer in nature is used to treat AD and PD	Akram and Nawaz (2017); Andrade (1996)
Pomegranate	*Punica granatum*/ Punicaceae	Flower	Corilagin, granatin, punicacortein A, pedunculagin and punicafolin	Powdered flowers tend to decrease oxidative stress and increases learning power, hence can be used to treat AD	Akram and Nawaz (2017)
Velvet leaf	*Cissampelo spareira*/ Menispermaceae	Leaves	Flavonoids, alkaloids, tannins, volatile oils, glycosides	The leaf extract shows the nootropic effect by decreasing the activity of acetylcholinesterase enzyme so used to treat AD	Akram and Nawaz (2017); Arora et al. (2012)

TABLE 17.1 *(Continued)*

Common name	Biological name/ family	Part used	Active constituents	Therapeutic applications	References
Lemon balm	*Mellisa officinalis*/ Lamiaceae	Leaves	Rosmarinic acid	Lemon balm leaves act as anxiolytic, anti-inflammatory and antidepressant agent, it is also used to treat AD	Akram and Nawaz (2017); Singhal et al. (2012)
Common sage	*Salvia officinalis*/ Lamiaceae	Leaves	Camphor, α-thujone, 1,8-cineole, viridiflorol, β-thujone and β-caryophyllene	The leaf extract serves as a memory enhancer via interacting with the muscarinic and cholinergic pathways. It is used to treat AD.	Akram and Nawaz (2017); Singhal et al. (2012); Khedher et al. (2017)
Nutmeg	*Myristica fragrans*/ Myristicaceae	Seed	Camphene, b-pinene, sabinene, cymene, garaniol, d-borneol, linolool, terpineol, safrol, elemicin, myristicins, phenylpropane derivatives, lauric acid, myristic acid, pentadecanoic acid, palmitic acid, heptadecanoic acid, stearic acid, oleic acid and b-sitosterol.	The powdered extract of seeds helps to manage the symptoms of AD and enhance memory	Akram and Nawaz (2017)
Early purple orchid	*Orchis mascula*/ Orchidaceae	Flower	Glucomannan	Enhance cognition which ultimately enhances dopamine levels, hence used to treat PD	Andrade (1996)

TABLE 17.1 *(Continued)*

Common name	Biological name/ family	Part used	Active constituents	Therapeutic applications	References
Clove	*Syzygium aromaticum*/ Myrtaceae	Fruit	Acetyl eugenol, beta-caryophyllene and vanillin, crategolic acid	Oily extracts elevate the cognition, increase dopamine postsynaptic receptor functioning, hence used to treat PD.	Andrade (1996)

Abbreviations: *AD, Alzheimer's disease; PD, Parkinson's disease; HD, Huntington's disease; and ADHD, Attention deficient hyperactivity disorder.

17.5.2 MECHANISM OF ACTION OF HERBAL MEDICATIONS

Herbal medicines tend to show specific as well as potent mechanism of actions. Most common mechanism of action of herbs is being antioxidant in nature. However, apart from the reducing oxidative stress in the brain, herbs also show various mechanisms to provide the particular therapeutic responses (Table 17.2).

17.5.3 ADVERSE EFFECTS OF HERBAL MEDICATIONS

Ayurveda is mainly connected with the cure accessible from nature and deals with the root cause of the disease and provides a permanent cure in most of the cases. Normally, a patient treated with Ayurvedic medicines, not only gets cured, but also achieve the permanent immunity. The main advantage that Ayurveda over Allopathy is that the former uses only natural means to cure a disease, and is the most eco-accommodating approach to get everlasting cure. It is well accepted that the Ayurveda not only treats a patient with mental diseases, but also increases the overall mental capability by strengthening immunity, thus keeping the mind and the body free from further damages. Ayurvedic medicines improve the concentration and other mental capabilities. Although herbal plants are known for their less or none side effects or adverse effects, but still some herbs may have certain life-threatening side effects which turn out to be adverse effects. Major adverse effects associated with herbal medications are presented in Table 17.3.

17.6 CONCLUSIONS

The principles of Allopathic and Ayurvedic systems of medicine are very different from each other. Allopathic drugs are prescribed on symptomatic principle, while Ayurvedic through the balance of three energies (vata, pita, and kapha) required for maintaining good health. However, it is well understood that in most of the cases, the synthetic drugs generally bring relief through a symptomatic treatment and hardly promise permanent cure. Since more than sixty million Indians are suffering from mental disorders and the country lags far behind the world for treatment and spending in the hospitals for mental cure, it is high time to look for the established alternative system of medicine. It has been estimated that nearly 1–2% Indian population is suffering from schizophrenia and bipolar disorder, whereas, 5% population

TABLE 17.2 Mechanism of Action of Herbal Medications.

Neurodegenerative disorders	Mechanism of action	Plant	References
Alzheimer's	Enhanced cholineacetyl transferase activity	Ashwagandha	Rao et al. (2012)
	Inhibition of lipid peroxidation	Curcumin	Butterfield et al. (2002)
	Antioxidant	Curcumin	Lim et al. (2001)
	Suppression of acetylcholinesterase activity	Brahmi	Limpeanchob et al. (2008)
	Inhibition of beta-amyloid cell death	Gotu kola	Dhanasekaran et al. (2009)
Parkinson's	Anti-inflammatory action by Inhibition of the production of IL-12p40	Grapes (resveratrol)	Renaud et al. (2014)
	Anti-inflammatory action by inhibition of NF-κB translocation	Ginseng	Liu et al. (2011)
	Antiapoptosis by reducing activity of caspase-3	Curcumin, Ginseng	Renaud et al. (2014)
	Antioxidant activity by activation of PPAR-γ, AMPK, and SIRT1 receptors	Valerian, grapes	Renaud et al. (2014)
Huntington's	Antioxidant activity by inactivation of succinate dehydrogenase	Brahmi	Coles et al. (1979)
	Anti-inflammatory action by inhibiting lymphocyte proliferation	Ashwagandha	Choudhary et al. (2013)
Attention deficient hyperactivity disorder	Neuroprotection by regulating dopamine levels and inhibiting the cholinesterase enzyme	Brahmi	Ahn et al. (2016)
	Reversal of 5-HT1 receptor, reverse the inhibition of MAO-A and MAO-B receptors	Ginko	Ahn et al. (2016)
	Enhanced dopamine and norepinephrine levels	Ginseng	Ahn et al. (2016)
	Inhibition of breakdown of GABA in CNS	Valerian	Ahn et al. (2016)

TABLE 17.3 Major Adverse Effects Associated with Herbal Medications.

Herbs/plants	Adverse effects	References
Hypericum perforatum (St. John's wort)	Due to its phototoxic, at high doses photodermatitis can occur. Human lens epithelial cells and retinal pigment epithelial cells can get damaged by exposure to a combination of hypericin and light in the visible or UV range. It can cause serotonin syndrome in sensitive patients and hair loss.	Parker et al. (2001)
Zingiber officinale (Ginger)	During pregnancy ginger can cause abortion as it acts as an anticoagulant. It can also cause co-morbidities, cardiac arrhythmias; it can lower blood sugar levels, duodenal ulcers and can enhance secretion of bile acids in the case of people with a history of gallstones.	Shawahna and Taha (2017)
Passiflora incarnata (Clove)	Smoking clove cigarettes can cause pneumonia after lung abscess. It can also cause acute hemorrhagic pulmonary edema and diminished lymphocytes responses.	Guidotti et al. (1989)
Passiflora incarnata (Passion flower)	The flower can cause asthma, sinus irritation, dermatitis, tachycardia, excessive sedation and abnormal bleeding.	Nojoumi et al. (2016)
Glycyrrhiza glabra (Liquorice)	It can cause cardiovascular complications such as hypertension, hypertensive encephalopathy, cardiac arrhythmias etc. It can also cause hypokalaemia myopathy stroke and rhabdomyolysis.	Omar et al. (2012)
Commiphora wightii (Gugglu)	Gugglu can cause gastric discomfort and allergic rashes. It should be avoided in pregnant or breastfeeding women and in children. It can cause irregular menstrual cycles.	Leiva et al. (2017)
Curcuma longa (Turmeric)	High doses and long term use of turmeric may cause nausea, diarrhea, increased serum alkaline phosphatase and lactate dehydrogenase contents.	Hewlings and Kalman (2017)
Cannabis sativa (Bhang)	It can cause addiction in the patient, at high dose tolerance can be developed leading to impaired short term memory, making it difficult to learn or retain information. It can also interfere with driving skills and can increase the risk of injury.	Volkow et al. (2014)

showed common mental disorders like depression, anxiety, convulsion, etc. The Ayurvedic prescriptions have been proven to be very useful against such disorders. The present review clearly explains that the Ayurvedic system of medicine is very well developed for treating most of the brain related disorders. This review includes some of the herbal medications, which have been described for mental disorders and are currently part of the Ayurveda. Thus, it could be concluded that the Ayurvedic system of herbal medicine can be regarded as a hope for the complete and permanent treatment of mental disorders through natural means with minimum side effects as compared with the Allopathic drugs.

KEYWORDS

- **Alzheimer's disease**
- **herbal therapeutics**
- **Huntington's disease**
- **neurodegenerative disorders**
- **Parkinson's disease**

REFERENCES

Ahmad, M.; Saleem, S.; Ahmad, A. S.; Ansari, M. A.; Yousuf, S.; Hoda, M. N.; Islam, F. Neuroprotective Effects of *Withania somnifera* on 6-Hydroxydopamine Induced Parkinsonism in Rats. *Hum. Exp. Toxicol.* **2005,** *24* (3), 137–147.

Ahmad, M.; Yousuf, S.; Khan, M. B.; Hoda, M. N.; Ahmad, A. S.; Ansari, M. A.; Ishrat, T.; Agrawal, A. K.; Islam, F. Attenuation by *Nardostachys jatamansi* of 6-Hydroxydopamine-Induced Parkinsonism in Rats: Behavioral, Neurochemical, and Immunohistochemical Studies. *Pharmacol. Biochem. Behav.* **2006,** *83* (1), 150–160.

Ahn, J.; Ahn, H. S.; Cheong, J. H.; Dela Peña, I. Natural Product-Derived Treatments for Attention-Deficit/Hyperactivity Disorder: Safety, Efficacy, and Therapeutic Potential of Combination Therapy. *Neural Plasticity* **2016,** *2016.* DOI: 10.1155/2016/1320423.

Akram, M.; Nawaz, A. Effects of Medicinal Plants on Alzheimer's Disease and Memory Deficits. *Neural Regen Res.* **2017,** *12* (4), 660.

Ali, S. K.; Hamed, A. R.; Soltan, M. M.; Hegazy, U. M.; Elgorashi, E. E.; El-Garf, I. A.; Hussein, A. A. In Vitro Evaluation of Selected Egyptian Traditional Herbal Medicines for Treatment of Alzheimer Disease. *BMC Complement Altern. Med.* **2013,** *13* (1), 121.

Andrade, C. The Herbal Treatment of Parkinson's Disease: A Possible Role for BR-16A (Mentat). *Ind. J. Psychol. Med.* **1996,** *19* (2), 82–88.

Arora, M.; Sharma, T.; Devi, A.; Bainsal, N.; Siddiqui, A. A. An Inside Review of *Cissampelos pareira* Linn: A Potential Medicinal Plant of India. *Int. Res. J. Pharm.* **2012,** *3* (12), 38–41.

Aso, E.; Ferrer, I. CB2 Cannabinoid Receptor as Potential Target Against Alzheimer's Disease. *Front. Neurosci.* **2016,** *10*, 243.

Bassi, S. M.; Sancesario, A.; Morace, R.; Centonze, D.; Iezzi, E. Cannabinoids in Parkinson's Disease. *Cannabis Cannabinoid Res.* **2017,** *2* (1), 21–29.

Bhangale, J. O.; Acharya, S. R. Anti-Parkinson Activity of Petroleum Ether Extract of *Ficus religiosa* (L.) leaves. *Adv. Pharmacol. Sci.* **2016,** *2016*. DOI: 10.1155/2016/9436106.

Blum, D.; Chern, Y.; Domenici, M. R.; Buée, L.; Lin, C. Y.; Rea, W.; Ferré, S.; Popoli, P. The Role of Adenosine Tone and Adenosine Receptors in Huntington's Disease. *J. Caffeine Adenosine Res.* **2018,** *8* (2), 43–58.

Butterfield, D. A.; Castegna, A.; Pocernich, C. B.; Drake, J.; Scapagnini, G.; Calabrese, V. Nutritional Approaches to Combat Oxidative Stress in Alzheimer's Disease. *J. Nutr. Biochem.* **2002,** *13* (8), 444–461.

Chakravarthi, K. K.; Avadhani, R. Beneficial Effect of Aqueous Root Extract of *Glycyrrhiza glabra* on Learning and Memory Using Different Behavioral Models: An Experimental Study. *J. Nat. Sci. Biol. Med.* **2013,** *4* (2), 420.

Cho, I. H. Effects of *Panax ginseng* in Neurodegenerative Diseases. *J. Ginseng Res.* **2012,** *36* (4), 342.

Chou, K. L. Adverse events from the Treatment of Parkinson's Disease. *Neurol Clin.* **2008,** *26* (3), S65-S83.

Choudhary, S.; Kumar, P.; Malik, J. Plants and Phytochemicals for Huntington's Disease. *Pharmacogn. Rev.* **2013,** *7* (14), 81.

Claeson, U. P.; Malmfors, T.; Wikman, G.; Bruhn, J. G. Adhatoda vasica: A Critical Review of Ethnopharmacological and Toxicological Data. *J. Ethnopharmacol.* **2000,** *72* (1–2), 1–20.

Coles, C. J.; Edmondson, D. E.; Singer, T. P. Inactivation of Succinate Dehydrogenase by 3-Nitropropionate. *J. Biol. Chem.* **1979,** *254* (12), 5161–5167.

Cummings, J. L.; Tong, G.; Ballard, C. Treatment Combinations for Alzheimer's Disease: Current and Future Pharmacotherapy Options. *J. Alzheimer's Dis.* **2019,** *67* (3), 779–794.

Curatolo, P.; D'Agati, E.; Moavcro, R. The Neurobiological Basis of ADHD. *Italian J. Pediatrics* **2010,** *36* (1), 79.

De Sousa, A.; Kalra, G. Drug Therapy of Attention Deficit Hyperactivity Disorder: Current Trends. *Mens Sana Monographs* **2012,** *10* (1), 45.

Dhanasekaran, M.; Holcomb, L. A.; Hitt, A. R.; Tharakan, B.; Porter, J. W.; Young, K. A.; Manyam, B. V. *Centella asiatica* Extract Selectively Decreases Amyloid β Levels in Hippocampus of Alzheimer's Disease Animal Model. *Phytother. Res.* **2009,** *23* (1), 14–19.

Fahey, J. W. *Moringa oleifera*: A Review of the Medical Evidence for Its Nutritional, Therapeutic, and Prophylactic Properties. Part 1. *Trees Life J.* **2005,** *1* (5), 1–5.

Finkbeiner S. Huntington's Disease. *Cold Spring Harb Perspect Biol.* **2011,** *3* (6), a007476.

Frank S. Treatment of Huntington's Disease. *Neurotherapeutics* **2014,** *11* (1), 153–160.

Godkar, P.; Gordon, R. K.; Ravindran, A.; Doctor, B. P. *Celastrus paniculatus* Seed Water Soluble Extracts Protect Cultured Rat Forebrain Neuronal Cells from Hydrogen Peroxide-Induced Oxidative Injury. *Fitoterapia* **2003,** *74* (7–8), 658–669.

Guidotti, T. L.; Laing, L. O.; Prakash, U. B. Clove Cigarettes. The Basis for Concern Regarding Health Effects. *West J. Med.* **1989,** *151* (2), 220–228.

Hassan, M. A. G.; Balasubramanian, R.; Masoud, A. D.; Burkan, Z. E.; Sughir, A.; Kumar, R. S. Role of Medicinal Plants in Neurodegenerative Diseases with Special Emphasis to Alzheimer's. *Int. J. Phytopharmacol.* **2014,** *5* (6), 454–462.

Hewlings, S. J.; Kalman, D. S. Curcumin: A Review of Its' Effects on Human Health. *Foods* **2017,** *6* (10), 92.

Hwang, C. K.; Chun, H. S. Isoliquiritigenin Isolated from Licorice *Glycyrrhiza uralensis* Prevents 6-Hydroxydopamine-Induced Apoptosis in Dopaminergic Neurons. *Biosci. Biotechnol. Biochem.* **2012,** *76* (3), 536–43.

Jaafaru, M. S.; Nordin, N.; Shaari, K.; Rosli, R.; Razis, A. F. Isothiocyanate from *Moringa oleifera* Seeds Mitigates Hydrogen Peroxide-Induced Cytotoxicity and Preserved Morphological Features of Human Neuronal Cells. *PloS One* **2018,** *13* (5), e0196403.

Jadiya, P.; Khan, A.; Sammi, S. R.; Kaur, S.; Mir, S. S.; Nazir, A. Anti-Parkinsonian Effects of *Bacopa monnieri*: Insights from Transgenic and Pharmacological *Caenorhabditis elegans* Models of Parkinson's Disease. *Biochem. Biophys. Res. Commun.* **2011,** *413* (4), 605–610.

Jain, N. N.; Ohal, C. C.; Shroff, S. K.; Bhutada, R. H.; Somani, R. S.; Kasture, V. S.; Kasture, S. B. *Clitoria ternatea* and the CNS. *Pharmacol Biochem. Behav.* **2003,** *75* (3), 529–536.

Jankovic, J.; Aguilar, L. G. Current Approaches to the Treatment of Parkinson's Disease. *Neuropsychiatr Dis. Treat* **2008,** *4* (4), 743–757.

Jansen, R. L.; Brogan, B.; Whitworth, A. J.; Okello, E. J. Effects of Five Ayurvedic Herbs on Locomotor Behaviour in a Drosophila Melanogaster Parkinson's Disease Model. *Phytother. Res.* **2014,** *28* (12), 1789–95.

Janssen, I. M.; Sturtz, S.; Skipka, G.; Zentner, A.; Garrido, M. V.; Busse, R. *Ginkgo biloba* in Alzheimer's Disease: A Systematic Review. *Wiener Medizinische Wochenschrift* **2010,** *160* (21–22), 539–546.

Joy, J. An Insight from the Ayurvedic Perspective of Neurodegeneration. *Parkinsonism Related Disorders* **2016,** *22*, e88.

Joy, J. The Ayurvedic Perspective on the Etiopathogenesis of Neurodegeneration. *J. Health Edu. Res. Dev.* **2015,** *3*, 137.

Kelly, C.; Castellanos, F. X.; Tomaselli, O.; Lisdahl, K.; Tamm, L.; Jernigan, T.; Newman, E.; Epstein, J. N.; Molina, B. S.; Greenhill, L. L.; Potkin, S. G. Distinct Effects of Childhood ADHD and Cannabis Use on Brain Functional Architecture in Young Adults. *NeuroImage: Clin.* **2017,** *13*, 188–200.

Khazdair, M. R.; Boskabady, M. H.; Hosseini, M.; Rezaee, R.; Tsatsakis, A. M. The Effects of *Crocus sativus* (saffron) and Its Constituents on Nervous System: A Review. *Avicenna J. Phytomed.* **2015,** *5* (5), 376–391.

Khedher, M. R.; Khedher, S. B.; Chaieb, I.; Tounsi, S.; Hammami, M. Chemical Composition and Biological Activities of *Salvia officinalis* Essential Oil from Tunisia. *EXCLI J.* **2017,** *16*, 160.

Khurana, N.; Gajbhiye, A. Ameliorative Effect of *Sida cordifolia* in Rotenone Induced Oxidative Stress Model of Parkinson's Disease. *Neurotoxicology* **2013,** *39*, 57–64.

Kieburtz, K.; Reilmann, R.; Olanow, C. W. Huntington's Disease: Current and Future Therapeutic Prospects. *Movement Disorders* **2018,** *33* (7), 1033–1041.

Kou, X.; Li, B.; Olayanju, J. B.; Drake, J. M.; Chen, N. Nutraceutical or Pharmacological Potential of *Moringa oleifera* Lam. *Nutrients* **2018,** *10* (3), 343.

Kumar, P.; Kumar, A. Possible Neuroprotective Effect of *Withania somnifera* Root Extract Against 3-Nitropropionic Acid-Induced Behavioral, Biochemical, and Mitochondrial Dysfunction in an Animal Model of Huntington's Disease. *J. Med. Food* **2009,** *12* (3), 591–600.

Lampariello, L. R.; Cortelazzo, A.; Guerranti, R.; Sticozzi, C.; Valacchi, G. The Magic Velvet Bean of *Mucuna pruriens*. *J. Tradit. Complement. Med.* **2012,** *2* (4), 331–339.

Leiva, A.; Contreras-Duarte, S.; Amigo, L.; Sepúlveda, E.; Boric, M.; Quiñones, V.; Busso, D.; Rigotti, A. Gugulipid Causes Hypercholesterolemia Leading to Endothelial Dysfunction, Increased Atherosclerosis, and Premature Death by Ischemic Heart Disease in Male Mice. *PloS One* **2017,** *12* (9), e0184280.

Lim, G. P.; Chu, T.; Yang, F.; Beech, W.; Frautschy, S. A.; Cole, G. M. The Curry Spice Curcumin Reduces Oxidative Damage and Amyloid Pathology in an Alzheimer Transgenic Mouse. *J. Neurosci.* **2001,** *21* (21), 8370–8377.

Limpeanchob, N.; Jaipan, S.; Rattanakaruna, S.; Phrompittayarat, W.; Ingkaninan, K. Neuroprotective Effect of *Bacopa monnieri* on Beta-Amyloid-Induced Cell Death in Primary Cortical Culture. *J. Ethnopharmacol.* **2008,** *120* (1), 112–117.

Liu, Q.; Kou, J. P.; Yu, B. Y. Ginsenoside Rg1 Protects Against Hydrogen Peroxide-Induced Cell Death in PC12 Cells via Inhibiting NF-κB Activation. *Neurochem. Int.* **2011,** *58* (1), 119–125.

Malik, J.; Karan, M.; Dogra, R. Ameliorating Effect of *Celastrus paniculatus* Standardized Extract and Its Fractions on 3-Nitropropionic Acid Induced Neuronal Damage in Rats: Possible Antioxidant Mechanism. *Pharm. Biol.* **2017,** *55* (1), 980–990.

Margret, A. A.; Begum, T. N.; Parthasarathy, S.; Suvaithenamudhan, S. A Strategy to Employ *Clitoria ternatea* as a Prospective Brain Drug Confronting Monoamine Oxidase (MAO) Against Neurodegenerative Diseases and Depression. *Nat. Prod. Bioprospect* **2015,** *5* (6), 293–306.

Michel, H. E.; Tadros, M. G.; Abdel-Naim, A. B.; Khalifa, A. E. Prepulse Inhibition (PPI) Disrupting Effects of *Glycyrrhiza glabra* Extract in Mice: A Possible Role of Monoamines. *Neurosci. Lett.* **2013,** *544*, 110–114.

Mythri, R. B.; Bharath, M. M. Curcumin: A Potential Neuroprotective Agent in Parkinson's Disease. *Curr. Pharm. Des.* **2012,** *18* (1), 91–99.

Nojoumi, M.; Ghaeli, P.; Salimi, S.; Sharifi, A.; Raisi, F. Effects of Passion Flower Extract, as an Add-on Treatment to Sertraline, on Reaction Time in Patients with Generalized Anxiety Disorder: A Double-Blind Placebo-Controlled Study. *Iran J. Psych.* **2016,** *11* (3), 191–197.

Omar, H. R.; Komarova, I.; El-Ghonemi, M.; Fathy, A.; Rashad, R.; Abdelmalak, H. D.; Yerramadha, M. R.; Ali, Y.; Helal, E.; Camporesi, E. M. Licorice Abuse: Time to Send a Warning Message. *Ther. Adv. Endocrinol. Metab.* **2012,** *3* (4), 125–138.

Panday, D. R.; Rauniar, G. P. Effect of Root-Extracts of *Ficus benghalensis* (Banyan) in Memory, Anxiety, Muscle Co-Ordination and Seizure in Animal Models. *BMC Complement Altern. Med.* **2016,** *16* (1), 429.

Parker, V.; Wong, A. B.; Boon, H. S.; Seeman, M. V. Adverse Reactions to St John's wort. *Can. J. Psychiatry* **2001,** *46* (1), 77–79.

Perry, E.; Howes, M. J. Medicinal Plants and Dementia Therapy: Herbal Hopes for Brain Aging? *CNS Neurosci Ther* **2011,** *17* (6), 683–698.

Pinho, B. R.; Ferreres, F.; Valentão, P.; Andrade, P. B. Nature as a Source of Metabolites with Cholinesterase-Inhibitory Activity: An Approach to Alzheimer's Disease Treatment. *J. Pharm Pharmacol.* **2013,** *65* (12), 1681–1700.

Pitsikas, N. The effect of *Crocus sativus* L. and Its Constituents on Memory: Basic Studies and Clinical Applications. *Evid. Based Complement Alternat. Med.* **2015,** *2015.* DOI: 10.1155/2015/926284.

Rao, R. V.; Descamps, O.; John, V.; Bredesen, D. E. Ayurvedic Medicinal Plants for Alzheimer's Disease: A Review. *Alzheimer's Res. Ther.* **2012,** *4* (3), 22.

Rasool, M.; Malik, A.; Qureshi, M. S.; Manan, A.; Pushparaj, P. N.; Asif, M.; Qazi, M. H.; Qazi, A. M.; Kamal, M. A.; Gan, S. H.; Sheikh, I. A. Recent Updates in the Treatment of

Neurodegenerative Disorders Using Natural Compounds. *Evid. Based Complement. Altern. Med.* **2014,** *2014*.

Renaud, J.; Bournival, J.; Zottig, X.; Martinoli, M. G. Resveratrol Protects DAergic PC12 Cells from High Glucose-Induced Oxidative Stress and Apoptosis: Effect on p53 and GRP75 Localization. *Neurotox Res.* **2014,** *25* (1), 110–123.

Rios, J. L.; Onteniente, M.; Picazo, D.; Montesinos, M. C. Medicinal Plants and Natural Products as Potential Sources for Antiparkinson Drugs. *Planta Med* **2016,** *82* (11/12), 942–951.

Sagredo, O.; Ruth Pazos, M.; Valdeolivas, S.; Fernández-Ruiz, J. Cannabinoids: Novel Medicines for the Treatment of Huntington's Disease. *Recent Patents CNS Drug Discov.* **2012,** *7* (1), 41–48.

Salehi, B.; Imani, R.; Mohammadi, M. R.; Fallah, J.; Mohammadi, M.; Ghanizadeh, A.; Tasviechi, A. A.; Vossoughi, A.; Rezazadeh, S. A.; Akhondzadeh, S. *Ginkgo biloba* for Attention-Deficit/Hyperactivity Disorder in Children and Adolescents: A Double Blind, Randomized Controlled Trial. *Prog. Neuropsychopharmacol. Biol. Psych.* **2010,** *34* (1), 76–80.

Sarris, J.; Kean, J.; Schweitzer, I.; Lake, J. Complementary Medicines (Herbal and Nutritional Products) in the Treatment of Attention Deficit Hyperactivity Disorder (ADHD): A Systematic Review of the Evidence. *Complement Ther. Med.* **2011,** *19* (4), 216–227.

Sehgal, N.; Gupta, A.; Valli, R. K.; Joshi, S. D.; Mills, J. T.; Hamel, E.; Khanna, P.; Jain, S. C.; Thakur, S. S.; Ravindranath, V. *Withania somnifera* Reverses Alzheimer's Disease Pathology by Enhancing Low-Density Lipoprotein Receptor-Related Protein in Liver. *Proc. Natl. Acad. Sci. USA* **2012,** *109* (9), 3510–3515.

Shawahna, R.; Taha, A. Which Potential Harms and Benefits of Using Ginger in the Management of Nausea and Vomiting of Pregnancy Should Be Addressed? A Consensual Study Among Pregnant Women and Gynecologists. *BMC Complement Altern. Med.* **2017,** *17* (1), 204.

Singhal, A. K.; Naithani, V.; Bangar, O. P. Medicinal Plants with a Potential to Treat Alzheimer and Associated Symptoms. *Int. J. Nutr. Pharmacol. Neurol. Dis.* **2012,** *2* (2), 84.

Singhal, H. K.; Neetu, A. K.; Rai, M. Ayurvedic Approach for Improving Reaction Time of Attention Deficit Hyperactivity Disorder Affected Children. *Ayu* **2010,** *31* (3), 338.

Stella, F.; Radanovic, M.; Canineu, P. R.; de Paula, V. J.; Forlenza, O. V. Anti-Dementia Medications: Current Prescriptions in Clinical Practice and New Agents in Progress. *Therap. Adv. Drug Saf.* **2015,** *6* (4), 151–165.

Stockler-Pinto, M. B.; Mafra, D.; Moraes, C.; Lobo, J.; Boaventura, G. T.; Farage, N. E.; Silva, W. S.; Cozzolino, S. F.; Malm, O. Brazil Nut (*Bertholletia excelsa*, HBK) Improves Oxidative Stress and Inflammation Biomarkers in Hemodialysis Patients. *Biol. Trace Elem. Res.* **2014,** *158* (1), 105–112.

Sutalangka, C.; Wattanathorn, J.; Muchimapura, S.; Thukham-mee, W. *Moringa oleifera* Mitigates Memory Impairment and Neurodegeneration in Animal Model of Age-Related Dementia. *Oxid. Med. Cell Longev*. **2013,** *2013*. DOI: 10.1155/2013/695936.

Talpate, K. A.; Bhosale, U. A.; Zambare, M. R.; Somani, R. S. Neuroprotective and Nootropic Activity of *Clitorea ternatea* Linn. (Fabaceae) Leaves on Diabetes Induced Cognitive Decline in Experimental Animals. *J. Pharm. Bioallied. Sci.* **2014,** *6* (1), 48–55.

Tanaka, A.; Hamada, N.; Fujita, Y.; Itoh, T.; Nozawa, Y.; Iinuma, M.; Ito, M. A Novel Kavalactone Derivative Protects Against H_2O_2-Induced PC12 Cell Death via Nrf2/ARE Activation. *Bioorg. Med. Chem.* **2010,** *18* (9), 3133–3139.

Tanaka, K.; S-Galduroz, R. F.; Gobbi, L. T.; Galduróz, J. C. *Ginkgo biloba* Extract in an Animal Model of Parkinson's Disease: A Systematic Review. *Curr. Neuropharmacol.* **2013,** *11* (4), 430–435.

Tzeng, Y. M.; Lee, M. J. Neuroprotective Properties of Kavalactones. *Neural Regen. Res.* **2015,** *10* (6), 875–877.

Vaidya, A. D. B.; Devasagayam, T. P. A. Current Status of Herbal Drugs in India: An Overview. *J. Clin. Biochem. Nutr.* **2007,** *41* (1), 1–1.

Van Bulck, M.; Sierra-Magro, A.; Alarcon-Gil, J.; Perez-Castillo, A.; Morales-Garcia, J. A. Novel Approaches for the Treatment of Alzheimer's and Parkinson's Disease. *Int. J. Mol. Sci.* **2019,** *20* (3), E719.

Van Kampen, J. M.; Baranowski, D. B.; Shaw, C. A.; Kay, D. G. *Panax ginseng* Is Neuroprotective in a Novel Progressive Model of Parkinson's Disease. *Exp. Gerontol.* **2014,** *50*, 95–105.

Vergara-Jimenez, M.; Almatrafi, M.; Fernandez, M. Bioactive Components in *Moringa oleifera* Leaves Protect Against Chronic Disease. *Antioxidants (Basel)* **2017,** *6* (4), 91.

Videnovic, A. Treatment of Huntington Disease. *Curr. Treat Options Neurol.* **2013,** *15* (4), 424–438.

Volkow, N. D.; Baler, R. D.; Compton, W. M.; Weiss, S. R. Adverse Health Effects of Marijuana Use. *N. Eng. J. Med.* **2014,** *370* (23), 2219–2227.

Yiannopoulou, K. G.; Papageorgiou, S. G. Current and Future Treatments for Alzheimer's Disease. *Therap. Adv. Neurol. Disorders* **2013,** *6* (1), 19–33.

CHAPTER 18

Ethnomedicinal Practices and the Role of Ayurveda in the Management of Oral Health and Hygiene

PRIYA PRADEEP[1], PRADEEP KUMAR K.[2], and BHAGYA B. SHARMA[3]

[1]*Department of Roganidana, Yenepoya Ayurveda Medical College and Hospital, Yenepoya (Deemed to be University), Derlakatte, Mangalore, Karnataka, India*

[2]*Deptartment of Shalakya Tantra, Yenepoya Ayurveda Medical College and Hospital, Yenepoya (Deemed to be University), Derlakatte, Mangalore, Karnataka, India*

[3]*Centre for Environmental Studies, Yenepoya (Deemed to be University), Derlakatte, Mangalore, Karnataka, India*

ABSTRACT

Oral diseases are most prevalent globally and needs primary health care services as concern of public health. Use of ethnophytotherapeutic remedies for routine oral care and to treat or cure oral ailments have a long-recorded history. India is rich in ethnofloral diversity with many medicinal plants used in ethnomedicinal practices. For routine oral health care, up to 74 plant species (57 genera) have been recommended with parts used, medicinal value and methods to be adapted. Most commonly used genera of plant species for routine oral care include *Citrus*, *Garcinia*, *Syzygium*, and *Terminalia*. A maximum of 80% of twig/stem/branch are used, while use of root, leaves,

Ethnic Knowledge and Perspectives of Medicinal Plants, Volume 1: Curative Properties and Treatment Strategies. Munir Ozturk, Kandikere R. Sridhar, Maryam Sarwat, Volkan Altay, & Francisco Martín Huerta-Martínez (Eds.)

bark, and latex ranges from 38%. Use of plant materials as toothbrush is as high as 90%. About 142 plant species (110 genera) have been recommended for treatment or cure of oral diseases. Most commonly used genera include *Acacia, Ficus, Jatropha,* and *Solanum*. Up to 53% of twig/stem/branch/root and 24% leaves and 11% of latex are used. Plant material used as toothbrush was up to 34% followed by chewing and latex/gum/ash/decoction/juice. Up to 57% of plant materials are useful for overall teeth care, followed by mouth ulcer and gingivitis. The present review provides an overview with database of plant species used toward oral health and hygiene.

18.1 INTRODUCTION

The flora in India is a wealth of valuable medicinal plants used in human health care. Among the hygiene, oral health care is the most important concern for overall human well-being. The use of plants in treating human oral ailments has been an integral part of our culture. India has a rich heritage of traditional or ethnic healing systems. Traditional use of plants as medicine in folklore practice is well established in Ayurveda and Siddha since ancient days for treating various ailments including oral hygiene. Ethnomedicinal knowledge of plants and their applications are inborn cultural practices and these are besides useful for preservation of cultural customs also restore healthcare of community at large and useful in development of drugs. The tribal population distributed across various parts of the country still use plants and various herbal formulations for maintenance of oral health and hygiene.

Azadirachta indica has been widely used by traditional practitioners in the management of oral-related complaints like stomatitis, gingivitis, dental caries, and toothache (pain relief). Neem is potent against oral acidogenic bacteria and periodontal pathogens. Leaves possess immunomodulatory, anti-inflammatory, antibacterial, antiviral, antioxidant, and anticarcinogenic properties. Venugopal et al. (1998) analyzed 2000 children (age group, 1–14 years) for incidence of dental caries in Mumbai. Among them, the children who were using neem stick toothbrush were less affected with the dental caries. In Indian folk remedy, oil pulling has been widely used to prevent dental caries, bad breath, and strengthen teeth and gum (Singh and Purohit, 2011). The oils such as coconut oil, sesame oil, sunflower oil, and gingelly oil are used in oil-pulling therapy for the maintenance of oral health and hygiene.

Tender twigs or tender stem or leaves of various plant species such as *Acacia arabica, A. indica, Ficus benghalensis, Jatropha curcas, Mangifera indica,* and *P. guajava* are extensively used for cleaning of teeth as toothbrush as well as to massage the gum, which cure gingival-related complaints, prevent dental carries, and dental plaque formation. In South India, commonly mango leaf (*M. indica*) is used for cleaning the teeth. To perform that, fresh mango leaf, free from disease is washed, its midrib is removed, folded, and tightly rolled. One side of the roll is crushed by biting the end, which is rubbed on the teeth. The midrib part of the leaf can serve as a tongue cleaner. Bairy et al. (2002) evaluated the antibacterial activity of *M. indica* on anaerobic dental microbiota based on in vivo studies, which revealed significant decrease in the proportion of *Prevotella intermedia* and *Prevotella gingivalis* in mango leaf users compared to toothbrush users (Bairy et al., 2002). This review provides a brief account on oral microbiome, diseases of oral cavity, and insight on the ethnic knowledge on use of different plant species for routine oral care as well as in treatment of oral diseases.

18.2 ORAL MICROBIOME

Oral microbiome is a collection of microorganisms that reside in the oral cavity. When compared to gut, oral cavity is the second largest microbial complex in humans. The composition of microbiome varies depending upon the habitat in the oral cavity (Yamashita and Takeshita, 2017). Oral bacteria exhibit specificity in the colonization, for instance *Rothia* species colonize over the tongue or tooth, *Simonsiella* colonize at the hard palate, *Streptococcus salivarius* colonizes the tongue and *Treponema* colonizes the sub-gingival crevice. Such colonization of bacteria in the oral cavity is associated with various health and disease conditions (Krishnan et al., 2017). The oral microbiome plays a major role in maintaining the health of oral cavity as well as prevent the development of oral diseases. Lifestyle and diet including consumption of spicy food, drinking alcohol, smoking, and also antibiotic treatments can constantly change the commensal microbial communities, resulting in disturbances of normal microbiota and may increase the susceptibility to pathogens (Jia et al., 2018).

18.2.1 BACTERIAL COMPOSITION

Human oral microbiome comprises of core and variable microbes. The core microbes are found in all individuals and exists at different sites of the body under healthy conditions. The variable microbes depends on unique lifestyle and physiological differences of the individuals (Deo and Deshmukh, 2019). The surfaces of the oral cavity are coated with a plethora of bacteria and they form biofilms (Deo and Deshmukh, 2019). The bacteria colonize on the two kinds of surfaces in the oral cavity: soft mucosal surface (shedding) and hard solid surface of the teeth (He et al., 2015). Microbes in oral cavity flourish on the teeth, tongue, cheeks, sulcus, tonsils, gingival, and palate of oral cavity (hard and soft surfaces).

The microbiome in oral cavity has a complex environment with about 750 different types of microorganisms. *Actinomyces, Neisseria, Streptococcus,* and *Veillonella* are the prevailing microbial populations in the mouth. These microorganisms help maintaining the oral hygiene by prevention of pathogenic strains from attachment to the mucosal surfaces (Mosaddad et al., 2019). Normal pH of oral cavity ranges between 6.5 and 7 and the normal temperature in an average has 37°C, which provides the bacteria a stable environment to thrive and grow (Deo and Deshmukh, 2019). The major Gram-positive bacteria found in the oral cavity are *Abiotrophia, Actinomyces, Bifidobacterium, Corynebacterium, Eubacterium, Lactobacillus, Peptostreptococcus, Propionibacterium, Pseudoramibacter, Rothia Streptococcus,* and *Stomatococcus* (Deo and Deshmukh, 2019). Gram-negative bacteria in oral cavity include *Capnocytophaga, Campylobacter, Desulfobacter, Desulfo vibrio, Eikenella, Fusobacterium, Hemophilus, Leptotrichia, Moraxella, Neisseria, Prevotella, Selemonas, Simonsiella, Treponema, Veillonella,* and *Wolinella*. Microorganisms those are often isolated in patient with oral infection are *Aerobacter aeruginosa*, *Candida, Clostridium* spp., *Eubacteria, Fusobacterium nucleatum*, *Peptococci*, *Peptostreptococci, Staphylococcus aureus,* and *Streptococcus viridians*. Other Gram-positive bacteria found in oral cavity include *Spirochetes* and *Veillonella*, while the Gram-negative bacteria include *Escherichia coli, Haemophilus influenza, Klebsiella* spp., *Neisseria* spp., and *Pseudomonas* spp. (Patil et al., 2013).

18.2.2 NONBACTERIAL COMPOSITION

Diverse nonbacterial microbes in the oral cavity include the fungi, protozoa, and viruses. Protozoas such as *Entamoeba gingivalis* and *Trichomonas tenax* are commonly found as saprophytes. Among the fungi, *Aspergillus, Aureobasidium, Candida, Cladosporium, Cryptococcus Fusarium,* and *Saccharomycetes* are most common in the oral cavity (Deo and Deshmukh, 2019).

18.3 DISEASES OF THE ORAL CAVITY

Diseases of the oral cavity mainly originate due to poor hygiene of oral cavity and by the nutritional factors, which affect the oral microbiota. Thorough understanding of environment of the oral cavity and related microbial interactions reveals the causative factors responsible for diseases. Among the diseases of oral cavity, dental caries, and periodontal diseases are prevalent worldwide and lead to destruction of teeth. Other oral cavity disorders are oral carcinoma, oral manifestations of HIV, fluorosis of teeth, and developmental disorders (Bratthall et al., 2006). These diseases can be preventable and different measures have been formulated to control them.

18.3.1 DENTAL CARIES

Dental caries is an interaction between microbial biofilm established on the teeth and fermentable carbohydrates. Caries is a multifactorial disease resulting in demineralization and remineralization of tooth. It may affect child as well as adult dentitions (Pitts et al., 2017). Most of the evidence on the dental caries epidemiology advocates *Streptococcus mutans* is one of the most effective cariogenic bacteria in the initiation of dental caries. The use of antibiotics is a proven method to prevent dental caries. In rural areas, the herbal therapies are the important source of medicine. Thus, the antibacterial, antiviral and anti-inflammatory functions of herbs and herbal products entered into the dentistry (Karadağlıoğlu et al., 2019).

18.3.2 PERIAPICAL PERIODONTITIS

Periapical periodontitis is an inflammatory disease that occurs in the periapical area (tissues around the apex of the root of tooth). It is caused by pulpal infection results in resorption of apical alveolar bone and tooth loss (Siddiqui et al., 2019). Under etiology, 80% of the factors are contributed by environmental determinants and individual genetic variation and remaining 20% contributed by the plaque deposits (Bartold and Van Dyke, 2019). Common pathogenic bacteria of periodontal diseases are *Cryptobacterium curtum, Dialister pneumosintes, Filifactor alocis, Mitsuokella dentalis, Selenomonas sputigena, Slackia exigua, Solobacterium moorei,* and *Treponema lecithinolyticum* (Hiranmayi et al., 2009).

18.3.3 GINGIVITIS

The inflammation of the gum is known as gingivitis, it is usually caused by a film of plaque or bacteria on the tooth surface. It affects soft tissues and leads to gingival edema, bleeding, and hypertrophy. If left unattended it may lead to severe infection of gum and loss of tooth. Gingivitis has been classified into two types: 1) Plaque induced gingivitis; 2) Nonplaque induced gingivitis. The plaque-induced gingivitis caused by bacterial infection located on the gingival margin (Asokan et al., 2009; Highfield, 2009), while the nonplaque-induced gingivitis are uncommon and often it is manifest secondary to systemic diseases or genetic or developmental disorders (Holmstrup et al., 2018). In different clinical trials, it was proved that the use of herbal products in the form of mouthwash or dentifrices in gingivitis was found equally effective as a control commercial product Sensodyne in improving gingival index and plaque index (Safiaghdam et al., 2018).

18.3.4 ORAL LICHEN PLANUS

The lichen planus in oral cavity is one of the chronic inflammatory disease of mucosa. It affects tongue, buccal mucosa, gingiva, lip, and palate (Casparis et al., 2015). Oral lichen planus found in approximately 1–2% of the population, which commonly affects middle-aged adults with a slight female predominance (Weston and Payette, 2015). It appears as white papules annular or plaque, erythema, blister or erosion-like pattern. Lichen planus may also undergo malignant transformation (Carrozzo et al, 2000).

18.3.5 LEUKOPLAKIA

Leukoplakia is the common premalignant lesion and is reported to undergo malignant changes to oral squamous cell carcinoma. Leukoplakia is common in smokers and usually appears in the fourth decade of life. The common site of leukoplakia is buccal mucosa and tongue (Van der Waal et al., 1997; Bairy et al., 2002).

18.4 ORAL HEALTH AND HYGIENE

Ayurveda the Indian system of medicine under the heading of *Dinacharya* has elucidated various daily regimes that one should follow every day to maintain healthy body and mind. The procedures like *Dantadavana* (brushing teeth), *Kavala* (mouthwash), and *Gandusha* (throat gargle) to maintain oral hygiene and prevent oral disorders are explained. As a preventive measure, Ayurveda recommends brushing the teeth in morning as well as after each meal. For brushing, twigs should be collected from healthy tree, which is crushed at one end, having nine inches long, and thickness of little finger. The plants selected for brush should have astringent and bitter or acrid taste (Singh and Purohit, 2011).

18.4.1 PLANTS USED FOR ROUTINE ORAL CARE

The twigs of plants like *Acacia catechu, Acacia farnisiana, Achyranthus aspera, Aegle marmelos, Albezzia lebback, Anthouphalus cadamba, Azadirecta indica, Calotropis gigantea, Ficus bengalensis, Ficus recemosa, Glycyrrhiza glabra, Jasminum grandiflorum, M. indica, Michelia champaca, Nerium oleander, Pongamia pinnata, Pterocarpus marsupium, Purerasia tuberra Terminalia arjuna*, and *Vateria indica* are used to prepare toothbrush (Figure 18.1). The fine powders of *Triphala* (prepared by *Emblica officinalis, Terminalia chebula* and *T. bellerica*), *Trikatu* (consists of *Piper longum, Piper nigrum*, and *Zingiber officinale*) and *Trijata* (composed of *Cinnamomum tamala, C. verum*, and *Elettaria cardamomum*) mixed with honey is used as toothpaste (Figure 18.2).

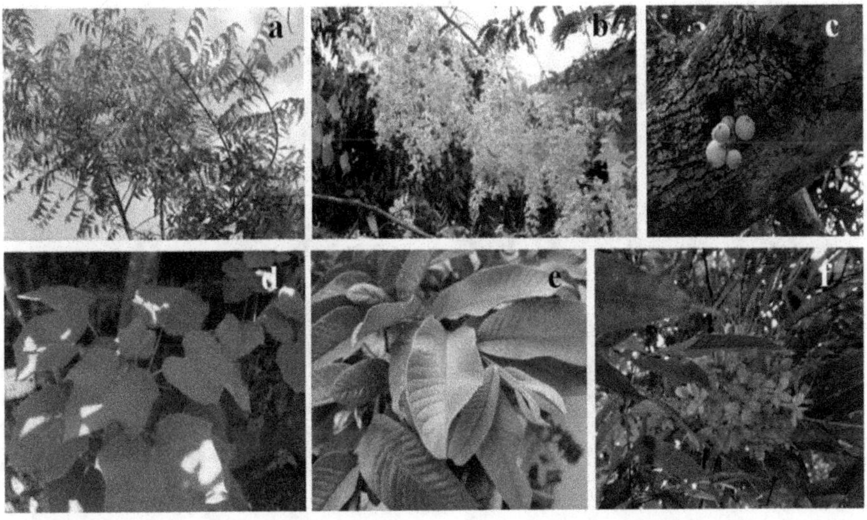

FIGURE 18.1 Selected plant species used in routine oral care: *Azadirachta indica* (a), *Cassia fistula* (b), *Ficus racemosa* (c), *Jatropha curcas* (d), *Psidium gujava* (e), and *Saraca asoca* (f).

For mouthwash, herbal decoction of *Triphala*, *Mimusopus elengi*, or *Tephrosia purpurea*, *Pongamia glabra* and honey are used. The oil processed with medicinal herbs like *Arimedadi taila*, *Murchita tila taila* are indicated for oil pulling in mouth ulcer, dental carries, sensitivity of teeth, bad breath, and periodontal diseases (swollen gum, hyperemia of gum, bleeding gum and pyorrhoea) (Peiris et al., 2019). The in vitro microbiological study on *Gandusha* (indigenous mouthwash) for periodontal disease showed significant antifungal activity against tested fungi (Peiris et al., 2019). To cleanse the throat and oral cavity Ayurveda advocates *Kavala* (gargle), wherein three-fourth of mouth is filled with the medicated decoction or oil, the liquid is swished in the mouth for specific duration and then spat out (Amruthesh, 2008). These procedures could be adopted as a preventive or curative measure.

As many as 74 plant species (57 genera) could be recommended for routine oral health care. Uses of various plant species in oral care with parts used, medicinal value, and methods need to be adapted are presented in Table 18.1. Among the 75 plant species, most commonly used genera for routine oral care include *Citrus*, *Garcinia* (5 spp. each), *Syzygium*, and *Terminalia* (4 spp. each). From 74 plant species, a total of 84 plant materials are used for oral health care, which consist of a maximum of 80% of twig/stem/branch followed by root (8%), leaves (5%), bark (4%), and latex (3%) (Figure 18.3). Among 69 mode of uses, use as toothbrush was as high as 90% followed by powder (5%), latex (4%), and ash (1%). Regarding oral care, 62% of plant materials are used for teeth care, while 38% serve dual purpose of teeth and gum care.

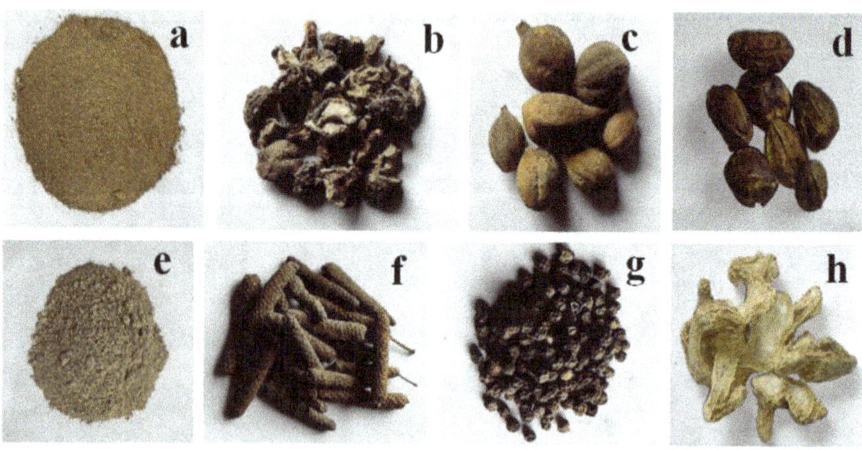

FIGURE 18.2 Components of Ayurvedic product *Triphala* (a): *Emblica officinalis* (b), *Terminalia bellerica* (c), *Terminalia chebula* (d); Components of Ayurvedic product *Trikatu* (e): *Piper longum* (f), *Piper nigrum* (g) and *Zingiber officinalis* (h).

TABLE 18.1 Plant Species Used in Routine Oral Care.

	Botanical name	Family	Oral care	Part used	Mode of use
1	*Abrus precatorius* L.	Fabaceae	Teeth and gum health	Leaves	Powder used for brushing, and chewing the leaves to cure mouth ulcer and toothache
2	*Albizia lebbeck* (L.) Benth.	Fabaceae	Strengthens teeth and gum	Bark	Dried bark powder used as toothpowder
3	*Azadirachta indica* A. Juss.	Meliaceae	Teeth and gum health	Leaves and twigs	Leaves to clean teeth and twigs used as toothbrush
4	*Bambusa balcooa* Roxb.	Poaceae	Strengthens teeth and gum	Tender stem	Toothbrush
5	*Bambusa tulda* Roxb.	Poaceae	Cleaning teeth	Tender stem	Toothbrush
6	*Cajanus cajan* (L.) Millsp.	Fabaceae	Strengthen teeth and gum	Tender stem	Toothbrush
7	*Callicarpa arborea* Roxb.	Lamiaceae	Cleans teeth, strengthens teeth and gum	Tender stem	Toothbrush
8	*Calotropis gigantea* (L.) Dryand	Apocynaceae	Clean teeth	Tender stem and root	Stem used as toothbrush and ash of root used as remedy against pyorrhoea
9	*Camellia sinensis* (L.) Kuntze	Theaceae	Strengthens teeth and gum	Tender stem	Toothbrush
10	*Cassia fistula* L.	Fabaceae	Cleaning teeth	Tender stem	Toothbrush
11	*Cinnamomum bejolghota* (Buch.-Ham.) Sweet.	Lauraceae	Cleaning teeth	Stem	Toothbrush
12	*Cinnamomum verum* J. Presl	Lauraceae	Cleaning teeth	Stem	Toothbrush
13	*Citrus acida* Pers.	Rutaceae	Teeth and gum health	Stem	Toothbrush

TABLE 18.1 *(Continued)*

	Botanical name	Family	Oral care	Part used	Mode of use
14	*Citrus assamensis* Dutta & Bhattacharya	Rutaceae	Cleaning teeth	Stem	Toothbrush
15	*Citrus aurantiifolia* (Christm) Swingle.	Rutaceae	Cleaning teeth	Stem	Toothbrush
16	*Citrus maxima* (Burm.) Merr.	Rutaceae	Cleaning teeth	Stem	Toothbrush
17	*Citrus medica* L.	Rutaceae	Cleaning teeth	Stem	Toothbrush
18	*Crateva nurvala* Buch-Ham	Capparaceae	Strengthens teeth and gum	Tender stem	Toothbrush
19	*Datura innoxia* Mill.	Solanaceae	Cleaning teeth	Root	Toothbrush
20	*Dicoma tomentosa* Cass.	Asteraceae	Teeth and gum health	Roots and branches	Toothbrush
21	*Ehretia laevis* Roxb.	Boraginaceae	Teeth and gum health	Tender branch	Toothbrush
22	*Elaeocarpus floribundus* Blume	Elaeocarpaceae	Cleaning teeth	Tender stem	Toothbrush
23	*Ficus racemosa* L.	Moraceae	Cleaning teeth	Tender stem	Toothbrush
24	*Flacourtia jangomas* (Lour.) Raeusch.	Salicaceae	Cleaning teeth	Tender branch	Toothbrush
25	*Garcinia lanceifolia* Roxb.	Clusiaceae	Cleaning teeth	Twigs	Toothbrush
26	*Garcinia oxyphylla* Miq.	Clusiaceae	Teeth and gum health	Tender branches	Toothbrush
27	*Garcinia pedunculata* Roxb. ex Buch.-Ham.	Clusiaceae	Cleaning teeth	Tender branches	Toothbrush
28	*Garcinia sopsopia* (BuchHam) D. J. Mabberley	Clusiaceae	Strengthens teeth and gum	Branches	Toothbrush
29	*Garcinia xanthochymus* Hook. f. ex T. Anderson	Clusiaceae	Cleaning teeth	Branches	Toothbrush

TABLE 18.1 *(Continued)*

	Botanical name	Family	Oral care	Part used	Mode of use
30	*Glycosmis pentaphylla* (Retz.) DC.	Rutaceae	Strengthens teeth and gum	Branches	Toothbrush
31	*Glycyrrhiza glabra* L.	Fabaceae	Cleaning teeth	Root	Toothbrush
32	*Grewia sapida* Roxb.	Malvaceae	Cleaning teeth	Stem	Toothbrush
33	*Haldina cordifolia* (Roxb.) Ridsdale	Rubiaceae	Cleaning teeth	Twigs	Toothbrush
34	*Hibiscus rosa sinensis* L.	Malvaceae	Cleaning teeth	Stem	Toothbrush
35	*Jatropha curcas* L.	Euphorbiaceae	Cleaning teeth	Stem and latex	Stem serves as toothbrush and latex maintains oral hygiene
36	*Lantana camara* L.	Verbenaceae	Cleaning teeth	Tender stem	Toothbrush
37	*Litsea salcifolia* (J. Roxb. ex Nees) Hook. f.	Lauraceae	Cleaning teeth	Tender stem	Toothbrush
38	*Madhuca longifolia* (J. König ex L.) J. F. Macbr.	Sapotaceae	Strengthens teeth and gum	Stem	Toothbrush
39	*Magnolia hodgsonii* (Hook. f. & Thomson) H. Keng	Magnoliaceae	Cleaning teeth	Branch	Toothbrush
40	*Mangifera indica* L.	Anacardiaceae	Cleaning teeth	Twigs and latex	Twigs serve as toothbrush and latex used for gingivitis
41	*Melastoma malabathricum* L.	Melastomeaceae	Cleaning teeth	Tender stem	Toothbrush
42	*Mimusops elengi* L.	Sapotaceae	Cleaning teeth	Stem and bark	Toothbrush
43	*Morus alba* L.	Moraceae	Cleaning teeth	Tender stem	Toothbrush
44	*Murraya koenigii* (L.) Sprengel	Rutaceae	Cleaning teeth	Tender branch	Toothbrush
45	*Naravelia zeylanica* (L.) DC.	Ranunculaceae	Cleaning teeth	Tender stem	Toothbrush

TABLE 18.1 *(Continued)*

	Botanical name	Family	Oral care	Part used	Mode of use
46	*Neolamarckia cadamba* (Roxb.) Bosser.	Rubiaceae	Strengthens teeth and gum	Tender stem	Toothbrush
47	*Nyctanthes arbor-tristis* L.	Oleaceae	Cleaning teeth	Twigs	Toothbrush
48	*Phanera vahlii* (Wight & Arn.) Benth.	Fabaceae	Cleans teeth, strengthens teeth and gum	Root	Toothbrush
49	*Piper betle* L.	Piperaceae	Strengthens teeth and gum	Leaves	Chewed to prevent bad breath
50	*Pongamia pinnata* (L.) Pierre	Fabaceae	Cleaning teeth	Tender branch	Toothbrush
51	*Psidium guajava* L.	Myrtaceae	Cleaning teeth	Tender stem	Toothbrush
52	*Punica granatum* L.	Lythraceae	Strengthens teeth and gum	Leaves and tender twigs	Leaves chewed to prevent ulcer and twigs serve as toothbrush
53	*Saraca indica* L.	Fabaceae	Cleaning teeth	Tender stem	Toothbrush
54	*Smilax perfoliata* Lour.	Smilaceae	Cleaning teeth	Stem	Toothbrush
55	*Smilax zeylanica* L.	Smilaceae	Strengthens teeth and gum	Tender Stem	Toothbrush
56	*Solanum torvum* Sw.	Solanaceae	Cleaning teeth	Root	Toothbrush
57	*Streblus asper* Lour	Moraceae	Cleaning teeth	Stem	Toothbrush
58	*Syzygium balsameum* (Wight) Wall. ex Walp.	Myrtaceae.	Strengthens teeth and gum	Stem	Toothbrush
59	*Syzygium cumini* (L.) Skeels.	Myrtaceae	Cleaning teeth	Tender twigs	Toothbrush
60	*Syzygium fruticosum* DC.	Myrtaceae	Cleans teeth, strengthens teeth and gum	Twig	Toothbrush
61	*Syzygium jambos* (L.) Alston	Myrtaceae	Strengthens gum and teeth	Branch	Toothbrush

TABLE 18.1 *(Continued)*

	Botanical name	Family	Oral care	Part used	Mode of use
62	*Tabernaemontana divaricata* (L.) R. Br. ex Roem. & Schult.	Apocynaceae	Cleaning teeth	Stem, root and latex	Stem and roots serve as toothbrush, and latex prevent pain in tooth
63	*Tamarindus indica* L.	Fabaceae	Strengthens teeth and gum	Bark	Bark powder used as toothpowder
64	*Tephrosia purpurea* (L) Pers.	Fabacea	Cleaning teeth	Stem	Toothbrush
65	*Terminalia arjuna* (Roxb.) Wight & Arn.	Combretaceae	Strengthens teeth and gum	Twig	Toothbrush
66	*Terminalia bellirica* (Gaertn.) Roxb.	Combretaceae	Cleaning teeth	Twig	Toothbrush
67	*Terminalia chebula* Retz.	Combretaceae	Strengthen teeth and gum	Twig	Toothbrush
68	*Terminalia citrina* (Gaertn.) Roxb. ex Flem.	Combretaceae	Cleaning teeth	Twig	Toothbrush
69	*Toddalia asiatica* (L.) Lam.	Rutaceae	Strengthens teeth and gum	Stem	As toothpowder to prevent toothache
70	*Urena lobata* L.	Malvaceae	Cleaning teeth	Stem	Toothbrush
71	*Vachellia farnesiana* (L.) Wight & Arn.	Fabaceae	Strengthens gum and teeth	Tender twigs	Toothbrush
72	*Vitex negundo* L.	Lamiaceae	Cleaning teeth and remedy for toothache	Stem	Toothbrush
73	*Zanthoxylum americanum* Mill.	Rutaceae	Cleaning teeth	Stem and twig	Toothbrush
74	*Ziziphus mauritiana* Lam.	Rhamnaceae	Cleaning teeth	Stem	Toothbrush

18.4.2 PLANTS USED FOR TREATMENT OF ORAL DISEASES

The medicinal plants are the main source of active biological components. These phytochemicals serve as effective substitute to antibiotics and represent an improved approach in dental caries and other oral infections. In a study carried out by Deshmukh et al. (2017) on the evaluation of formulations and herbal toothpaste, they concluded that herbal toothpastes are more acceptable, safer with minimum side effects compared to synthetic preparations in the market. The herbal oral health products are easily available, acceptable, cost effective and restore oral health with minimal side effects with maximum efficiency. The use of herbal products is an easy remedy for promote and maintain oral health. Selected plant species useful in treatment of oral diseases are given in Figure 18.4.

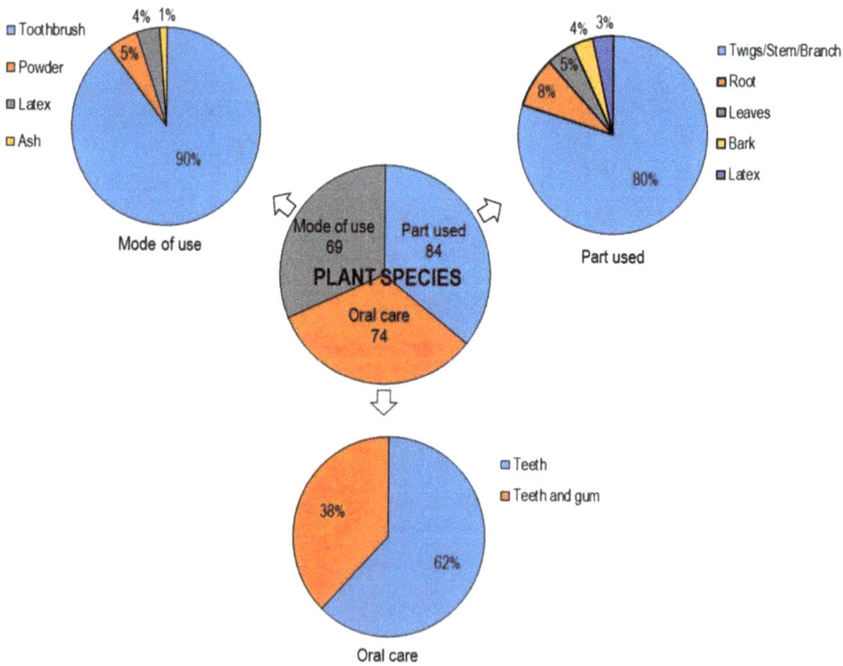

FIGURE 18.3 Uses of plant species in routine oral health and hygiene.

As many as 142 plant species (110 genera) have been recommended for treatment of oral diseases. Applications of various plant species in treatment or cure of oral ailments, parts used, medicinal value, and methods of use are documented in Table 18.2. Among 142 plant species, most commonly used genera of plant species to treat or cure oral ailments include *Solanum* (7 spp.), *Acacia* (5 spp.), *Ficus,* and *Jatropha* (4 spp. each). From 142 plant species, a total of 213 plant materials are used to treat or cure the oral diseases, which consists of a maximum of 53% of twig/stem/branch/root followed by leaves (24%), latex (11%), bark (7%), whole plant (4%), and rhizome (1%) (Figure 18.5). Among 144 mode of uses, use as toothbrush was as high as 34% followed by Chewing (19%), latex/gum/ash, decoction/juice (11% each), crushing (7%), paste (6%), powder (4%), mouthwash (3%), dentifrice (3%), and smoke (2%). Regarding oral disease treatment or care, 57% of plant materials are useful in teeth care, followed by mouth ulcer (12%), gingivitis (11%), tooth decay, helitosis, pyorrhoea (5% ach), dental caries (2%), child teething, gum bleeding, and pharyngitis (1% each).

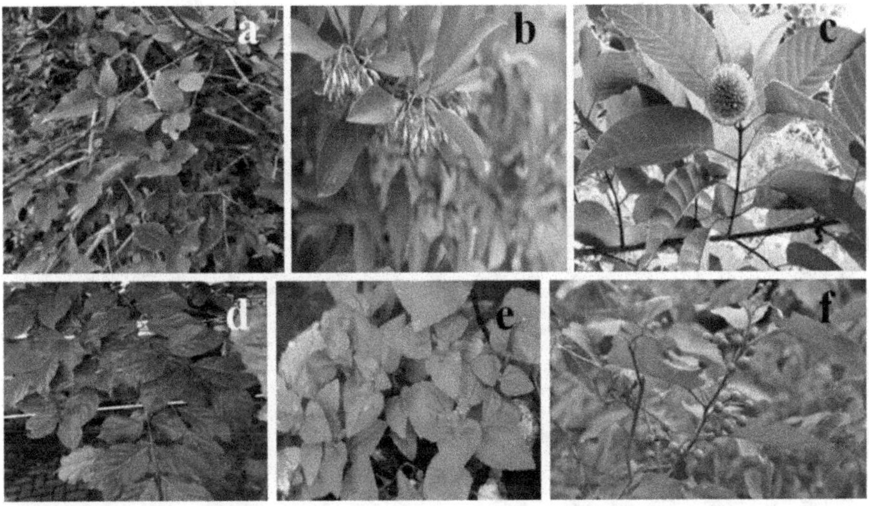

FIGURE 18.4 Selected plant species used in treatment of oral diseases: *Aegle marmelos* (a), *Mimusops elengi* (b), *Neolamarckia cadamba* (c), *Pongamia pinnata* (d), *Solanum torvum* (e), and *Spilanthes paniculata* (f).

18.5 CONCLUSIONS

Traditional practices regarding the use of plant parts for oral health and ailments is rooted in most of rural and ethnic communities. Use of ethno-medicinal practices for oral care as well as to cure or treatment of oral

TABLE 18.2 Plant Species Used in Treating or Curing Oral Diseases.

	Botanical name	Family	Treatment	Part used	Mode of use
1	*Abrus precatorius* Linn.	Fabaceae	Mouth ulcer	Leaves	Chewed for mouth ulcer and toothache
2	*Abutilon indicum* L. Sweet	Malvaceae	Toothache and tooth decay	Leaves	Chewed and swallow the juice
3	*Acacia arabica* (Lam.) Willd.	Mimosaceae	Mouth ulcer, gingivitis, pharyngitis and toothache	Tender stem, leaves, bark and gum	Stem serves as toothbrush, leaves as dentifrice, bark decoction as mouthwash and gum to prevent toothache
4	*Acacia catechu* (L. f.) Willd.	Fabaceae	Toothache	Bark	Dentifrice
5	*Acacia farnesiana* Wild.	Mimosaceae	Pyorrhoea	Tender twigs	Toothbrush
6	*Acacia leucophloea* (Roxb.)' Willd.	Mimosaceae	Toothache and gingivitis	Bark	Bark decoction gargled in toothache and gingivitis
7	*Acacia nilotica* (L.) Delile	Mimosaceae	Toothache and dental caries	Twigs	Toothbrush
8	*Acalypha indica* L.	Euphorbiacea	Toothache and gingivitis	Whole plant	Whole plant decoction given orally in toothache and gingivitis
9	*Achyranthes aspera* Linn.	Amaranthaceae	Toothache and periodontitis	Stem and whole plant ash	Stem used as toothbrush and ash used as toothpowder
10	*Achillea millefolium* L.	Asteraceae	Halitosis and toothache	Leaves	Chewed in halitosis and crushed leaves relieves pain in tooth
11	*Acorus calamus* L.	Acoraceae	Toothache and gingivitis	Rhizome	Paste of the rhizome is applied for toothache and gum
12	*Aegle marmelos* (L.) Corr.	Rutaceae	Toothache and teeth whitening	Twigs	Toothbrush
13	*Ageratum conyzoides* L.	Asteraceae	Mouth ulcer	Leaves	Chewed in mouth ulcer

TABLE 18.2 *(Continued)*

	Botanical name	Family	Treatment	Part used	Mode of use
14	*Agave americana* L.	Agavaceae	Toothache	Leaves	Crushed leaves poultice used for toothache
15	*Alangium salviifolium* (L. f.) Wangerin	Alangiaceae	Halitosis and dental caries	Tender stem	Toothbrush
16	*Albizia amara* (Roxb.) B. Boivin	Mimosaceae	Mouth ulcer	Leaves and bark	Leaf or bark decoction used for mouthwash in mouth ulcer
17	*Albizia lebbeck* (L.) Benth.	Mimosaceae	Toothache	Bark	Dried bark powder used as toothpowder
18	*Allium sativum* L.	Amaryllidaceae	Tooth decay	Bulb	Paste of the bulb applied to the gum and cavities
19	*Ampelocissus latifolia* (Roxb.) Planch.	Vitaceae	Toothache	Leaf	Chewed in toothache
20	*Anacardium occidentale* L.	Asteraceae	Toothache, pyorrhoea, and pharyngitis	Root	Dentifrices
21	*Anacyclus pyrethrum* (L.) Lag.	Lamiaceae	Child teething problems	Leaves	Decoction given orally for child teething problems
22	*Anisomeles malabarica* (L.) R. Br.	Annonaceae	Toothache and gingivitis	Tender stem and leaves	Toothbrush
23	*Annona squamosa* L.	Arecaceae	Dental caries	Seed	Dentifrice
24	*Areca catechu* L.	Boraginaceae	Toothache	Root	Crushed paste applied over painful tooth
25	*Arnebia euchroma* (Royle) I. M. Johnst.	Moraceae	Mouth ulcer	Tender branch	Toothbrush
26	*Artocarpus heterophyllus* Lam.	Liliaceae	Mouth ulcer	Root	Powder with milk consumption orally in recurrent mouth ulcer
27	*Asparagus racemosus* Willd.	Meliaceae	Pyorrhoea	Leaves and twigs	Leaves for teeth cleaning and twigs serve as toothbrush

TABLE 18.2 *(Continued)*

	Botanical name	Family	Treatment	Part used	Mode of use
28	*Azadirachta indica* A. Juss.	Euphorbiaceae	Toothache	Tender twigs	Toothbrush
29	*Baccaurea sapinda* (Roxb.) Müll.-Arg.	Acanthaceae	Toothache and tooth decay	Root and leaves	Tender leaves and root chewed for tooth decay
30	*Barleria prionitis* L.	Caesalpiniacea	Toothache	Twigs	Toothbrush
31	*Bauhinia variegate* L.	Burseraceae	Toothache and gingivitis	Latex and bark	Used as applicant in gingivitis and toothache
32	*Bombax ceiba* L.	Bombacaceae	Toothache	Gum	Gum applied to the cavities of tooth
33	*Bombax ceiba* L.	Rubiaceae	Toothache	Whole plant	Boiled and its steam inhaled in toothache
34	*Borreria articularis* (L. f.) F.N. Williams	Anacardiaceae	Toothache	Gum	Applied over affected area
35	*Buchanania lanzan* Spreng.	Fabaceae	Toothache	Tender stem	Toothbrush
36	*Butea monosperma* (Lam.) Taub.	Asteraceae	Mouth ulcer	Roots	Chewed in mouth ulcer
37	*Caesulia axillaris* Roxb.	Asclepidaceae	Toothache and pyorrhoea	Tender stem and root	Stem used as toothbrush and ash of root applied in pyorrhoea
38	*Calotropis gigantea* (L.) Dryand. Ex T. Aiton	Burseraceae	Gingivitis and mouth ulcer	Latex	Applied in gingivitis and mouth ulcer
39	*Canarium bengalense* Roxb.	Caricaceae	Toothache and mouth ulcer	Latex	Applied for mouth ulcer and toothache
40	*Carica papaya* L.	Caesalpiniaceae	Halitosis	Leaves	Chewed for bad breath
41	*Cassia javanica* L.	Caesalpiniaceae	Toothache	Leaves	Chewed to relive toothache
42	*Cassia occidentalis* L.	Caesalpiniaceae	Child teething problems	Leaves	Decoction given in child teething problems

TABLE 18.2 *(Continued)*

	Botanical name	Family	Treatment	Part used	Mode of use
43	*Cassia tora* Linn.	Asteraceae	Tooth decay	Leaves and twigs	Paste of leaves applied for toothache and twigs serve as toothbrush
44	*Centipeda minima* (L.) A. Braun & Asch.	Lauraceae	Gingivitis, pyorrhoea and halitosis	Branch and leaves	Branch used as toothbrush and leaves chewed to avoid bad breath
45	*Cinnamomum tamala* (Buch.-Ham.) Nees & Eberm.	Lauraceae	Inflammation of gum	Stem	Toothbrush
46	*Cinnamomum verum* J. Presl	Cleomaceae	Toothache	Leaves	Chewed and placed over painful tooth
47	*Cleistanthus collinus* (Roxb.) Benth. ex Hook. f.	Capparidaceae	Toothache	Tender stem	Toothbrush
48	*Crateva nurvala* Buch.-Ham.	Fabaceae	Mouth ulcer	Whole plant	Decoction used as mouthwash in mouth ulcer
49	*Crotalaria retusa* L.	Apiaceae	Mouth ulcer	Seeds	Chewed for mouth ulcer
50	*Cuminum cyminum* L.	Solanaceae	Toothache	Root	Toothbrush
51	*Datura innoxia* Mill.	Solanaceae	Toothache	Seed	Paste applied for toothache
52	*Datura stramonium* L.	Poaceae	Toothache and gingivitis	Root	Decoction as mouth rinse for toothache and gingivitis
53	*Desmostachya bipinnata* (L.) Stapf.	Fabaceae	Toothache	Root	Chewed in toothache
54	*Desmodium gangeticum* (Linn.) DC.	Fabaceae	Toothache	Whole plant	Chewed for toothache
55	*Desmodium triflorum* L. DC.	Fabaceae	Toothache	Tender branches	Chewed for toothache
56	*Desmodium velutinum* (Willd.) DC	Ebenaceae	Toothache and dental caries	Tender branch	Toothbrush

TABLE 18.2 *(Continued)*

	Botanical name	Family	Treatment	Part used	Mode of use
57	*Diospyros montana* Roxb.	Elaeocarpaceae	Toothache and clean teeth	Tender stem	Toothbrush
58	*Elaeocarpus floribundus* Blume	Asteraceae	Toothache	Leaves	Cleaning teeth and for toothache
59	*Elephantopus scaber* L.	Euphorbiacea	Toothache and mouth ulcer	Leaves	Juice instilled into ear for toothache mouth ulcer
60	*Emblica officinalis* Gaertn.	Asteraceae	Toothache	Leaves	Crushed and applied painful tooth
61	*Emilia sonchifolia* (L.) DC. ex DC.	Apiaceae	Toothache	Dried latex	Applied over cavity for instant pain relief
62	*Ferula asafetida* L.	Moraceae	Gingivitis and pyorrhoea	Aerial roots and latex	Roots as toothbrush and latex applied over bleeding gum and for gingivitis
63	*Ficus benghalensis* L.	Moraceae	Gingivitis and clean teeth	Tender stem	Toothbrush
64	*Ficus glomerata* Roxb.	Moraceae	Toothache	Tender and leaves and twigs	Chewed in toothache
65	*Ficus religiosa* L.	Moraceae	Mouth ulcer	Bark	Decoction used as mouthwash for mouth ulcer
66	*Ficus virens* W.T. Aiton	Salicaceae	Clean teeth	Tender branch	Toothbrush
67	*Flacourtia jangomas* (Lour.) Raeusch.	Guttiferae	Toothache	Twigs	Toothbrush
68	*Garcinia lanceifolia* Roxb.	Guttiferae	Dental caries	Tender branches	Toothbrush
69	*Garcinia oxyphylla* Miq.	Guttiferae	Pyorrhoea	Branches	Toothbrush
70	*Garcinia sopsopia* (Buch.-Ham.) Mabb.	Fabaceae	Mouth ulcer and toothache	Root	Toothbrush

TABLE 18.2 *(Continued)*

	Botanical name	Family	Treatment	Part used	Mode of use
71	*Glycyrrhiza glabra* L.	Malvaceae	Toothache	Seed	Ash used for toothache
72	*Gossypium herbaceum* L.	Achariaceae	Tooth decay	Leaves	Chewed for tooth decay
73	*Gynocardia odorata* R. Br.	Perplocaceae	Mouth ulcer	Root	Paste applied over mouth ulcer
74	*Hemidesmus indicus* (L) R. Br. ex Schult	Elaeagnaceae	Halitosis	Root	Chewed in bad breath
75	*Hippophae salicifolia* D. Don	Linaceae	Toothache	Root	Powder applied on painful tooth
76	*Hugonia mystax* L.	Solanaceae	Toothache	Seed	Smoke exposed to affected tooth in toothache
77	*Hyoscyamus niger* Linn.	Fabaceae	Tooth decay	Root	Powder used for brushing for toothache
78	*Indigofera aspalathoides* DC.	Euphorbiaceae	Gingivitis and toothache	Stem	Toothbrush
79	*Jatropha curcas* L.	Euphorbiaceae	Gingivitis and toothache	Tender stem and latex	Stem serves as toothbrush and latex application for gingivitis
80	*Jatropha glandulifera* Roxb.	Euphorbiacea	Mouth ulcer	Latex	Applied for mouth ulcer
81	*Jatropha gossypiifolia* L.	Euphorbiacea	Toothache and gingivitis	Latex	Applied for gingivitis and toothache
82	*Jatropha villosa* Wight	Acanthaceae	Halitosis and pyorrhoea	Tender stem	Toothbrush
83	*Justicia adhatoda* L.	Lamiaceae	Toothache	Leaf	Paste applied on gum for toothache
84	*Lavandula bipinnata* (Roth) Kuntze	Lythraceae	Toothache	Stem and bark	Toothbrush to relive toothache
85	*Lawsonia alba* Lam.	Lythraceae	Mouth ulcer	Leaves	Gargle with leaf juice for mouth ulcer

TABLE 18.2 *(Continued)*

	Botanical name	Family	Treatment	Part used	Mode of use
86	*Lawsonia inermis* L.	Lauraceae	Gingivitis and pyorrhoea	Tender stem	Toothbrush
87	*Litsea citrata* Blume	Lamiaceae	Toothache and gingivitis	Leaves	Chewed for toothache and gingivitis
88	*Leucas aspera* (Willd.) Link	Magnoliaceae	Toothache	Branch	Toothbrush
89	*Magnolia hodgsonii* (Hook. f & Thomson) H. Keng	Anacardiaceae	Toothache and gingivitis	Twigs and latex	Twigs used as toothbrush and latex applied for gingivitis
90	*Mangifera indica* L.	Melastomeaceae	Gingivitis	Tender stem	Toothbrush
91	*Melastoma malabathricum* L.	Meliaceae	Toothache	Twigs	Toothbrush
92	*Melia azedarach* L.	Sapotaceae	Gingivitis	Stem an bark	Toothbrush
93	*Mimusops elengi* L.	Moringaceae	Tooth decay	Root	Crushed and directly applied over tooth cavity
94	*Moringa oleifera* Lam.	Cucurbitaceae	Toothache	Root	Chewed or gargle with root decoction relives toothache
95	*Mukia maderaspatana* (L.) M. Roem.	Spreng Rutaceae	Toothache	Tender branch	Toothbrush
96	*Murraya koenigii* (L.) Spreng.	Rutaceae	Toothache	Stem	Toothbrush
97	*Murraya paniculata* (L.) Jack	Myricaceae	Toothache	Bark	Chewed for toothache
98	*Myrica esculenta* Buch.-Ham. ex D. Don	Oleaceae	Gingivitis	Twigs	Toothbrush

TABLE 18.2 *(Continued)*

	Botanical name	Family	Treatment	Part used	Mode of use
99	*Nyctanthes arbor-tristis* L.	Lamiaceae	Halitosis	Leaves	Chewed for bad breath.
100	*Ocimum basilicum* L.	Piperaceae	Toothache	Leaves	Crushed and applied over painful tooth
101	*Pedalium murex* L.	Euphorbiacea	Tooth decay and toothache	Twigs and fruits	Twigs used as toothbrush and fruits chewed for bad breath
102	*Phyllanthus amarus* Schum. & Thonn.	Piperaceae	Halitosis	Leaves	Chewed for bad breath
103	*Phyllanthus emblica* L.	Euphorbiacea	Mouth ulcer	Leaves	Chewed in mouth ulcer
104	*Piper betle* Linn.	Plantaginaceae	Toothache and gum bleeding	Leaves	Crushed and applied over affected tooth and gum
105	*Plantago major* L.	Apocynaceae	Mouth ulcer	Latex	Applied over mouth ulcer
106	*Plumeria obtusa* L.	Apocynaceae	Mouth ulcer	Latex	Latex applied over mouth ulcer
107	*Plumeria acutifolia* Mull. Arg.	Ceasalpineaceae	Toothache	Tender branch	Toothbrush
108	*Pongamia pinnata* (L.) Pierre	Rosaceae	Toothache and gum diseases	Root and leaves	Decoction of root and leaves used as gargle in toothache and gum ailments
109	*Potentilla fulgens* Wall. ex Hook.	Rosaceae	Tooth decay	Root	Paste used for tooth decay
110	*Potentilla lineata* Trevir.	Myrtaceae	Mouth ulcer	Tender stem	Toothbrush
111	*Psidium guajava* L.	Onagraceae	Mouth ulcer	Leaves	Chewed in mouth ulcer
112	*Punica granatum* L.	Euphorbiacea	Toothache	Seeds	Crushed seeds fried in mustered oil till it emit smoke and the smoke is directed toward effected tooth
113	*Ricinus communis* L.	Rubiaceae	Gingivitis	Leaves	Paste applied over swollen gum
114	*Rubia cordifolia* L	Caesalpinaceae	Gingivitis	Tender stem	Toothbrush

TABLE 18.2 *(Continued)*

	Botanical name	Family	Treatment	Part used	Mode of use
115	*Saraca indica* L.	Asteracea	Toothache	Tuber	Decoction used to gargle mouth in toothache
116	*Saussurea costus* (Falc.) Lipsch.	Scrophullariaceae	Toothache	Whole plant	Decoction used for gargle for toothache
117	*Scoparia dulcis* L.	Verbenaceae	Toothache	Leaf	Crushed leaf placed over painful tooth
118	*Semecarpus anacardium* Linn.	Papilionaceae	Mouth ulcer	Leaf	Decoction used as mouthwash for mouth ulcer
119	*Sesbania grandiflora* (L.) Pers.	Solanaceae	Tooth decay	Seeds and flower	Dried seeds or flower kept in mouth for tooth decay
120	*Solanum ferox* L.	Solanaceae	Toothache	seeds	Dried seeds kept in mouth for toothache
121	*Solanum khasianum* Clarke	Solanaceae	Mouth ulcer	Leaves and fruit	Leaves and fruits chewed for mouth ulcer
122	*Solanum nigrum* L.	Solanaceae	Toothache	Fruit	Dried fruit smoke exposed to effected tooth relives toothache
123	*Solanum surattense* Burm. f.	Solanaceae	Toothache	Root	Toothbrush
124	*Solanum torvum* Sw.	Solanaceae	Tooth decay	Fruit	Ash applied for the dental caries
125	*Solanum virginianum* L.	Solanaceae	Toothache	Fruit	Smoke of burnt fruit exposed to effected tooth relives toothache
126	*Solanum xanthocarpum* Schrad. & H. Wendl.	Asteraceae	Toothache	Flower	Crushed and applied over painful tooth
127	*Spilanthes acmella* Murr.	Asteraceae	Toothache	Flower	Crushed and applied over painful tooth
128	*Spilanthes clava* DC.	Asteraceae	Toothache	Leaves and roots	Chewed for toothache
129	*Spilanthes paniculata* Wall. ex DC.	Moraceae	Toothache and gingivitis	Stem	Toothbrush

TABLE 18.2 *(Continued)*

	Botanical name	Family	Treatment	Part used	Mode of use
130	*Streblus asper* Lour	Apocyanaceae	Toothache	Stem root and latex	Stem as toothbrush and latex applied over painful tooth
131	*Tabernaemontana divaricata* (L.) R. Br. ex Roem. & Schult.	Combretaceae	Mouth ulcer and pyorrhoea	Twig	Toothbrush
132	*Terminalia citrina* Roxb. ex Flem.	Apocynaceae	Toothache	Latex	Latex applied over cavities for toothache
133	*Thevetia peruviana* (Pers.) K. Schum.	Poaceae	Mouth ulcer	Root	Decoction used to gargle for mouth ulcer
134	*Thysanolaena maxima* (Roxb.) Kuntze	Rutaceae	Toothache	stem	Stem powder used as toothpowder for toothache
135	*Toddalia asiatica* (L.) Lam.	Malvaceae	Toothache	Stem	Toothbrush
136	*Urena lobata* L.	Verbenaceae	Toothache	Stem	Toothbrush
137	*Vitex negundo* L.	Apocynaceae	Toothache	Leaves	Chewed and placed over painful tooth
138	*Wrightia tinctoria* (Roxb.) R. Br.	Rutaceae	Toothache	Seeds	Chewed for toothache
139	*Zanthoxylum alatum* Roxb.	Rutaceae	Toothache, Pyorrhoea	Stem and twig	Toothbrush
140	*Zanthoxylum hamiltonianum* Wall. ex Hook. f.	Zingiberaceae	Toothache and tooth decay	Rhizome	Paste applied for painful tooth and tooth decay
141	*Zingiber officinale* Roscoe	Rhamnaceae	Halitosis	Stem	Toothbrush
142	*Zizyphus mauritiana* Lam.	Rhamnaceae	Halitosis	Stem	Toothbrush

diseases has gained more importance due to less adverse health effects. This treasure of knowledge is not well practiced owing to transfer of such information orally from generation to generation. Some plants those are useful for dental care are difficult to find (especially in urban areas) and some geographic zones due to anthropogenic interference such as deforestation and increased pollution levels. Attempts should be made to integrate these traditional practices along with conventional treatments in a conscientious manner. Considerable evidences are available to demonstrate the potential of herbal materials or their extracts as natural products to alleviate oral health and hygiene. This study provides a database on usefulness of ethnic knowledge on plant species useful for oral health. Further, research on methods of use, advantages, and active compounds of these plant species have high potential to tackle the oral diseases more precisely.

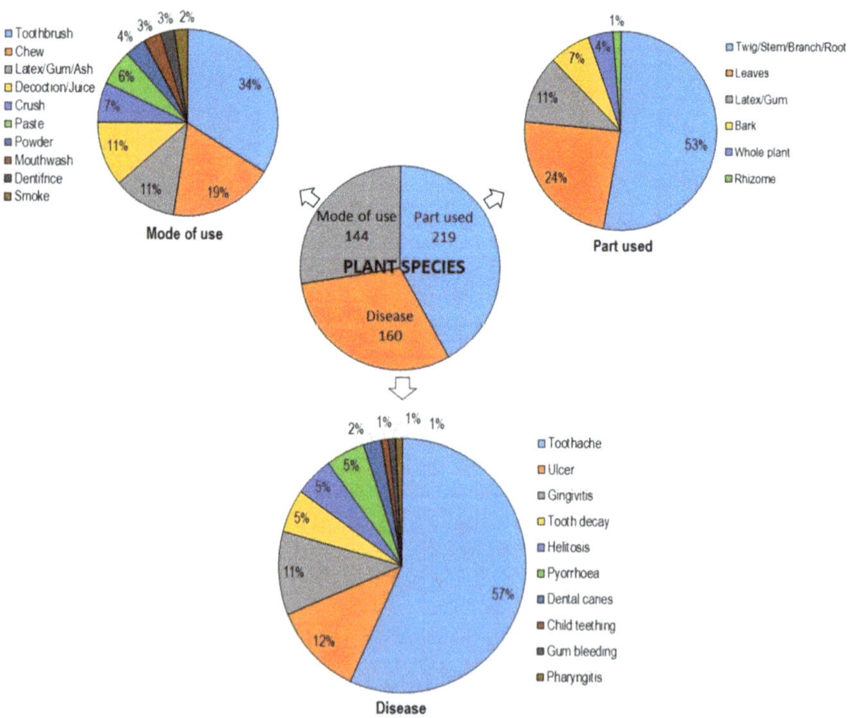

FIGURE 18.5 Uses of plant species in treatment or cure of oral diseases.

KEYWORDS

- **ethnomedicine**
- **medicinal plants**
- **oral care**
- **oral diseases**
- **traditional knowledge**

REFERENCES

Amruthesh, S. Dentistry and Ayurveda–IV: Classification and Management of Common Oral Diseases. *Ind. J. Dent. Res.* **2008,** *19*, 52–61.

Asokan, S.; Emmadi, P.; Chamundeswari, R. Effect of Oil Pulling on Plaque Induced Gingivitis: A Randomized, Controlled, Triple-Blind Study. *Ind. J. Dent. Res.* **2009,** *20*, 47–51.

Bairy, I.; Reeja, S.; Siddharth et al. Evaluation of Antibacterial Activity of Mangifera indica on Anaerobic Dental Microflora Based on In Vivo Studies. *Ind. J. Pathol. Microbiol.* **2002,** *45*, 307–310.

Bartold, P. M.; Van Dyke, T. An appraisal of the Role of Specific Bacteria in the Initial Pathogenesis of Periodontitis. *Clin. Periodontol.* **2019,** 6–11.

Bratthall, D.; Petersen, P. E.; Stjernswärd, J. R. et al. Oral and Craniofacial Diseases and Disorders. In *Disease Control Priorities in Developing Countries*, 2nd ed.; The World Bank: Washington DC, 2006; pp 723–736.

Carrozzo, M.; Porter, S.; Mercadante, V.; Fedele, S. Oral Lichen Planus: A Disease or a Spectrum of Tissue Reactions? Types, Causes, Diagnostic Algorhythms, Prognosis, Management Strategies. *Periodontol.* **2000,** *80*, 105–125.

Casparis, S.; Borm, J. M.; Tektas, S. et al. Oral Lichen Planus (OLP), Oral Lichenoid Lesions (OLL), Oral Dysplasia, and Oral Cancer: Retrospective Analysis of Clinicopathological Data from 2002–2011. *Oral Max. Surg.* **2015,** *19*, 149–156.

Deo, P.; Deshmukh, R. Oral Microbiome: Unveiling the Fundamentals. *J. Oral Max. Pathol.* **2019,** *23*, 122–128.

Deshmukh, P.; Telrandhe, R.; Gunde, M. Formulation and Evaluation of Herbal Toothpaste: Compared with Marketed Preparation. *Int. J. Pharm. Drug Anal.* **2017,** *5*, 406–410.

He, J.; Li, Y.; Cao, Y. et al. The Oral Microbiome Diversity and Its Relation to Human Diseases. *Folia Microbiol.* **2015,** *60*, 69–80.

Highfield, J. Diagnosis and Classification of Periodontal Disease. *Aust. Dent. J.* **2009,** *54* (Suppl 1), S11–S26.

Hiranmayi, K. V.; Sirisha, K.; Rao, M. R.; Sudhakar, P. Novel Pathogens in Periodontal Microbiology. *J. Pharm. Bioallied Sci.* **2009,** *9*, 155–163.

Holmstrup, P.; Plemons, J.; Meyle, J. Non–Plaque-Induced Gingival Diseases. *J. Clin. Periodontol.* **2018,** *45*, S28–S43.
Jia, G.; Zhi, A.; Lai, A. et al. The Oral Microbiota—A Mechanistic Role for Systemic Diseases. *Br. Dent. J.* **2018,** *224*, 447–455.
Karadağlıoğlu, Ö. İ.; Ulusoy, N.; Başer, K. H. C. et al. Antibacterial Activities of Herbal Toothpastes Combined with Essential Oils Against *Streptococcus mutans*. *Pathogens* **2019,** *8*, 20.
Krishnan, K.; Chen, T.; Paster, B. J. A Practical Guide to the Oral Microbiome and Its Relation to Health and Disease. *Oral Dis.* **2017,** *23*, 276–286.
Mosaddad, S. A.; Tahmasebi, E.; Yazdanian, A. et al. Oral Microbial Biofilms: An Update. *Eur. J. Clin. Microbiol. Infect. Dis.* **2019,** *38*, 2005–2019.
Patil, S.; Rao, R. S.; Sanketh, D. S.; Amrutha, N. Microbial Flora in Oral Diseases. *J. Contemp. Dent. Pract.* **2013,** *14*, 1202–1208.
Peiris, K. P. P.; Samaranayake, G. V. P.; Dewasurendra, D. M. In Vitro Microbiological Study on an Indigenous Mouthwash (Gandusha) for Periodontal Disease. *Int. J. Rec. Sci. Res.* **2019,** 31610–31613.
Pitts, N. B.; Zero, D. T.; Marsh, P. D. et al. Dental Caries. *Nat. Rev. Dis. Primers* **2017,** *3*, 1–16.
Safiaghdam, H.; Oveissi, V.; Bahramsoltani, R. et al. Medicinal Plants for Gingivitis: A Review of Clinical Trials. *Iran. J. Basic Med. Sci.* **2018,** *21*, 978–991.
Siddiqui, Y. D.; Omori, K.; Ito, T. et al. Resolvin D2 Induces Resolution of Periapical Inflammation and Promotes Healing of Periapical Lesions in Rat Periapical Periodontitis. *Front. Immunol.* **2019,** *10*, 307. DOI: 10.3389/fimmu.2019.00307
Singh, A.; Purohit, B. Tooth Brushing, Oil Pulling and Tissue Regeneration: A Review of Holistic Approaches to Oral Health. *J. Ayur. Integr. Med.* **2011,** *2*, 64–68.
Van der Waal, I.; Schepman, K. P.; Van der Meij, E. H.; Smeele, L. E. Oral Leukoplakia: A Clinicopathological Review. *Oral Oncol.* **1997,** *33*, 291–301.
Venugopal, T.; Kulkarni, V. S.; Nerurker, R. A. et al. Epidemiological Study of Dental Caries. *Ind. J. Pediatr.* **1998,** *65*, 883–889.
Weston, G.; Payette, M. Update on Lichen Planus and Its Clinical Variants. *Int. J. Womens Dermatol.* **2015,** *1*, 140–149.
Yamashita, Y.; Takeshita, T. The Oral Microbiome and Human Health. *J. Oral Sci.* **2017,** *59*, 201–206.

PART VI

Other Applications Related to Health

CHAPTER 19

Ethnomedicinal Applications of 100 Wild Mushrooms of the Indian Subcontinent

SHIVANNEGOWDA MAHADEVAKUMAR[1], CHANDAGALU R. SANTHOSH[2], BETTADAPURA R. NUTHAN[2], KANDIKERE R. SRIDHAR[3,4] SREEDHARAMURTHY SATISH[2], and KESTUR N. AMRUTHESH[1]

[1]*Department of Studies in Botany, University of Mysore, Manasagangotri, Mysore, Karnataka, India*

[2]*Department of Studies in Microbiology, University of Mysore, Manasagangotri, Mysuru, Karnataka, India*

[3]*Department of Biosciences, Mangalore University, Mangalagangotri, Mangalore, Karnataka, India*

[4]*Centre for Environmental Studies, Yenepoya (deemed to be) University, Mangalore, Karnataka, India*

ABSTRACT

The Indian subcontinent embraced about 550 tribal communities with nearly 50 million population. They are intimately associated with the natural resources such as flora, fauna, and forest products in their vicinity for their nutrition, health, agriculture, and shelter. In addition to nutrition, several wild or ethnomedicinal mushrooms are used by many tribals for medicinal, nutraceutical, and health-promoting purposes. Tribal knowledge on the medicinal mushrooms is one of the main phases to go forward to authenticate the pharmaceutical values. This review sheds light on the use

Ethnic Knowledge and Perspectives of Medicinal Plants, Volume 1: Curative Properties and Treatment Strategies. Munir Ozturk, Kandikere R. Sridhar, Maryam Sarwat, Volkan Altay, & Francisco Martín Huerta-Martínez (Eds.)

of 100 wild mushrooms (belong to 61 genra) toward medicinal or health care purposes by the ethnic groups mainly from the northern region of India. Among the 12 states of the Indian subcontinent, the highest number of ethnomedicinal mushrooms occur in Jammu and Kashmir (42 spp.) followed by Uttar Pradesh (36 spp.) and West Bengal (20 spp.). The highest number of medicinal mushrooms are used for single ailment (35 spp.) followed by two (28 spp.) and three (20 spp.) diseases. Among the 21 ailments, as high as 42 mushrooms are used to tackle dermatological problems followed by respiratory (20 spp.) and hematological (18 spp.) diseases. Up to 16 mushrooms are used as food or as health drink (or tonic). A maximum of six species each of *Russula* and *Termitomyces* are used in ethnomedicine, followed by five species of *Morchella*. Different facets discussed include wild mushrooms, ethnomedicinal mushrooms, current developments, and future challenges on the ethnomedicinal mushrooms of India.

19.1 INTRODUCTION

Tribals in India are confined to a specific geographic area and have their own unique practices of utilizing the available natural resources for their day-to-day needs. They are usually isolated from the mainstream of population, dwell in forests, and occupies a dominant position in the tribal society (Tribal Health Bulletin, 2014). The knowledge and practices of utilization of the natural resources available in their tribal locality will be transmitted to their kins from generation to generation (Panda and Tayung, 2015; Ozturk et al., 2020, 2021a, b). However, tribals are being away from the urban locations, there will be a clear knowledge gap of ethnic know how on the natural resources (e.g., wild plants, animals, and mushrooms) around them to treat various ailments. Documentation of such knowledge is the primary step to follow new inventions to treat human ailments. Understanding the value of ethnic health practices expands the basic knowledge of the investigators (biologists and anthropologists) to gain precise insight. Understanding the traditional knowledge on usefulness of wild medicinal plants is the basis for the development of specific or new drugs and pharmaceuticals (Posey, 2002; Srinivas et al., 2019; Pleskanovskaya et al., 2019; Ozturk and Hakeem, 2018, 2019a, b; Ozturk et al., 2017a, b, c, 2018a, b, c, d, e, f, g, 2020; Masoodi et al., 2020; Younessi-Hamzekhanlu et al., 2020). Anthropologists and biologists will try to understand and connect the intricate relationship of tribals with the nature to gain precise knowledge to develop possible pharmaceutically valued products of health concern. Tribals occupy crucial position and serve as primary knowledge bank for sustainable human needs (diet, health, agriculture, and shelter). Samorini (2001) has pointed out that mushrooms are used in traditional medicine in the neolithic and paleolithic eras. Vikineswary and Chang (2013) have documented the importance of mushrooms in prevention of lifestyle diseases.

Tribals distributed in different regions of the Indian subcontinent utilize wild *mushrooms* for a variety of benefits especially for diet and health care. Use of macrofungi (or also called "mushrooms") as medicine goes back to the prehistoric times and it has become an integral part of socio-economic and cultural values of tribes (Charaya and Mehrotra, 1999). Ethnomycology was in practice in India during 17001100 BC (Wasson, 1971). According to Purkayastha and Chandra (1985), up to 283 mushrooms are used for consumption in India, likewise several mushrooms serve as nutraceuticals as well as medicines for common illness. The WHO (2002–2005) in its report has pointed out that ethnomedicine used in Arabic, Ayurveda, Chinese, and Unani has attracted the attention throughout the world. Traditional knowledge is the basis for scientific management, conservation, and sustainable practice of natural resources (Gadgil et al., 1993; Ozturk et al., 2021a, b). The Science, Technology, and Innovation Policy by the Department of Science and Technology, the Government of India has proposed to accelerate the ancient and contemporary knowledge for future scientific advancement (Patwardhan and Lakhotia, 2021). Ethnomedicinal uses of mushrooms have been distributed in various publications, are of immense value to test, and to develop specific useful pharmaceutical products. In view of documentation and bioprospecting of wild medicinal mushrooms used by the tribals of the Indian subcontinent, this review focuses to project the diversity of wild mushrooms, ethnomedicinal uses along with current developments and future challenges.

19.2 WILD MUSHROOMS

The global diversity of fungi although a black box, it has been cautiously estimated between 2.2 and 3.8 million species based on the ratio of angiosperms and fungi (Hawksworth and Lücking, 2017; Hawksworth, 2019). The current globally known fungi are about 144,000, while the Indian subcontinent possesses up to 29,000, which is close to 20% of known fungi (Manoharachary et al., 2005; Cannon et al., 2018; Niskanen et al., 2018; Wills, 2018; Hawksworth, 2019). Hawksworth (2001) estimated 140,000 mushrooms occur globally based on 10% of the global estimate of all fungi.

However, it has been revised recently as only 3.7–6.4% (Hawksworth, 2019). Based on the figures of expected number of species of all fungi in the Indian subcontinent (96,000), expected number of mushrooms will be around 15,300 species (Hawksworth, 2019).

India is rich in biodiversity of wild mushrooms owing to four mega biodiversity hotspots (Western Ghats, Western Himalayas, Eastern Himalayas, and Nicobar Islands) (Singh and Chaturvedi, 2017). Many mycologists significantly contributed to the diversity of wild mushrooms of the Indian subcontinent. Berkeley (1867) enhanced the knowledge on Agarics from Nilgiri Biosphere reserve of the Western Ghats (see Manjula, 1983 for more contributions of Barkeley). A large number of agarics (*Lepiota, Leucocoprinus,* and *Macrolepiota*) were reported by Butler and Bisby (1931). Purkayastha and Chandra (1985) in their manual of edible mushrooms described several mushrooms along with their pattern of distribution. Bilgrami et al. (1991) documented a wealth of mushrooms in their book *Fungi of India.* Later, Natarajan and coworkers enriched the knowledge on mushrooms of the Western Ghats (Natarajan and Manjula 1983; Natarajan, 1995; Natarajan et al., 2005).

The Western Ghats roughly possess about 700–750 species belonging to 70–75 genera, among them about 10% (70–80 spp.) are known by local communities in Maharashtra, Goa, Karnataka, Kerala, and Tamil Nadu to be safe for human consumption (Kamat, 1994). Sridhar (2019) consolidated selected literature on mushrooms of the Western Ghats (books/monographs, reviews, checklists, diversity, distribution, mycorrhizae, nutrition, and bioactive properties). A total of 550 mushrooms were documented (166 genera and 51 families of Basidiomycota and Ascomycota) from the forest regions of Kerala (Mohanan 2011).

Leelavathy and Ganesh (2000) documented polypore mushrooms of Kerala. Manimohan and his team contributed significantly toward the mushrooms of Kerala by adding several new taxa and focused mainly on the systematics (e.g., Manimohan et al., 2006; Farook et al., 2013; Aravindakhan and Manimohan, 2015; Latha and Manimohan, 2017). Up to 25 species of wild mushrooms are consumed by the tribals of Kerala and the most common species include *Lentinus, Pleurotus,* and *Termitomyces* (Varghese et al., 2010). Usha and Janardhana (2014) recorded a total of 134 mushrooms belonging to 56 genera and 34 families in Karnataka. From the forests and coffee agroforests, 157 species of mushrooms have been documented by Karun and Sridhar (2016). Up to 20 species of termitomycetes were recorded from the Western Ghats region (Karun and Sridhar, 2013). Karun and Sridhar (2014) also documented 79 species of mushrooms from the southwest coast of Karnataka. Among them 25 species were ectomycorrhizal, 17 species were edible and 10 species were medicinal.

Significant contributions on the taxonomy and diversity of mushrooms in northern India (Sarwal, 1984; Atri and Saini, 2000). Kaur et al. (2013) and Kumar et al. (2014) described 92 species under the genus *Lepiota*. Several mushrooms have been found in buffalo dung from Punjab (e.g., Amandeep et al., 2013). A 5 years inventory (2008–2012) in West Bengal revealed 34 wild mushrooms, among them 31 are edible (Dutta and Acharya, 2014). Khaund and Joshi (2013) have documented 11 edible wild mushrooms used by the Khasi tribe of Meghalaya. Bhatt et al. (2016) documented 219 species of mushrooms from the Garhwal Himalaya. Among them, *Cantharellus cibarius, Cantharellus minor, Grifola frondosa,* and *Morchella esculenta* are commonly consumed by the local people. Three tribal communities (*Biate, Karbi,* and *Khelma*) of Assam possess traditional knowledge on the edibility of about 19 wild mushrooms (Borah et al., 2018). Wild edible mushrooms of forests in northern Orissa have been studied by Panda et al. (2019) and reported 20 mushrooms. These mushrooms are of socioeconomic significance as they provide livelihoods for the rural and tribal people of Orissa. Atri (2020) has consolidated ecology, conservation, nutritional, nutraceutical, and sociobiological aspects of mushrooms of the northern India.

19.3 ETHNOMEDICINAL MUSHROOMS

The ethnomedicine (or traditional medicine) has been recognized as paramount importance and up to 80% of world's populations is dependent on ethnomedicine (Jian and Singh, 2010). In the developing countries like India, more than 65% of population in rural areas uses ethnic knowledge-based medicine to meet their primary health care. India has been inhabited up to 550 tribal communities with a population over 50 million in the Western Ghats, eastern India, eastern Himalayas, and other parts (Binu et al., 1992). These traditional medicinal practices have been conserved for several centuries and serve as an effective means toward identification of novel principles for modern value-added therapeutics or drugs (Jian and Singh, 2010; Ozturk et al., 2020, 2021a, b).

Practice of consuming mushrooms is as old as human civilization, but accurate documentation of such ethnic knowledge is deficient. Perceptions, concepts, and mode of utilization of mushrooms for disease treatment or control differ among cultural groups (Haro-Luna et al., 2019). Atri and Mridu (2018) has given a precise account of ethnomycological scenario in

India. Ethnomycological research carried out from various parts of India also documented such differences among the tribes. India is having a lot of variation in cultures, customs, and ethnic knowledge across and within the states about the use of mushrooms as diet and or medicine. Some of the states in India where mushrooms are used as medicine include Arunachal Pradesh, Assam, Manipur, Nagaland, Orissa, and West Bengal (Baruah et al., 1971; Sing and Sing, 1993; Sing et al., 2002; Sarma et al., 2010; Tanti et al., 2011).

Kamat (1994) has explored ethnomycology in Goa with special reference to termitomycetes, psychedelic, and other mushrooms. Diversity, distribution, ethnic value, and related attributes of 11 species of *Termitomyces* were recorded in Kodagu region of Western Ghats (Pahlevanlo et al., 2011; Pahlevanlo and Janardhana, 2012a, b). So far, 31 species of mushrooms have been reported from the elephant dung mainly in Karnataka and Kerala (Karun and Sridhar, 2015). Based on the tribal knowledge, 51 species of edible mushrooms have been identified in the Western Ghats of Karnataka (Karun and Sridhar, 2017). From the lateritic scrub jungles of southwest Karnataka, a new ectomycorrhizal *Amanita* species has been recorded (Karun and Sridhar, 2014). It is one of the delicacies of the coastal dwellers and it will be eaten in tender stage of growth (egg or dumble shape). Similar observation was made with respect to edibility of immature *Amanita bisporigera* in the West Bengal region (Singha et al., 2020). Similar to *Aminata*, another delicy mushroom is *Astraeus hygrometricus* from the foothills of the Western Ghats (Pavithra et al., 2015). The livelihood of some of the tribes' residing in the foothills of the Western Ghats depends on the trade of this mushroom in the local markets during the southwest monsoon season.

Varghese et al. (2010) have documented tribal importance of 21 wild mushrooms of Kerala. Paniya, Kattunaikkar, and Kuruma are aware of wild mushrooms used for edibility as well as medicinal. Tribal women are highly efficient in identifying the poisonous and non-poisonous mushrooms. Toxic and hallucinogenic mushrooms have also been reported from Vrinda and Pradeep (2011). Tamil Nadu has 36 tribal communities and six communities are living in Kanyakumari District depending on wild mushrooms for food and medicine, the majority of tribe called *Kaani* employs seven wild mushrooms as source of food (Sargunam et al., 2012). Venkatachalapathi and Paulsamy (2016) documented 30 wild medicinal mushrooms in the Walayar Valley of Tamil Nadu based on the knowledge by the *Irula* tribe. These medicinal mushrooms are used to treat eight human ailments (cardiovascular, dermatological, endocrinal, gastrointestinal, genitourinary, liver, respiratory, and skeletal-muscle disorders).

Ethnomedicinal uses of termitomycetes in Uttar Pradesh have been documented by Srivasthava et al. (2011). Twelve ethnic tribal groups in Nagaland possess extensive traditional mycological knowledge and they trade 13 edible wild mushrooms in Kohima Town (Tanti et al., 2011). It is interesting to note that although some of these edible fleshy mushrooms are sold in the markets during March through September, *Pleurotus ostreatus* owing to substantial availability sold afresh during April to August, while in dried form throughout the year. Further, the price of this dried mushroom is twice than the fresh mushrooms. In Sikkim, *Cordyceps* is one of the main medicinal mushrooms, which is usefulness to treat as many as 21 human ailments (e.g., cancer, asthama, tuberculosis, diabetes, jaundice, and hepatitis) (Panda and Swain, 2011). The Khasi tribal people of Meghalaya can distinguish edible and poisonous mushrooms based on morphological grounds (Khaund and Joshi, 2013).

It is interesting to note that the tribal population (*Santal*) live in fringes of forests (Bihar, Orissa, Chattisgarh, and Jarkhand) depend on about 18 wild edible mushrooms for their livelihood during monsoon season (Manna et al., 2014). The most prominent wild mushrooms preferred include *Amanita banningiana, A. hygrometricus, Russula nigricans,* and *Termitomyces microcarpus.* Tribes of Nagaland (*Aoo Naga*) utilize 20 edible wild mushrooms as food source (Kumar et al., 2014). Dutta and Acharya (2014) recognized five ethnically used medicinal mushrooms in a survey in West Bengal. Semwal et al. (2014) documented up to 23 species of edible and or medicinal wild mushrooms. Malik et al. (2017) documented 33 mushrooms (used by tribals as well as herbalists) and their ethnomedicinal uses of Kashmir. Up to 14 communities residing in Dehradun have been surveyed about their indigenous knowledge on medicinal mushrooms (Kumar et al, 2017). Indigenous people are well informed about the edible and poisonous mushrooms in their vicinity.

Bhatt et al. (2018) studied medicinal mushrooms of Uttarakhand and reported 15 mushrooms possess therapeutic potential. They have documented medicinal properties of these mushrooms with emphasis on their importance to treat different diseases and illness. Enthnomycological and sociobiological aspects of mushrooms of India along with different countries worldwide have been reviewed (Atri and Mridu, 2018; Atri et al., 2019; Atri, 2020). Debnath et al. (2019) have documented the uses of medicinal mushrooms by tribals for various diseases mainly in northern India. The tribal community in India used medicinal mushrooms as powder, powder mixed in drinks or other items (e.g., water, milk, tea, vegetables, chilli, sugar, oil, butter, and egg). Among the ethnomedicinal mushrooms, 18 genera are extensively used by ethnic tribes (*Agaricus, Astraeus, Auricularia, Bovista, Coprinus, Flammulina, Fomes, Ganoderma, Hericium, Phallus, Pisolithus, Pleurotus, Lactarius Lentinus, Lycoperdon, Morchella, Termitomyces,* and *Trametes*). It is predicted that such diversity of medicinal mushrooms occur due to climatic conditions as well as diverse vegetation. A survey of forest-dwelling tribes in Gurguripal (West Bengal) revealed 19 species of wild mushrooms are effectively used to treat human ailments by the traditional healers (Singha et al., 2020).

19.4 ETHNOMEDICINAL APPLICATIONS

Usefulness of mushrooms in the treatment of illnesses based on traditional medicinal systems have a long history. The Greek physician Dioscorides mentioned about the use of mushroom "*Fomitopsis officinalis*" (*Agaricum*), which was later known as Quinine conk, in his monumental work "*De Materia Medica*" (Pala et al., 2013). This fungus was used to treat the respiratory disease tuberculosis. It was evident from the literature that the *Pleurotus* species (e.g., *Pleurotus tuberregium*) are used to treat headache, stomach ailments, cold, fever, asthma, high blood pressure, and small pox. Similarly, there are reports on the use of mushrooms to cure epilepsy, burns, wounds, dermal problems, heart-related complaints, rheumatoid arthritis, cholera, and recurring fever.

Mushrooms have been proved by in vivo and in vitro tests that they have cytotoxic, antimicrobial, and hepatoprotective capacity, hence act against cancer aswell as diabetes (cf. Mortimer et al., 2021). Some of the potential medicinal mushrooms include: *Ganoderma lucidum* (antitumor, antioxidant, and antimicrobial), *Hericium erinaceus* (nerve damage repair and neuroregenerative), *Cordyceps* (against diabetes), and *Inonotus obliquus* (antitumor, against diabetes, and treat cardiovascular ailments). Mushrooms have been extensively used globally owing to their nutritional and medicinal attributes, mainly in some of the countries in Asia, North America, and Central America (Badalyan, 2014). Mushrooms serve as diet for many years due to their nutritional, aroma, therapeutic properties, and economic benefits.

Major studies on ethnomedicinal mushrooms of tribes of the Indian subcontinent comes from Jammu and Kashmir (Pala et al., 2013; Malik et al., 2017). Use of 35 medicinally valued mushrooms belonging to 28 genera and 20 familes by the tribals and herbal healers have been recorded (Pala et al., 2013). They were having broad spectrum medicinal applications including treating simple skin diseases to more complex disease like diabetes and cancer. Indigenous people having immense knowledge of mushrooms used in food and medicines by various tribes of *Chakrata* (Dehradun) were documented by Kumar et al. (2017). A total of 63 mushrooms documented from the tribes of *Chakrata* having food and medicinal value, among them only two and one mushrooms were used to treat burn (*A. hygrometricus* and *Geastrum triplex*) and pus remedy (*A. auricula-judae*), respectively.

Devi (2017) reported the use of four mushrooms from indigenous people of Assam (*Auricularia judae, G. lucidum, Lentinula edodes,* and *Bovista plumbea*). Although there were other macrofungal resources reported by Devi (2017), they were used mainly to serve as source of food. Ethnomycological knowledge from three indigenous people of Assam (*Karbi, Biate,* and *Khelma*) enlisted a total of 92 macrofungal resources (Borah et al., 2018). However, most of the knowledge reported were on food and nutraceuticals and not mentioned about mushrooms as medicines. Some of the other regions recorded tribal ethnomedicinal aspects of mushrooms include Assam, Madhya Pradesh, Nagaland, Uttar Pradesh, and West Bengal (Rai et al., 1993; Dutta and Acharya, 2014; Kumar et al., 2014, 2017; Devi et al., 2016; Devi, 2017; Singha et al., 2017, 2020; Vishwakarma and Tripathi, 2019). Debnath et al. (2019) provided a detailed review of ethnomedicinal mushrooms and their applications by various tribes mainly from northern India. Singha et al. (2017, 2020) recorded the macrofungal resources utilized by ethnic tribes of Gurguripal of West Bengal. In the year 2017, they have recorded a total of 32 mushrooms, among them, 19 were used for various medicinal uses by the tribes. Singha et al. (2020) recorded a total of 23 wild mushrooms from ethnic tribes in Gurguripal of West Bengal and the mushrooms documented were belonged to 16 families. Among 23 mushrooms documented 19 species were effectively used to treat various diseases.

Ethnomycological studies reported from Madhya Pradesh revealed that the tribes are also using wild mushrooms for medicinal applications. Rai et al. (1993) recorded the ethnomycological information on eight mushrooms from Jabalpur region to treat burns, bleedings cuts, eye disorders, fever, vomiting, typhoid, and also to induce lactation. Studies on potential use of tribal mushrooms of Madhya Pradesh was carried out (Rahi, 2002; Rajak and Rai, 2005). Further, Harsh et al. (1999) reported the ethnomycological experience of *Gond, Baigas,* and *Abujmariahs* tribes of Madhya Pradesh. They have reported a total of nine medicinal mushrooms used by the indigenous people to treat burns (*Agaricus hygrometricus*); wounds (*Bovista apedicellata*); to treat bleeding from deep cuts and wounds (*Lycoperdon pusillum*); typhoid and labor pains (*Phallus impudicus*); cataract, asthma and hydrocele (*G. lucidum*; to activate lactation after delivery (*Xylaria polymorpha*); to treat ear pain, fever, and vomiting (*Microporus xanthopus*); chronic cough (*Daldinia concentrica*) (Harsh et al., 1999).

Karwa and Rai (2010) reported a total of 153 species of edible and medicinal mushrooms from Melghat forest of Satpuda Tiger Reserve, Maharashtra. The major genera of mushrooms dominated in Melghat forests belong to *Agaricus, Auricularia, Cantharellus, Ganoderma, Morchella, Pleurotus, Schizophyllum,* and *Termitomyces*. Similarly, Sargunam et al. (2012) reported seven mushrooms involved in food culture of *Kaani* tribe in Kanyakumari (Tamil Nadu), which include *Aricularia auricula, Lentinus fusipes, L. tuberegium, Pleurotus sajor-caju, Termitomyces heimii, T. microcarpus,* and *Volvariella volvacea*. Thangaraj et al. (2017) recorded four mushrooms used by the tribes in Sirumali Hills of Tamil Nadu to cure various disease: *Calvatia gigantean* (to treat stomach upset), *Daldinia concentrica* (to treat skin irritations and wound), *Podoxis pistillaris* (to cure skin diseases and burns) and *T. microcarpus* (to treat male infertility). Through experimentation on animal models the wound-healing potential of *Daldinia concentrica* has been proved.

Applications of ethnomedicinal mushrooms to treat or cure various illness in different regions of the Indian subcontinent are given in Table 19.1. A total of 100 species belong to 61 genera have ethnomedicinal significance. A maximum of six species each of *Russula* and *Termitomyces* are used in ethnomedicine, followed by five species of *Morchella*. Four species each of *Agaricus, Coprinus,* and *Helvella* followed by three species each of *Ganoderma, Trametes,* and *Volvariella* are used in ethnomedicine. Two species each of 10 genera (*Bovista, Clavtia, Cyathus, Lentinus, Lycoperdon, Phallus, Pleurotus, Ramaria, Rhizopogon,* and *Xylaria*) serve in ethnomedicine. The rest one species each of 42 genera serve in ethnomedicine. Interestingly, poisonous mushroom *Amanita muscaria* is used to treat the rheumatoid arthritis in Jammu and Kashmir (Pala et al., 2013).

Distribution pattern of ethnomedicinal mushrooms in different states indicates the highest in the state of Jammu and Kashimr (42 spp.) followed by Uttar Pradesh (36 spp.) and West Bengal (20 spp.). In rest of the nine states, it ranged from 1 to 8 spp. (Figure 19.1). Sikkim and Tripura are represented by only one medicinal mushroom each. A maximum of 35 species of mushrooms are used to treat or cure single human ailment, followed by 28 and 20 species to treat or cure two and three ailments, respectively (Figure 19.2). Some medicinal mushrooms have the capacity to treat or cure as much as seven (e.g., *Daldinia concentrica,* and *Sparassis crispa*) and eight (*Auricularia auricula-judae*) ailments. As many as 21 ailments could treated or cured by ethnomedicinal mushrooms occurring in the Indian subcontinent

TABLE 19.1 Ethnomedicinal Uses of Mushrooms Used to Cure or Treat Different Human Ailments of the Tribals in India.

Mushroom	State	Medicinal use	References
Agaricus augustus Fr.	Jammu and Kashmir	Tonic as supplementary diet of patients suffering from asthma, stroke, diabetes and heart ailments	Malik et al. (2017)
Agaricus bisporus (J.E. Lange) Imbach	Jammu and Kashmir	Tonic for patients suffering from cardiovascular diseases; used to treat leucoderma, prescribed to diabetes patients and serve as immunomodulators	Pala et al. (2013); Malik et al. (2017)
Agaricus campestris L.	Jammu and Kashmir	Treatment of scalds and burns	Pala et al. (2013)
Agaricus sylvaticus Schaeff.	Orissa and Uttar Pradesh	Lowering of high fever	Sachan et al. (2013); Vishwakarma and Tripathi (2019)
Amanita muscaria (L.) Lam.	Jammu and Kashmir	Treatment for rheumatoid arthritis	Pala et al. (2013)
Astraeus hygrometricus (Pers.) Morgan	Madhya Pradesh, Himachal Pradesh and West Bengal	Treatment for burns	Rai et al. (1993); Kumar et al. (2017); Singha et al. (2020)
Auricularia auricula-judae (Bull.) Quél.	Himachal Pradesh, Uttar Pradesh, West Bengal and Assam	Used as ear pus remedy; to treat inflammation of throat, eye irritation, cough and tooth ache; cardiovascular diseases, diabetes; to heal wounds	Devi (2017); Kumar et al. (2017); Vishwakarma and Tripathi (2019); Singha et al. (2020)
Boletus edulis Bull.	Jammu and Kashmir	Used after delivery as expectorants, antidepressant; used to treat lumbago leg pain, limbs numbness and discomfort of tendon	Malik et al. (2017)
Bovista pusilla (Batsch) Pers.	Madhya Pradesh	Stops bleeding of cuts	Rai et al. (1993)
Bovista plumbea Pers.	Assam	Used in treating sores, immunity booster, ulcers, skin infection and health drink	Devi et al. (2016); Devi (2017)
Cantharellus cibarius Fr.	Jammu and Kashmir	Used to treat wounds, natural tonic for general weakness and bone related ailments	Malik et al. (2017)

TABLE 19.1 *(Continued)*

Mushroom	State	Medicinal use	References
Calvatia gigantea (Batsch) Lloyd	Tamil Nadu	Treatment for stomach upset and stomach ache in women during menstruation	Thangaraj et al. (2017)
Calvatia cyathiformis (Bosc) Morgan	Madhya Pradesh	Used for wound healing and to check pus formation	Rai et al. (1993)
Coprinellus micaceus (Bull.) Vilgalys, Hopple & Jacq. Johnson	Uttar Pradesh	Antimicrobial activity	Vishwakarma and Tripathi (2019)
Coprinopsis atramentaria (Bull.) Redhead, Vilgalys & Moncalvo	Uttar Pradesh	Antifungal and antitumour activities	Vishwakarma and Tripathi (2019)
Coprinus atramentarius (Bull.) Fr.	Jammu and Kashmir	Used in treat kidney problems, removal of gall stones and pus cells in urine	Pala et al. (2013)
Coprinus comatus (O.F. Müll.) Pers.	Gujarat, Uttar Pradesh and West Bengal	Used to treat skin-related diseases and wounds; antifungal, lowering cholesterol level and treating skin diseases	Lahiri et al. (2010); Vishwakarma and Tripathi (2019); Singha et al. (2020)
Coprinus disseminatus (Pers.) Gray	Uttar Pradesh	Antitumor activity	Vishwakarma and Tripathi (2019)
Coprinus micaceus (Bull.) Fr.	Jammu and Kashmir	Used to treat skin infections	Pala et al. (2013)
Cordyceps sinensis (Berk.) Sacc.	Sikkim	Remedy for diabetes, cancer and sexual potency	Panda et al. (2011)
Cyathus stercoreus (Schwein.) De Toni	Madhya Pradesh	To treat eye disorders like pain, redness and, conjunctivitis	Rai et al. (1993)
Cyathus limbatus Tul. & C. Tul.	Madhya Pradesh	To treat eye disorders	Rai et al. (1993)

TABLE 19.1 *(Continued)*

Mushroom	State	Medicinal use	References
Daldinia concentrica (Bolton) Ces. & De Not.	Uttar Pradesh, West Bengal and Tamil Nadu	Used to treat burns, itches and minor skin infections; used to treat skin irritation, wound healing, constipation, and to stop bleeding	Dutta and Acharya (2014); Singha et al. (2020); Thangaraj et al. (2017); Vishwakarma and Tripathi (2019)
Disciotis venosa (Pers.) Arnould	Jammu and Kashmir	Used to treat common cold	Malik et al. (2017)
Entoloma bloxami (Berk. & Broome) Sacc.	Nagaland	Used to treat skin diseases	Kumar et al. (2014)
Fistulina hepatica (Schaeff.) With.	Uttar Pradesh	Used against fever	Vishwakarma and Tripathi (2019)
Flammulina velutipes (Curtis) Singer	Jammu and Kashmir	Serve as tonic and immunomodulator	Malik et al. (2017)
Fomes fomentarius (L.) Fr.	Jammu and Kashmir and Uttar Pradesh	Disinfectant for wound, coagulates blood, anti-inflammatory and treat arthritis	Pala et al. (2013); Vishwakarma and Tripathi (2019)
Fomitopsis pinicola (Sw.) P. Karst.	Jammu and Kashmir, and Uttar Pradesh	Used against rheumatoid arthritis, to prevent bleeding of minor injuries and against inflammation of digestive tract	Pala et al. (2013); Vishwakarma and Tripathi (2019)
Ganoderma applanatum (Pers.) Pat.	Jammu and Kashmir; Uttar Pradesh and West Bengal	Used to reduce fever, to cure diabetes, high blood pressure and serve as immunomodulator	Pala et al. (2013); Singha et al. (2017); Vishwakarma and Tripathi (2019)
Ganoderma lucidum (Curtis) P. Karst.	Nagaland, Uttar Pradesh, Assam and West Bengal	Treatment for asthma, to treat dizziness, diabetes, toxic mushroom poisoning and to treat ulcers	Kumar et al., 2014; Devi (2017); Vishwakarma and Tripathi (2019); Singha et al. (2017, 2020)
Ganoderma tsugae Murrill	Uttar Pradesh	Used against cough and cold	Vishwakarma and Tripathi (2019)
Geastrum triplex Jungh.	Himachal Pradesh	Used as remedy for burns	Kumar et al. (2017)

TABLE 19.1 *(Continued)*

Mushroom	State	Medicinal use	References
Geopora sumneriana (Cooke ex W. Phillips) M. Torre	Jammu and Kashmir	Used as anti-cold, stimulant tonic and used as immunomodulator	Malik et al. (2017)
Gomphus floccosus (Schwein.) Singer	Jammu and Kashmir	Used to treat eczema and athlete's foot disease	Pala et al. (2013)
Grifola frondosa (Dicks.) Gray	Uttar Pradesh	Used against muscle pain, serve as immune booster and antihyperglycemic	Vishwakarma and Tripathi (2019)
Gyromitra sphaerospora (Peck) Sacc.	Jammu and Kashmir	Used for the treatment of goiter	Pala et al. (2013)
Helvella acetabulum (L.) Quél.	Jammu and Kashmir	Used to treat chronic cough	Malik et al. (2017)
Helvella crispa Bull.	Jammu and Kashmir	Used for the treat asthma, cough, intestinal inflammation and mouth ulcer	Malik et al. (2017)
Helvella lacunosa Fr.	Jammu and Kashmir	Used to treat piles	Pala et al. (2013)
Helvella macropus (Pers.) P. Karst.	Jammu and Kashmir	Used to treat asthma	Pala et al. (2013)
Humaria hemisphaerica (F.H. Wigg.) Fuckel	Jammu and Kashmir	Used to treat blisters on skin	Pala et al. (2013)
Hericium coralloides (Scop.) Pers.	Jammu and Kashmir	Used to lower the risk of cancer and heart diseases	Pala et al. (2013)
Hypsizygus tessulatus (Bull.) Singer	Nagaland	Used to treat skin diseases	Kumar et al. (2014)
Inonotus hispidus (Bull.) P. Karst.	Jammu and Kashmir	Serve as disinfectant for the treatment of boils	Pala et al. (2013)
Lactarius deliciosus (L.) Gray	Jammu and Kashmir and West Bengal	Used to treat frost bites and serve to enhance immunity	Pala et al. (2013); Singha et al. (2020)

TABLE 19.1 *(Continued)*

Mushroom	State	Medicinal use	References
Lentinula edodes (Berk.) Pegler	Assam	Used to increase strength and immunity	Devi (2017)
Lentinus sajor-caju (Fr.) Fr.	Orissa	Used to treat cold and cough	Sachan et al. (2013)
Lentinus tigrinus (Bull.) Fr.	Jammu and Kashmir	Used for the treat dry cough, asthma and serve as brain tonic against	Malik et al. (2017)
Lenzites betulinus (L.) Fr.	Uttar Pradesh	Antimicrobial	Vishwakarma and Tripathi (2019)
Lepiota cristata (Bolton) P. Kumm.	Gujarat and Uttar Pradesh	Used to treat boils and to cure skin infections	Lahiri et al. (2010); Vishwakarma and Tripathi (2019)
Lycoperdon perlatum Pers.	Jammu and Kashmir Uttar Pradesh and West Bengal	Used for wound healing, spores are sprinkled on wound to stop bleeding and used to intoxicate honey bee bite	Pala et al. (2013); Vishwakarma and Tripathi (2019); Singha et al. (2020)
Lycoperdon pyriforme Schumach.	Jammu and Kashmir and Uttar Pradesh	Used for wound healing, frost bites and to treat stomach pain	Malik et al. (2017); Vishwakarma and Tripathi (2019)
Macrolepiota rhacodes (Vittad.) Singer	Uttar Pradesh	Used to cure high blood pressure and diabetes	Vishwakarma and Tripathi (2019)
Microporus xanthopus (Fr.) Kuntze	Madhya Pradesh	Remedy for vomiting, fever and earache	Rai et al. (1993)
Morchella angusticeps Peck	Uttar Pradesh	Consumed as health protecting food	Vishwakarma and Tripathi (2019)
Morchella conica Krombh.	Jammu and Kashmir	Serve as brain tonic, used as sex stimulant, to treat heart ailment and arthritis	Malik et al. (2017)
Morchella esculenta (L.) Pers.	Jammu and Kashmir, and Uttar Pradesh	Used to treat sexual weakness in men	Pala et al. (2013); Vishwakarma and Tripathi (2019)
Morchella hybrid Pers.	Jammu and Kashmir	Used in heart ailments, brain tonic, treat weakness and arthritis	Malik et al. (2017)

TABLE 19.1 *(Continued)*

Mushroom	State	Medicinal use	References
Morchella vulgaris (Pers.) Gray	Jammu and Kashmir	Serve as brain tonic, used in heart ailments, to treat weakness and arthritis	Malik et al. (2017)
Panaeolus sphinctrinus (Fr.) Quél.	Jammu and Kashmir	Use as an anesthetic agent	Pala et al. (2013)
Peziza repanda Wahlenb. ex Fr.	Jammu and Kashmir	Used to treat diabetes, eczema and constipation	Pala et al. (2013)
Phallus rubicundus (Bosc) Fr.	Madhya Pradesh	Used for the treatment of typhoid and to relieve labour pain	Rai et al. (1993)
Phallus impudicus L.	Jammu and Kashmir	Heals wounds and burns	Pala et al. (2013)
Phellinus durissimus (Lloyd) A. Roy	Gujarat	Used against mumps and simple edema	Lahiri et al. (2010)
Pisolithus arhizus (Scop.) Rauschert	West Bengal	Used to treat wounds	Manna et al. (2014)
Pleurotus djamor (Rumph. ex Fr.) Boedijn	Tripura	Antibacterial	Das et al. (2017)
Pleurotus ostreatus (Jacq.) P. Kumm.	Orissa, Uttar Pradesh and West Bengal	Used to treat high blood pressure, asthma, fever, dysentery and hypocholesterolemic conditions	Sachan et al. (2013); Vishwakarma and Tripathi (2019); Singha et al. (2020)
Podaxis pistillaris (L.) Fr.	Tamil Nadu	Used to treat skin diseases and skin burns	Thangaraj et al. (2017)
Polyporus badius sensu Weinmann, Hymen.	West Bengal	Used to treat skin and to treat against poisonous insect bite	Singha et al. (2020)
Pycnoporus cinnabarinus (Jacq.) P. Karst.	Uttar Pradesh	Used against ear infections and wounds	Vishwakarma and Tripathi (2019)
Ramaria formosa (Pers.) Quél.	Jammu and Kashmir	Used to treat cardiac and diabetic patients	Pala et al. (2013)

TABLE 19.1 *(Continued)*

Mushroom	State	Medicinal use	References
Ramaria stricta (Pers.) Quél.	Jammu and Kashmir	Used to treat asthma, respiratory diseases, eye ailments, serve as blood purifier and skin colour enhancer	Malik et al. (2017)
Rhizopogon roseolus (Corda) Th. Fr.	Jammu and Kashmir	Used against urinary tract infection	Malik et al. (2017)
Rhizopogon villosulus Zeller	Jammu and Kashmir	Used to treat kidney stones, urinary tract infections and asthma	Malik et al. (2017)
Russula albonigra	West Bengal	Controls cold and cough	Singha et al. (2017, 2020)
Russula aquosa Leclair	Uttar Pradesh	Serve to heal wounds and serve as immunomodulator	Vishwakarma and Tripathi (2019)
Russula cyanoxantha	West Bengal	Controls low and high blood pressure	Singha et al. (2017, 2020)
Russula delica Fr.	Orissa and West Bengal	Used against nutritional disorders, malnutrition and weakness	Sachan et al. (2013); Singha et al. (2017, 2020)
Russula emetica (Schaeff.) Pers.	Uttar Pradesh and West Bengal	Serve to heal wounds, rheumatism and lowers blood pressure	Vishwakarma and Tripathi (2019); Singha et al. (2020)
Russula senecis	West Bengal	To treat wounds against microbial infection and cuts	Singha et al. (2020)
Schizophyllum commune Fr.	Uttar Pradesh and West Bengal	Used as tonic and enhance immune functions	Dutta and Acharya (2014), Singha et al. (2020); Vishwakarma and Tripathi (2019)
Sparassis crispa (Wulfen) Fr.	Jammu and Kashmir; Uttar Pradesh	Serve as general tonic; used as treat against memory loss, anger, depression, chest pain; serve as anticold and purify blood	Malik et al. (2017); Vishwakarma and Tripathi (2019)
Sparassis spathulata (Schwein.) Fr.	Jammu and Kashmir	Used as general tonic, serve as anticold and purify blood	Malik et al. (2017)

TABLE 19.1 *(Continued)*

Mushroom	State	Medicinal use	References
Stereum hirsutum (Willd.) Pers.	Uttar Pradesh	Serve in wound healing	Vishwakarma and Tripathi (2019)
Termitomyces clypeatus R. Heim	West Bengal	Used as antihelminthic, used to treat chicken pox and to control bleeding	Manna et al. (2014); Singha et al. (2020)
Termitomyces eurrhizus (Berk.) R. Heim	Orissa	Used to lower the high blood pressure, to treat against rheumatism and diarrhea	Sachan et al. (2013)
Termitomyces heimii Natarajan	Uttar Pradesh and West Bengal	Used as energy tonic and for wound healing	Vishwakarma and Tripathi (2019); Singha et al. (2020)
Termitomyces mammiformis R. Heim	Nagaland	Used to treat cough, whooping cough and abdominal discomfort	Kumar et al. (2014)
Termitomyces reticulatus Van der Westh. & Eicker	Orissa	To lower blood pressure and rheumatism.	Panda and Tayung (2015)
Termitomyces tylerianus Otieno	Gujarat	Used to protect against chicken pox	Lahiri et al. (2010)
Trametes gibbosa (Pers.) Fr.	Uttar Pradesh	Serve as antitumor, anti-inflammatory and antimicrobial	Vishwakarma and Tripathi (2019)
Trametes hirsuta (Wulfen) Lloyd	Uttar Pradesh	Used to cure wounds	Vishwakarma and Tripathi (2019)
Trametes versicolor (L.) Lloyd	Jammu and Kashmir, and Uttar Pradesh	Used to treat dermatitis and antimicrobial	Pala et al. (2013); Vishwakarma and Tripathi (2019)
Volvariella glandiformis (Berk. & Broome) Pegler	Orissa	Used for lowering of high blood pressure	Panda and Tayung (2015)
Volvariella indica M.K. Saini, N.J. Kaur & Atri	Uttar Pradesh	Used to lower high blood pressure	Vishwakarma and Tripathi (2019)

TABLE 19.1 *(Continued)*

Mushroom	State	Medicinal use	References
Volvariella volvacea (Bull.) Singer	Orissa, Uttar Pradesh and West Bengal	Used to lower high blood pressure and blood purifier	Sachan et al. (2013); Vishwakarma and Tripathi (2019); Singha et al. (2017, 2020)
Verpa bohemica (Krombh.) J. Schröt.	Jammu and Kashmir	Used against urinary disorders	Pala et al. (2013)
Xylaria hypoxylon (L.) Grev.	Uttar Pradesh	Antimicrobial	Vishwakarma and Tripathi (2019)
Xylaria polymorpha (Pers.) Grev.	Madhya Pradesh and Uttar Pradesh	Serve to induce lactation	Rai et al. (1993); Vishwakarma and Tripathi (2019)

(Figure 19.3). A maximum of 42 species of medicinal mushrooms are useful in treating or curing the dermatological ailments, followed by 20, 18, and 16 species to treat or cure respiratory, hematological and used as health food/drink, respectively. It is interesting to note that *Lycoperdon perlatum* has the capacity to intoxicate honey bee bite (Table 19.1).

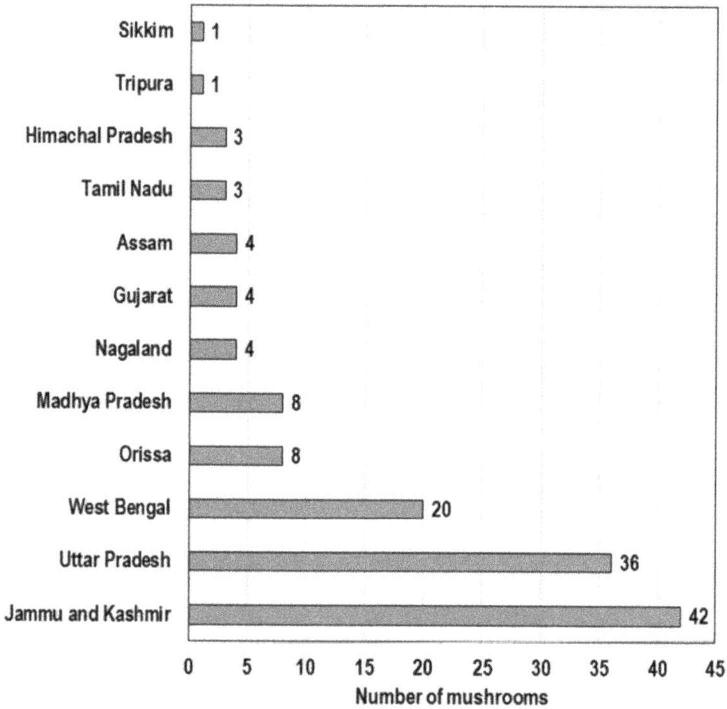

FIGURE 19.1 Distribution pattern of ethnomedicinal mushrooms in the Indian subcontinent.

19.5 RECENT DEVELOPMENTS

Ethnic knowledge on wild edible and medicinal mushrooms is highly essential for the transmission of knowledge related to their applications to the next generation. Majority of the tribal ethnomycological applications are not easily available to the scientific community. Many mushrooms reported to be used by various ethnic tribes and herbal practitioners will serve as an important source of biologically active compounds of medicinal interest (antioxidant, antimicrobial, anticancer, cytotoxic, and antimutagenic). In addition, they also serve as immunity boosters, assist in lowering high blood

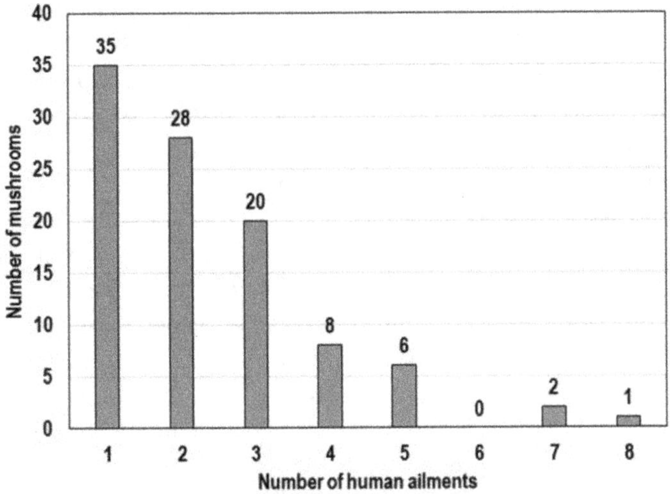

FIGURE 19.2 Applications of ethnomedicinal mushrooms against human ailments in the Indian subcontinent.

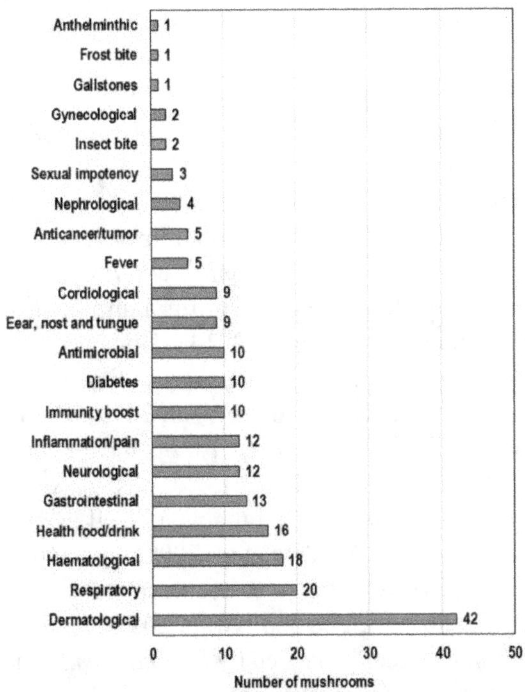

FIGURE 19.3 Use of ethnomedicinal mushrooms against various diseases in the Indian subcontinent.

pressure and increase defense against viral infections (Grüter et al., 1990; Barros et al., 2008; Cheung, 2008; Yang, 2011).

Sharma et al. (2017) provided statistics of mushroom production in the Indian subcontinent. Mushroom production in India is steadily increasing from 1970 onwards and the industry recorded a growth of 4.3% per annum during 2010–2017. The button mushroom (*Agaricus bisporus*) production was as high as 73%, the rest include 16% oyster mushroom (*Pleurotus* spp.), 7% paddy straw mushroom (*Volvariella volvacea*), 3% milk mushroom (*Lentinua edodes*), and other mushrooms (1%). There is as much as 8000–10,000 tons demand for mushrooms in India per annum. During 2016, 130,000 tons of mushrooms are produced in India with highest in Punjab (18,000 tons) followed by Orissa (16,000 tons), Haryana (15,100 tons), Maharashtra (12,000 tons), Gujarat (11,200 tons), Uttarakhand (10,200 tons), and Tamil Nadu (10,000 tons). Up to 10 small to medium scale mushroom producing industries are working in India. Most of these mushrooms are well known and also cultivated in other regions of the world. In view of nutritional, nutraceutical, and medicinal applications, indigenous mushrooms used by the tribes in India needs to be cultivated to boost the economy of the country toward developing strong foothold of traditional-based technology. This will help encouraging scientific investigations as well as to uplift the rural or tribal economy (Tibuhwa, 2012).

Biotechnological innovations of ethnomedicinal mushrooms boost the entrepreneur opportunities. To achieve such goals, scientific validation is required and some examples are available on these lines. One of the examples to explore the medicinal value of mushroom through scientific approach is *Lentinus* species. The white rot mushroom *Lentinus squarrosulus* has dual advantage as food as well as medicine in rural and or in tribal population of West Bengal (Dutta and Acharya, 2014). Updated nutritional qualities of uncooked and cooked wild *L. squarrosulus* collected from the forests of Western Ghats is available (Ghate and Sridhar, 2019). Bioactive compounds and bioactive potential of wild *L. squarrosulus* have been well established recently (Ravikrishnan et al., 2021a, b). Besides, *L. squarrosulus* is also known to treat the viral disease like mumps as well as cardiac ailments in Nigeria (Akpeja et al. 2003; Ayodele et al. 2009; Oyetayo 2011). Moreover, Nigerian folklore is also well known to use this mushroom to treat anaemia and infertility in humans (Okigbo and Nwatu 2015).

Two antibiotic substances produced by *L. squarrosulus* have been characterized (Sudirman et al., 1994; Isaka et al., 2011). Usha et al. (2016) reported a novel bioactive compound from *L. squarrosulus* from the Western Ghats has been designated as 2-chloro-1-(2-chlorocyclopropyl)-2-(4-nitrophenyl) ethanone. From the fermentation broth of *L. squarrosulus* (BCC22366), a new tetrahydrobenzofuran derivative, (6S,7S)-6,7-dihydroxy-3,6-dimethyl-2-isovaleroyl-4,5,6,7-tetrahydrobenzofuran, together with the known 1,2 dihydroxymintlactone was isolated (Isaka et al., 2011). Further, Singh et al. (2013) reported an intracellular lectin with 55 kDa having highest specificity for mucin and asialofetuin from *L. squarrosulus*. Roy et al. (2020) have demonstrated occurrence of 38 compounds (GC-MS and in silico analysis) for drug-likeness, bioactivity, and ADMET predictions showed 10 compounds are having drug-likeness and ADMET properties.

Datta and Das (2021) discussed strengthening entrepreneurship of mushrooms in sub-Himalayan region (e.g., West Bengal). They suggested 10 different strategies to strengthen the competitiveness and considered that the West Bengal is ideally suitable for environment friendly cultivation of mushrooms, which fetches strong livelihoods.

19.6 FUTURE CHALLENGES

According to Ponce et al. (2019), the wealth of ethnomycological knowledge in Guatemala is valuable to communities culturally and economically in spite of erosion of ethnic knowledge. They strongly point out that the tradition will continue from generation to generation for the thrust for nutrition, medicine, and nutraceuticals for survival of ethnic tribes. The detailed information on availability of literature and success stories of documentation of ethnomedicinally important mushrooms used to treat various ailments provide clues that there are many more documentation needed with close interaction and working relationship with the native tribes. Besides, traditional healers and herbal specialists are highly valuable to extract authentic information. Perception among the tribals and healers need to be triggered that such information will benefit the tribals' economy and livelihood through the local governments.

Other major challenges about documentation of ethnic mycological knowledge is lack of skilled tribal people. However, the herbalists and healers among the tribals or others are immense importance to unlock the precise way of utilization of mushrooms for specific ailment. The most important aspect to be understood by the tribals about how they sort out or identify edible from poisonous mushrooms in the field. If they use poisonous mushrooms in medicine, in what way they process and route of administration become important. Institutions (e.g., forest departments, NGOs, and universities) close to the tribal camps are highly valuable as they know the forest nearby as well as knowledge about the tribals (e.g., language, habits, and local markets). Such activities should be given major prominence to the ethnobiologists with sufficient grants to run such projects.

Institutions and universities should develop program to educate the tribals as well as youngsters to move forward to understand the importance of enthnomedicinal mushrooms in their vicinity. The National Biodiversity Authority of India has developed a unique program called People Biodiversity Register, where a coordinator along with a group of three technical experts visit a village and document the natural resources used by them and their culture. Similar teams need to be framed to collect and verify the collected data through sceintific validation via in vivo and in vitro experimentation. Such actions maximize the conventional use of biodiversity of a specific region.

19.7 CONCLUSIONS

The Indian subcontinent is well known for its strategic geographic setup encompassing tropical, subtropical, and temperate climatic conditions. Being embrased four hotspots of biodiversity, the mushroom wealth has to be studied in greater detail. Tribles throughout the country used mushrooms for nutrition and medicinal purposes, it provides unique opportunity to the scientific personnel as well as tribals to focus deeply toward utilization of mushroom diversity for various purposes. The socioeconomic status of tribes and cottage industries in many parts of the country is dependent on the mushroom diversity. Most important aspect is to understand the tribal knowledge in identification of edible, medicinal, and poisonous mushrooms. Tribals have their own folk morphology and taxonomy, which needs to be followed for scientific validation.

In most of the situation, the wild edible or medicinal mushrooms are fetched from the forests. Many edible or medicinal mushrooms being ecto-mycorrhizal, specific tree species is important to perpetuate desired mush-room (Sridhar and Karun, 2019). Such studies help understanding the extent of ectomycorrhizal association and protection or reforestation of specific tree species support specific mushrooms of interest toward edibility or medicine. Similarly, several value-added psychedelic (or hallucinogenic) mushrooms are associated with insects and dung (e.g., cow, bison, and elephant; rumi-nents and nonruminents) in the forests. Again such connotation depends on tripartite association among plans, insects (or animal), and mushrooms. There are several instances that *Cordyceps* and *Ganoderma* are used for medicinal purposes. This will project new avenues to the scientific personnel as well as the students to involve in various multidisciplinary and interdisciplinary aspects pertain to botany, zoology, microbiology, mycology, entomology, forestry, pharmacology, nutrition, management, and biotechnology.

ACKNOWLEDGMENTS

Mahadevakumar is grateful to the Council of Scientific and Industrial Research, New Delhi for the award of Research Associate Fellowship. Nuthan acknowledges the Indian Council of Medical Research, New Delhi for the award of Senior Research Fellowship.

KEYWORDS

- **ethnomedicine**
- **medicinal mushrooms**
- **nutraceuticals**
- **tribal knowledge**
- **wild mushrooms**

REFERENCES

Akpeja, E. O.; Isikhuemhen, O. S.; Okhuoya, J. A. Ethnomycology and Usage of Edible and Medicinal Mushrooms Among the Igbo People of Nigeria. *Int. J. Med. Mush.* **2003,** *5*, 313–319.

Amandeep, K.; Atri, N. S.; Munruchi K. Diversity of Species of the Genus *Bolbitius* (Bolbitiaceae, Agaricales) Collected on Dung from Punjab, India. *Mycosphere* **2013,** *4*, 1053–1064.

Aravindakhan, D.; Manimohan, P. *Mycenas of Kerala*; SporePrint Books: Calicut, Kerala, India, 2015; p 213.

Atri, N. S. Exploration, Sociobiology and Conservation of Mushrooms—My Experience. *KAVAKA—Trans. Mycol. Soc. India* **2020,** *54*, 1–9.

Atri, N. S.; Mridu. Mushrooms—Some Ethnomycological and Sociobiological Aspects. *KAVAKA—Trans. Mycol. Soc. India* **2018,** *51*, 11–19.

Atri, N. S.; Saini, S. S. Collection and Study of Agarics—An Introduction. *Ind. J. Mush.* **2000,** *18*, 1–5.

Atri, N. S.; Sharma, Y. P.; Kaul, S. K.; Mridu. Wild Edible Mushrooms of North West Himalaya—Their Nutritional and Sociobiological Aspects. In *Microbial Diversity:*

Ecosystem Sustainability and Biotechnological Applications; Satyanarayana, T.; Das, S. K.; Johri, B. N., Ed.; Springer Nature: Singapore Pte. Ltd., 2019; pp 533–563.

Ayodele, S. M.; Akpaja, E. O.; Adamu, Y. Some Edible and Medicinal Mushrooms Found in Igala Land in Nigeria and Their Sociocultural and Ethnomycological Uses. In *Proceeding of the 5th International Medicinal Mushroom Conference*; Nantong, China, 2009; pp 526–531.

Badalyan, S. Potential of Mushroom Bioactive Molecules to Develop Healthcare Biotech Products. In *Proceedings of the 8th International Conference on Mushroom Biology and Mushroom Products*; Mushroom Society of India: New Delhi, 2014; pp 373–378.

Barros, L.; Telma, C.; Paula, B.; Leticia M. E.; Isabel, C. F. R. F. Wild and Commercial Mushrooms as Source of Nutrients and Nutraceuticals. *Food Chem. Toxicol.* **2008,** *46*, 2742–2747.

Baruah, H. K.; Sing, D. K.; Islam, M. On the Distribution of Higher Basidiomycetes in the Sibsagar District, Assam. *Bull. Bot. Surv. India* **1971,** *13*, 285–289.

Berkeley, M. J. Fungi of the Plains of India. *Intell. Observ.* **1867,** *12*, 18–21.

Bhatt, R. P.; Singh, U.; Stephenson, S. L. Wild Edible Mushrooms from High Elevations in the Garhwal Himalaya–I. *Curr. Res. Environ. Appl. Mycol.* **2016,** *6*, 118–131

Bhatt, R. P.; Singh, U.; Uniyal, P. Healing Mushrooms of Uttarakhand Himalaya, India. *Curr. Res. Environ. Appl. Mycol.* **2018,** *8*, 1–23.

Bilgrami, K. S.; Jamaluddin, S.; Rizwi, A. M. *Fungi of India*; Today and Tomorrow's Printers and Publishers: India, 1991; p 798.

Binu, S.; Nayar, T. S.; Pushpangadan, P. An Outline of Ethnobotanical Research in India. *J. Econ. Tax. Bot.* **1992,** *10*, 405–428.

Borah, N.; Semwal, R. L.; Garkoti, S. C. Ethnomycological Knowledge of Three Indigenous Communities of Assam, India. *Ind. J. Trad. Know.* **2018,** *17*, 327–335.

Butler, E. J.; Bisby, G. R. *The Fungi of India*. Imperial Council of Agricultural Research India. *Sci. Monograph* **1931,** *18*, p 237.

Cannon, P. F.; Aguirre-Hudson, B.; Aime, M. C.; Ainsworth, A. M.; Bldartondo, M. I. et al. Definition and Diversity. In *State of the World's Fungi*; Willis, K. J., Ed., Royal Botanic Gardens: Kew, 2018; pp 4–11.

Charaya, M. U.; Mehrotra, R. S. From Ethnomycology to Fungal Biotechnology: A Historical Perspective. In *From Ethnomycology to Fungal Biotechnology: Exploiting Fungi from Natural Resources for Novel Products*; Singh, J.; Aneja, K. R., Ed.; Springer: New York, 1999; pp 1–10.

Cheung, P. C. K. Nutritional Value and Health Benefits of Mushrooms. In *Mushrooms as Functional Foods*; Peter, C. K., Ed.; John Wiley & Sons, Inc.: Hoboken, 2008; pp 71–110.

Das, A. R.; Saha, A. K.; Joshi, S. R.; Das, P. Wild Edible Macrofungi Consumed by Ethnic Tribes of Tripura in Northeast India with Special Reference to Antibacterial Activity of *Pleurotus djamor* (Rumph. ex Fr.) Boedijn. *Int. Food Res. J.* **2017,** *24*, 834–838.

Datta, P.; Das, S. Model-Based Strategic Planning for Strengthening Mushroom Entrepreneurship: Insights from a Sub-Himalayan Region of West Bengal, India. *Geo J.* **2021,** *86*, 145–158.

Debnath, S.; Debnath, B.; Das, P.; Saha, K. Review on an Ethnomedicinal Practices of Wild Mushrooms by the Local Tribes of India. *J. Appl. Pharm. Sci.* **2019,** *9*, 144–156.

Devi, K. Ethnomycological Studies of Some Wild Edible and Medicinal Mushrooms in Kamrup District of Assam, India. *Int. J. Curr. Adv. Res.* **2017,** *6*, 3954–3959.

Devi, K.; Brahma, J.; Shrivastava, K. Documentation of Four Hitherto Unreported Wild Edible Macro Fungi from Chirang District of Assam, North-East India. *Int. J. Cons. Sci.* **2016,** *7*, 709–718.

Dutta, A. K.; Acharya, K. Traditional and Ethno-Medicinal Knowledge of Mushrooms in West Bengal, India. *Asian J. Pharm. Clin. Res.* **2014,** *7*, 36–41.

Farook, V. A.; Khan, S. S.; Manimohan, P. A. Checklist of Agarics (Gilled Mushrooms) of Kerala State, India. *Mycosphere* **2013,** *4*, 97–131.

Gadgil, M.; Berkes, F.; Folke, C. Indigenous Knowledge for Biodiversity Conservation. *Ambio* **1993,** *22*, 151–156.

Ghate, S. D.; Sridhar, K. R. Nutritional Attributes of Two Wild Mushrooms of Southwestern India. In *Advances in Macrofungi: Diversity, Ecology and Biotechnology*; CRC Press Taylor & Francis: Boca Raton, 2019; pp 105–120.

Grüter, A.; Friederich, U.; Würgler, F. E. Antimutagenic Effects of Mushrooms. *Mutation Res.* **1990,** *231*, 243–249.

Haro-Luna, M. X.; Ruan-Soto, F.; Guzmán-Dávalos, L. Traditional Knowledge, Uses, and Perceptions of Mushrooms Among the Wixaritari and Mestizos of Villa Guerrero, Jalisco, Mexico. *IMA Fungus* **2019,** *10*, 16. 10.1186/s43008-019-0014-6

Harsh, N. S. K.; Rai, B. K.; Soni, V. K. Some ethnomycological studies from Madhya Pradesh, India. In *From Ethnomycology to Fungal Biotechnology*; Singh, J.; Aneja, K. R., Ed.; Platinum Press: New York, 1999; pp 19–31.

Hawksworth, D. L. *Advances in Macrofungi: Diversity, Ecology and Biotechnology*; CRC Press, 2019; pp 1–9.

Hawksworth, D. L. The Magnitude of Fungal Diversity: The 1.5 Million Species Estimate Revisited. *Microbiol. Res.* **2001,** *105*, 1422–1432.

Hawksworth, D. L.; Lücking, R. Fungal Diversity Revisited: 2.2 to 3.8 Million Species. *Microbiol. Spectrum* **2017,** *5*, FUNK-0052-2016.

Isaka, M.; Sappan, M.; Rachtawee, P.; Boonpratuang, T. A Tetrahydrobenzofuran Derivative from the Fermentation Broth of *Lentinus squarrosulus* BCC 22366. *Phytochem. Lett.* **2011,** *4*, 106–108.

Jian, S. P.; Singh. J. Traditional Medicinal Practices Among the Tribal People of Raigarh (Chhattisgarh), India. *Ind. J. Nat. Prod. Resour.* **2010,** *1*, 109–115.

Kamat, N. K. 1994. file:///C:/Users/User1/Downloads/MUSHROOM_BIODIVERSITY_OF_GOA.pdf

Karun, N. C.; Sridhar, K. R. A Preliminary Study on Macrofungal Diversity in an Arboretum and Three Plantations of the Southwest Coast of India. *Curr. Res. Environ. Appl. Mycol.* **2014,** *4*, 173–187.

Karun, N. C.; Sridhar, K. R. Edible Wild Mushrooms in the Western Ghats: Data on the Ethnic Knowledge. *Data in Brief* 2017, *14*, 320–328.

Karun, N. C.; Sridhar, K. R. Elephant Dung-Inhabiting Macrofungi in the Western Ghats. *Curr. Res. Environ. Appl. Mycol.* **2015,** *5*, 60–69.

Karun, N. C.; Sridhar, K. R. Occurrence and Distribution of Termitomyces (Basidiomycota, Agaricales) in the Western Ghats and on the West Coast of India. *Czech Mycol.* **2013,** *65*, 233–254.

Karun, N. C.; Sridhar, K. R. Spatial and Temporal Diversity of Macrofungi in the Western Ghat Forests of India. *Appl. Ecol. Environ. Res.* 2016, *14*, 1–21.

Karwa, A.; Rai, M. K. Tapping into the Edible Fungi Biodiversity of Central India. *Biodiversitas* **2010,** *11*, 97–101.

Kaur, A.; Atri, N. S.; Kaur, M. A New Variety of *Rhodocybe popinalis* (*Entolomataceae, Agaricales*) from Coprophilous Habitats of India. *J. New Biol. Rep.* **2013,** *2*, 260–263.

Khaund, P.; Joshi, S. R. Wild Edible Macrofungal Species Consumed by the Khasi Tribe of Meghalaya, India. *Ind. J. Nat. Prod. Resour.* **2013,** *4*, 197–204.

Kumar, M.; Harsh, N. S. K.; Prasad, R.; Pandey, V. V. An Ethnomycological Survey of Jaunsar, Chakrata, Dehradun, India. *J. Threat. Taxa* **2017,** *9*, 10717–10725.

Kumar, R.; Pandey, S.; Tapwal, A.; Rishi, R. R.; Giri, K.; Mishra, G. Ethnomycological Knowledge on Wild Mushrooms by Tribes of Mokokchung, Nagaland, North East India. *J. Ethnobiol. Trad. Med. Photon.* **2014,** *122*, 890–899.

Lahiri, S. S.; Shukla, M. D.; Shah, M. B.; Modi, H. A. Documentation and Analysis of Certain Macrofungal Traditional Practices from Western India (Gujarat). *Ethnobot. Leaflets* **2010,** *2010*, 9.

Latha, K. P. D.; Manimohan, P. *Inocybes of Kerala*; SporePrint Books: Calicut, Kerala, India, 2017; p 181.

Leelavathy, K. M.; Ganesh, P. N. *Polypores of Kerala*; Daya Publishing House: New Delhi, 2000; p 165.

Malik, A. R.; Wani, A. H.; Bhat, M. Y.; Parveen, S. Ethnomycological Knowledge of Some Wild Mushrooms of Northern Districts of Jammu and Kashmir, India. *Asian J. Pharm. Clin. Res.* **2017,** *10*, 399–405.

Manimohan, P.; Noordeloos, M. E.; Dhanya, A. M. Studies on the Genus Entoloma (Basidiomycetes, Agaricales) in Kerala State, India. *Personia* **2006,** *19*, 45–93.

Manjula, B. A Revised List of the Agaricoid and Boletoid Basidiomycetes from India and Nepal. *Proc. Pl. Sci.* **1983,** *92*, 81. DOI: 10.1007/BF03052975

Manna, S.; Ray, D.; Roy, A. Tribal Relation to Spatio-Temporal Variation of Wild Mushrooms in Eastern Lateritic Part of India. *Ethnobot. Res. Appl.* **2014,** *12*, 15–24.

Manoharachary, C.; Sridhar, K. R.; Singh, R.; Adholeya, A.; Suryanarayanan, T. S. et al. Fungal Biodiversity: Distribution, Conservation and Prospecting of fungi From India. *Curr. Sci.* **2005,** *89*, 58–71.

Masoodi, K. Z.; Amin, I.; Mansoor, S. et al. Botanicals from the Himalayas with Anticancer Potential—An Emphasis on Kashmir Himalayas. In *Biodiversity and Biomedicine—Our Future*; Ozturk, M.; Egamberdieva, D.; Pešić, M., Eds., Chapter 11; Academic Press, 2020; pp 189–234.

Mohanan, C. *Macrofungi of Kerala*; Kerala Forest Research Institute, Hand Book # 27, Kerala, India, 2011; p 597.

Mortimer, P. E.; Boa, E.; Hude, K. D.; Li, H. Macrpfimgo as Food. *Encylop. Mycol.* **2021,** 10.1016/B978-0-12-819990-9.00071-8

Natarajan, K. Mushroom Flora of South India (Except Kerala). In *Advances in Horticulture*; Chadha, K. L.; Sharma, S. R., Ed.; Malhotra Publishing House: New Delhi, 1995; pp 381–397.

Natarajan, K.; Kumaresan, V.; Narayanan, K. A Checklist of Indian Agarics and Boletes (1984–2002). *KAVAKA—Trans. Mycol. Soc. India*, **2005,** *33*, 61–128.

Natarajan, K.; Manjula, B. South Indian Agaricales XII Lepiota. *Biblio. Mycol.* **1983,** *91*, 568–681.

Niskanen, T.; Douglas, B.; Kirk, P.; Crous, P. W.; Lücking R. et al. New Discoveries: Species of Fungi Described in 2017. In *State of the World's Fungi*. Willis, K. J., Ed.; Royal Botanic Gardens: Kew, 2018; pp 18–23.

Okigbo, R. N.; Nwatu, C. M. Ethnostudy and Usage of Edible and Medicinal Mushrooms in Some Parts of Anambra State, Nigeria. *Nat. Resour.* **2015,** *6*, 79–89.

Oyetayo, O. V. Medicinal Uses of Mushrooms in Nigeria: Towards Full and Sustainable Exploitation. *Afr. J. Trad. Compl. Alt. Med.* **2011,** *8*, 267–274.

Ozturk, M.; Altay, V.; Altundağ, E.; Ibadullayeva, S. J.; Aslanipour, B.; Gönenç, T. M. Herbals in Iğdır (Turkey), Nakhchivan (Azerbaijan), and Tabriz (Iran). In *Plant and Human Health*; Ozturk, M.; Hakeem, K. R., Eds., Vol. 1; Springer: Cham, Chapter 6, 2018c; pp 197–266.

Ozturk, M.; Altay, V.; Efe, R. *Biodiversity, Conservation and Sustainability in Asia: Volume I: Prospects and Challenges in West Asia and Caucasus*; Springer Nature: Switzerland AG, 2021a. DOI: 10.1007/978-3-030-59928-7

Ozturk, M.; Altay, V.; Gonenç, T. M. Herbal from High Mountains in the East Mediterranean. In *Drug Discovery from Herbs-Approaches and Applications*; Bhojraj, S. et al., Eds.; NAM S & T Centre, DAYA Publishing House: New Delhi-India, Chapter 24, 2017b; pp 327–367.

Ozturk, M.; Altay, V.; Gucel, S.; Altundağ, E. Plant Diversity of the Drylands in Southeast Anatolia-Turkey: Role in Human Health and Food Security. In *Plant Biodiversity: Monitoring, Assessment and Conservation*; Ansari, A. A.; Gill, S. S., Eds., Chapter 5, CABI UK, 2017c; pp 83–124.

Ozturk, M.; Altay, V.; Hakeem, K. R.; Akçiçek, E. *Liquorice from Botany to Phytochemistry*; SpringerBriefs in Plant Science, 2017a. https://doi.org/10.1007/978-3-319-74240-3

Ozturk, M.; Altay, V.; Latiff, A. et al. A Comparative Analysis of the Medicinal Pteridophytes in Turkey, Pakistan, and Malaysia. In *Plant and Human Health*; Ozturk, M.; Hakeem, K. R., Eds., Vol. 1; Springer: Cham, Chapter 9, Springer International Publishing AG, 2018d; pp 349–390.

Ozturk, M.; Altay, V.; Latiff, A. et al. A Comparative Analysis of the Medicinal Plants Used for Diabetes Mellitus in the Traditional Medicine in Turkey, Pakistan, and Malaysia. In *Plant and Human Health*; Ozturk, M.; Hakeem, K. R., Eds., Vol. 1; Springer: Cham, Chapter 11, Springer International Publishing AG, 2018e; pp 409–461.

Ozturk, M.; Altay, V.; Latiff, A. et al. Potential Medicinal Plants Used in the Hypertension in Turkey, Pakistan, and Malaysia. In *Plant and Human Health*; Ozturk, M.; Hakeem, K. R., Eds., Vol. 1; Springer: Cham, Chapter 16, Springer International Publishing AG, 2018f; pp 595–618.

Ozturk, M.; Altay, V.; Orçen, N. et al. A Little Known and a Little Consumed Natural Resource: *Salicornia*. In *Global Perspectives on Underutilized Crops;* Ozturk, M. et al., Eds., Chapter 3; Springer International Publishing AG, 2018a; pp 83–108.

Ozturk, M.; Altundağ, E.; Ibadullayeva, S. J.; Altay, V.; Aslanıpour, B. A Comparative Analysis of Medicinal and Aromatic Plants Used in the Traditional Medicine of Iğdır (Turkey), Nakhchivan (Azerbaijan), and Tabriz (Iran). *Pak. J. Bot.* **2018b**, *50* (1), 337–343.

Ozturk, M.; Egamberdieva, D.; Milica, P. *Biodiversity and Biomedicine-Our Future*; Academic Press, Elsevier Inc.: UK, USA, 2020.

Ozturk, M.; Gökler, I.; Altay, V. Medicinal Bryophytes Distributed in Turkey. In *Plant and Human Health*; Ozturk, M.; Hakeem, K. R., Eds., Vol. 1; Springer: Cham, Chapter 8, Springer International Publishing AG, 2018g; pp 323–348.

Ozturk, M.; Hakeem, K. R. *Plant and Human Health—Vol. 1—Ethnobotay and Physiology*; Springer Science + Business Media: New York, 2018.

Ozturk, M.; Hakeem, K. R. *Plant and Human Health—Vol. 2—Phytochemistry and Molecular Aspects*; Springer Science + Business Media: New York, 2019a.

Ozturk, M.; Hakeem, K. R. *Plant and Human Health—Vol. 3—Phytochemistry and Therapeutic Uses*; Springer Science + Business Media: New York, 2019b.

Ozturk, M.; Khan, S. M.; Altay, V.; Efe, R.; Egamberdieva, D.; Khassanov, F. *Biodiversity, Conservation and Sustainability in Asia: Volume II: Prospects and Challenges in South and Middle Asia*; Springer Nature: Switzerland AG, 2021b. DOI: 10.1007/978-3-030-73943-0

Pahlevanlo, A.; Janardhana, G. R. Diversity of Termitomyces in Kodagu and Need for Conservation. *J. Adv. Laborat. Res. Biol.* **2012a**, *3*, 54–57.
Pahlevanlo, A.; Janardhana, G. R. First Record of *Sinotermimyces taiwanensis* from India. *J. Mycol. Pl. Path.* **2012b**, 41, 636–638.
Pahlevanlo, A.; Mahadevakumar, S.; Janardhana, G. R. Diversity and Cultural Characteristics of *Termitomyces* Species from Kodagu Region of Karnataka (India). *International Conference on Microbial Biotechnology for Sustainable Development*, 2011; pp EM 81–68.
Pala, S. A.; Wani, A. H.; Bhat, M. Y. Ethnomycological Studies of Some Wild Medicinal and Edible Mushrooms in the Kashmir Himalayas (India). *Int. J. Med. Mush.* **2013,** *15*, 211–220.
Panda, A. K.; Swain, K. C. Traditional Uses and Medicinal Potential of *Cordyceps sinensis* of Sikkim. *J. Ayurv. Integr. Med.* **2011,** *2*, 9–13.
Panda, M. K.; Tayung, K. Documentation and Ethnomedicinal Knowledge on Wild Edible Mushrooms Among Ethnic Tribes of Northern Odisha, India. *Asian J. Pharm. Clin. Res.* **2015,** *8*, 139–143.
Panda, M. K.; Thatoi, H. N.; Sahu, S. C.; Tayung, K. Wild Edible Mushrooms of Northern Odisha, India: Data on Distribution and Utilization by Ethnic Communities. Res. *J. Life Sci., Bioinform. Hamaceut. Chem. Sci.* **2019,** *5*, 268.
Patwardhan, B.; Lakhotia, S. C. Traditional Knowledge Systems and New Science Policy Thrust. *Curr. Sci.* **2021,** *120*, 603–604.
Pavithra, M.; Greeshma, A. A.; Karun, N. C.; Sridhar, K. R. Observations on the *Astraeus* spp. of Southwestern India. *Mycosphere* **2015,** *6*, 421–432.
Pleskanovskaya, S. A.; Mamedova, M. A.; Ashıralıyeva, M. A. et al. *Glycyrrhiza glabra* (Liquorice) in Turkmenistan—Medicinal and Biological Aspects. In *Plant and Human Health,—Pharmacology and Therapeutic Uses*; Ozturk, M.; Hakeem, K. R., Eds., Vol. 3, Chapter 2; Springer Nature: Switzerland, 2019; pp 23–35.
Ponce, J. P. M.; Calderón, M. A. H.; Comandini, O.; Rinaldi, A. C.; Arzú, R. F. Ethnomycological Knowledge Among Kaqchikel, Indigenous Maya People of Guatemalan Highlands. *J. Enthnobiol. Ethnomed.* **2019,** *15*, 36. DOI: 10.1186/s13002-019-0310-7
Posey, D. A. Kayapó Ethnoecology and Culture. In *Studies in Environmental Anthropology*; Plenderleith, K., Ed.; Routledge: London and New York, 2002; p 285.
Purkayastha, R. P.; Chandra, A. *Manual of Indian Edible Mushrooms*; Today and Tomorrow's Printers and Publishers: India, 1985; p 267.
Rahi, D. K. *Cultivation of Wild Mushrooms of Central India, Using Different Agrowastes*; Ph.D. Dissertation, Rani Durgawati University, Madhya Pradesh, India, 2002; pp 33–45.
Rai, B. K.; Ayachi, S. S.; Rai, A. A Note on Ethno-Myco-Medicines from Central India. *Mycologist* **1993,** 192–193.
Rajak, R. C.; Rai, M. K. Edible Tribal Mushroom Resources of Central India and Their Ethnological Aspects. *Int. J. Med. Mush.* **2005,** *7*, 1–458.
Ravikrishnan, V.; Sridhar, K. R.; Rajashekhar, M. Bioactive Attributes of Edible Wild Mushrooms of the Western Ghats. In *Advances in Macrofungi: Pharmaceuticals and Cosmeceuticals*; CRC Press, Taylor & Francis Group: Boca Raton, 2021a; pp 20–38.
Ravikrishnan, V.; Sridhar, K. R.; Rajashekhar, M. Biochemical Profile of Six Edible Wild Mushrooms of the Western Ghats. In *Advances in Macrofungi: Industrial Avenues and Prospects*; CRC Press, Taylor & Francis Group: Boca Raton, 2021b; pp 142–162.
Roy, R. R.; Kandagalla, S.; Krishnappa, M. Exploring the Ethnomycological Potential of Lentinus squarrosulus Mont. through GC-MS and Chemoinformatics Tools. *Mycology* **2020,** *11*, 78–89.

Sachan, S. K. S.; Patra, J. K.; Thatoi, H. N. Indigenous Knowledge of Ethnic Tribes for Utilization of Wild Mushrooms as Food and Medicine in Similipal Biosphere Reserve, Odisha, India. *India. J. Agr. Tech.* **2013,** *9*, 403–416.

Samorini G. *Fungi Hallucinogeni. Studi etnomicologici*; Dozza, T., Ed.; Bologna, Italy, 2001; p 250.

Sargunam, D.; Johnsy, G. Samuel, A. S.; Kaviyarasan, V. Mushrooms in the Food Culture of the Kaani Tribe of Kanyakumari District. *Ind. J. Trad. Know*. **2012,** *11*, 150–153.

Sarma, T. C.; Sarma, I.; Patiri, B. N. Wild Edible Mushrooms Used by Some Ethnic Tribes of Western Assam. Bioscan **2010,** *10*, 613–625.

Sarwal, B. M. Taxonomic Studies on Indian Agarics–II B. *Ind. Phytopath.* **1984,** *37*, 228–233.

Semwal, K. C.; Stephenson, S. L.; Bhatt, V. K.; Bhatt, R. P. Edible Mushrooms of the Northwestern Himalaya, India: A Study of Indigenous Knowledge, Distribution and Diversity. *Mycosphere* **2014,** *5*, 440−461.

Sharma, V. P.; Annepu, S. K.; Gautam, Y.; Singh, M.; Kamal, S. Status of Mushroom Production in India. *Mush. Res.* **2017,** *26*, 111−120.

Sing, N. I.; Sing, S. M. Wild Edible Fleshy Fungal Flora of Manipur. *Bioveel* **1993,** *4*, 153−158.

Sing, N. I.; Sing, S. M.; Th, C. Fleshy Fungi of Manipur. In *Plant Genetic Diversity: Exploration, Evaluation and Conservation*; Affiliated East West Press Pvt. Ltd.: New Delhi, 2002; pp 9–13.

Singh, J. S.; Chaturvedi, R. K. Diversity of Ecosystem Types in India: A Review. *Proc. Ind. Nat. Sci. Acad.* **2017,** *83*, 569594.

Singh, R.; Kaur, H.; Kumar, P.; Kaur, H. Purification and Characterization of a Thermostable Mycelial Lectin from Basidiomycete *Lentinus squarrosulus*. *Biologia* **2013,** *8*, 1034–1040.

Singha, K.; Banerjee, A.; Mondal, K. S.; Pati, B. R.; Mohapatra, P. K. D. Eco-Diversity, Productivity and Distribution Frequency of Mushrooms in Gurguripal Eco-Forest, Paschim Medinipur, West Bengal, India. *Curr. Res. Environ. Appl. Mycol.* **2017,** *7*, 8–18.

Singha, K.; Sahoo, S.; Roy, A.; Banerjee, A.; Mondal, K. S. et al. Contributions of Wild Mushrooms in livelihood Management of Ethnic Tribes in Gurguripal, West Bengal, India. *Int. J. Pharm. Sci. Res.* **2020,** *11*, 3160–3171.

Sridhar, K. R. Expedition with Micro- and Macro-Fungi: New Perspectives to Bridge the Gaps. *KAVAKA—Trans. Mycol. Soc. India* **2019,** *52*, 1−19.

Sridhar, K. R.; Karun, N. C. Diversity and Ecology of Ectomycorrhizal Fungi in the Western Ghats. In *Microbial Interventions in Agriculture and Environment*; Springer Nature: Singapore Pte. Ltd., 2019; pp 479–507.

Srinivas, V.; Manjunatha, B. R.; Anjaneya, S. Traditional Knowledge on Medicinal Plants of Tribals Residing in Heggadadevanakote and Hunsur Taluks of Mysore District, Karnataka, India. *Int. J. Agri. Sci.* **2019,** *11*, 7966–7970.

Srivasthava, B.; Dwivedi, A. K.; Pandey, V. N. Morphological Characterization and Yield Potential of *Termitomyces* spp. Mushroom in Gorakhpur Forest Division. *Bull. Environ. Pharmacol. Life Sci.* **2011,** *1*, 54−56.

Sudirman, L. I.; Lefebvre, G.; Kiffer, E.; Botton, B. Purification of Antibiotics Produced by *Lentinus squarrosulus* and Preliminary Characterization of a Compound Active Against *Rigidoporus lignosus*. *Curr. Microbiol.* **1994,** *29*, 1–6.

Tanti, B.; Gurung, L.; Sharma, G. C. Wild Edible Fungal Resources Used by Ethnic Tribes of Nagaland, India. Indian *J. Tradit. Know*. **2011,** *10*, 512–515.

Thangaraj, R.; Raj, S.; Renganathan, K. Wound Healing Effect of King Alferd's Mushroom (*Daldinia concentrica*) Used by Tribes of Sirumalai hills, Tamil Nadu, India. *Int. J. Pharm. Pharm. Sci.* **2017,** *9*, 161–164.

Tibuhwa, D. D. Folk Taxonomy and Use of Mushrooms in Communities Around Ngorongoro and Serengeti National Park, Tanzania. *J. Ethnobiol. Ethnomed.* **2012,** *8*, 36.

Tribal Health Bulletin. Regional Medical Research Centre for Tribals (Indian Council of Medical Research) Jabalpur, 2014; p 72.

Usha, N.; Janardhana, G. R. Diversity of Macrofungi in the Western Ghats of Karnataka (India). *Indian Forester* **2014,** *140*, 531–536.

Usha, N.; Shashikanth, S.; Janardhana, G. R. Structural Elucidation of Novel Bioactive Compound (2-chloro-1-(2-chlorocyclopropyl)-2-(4-nitrophenyl)ethanone) from Basidiomycetous Fungus *Lentinus squarrosulus*. *Int. J. Pharmacol. Res.* **2016,** *6*, 62–67.

Varghese, S. P.; Pradeep, C. K.; Vrinda, K. B. Mushrooms of Tribal Importance in Wyanad Area of Kerala. *J. Mycopathol. Res.* **2010,** *48*, 311320.

Venkatachalapathi, A.; Paulsamy, S. Exploration of Wild Medicinal Mushroom Species in Walayar Valley, the Southern Western Ghats of Coimbatore District Tamil Nadu. *Mycosphere* **2016,** *7*, 118–130.

Vikineswary, S.; Chang, S. T. Edible and Medicinal Mushrooms for Sub-Health Intervention and Prevention of Lifestyle Diseases. *Tech Monitor* **2013,** July–September, 33–43.

Vishwakarma, P.; Tripathi, N. N. Ethnomacrofungal Study of Some Wild Macrofungi Used by Local Peoples of Gorakhpur District, Uttar Pradesh. *Ind. J. Nat. Prod. Resour.* **2019,** *10*, 81–89.

Vrinda, K. B.; Pradeep, C. K. Toxic and Hallucinogenic Mushrooms of Kerala. *J. Mycopathol. Res.* **2011,** *49*, 231–246.

Wasson, R. G. Soma: Divine Mushroom of Immortality, *Ethnomycology Studies # 1—Harvest Special*; Harcourt Brace Jovanovich: New York, 1971.

WHO. Traditional Medicine Strategy, World Health Organization, Geneva, 2002–2005. https://www.beovita.eu/pdf/WHO_EDM_TRM_2004.pdf

Wills, K. J. *State of the World's Fungi*; Royal Botanic Gardens: Kew, 2018; p 88.

Yang, Z. L. Mushrooms, Health and Nutrition. In *Mushrooms in Forests and Woodlands: Resource Management, Values and Local Livelihoods*; Cunningham, A. B., Yang, X., Eds.; Earthscan: London, 2011; pp 161–173.

Younessi-Hamzekhanlu, M.; Ozturk, M.; Altay, V. et al. Ethnopharmacological Study of Medicinal Plants from Khoy City of West Azerbaijan-Iran. *Indian J. Trad. Knowl* **2020,** *19* (2), 251–267.

CHAPTER 20

Ethnomedicinal Significance of Epiphytic Orchids and Their Fungal Endophytes

BETTADAPURA R. NUTHAN[1],
BETTADAPURA R. MEGHAVARSHINIGOWDA[2],
SHIVANNEGOWDA MAHADEVAKUMAR[2],
KUPPURU M. MARULASIDDASWAMY[3], DEVARAJU RAKSHITH[4],
KANDIKERE R. SRIDHAR[5,6], and SREEDHARAMURTHY SATISH[1]

[1]Department of Studies in Microbiology, University of Mysore, Manasagangotri, Mysore, Karnataka, India

[2]Department of Studies in Botany, University of Mysore, Manasagangotri, Mysore, Karnataka, India

[3]Department of Studies in Biotechnology, University of Mysore, Manasagangotri, Mysore, Karnataka, India

[4]Department of Microbiology, Yuvaraja's College, University of Mysore, Mysore, Karnataka, India

[5]Department of Biosciences, Mangalore University, Mangalagangotri, Karnataka, India

[6]Centre for Environmental Studies, Yenepoya (Deemed to be University), Mangalore, Karnataka, India

ABSTRACT

Ethnic familiarity about the use of medicinal plants is part and parcel of human civilization. Among various plant species, epiphytic orchids gained importance owing to their unique ecological niches, physiology and exceptional medicinal values tapped by the tribes across the globe. As on today, a

Ethnic Knowledge and Perspectives of Medicinal Plants, Volume 1: Curative Properties and Treatment Strategies. Munir Ozturk, Kandikere R. Sridhar, Maryam Sarwat, Volkan Altay, &
Francisco Martín Huerta-Martínez (Eds.)

large number of medicinal plants including orchids have been evaluated for their association with endophytic fungal communities and their application in production of pharmaceutically valued secondary metabolites. A plethora of bioactive molecules have been isolated and screened from the epiphytic orchids for their antimicrobial, anticancer, anti-inflammatory and antiaging potential. This chapter encompasses distribution and ethnomedicinal significance of epiphytic orchids distributed mainly in the Asian region. Bioactive principles of orchids and their activity have been documented along with endophytic fungal diversity of selected orchid species as baseline data.

20.1 INTRODUCTION

Human civilization is inseparable from the ethnic knowledge of nutritional and medicinal potential of surrounding vegetation (Ozturk et al., 2020, 2021a, b). Vegetation around us has prime role in human nutrition and medicine in general for human survival and perpetuation. The primeval human might have had the therapeutic indications of plants as nutritional source and or healing properties of different ailments (Raghunathan, 1995; Ozturk et al., 2020, 2021a, b). Ethnic knowledge on use of medicinal plants is as old as humanity and the existing folk knowledge is being passed from one generation to another. Ethnic groups have practiced conservation of plant species those possess pharmacological applications. Many medicinal plants used in systems of "primitive medicine" by primates and humans are now recognized to have specific beneficial pharmacological benefits. Indeed, much of the basic armamentarium of pharmacology today has been built through long-term traditional knowledge on the herbal remedies (Dunn, 1976; Ozturk et al., 2017; Pleskanovskaya et al., 2019; Younessi-Hamzekhanlu et al., 2020).

Exploration carried out under ethnobotany with pharmacological perspectives depends on the potential of plant species used by indigenous people in a systematic way (e.g., Ayurveda). Many of the epiphytic orchids are used in ethnomedicines across the globe to treat several kinds of diseases or illnesses such as stomach ache, anemia, earache, bronchitis, fever, asthma, tumors, skin diseases, and others (Wiart, 2006; Hossain, 2011; Yonzone et al., 2012; Nongdam, 2014; Rahamtulla et al., 2020). A plethora of valuable bioactive molecules have been isolated and screened for their antimicrobial, anticancer, antiaging, anti-inflammatory activities from epiphytic orchids using modern techniques, which substantiate the evidence for ethnomedicinal properties. Pooling the knowledge of medicinal practices of various ethnic groups along with the available well-documented medicinal literature with the aid of advanced scientific approaches leads to discover novel bioactive principles that can be beneficial to mankind (Raghunathan, 1995).

Orchids (family Orchidaceae) are nonwoody perennial plant species known to possess unique fascinating flowers consist of more than 25,000 species accounting up to 10% of angiosperms (Pillon and Chase, 2007). They are terrestrial or epiphytic in habitat with about half of the species being epiphytic. The general characteristic features of orchids that enable to distinguish from other plants include velamen tissue around the aerial roots, a column formed from the joining of stamen and pistil, a coherent mass of pollen (called pollinia), and minute seeds devoid of the endosperm (Banarji, 1978; Arditti, 1992). The habit of orchids varies from the leafless, achlorophyllous, and myco-heterotrophic plants. Orchids exhibit extensive ecological tolerance and have adapted to survive in desert, semiaquatic, arctic circles, mangrove, and lithophytic conditions (Stewart and Zettler, 2002; Blinova, 2011).

Orchids have cosmopolitan distribution and they are primarily dominated in tropical as well as subtropical regions. Andes of Colombia, Ecuador has the richest orchid diversity on the earth. Countries with humid tropical forests such as Central and South America, India, Nepal, Southern China, Thailand, Malaysia, Burma, Ceylon, Philippines, Mexico, Australia, Sumatra, Borneo, Madagascar, and New Guinea also have rich in orchid biodiversity (Hagsater and Dumont, 1996). India is one of the biodiversity hotspots for orchids and harbors more than 1300 species, which makes up to 9% of the total flora of the country. Majority of these orchids are endemic to the Himalayas, Western Ghats, Eastern Ghats and Northeast states of India (Medhi and Chakraborti, 2012; De and Medhi, 2015). Orchids have fascinated humankind by their unique flowers, therapeutic properties, and challenges they pose in cultivation. Orchids are a good source of numerous phytochemicals and have proved to be a potent reservoir of novel drugs that make them medicinally important and have been used as medicine throughout the world (Kong et al., 2003).

Epiphytic orchids (epi = on top; phyte = plant; tramslated from the Greek) grow harmlessly on a tree trunk, branches, or on the twig of a phorophyte. They are slow growing, produce thick and hard leaves with prominent, tremendous roots enabling the plant to firmly anchor and effectively absorb the nutrients from the atmosphere, materials leached or dripping from leaves, branches, and bark. Several factors such as luminous intensity, temperature, humidity, and slope of the branches of the trees determine the position of an epiphytic orchids on the phorophyte (Steege and Cornelissen, 1989;

Freiberg, 1996). They are extreme specialists adapted to climatically and ecologically harsh conditions in the tree canopy, represent an essential and exciting plant group (Biedinger and Fischer, 1996). Epiphytic orchids are abundant in cloud forests where saturated air and continuous dipping are observed and they are also present in tropical habitats. Some of the epiphytic orchids have successfully been established in dry forests with the aid of modified plant parts, altered physiology, and life cycle. Some orchids avoid the harsh environment by completing a major part of their life cycle during the favorable conditions and during the unfavorable conditions undergo dormancy, sustaining life with water and reserve food stored in tuber or pseudobulb. Other epiphytic orchids endure with the help of pseudobulbs, succulent leaves, velamentous roots, fat roots, and by adapting Crassulacean acid metabolism through the photosynthetic pathway (Zhang et al., 2016, 2018; Ng and Hew, 2000).

Epiphytic orchids have gained importance for their exceptional ethnomedicinal values and being used by various tribes across the world to overcome health risks and also they serve as a reservoir of various endophytic fungi, which are known to produce novel pharmaceutically significant bioactive molecules. In this chapter, diversity, distribution, and ethnomedicinal significance of epiphytic orchids are described to gain some insight into the pharmaceutically important bioactive principles. Further, diversity and distribution of endophytic fungi associate with epiphytic orchids have been documented.

20.2 DISTRIBUTION

The ethnomedicinally important epiphytic orchids show a greater degree of variation in distribution across the continents. They have been reported from all the continents except for Europe and Antarctica. It can be noted that a few species are used as medicine in more than one continent. More than three-quarters (82%) of the total epiphytic orchids listed in Table 20.1 are found to be located in the Asian Continent (Figure 20.1). The prresence of dense tropical forest with a wide range of climatic conditions and distinct seasons in South Asia (India, Nepal, Bhutan, Bangladesh, Tibet, Sri Lanka, Bangladesh, Pakistan, and Afghanistan) has favored the diversity and distribution of 21% of epiphytic orchids in Asia with prominence of the genera *Dendrobium*, *Cymbidium*, *Bulbophyllum*, *Coelogyne* and *Pleione*. East Asia (Northeastern Tibet, China, Taiwan, and Korea) contributes up to 7% epiphytic orchids of Asia. The major epiphytic orchid genera of this region include *Cymbidium*,

TABLE 20.1 Ethonomedicinal Value of Epiphytic Orchids (Part Used: Wp, Whole Plant; LF, Leaf; PSB, Pseudobulb; RT, Root; ST, Stem; FL, Flower; SE, Seeds; TU, Tuber, RH, Rhizome; BU, Bulb; FR, Fruit; SH, Sheath).

Epiphytic orchids	Distribution	Parts used	Ethnomedicinal uses	References
Acampe carinata (Griff.) Pantl.	South and Southeast Asia	RT, LF, WP	Used to treat snake and scorpion bites, to relieve chest pain and hyperacidity.	Dash et al. (2008)
Acampe papillosa (Lindl.) Lindl.	South Asia	RT	To treat secondary Syphilis, mild uterine diseases, eye diseases, and to control asthma and bronchitis.	Hossain (2009); Nongdam (2014)
Acampe praemorsa (Roxb.) Blatt. & McCann	South Asia	LF, SE, RT, WP	Used to treat rheumatism, arthritis, cough, stomach ache, earache, applied on the wound as an antibiotic and also used as a tonic.	Dash et al. (2008); Subedi et al. (2013)
Acampe rigida (Buch. -Ham. ex Sm.) P.F. Hunt	East, South, and Southeast Asia	WP	Used to treat jaundice	Rahamtulla et al. (2020)
Acriopsis liliifolia (J.Koenig) Seidenf.	Australia, South, and Southeast Asia	LF, RT	Used to treat fever	Sulistiarini (2003)
Aerides multiflora Roxb.	South and Southeast Asia	LF, TU, PSB, WP	Used to treat body ache, cuts, and wounds, also has antibacterial property	Joshi et al. (2009); Rahamtulla et al. (2020)
Aerides crispum Lindl.	South Asia	WP	To cure ear pain and deafness	Rajendran et al. (1997)
Aerides odorata Lour.	East, South, and Southeast Asia	LF, RT	Used to treat wounds, tuberculosis and to reduce joint pain and swellings	Nongdam (2014)
Anoectochilus formosanus Hayata	East Asia	WP	Used to treat fever, diabetes, liver disorder, chest and abdominal pain and have anti-inflammatory property	Shyur et al. (2004); Wang et al. (2002)
Anoectochilus roxburghii (Wall.) Lindl.	East, South, and Southeast Asia	WP	Used to treat fever, snake bite, lung and liver diseases, hypertension and to cure child malnutrition	Zhang et al. (2007a); Cui et al. (2013)

TABLE 20.1 *(Continued)*

Epiphytic orchids	Distribution	Parts used	Ethnomedicinal uses	References
Ansellia Africana Lindl.	Africa	PSB, ST, RT	Used to treat aphrodisiac, madness, coughs, pulmonary tuberculosis, reduce fever, acts as a hemostatic agent	Watt and Brandwijk (1962); Chinsamy et al. (2011)
Bulbophyllum careyanum (Hook.) Spreng.	East, South, and Southeast Asia	LF, PSB	Used to treat burned skin and it is an abortion stimulate and also helps to childbirth recovery	Subedi et al. (2013)
Bulbophyllum cariniflorum Rchb. F.	South Asia	RT	Used to treat inducing abortion	Dash et al. (2008)
Bulbophyllum flabellum-veneris (J.Koenig) Aver.	East, South, and Southeast Asia	WP	Used to enhance congeniality	Teoh (2019a, b)
Bulbophyllum guttulatum (Hook.f.) N.P.Balakr.	South and Southeast Asia	PSB	Used to treat burn wounds	Rahamtulla et al. (2020)
Bulbophyllum kwangtungense Schltr.	East Asia	TU	Used to treat pulmonary tuberculosis, reduce fever, and acts as a hemostatic agent	Wu et al. (2006)
Bulbophyllum leopardinum (Wall.)	East, South, and Southeast Asia	LF, PSB, WP	Used to treat burns and bone fracture	Subedi et al. (2013); Rahamtulla et al. (2020)
Bulbophyllum lilacinum Ridl.	South and Southeast Asia		Used to remove fatigue, restlessness	Hossain (2009)
Bulbophyllum neilgherrense	India	PSB	To treat leucoderma	Rajendran et al. (1997)
Bulbophyllum odoratissimum (Sm.) Lindl. ex Wall.	East, South, and Southeast Asia	WP	Used to treat tuberculosis, chronic inflammation, and bone fractures	Chen et al. (2007); Chen et al. (2008)
Bulbophyllum sterile (Lam.) Suresh	South Asia (India)	PSB	Used to treat rheumatism	Hossain (2009); Shanavaskhan et al. (2012)

TABLE 20.1 *(Continued)*

Epiphytic orchids	Distribution	Parts used	Ethnomedicinal uses	References
Bulbophyllum vaginatum (Lindl.) Rchb.f.	Southeast Asia	WP	Used to treat earache	Wiart (2006)
Camaridium densum (Lindl.) M.A. Blanco.	Central America	WP	Used as analgesic and relaxant	Déciga-Campos et al. (2007a, b)
Catasetum barbatum (Lindl.) Lindl.	South America and East Asia	WP	Used as a febrifuge and anti-inflammatory agent	Shimizu et al. (1988)
Coelogyne corymbosa Lindl.	East, and South Asia	PSB	Used to treat headache	Jana et al. (1997)
Coelogyne cristata Lindl.	South Asia	PSB	Taken during constipation. Used as an aphrodisiac. The juice is applied to wounds and boils. Pseudobulb gum is used for sores	Majumder et al. (2001); Pramanick (2016); Rahamtulla et al. (2020)
Coelogyne flaccida Lindl.	East, South, and Southeast Asia	PSB	Used to treat indigestion	Manandhar (2002)
Coelogyne fuscescens Lindl.	South and Southeast Asia	PSB	Used to treat indigestion	Manandhar (2002)
Coelogyne ovalis Lindl.	East, South, and Southeast Asia	PSB, WP	Used to treat fever, headache, and urinary tract problems	Yonzone et al. (2012)
Coelogyne prolifera Lindl.	East, South, and Southeast Asia	PSB	Used to treat fever, headache, burnt skin, boils, and backache	Pant and Raskoti (2013)
Coelogyne punctulata Lindl.	East, South, and Southeast Asia	PSB	Used to treat burn spots, reduce pain, headache, and fever	Yonzone et al. (2012)
Coelogyne stricta (D. Don) Schltr.	East, South, and Southeast Asia	PSB	Used to treat headache and fever	Baral and Kurmi (2006)
Conchidium muscicola (Lindl.) Rauschert	East, South, and Southeast Asia	WP	Used to treat the respiratory, cardiac, and nervous disorder	Pant and Raskoti (2013)

TABLE 20.1 *(Continued)*

Epiphytic orchids	Distribution	Parts used	Ethnomedicinal uses	References
Corymborkis veratrifolia (Reinw.) Blume	East, South, and Southeast Asia		Used to treat fever in children	Hossain (2009)
Crepidium acuminatum (D. Don) Szlach.	East, South, and Southeast Asia	ST, PSB, RT	Used to treat burns, bronchitis, fever, tuberculosis, and weakness. It is also used for the preparation of "Astavarga" in Ayurveda	Panda and Mandal (2013)
Cymbidium aloifolium (L.) Sw.	East, South, and Southeast Asia	RT, SE, LF, PSB	Used to treat diarrhea, fever, and inflammations, paralysis, otitis, dislocation, and fracture, and acts as a hemostatic agent	Rajendran et al. (1997); Gewali and Awale (2008); Nongdam (2014); Rahamtulla et al. (2020)
Cymbidium canaliculatum R.Br	Australia	PSB	Used to treat dysentery, boils, sores, wounds, itchy skin, and fractured arms	Webb (1960)
Cymbidium devonianum Paxton	East, South, and Southeast Asia	WP	Used to treat boils, cough, and cold	Pant and Raskoti (2013)
Cymbidium eburneum Lindl.	East, South, and Southeast Asia	SE, LF	Used to treat ptosis, facial paralysis, ulcers, headache, and tumors	Panda and Mandal (2013)
Cymbidium elegans Lindl.	East, South, and Southeast Asia	LF, RT, PSB	Used to treat fever	Thakur et al. (2010)
Cymbidium ensifolium (L.) Sw.	East, South, and Southeast Asia	RH, FL	Used to treat gonorrhea, eyesores, cough, lung, gastrointestinal problems, and sedative	Hossain (2011)
Cymbidium goeringii (Rchb.f.) Rchb.f.	East, South, and Southeast Asia	WP	Used to treat hypertension and used as a diuretic agent	Watanabe et al. (2007)
Cymbidium hookerianum Rchb. F.	East, South, and Southeast Asia	SE	Used to treat cuts as hemostatic	Yonzone et al. (2012)
Cymbidium iridioides D. Don	East, South, and Southeast Asia	PSB, LF	Used as a tonic and to clot blood	Vaidya et al. (2000)

TABLE 20.1 *(Continued)*

Epiphytic orchids	Distribution	Parts used	Ethnomedicinal uses	References
Cymbidium longifolium D Don.	South Asia	PSB	Used as emetic	Nongdam (2014)
Cymbidium macrorhizon Lindl.	East, South, and Southeast Asia	RH	Used to treat boils	Hossain (2011)
Cymbidium madidum Lindl.	Australia	PSB	Used to treat dysentery	Yonzone et al. (2012)
Dendrobium affine (Decne.) Steud.	Australia	PSB	Used to treat itchy skins, infected skin lesion, boils, and minor burns	Teoh (2019a, b)
Dendrobium aloifolium (Blume) Rchb.f.	Southeast Asia	LF	Used to treat headache	Giesen et al. (2007)
Dendrobium amoenum Wall. ex Lindl.	South Asia	PSB, LF	Used to treat burnt skin and dislocated bones	Venkateswarlu et al. (2002); Subedi et al. (2013)
Dendrobium aphyllum (Roxb.) C.E.C. Fisch	East, South, and Southeast Asia	LF, WP	Used to treat new-borns deformed body parts to reshape into normal	Hossain (2011); Rahamtulla et al. (2020)
Dendrobium canaliculatum var. foelschei (F.Muell.) Rupp & T.E. Hunt	Australia	PSB	Used to treat infected skin and cuts	Teoh (2019a, b)
Dendrobium candidum Wall. ex Landl.	China	LF	To treat diabetes	Nongdam (2014)
Dendrobium catenatum Lindl.	East Asia	LF	Used to treat anxiety and panic	Lo et al. (2004)
Dendrobium chryseum Rolfe	Australia	LF	Used to treat diabetes	Yang et al. (2006a, b)
Dendrobium chrysanthum Wall. ex Lindl.	East, South, and Southeast Asia	LF	Used to treat skin diseases and fever	Li et al. (2001); Nongdam (2014)

TABLE 20.1 *(Continued)*

Epiphytic orchids	Distribution	Parts used	Ethnomedicinal uses	References
Dendrobium chrysotoxum Lindl.	East, South, and Southeast Asia		Used as a tonic and antipyretic, have anti-inflammatory activities	Nongdam (2014); Ramesh et al. (2019)
Dendrobium crepidatum Lindl. & Paxton	East, South, and Southeast Asia	PSB	Used to treat fractured bones	Pant and Raskoti (2013)
Dendrobium densiflorum Lindl.	East, South, and Southeast Asia	PSB	Used to treat cataract development, to relieve fatigue, strengthen the stomach, prevent pimples, and boost body immune system	Fan et al. (2001); Thakur et al. (2010)
Dendrobium denudans D.Don	South Asia	ST	Used to treat cough, cold, nasal block, and tonsillitis and used as a tonic	Panda and Mandal (2013)
Dendrobium eriiflorum Griff.	South Asia	PSB	Used to treat bone dislocation and fracture	Subedi et al. (2013)
Dendrobium faciferum J.J.Sm	Southeast Asia	ST	Used to treat the bone dislocation	Heyne (1950)
Dendrobium farmeri Paxton	South Asia	WP	Have some antibacterial property	Hossain (2011)
Dendrobium fimbriatum Hook.	East, South, and Southeast Asia	LF, FL	Used to treat the liver problem, nervous breakdown and as a plaster to set crack bones	Bi et al. (2003); Baral and Kurmi (2006); Nongdam (2014); Rahamtulla et al. (2020)
Dendrobium fugax Rchb.f.	South and Southeast Asia	WP	Used as a tonic against weakness and as a stimulant	Tsering et al. (2017)
Dendrobium heterocarpum Wall. ex Lindl.	East, South, and Southeast Asia	PSB	Used to treat bone dislocation and fracture	Subedi et al. (2013)
Dendrobium longicornu Lindl.	East, South, and Southeast Asia	PSB, RT	Used to treat fever	Manandhar (2002)

TABLE 20.1 *(Continued)*

Epiphytic orchids	Distribution	Parts used	Ethnomedicinal uses	References
Dendrobium loddigesii Rolfe	East and Southeast Asia	LF	Used to treat fever and an anticancer agent	Ho and Chen (2003)
Dendrobium macraei Lindl.	South Asia	TU, WP	Used as a stimulant, demulcent, lowers the blood pressure, to treat skin allergy, snakebites, and eczema	Karnick (1996)
Dendrobium macrostachyum Lindl.	South, Southeast Asia, and Australia	LF, ST	Used to treat earache	Hossain (2011)
Dendrobium moniliforme (L.) Sw.	East, South, and Southeast Asia	LF, ST, PSB	Used to treat cataract, throat inflammation, gastritis and acts as an antipyretic, analgesic, and aphrodisiac agent	Chen and Chen (1935); Shu et al. (2009); Gutiérrez (2010)
Dendrobium monticola P.F.Hunt & Summerh.	East, South, and Southeast Asia	WP	Used to treat boils and pimples	Singh (2001)
Dendrobium moschatum (Banks) Sw.	East, South, and Southeast Asia	LF, PSB	Used to treat earache, bone dislocation, and fracture	Pant (2013); Malla et al. (2015); Rahamtulla et al. (2020)
Dendrobium nobile Lindl.	East, South, and Southeast Asia	PSB, SE, WP	Used to treat pulmonary tuberculosis, dyspepsia, reduced salivation, night sweats, fever, anorexia, and wounds	Kong et al. (2003); Gutiérrez (2010); Nongdam (2014)
Dendrobium officinale	China	ST	Used to treat hyperglycemia, hyperlipidemia, chronic gastritis, and dim eyesight and to strengthen immunity, as an anticancer and antiaging agent	Tang et al. (2017)
Dendrobium pachyphyllum (Kuntze) Bakh.f.	South and Southeast Asia	WP	Used to treat hydropsy	Heyne (1950)
Dendrobium polyanthum Wall. ex Lindl.	East, South, and Southeast Asia	PSB	Used to boost the immune system	Joshi et al. (2017)

TABLE 20.1 *(Continued)*

Epiphytic orchids	Distribution	Parts used	Ethnomedicinal uses	References
Dendrobium purpureum Roxb.	Southeast Asia and Australia	LF	Used to treat nail fungal infection	Teoh (2019b)
Dendrobium salaccense (Blume) Lindl.	East, South, and Southeast Asia	LF	Used as a fragrance material	Teoh (2019b)
Dendrobium teretifolium R.Br.	South Pacific island	LF	Used to treat severe headache and other pains	Lassak and McCarthy (1983)
Dendrobium transparens Wall. ex Lindl.	South Asia		Used to treat bone dislocation and fracture	Subedi (2002)
Dendrobium utile J.J.Sm.	Southeast Asia	ST	Used to treat the bone dislocation	Teoh (2019b)
Dichaea muricata (Sw.) Lindl.	Central and South America	LF	Used to treat eye infection	Kong et al. (2003)
Epidendrum rigidum Jacq.	North and South America	ST	Used to replenish body fluid	Hernández-Romero et al. (2005)
Epidendrum strobiliferum Rchb.f.	East Asia	ST	Used as analgesic	Ferreira et al. (2000)
Eria lasiopetala (Willd.) Ormerod.	East, South, and Southeast Asia	LF, WP	Used to treat boils, cuts, and wounds	Hossain (2009); Rahamtulla et al. (2020)
Eria bamusifolia Lindl.	India	WP	To treat hyperacidity and stomach related problems	Nongdam (2014)
Eria spicata (D Don.) Hand.-Mazz	India	ST, WP	To treat headache and mild stomach ailments	Nongdam (2014)
Eriopsis biloba Lindl.	South America	ST	Used to treat sore gums and mouth membranes	Kong et al. (2003)
Erycina pusilla (L.) N.H.Williams & M.W.Chase	America	LF	Used to treat lacerations	Kong et al. (2003)

TABLE 20.1 *(Continued)*

Epiphytic orchids	Distribution	Parts used	Ethnomedicinal uses	References
Eulophia speciosa (R.Br.) Bolus	Indonesia	RT	Used as analgesic	Heyne (1950)
Grammatophyllum scriptum (L.) Blume	Southeast Asia and Australia	BU, ST	Used to treat dysentery, aphthae, sores, to expel worms, dropsy, snake bites, scorpions' and centipedes' stings	Yonzone et al. (2012)
Jumellea fragrans (Thouars) Schltr.	Africa	LF, ST	Used as an antispasmodic, antiasthmatic agent, to treat eczema, diarrhea	Gurib-Fakim and Brendler (2004)
Liparis condylobulbon Rchb.f.	East, South East Asia, and Australia	PSB, LF	Used to treat intestinal complaints and constipation	Teoh (2016)
Liparis nervosa (Thunb.) Lindl.	Africa, Central, and South America, East, South and Southeast Asia, and Australia	WP, TU	Used to stop internal/external bleeding and to treat snake bites	Tsering et al. (2017)
Luisia tristis (G. Forst.) Hook.f.	East, South, South East Asia, and Australia	WP	Used to treat wounds	Vaidya et al. (2000)
Lusia trichorhiza (Hook) Blume.	India	WP	To treat jaundice and it contains the antibacterial effect	Nongdam (2014)
Masdevallia uniflora Ruiz & Pav.	Central America	WP	Used to facilitate urination and reduce bladder inflammation	Kong et al. (2003)
Mycaranthes pannea (Lindl.) S.C.Chen & J.J.Wood	East, South, and Southeast Asia		Used to treat ague, malaria fever, fractures, bruises, skin complaints, swelling, dislocation, and fracture	Namsa et al. (2009)
Nidema boothii (Lindl.) Schltr.	Southeast Asia	WP	Used as relaxant agent	Hernández-Romero et al. (2004)

TABLE 20.1 *(Continued)*

Epiphytic orchids	Distribution	Parts used	Ethnomedicinal uses	References
Oberonia caulescens Lindl.	East, South, and Southeast Asia	TU	Used to treat liver problems	Pant (2013)
Oberonia falconeri Hook f.	East, South, and Southeast Asia	LF	Used to treat bone fractures	Tiwari et al. (2012)
Oberonia lycopodioides (J.Koenig) Ormerod	Southeast Asia, Malaysia	LF	Used to treat boils	Nurfadilah (2020)
Oberonia mucronata (D.Don) Ormerod & Seidenf.	East, South, and Southeast Asia	WP	Used to treat rheumatism, promote blood circulation, inflammation of the bladder/ureter, bruises, and fractures, detoxicant, a diuretic agent	Teoh (2016)
Oberonia pachyrachis Rchb. f. ex Hook. f.	East, South, and Southeast Asia	LF	Has antibacterial property	Hossain (2011)
Otochilus albus Lindl.	South Asia	WP	Used to make tonic	Subedi et al. (2013)
Otochilus fuscus Lindl.	East, South, and Southeast Asia	WP	Used to treat febrifuge for stomach inflammation, allays hyperdipsia, dehydration, bone fracture, and dislocation and used as antiemetic	Rajbhandari (2014)
Otochilus lancifolius Griff.	East, South, and Southeast Asia	WP	Used to treat fractured and dislocated bones	Rajbhandari (2014)
Otochilus lancilabius Seidenf.	East, South, and Southeast Asia	WP	Used as an antiemetic, febrifuge and to treat dehydration	Wangchuk et al. (2017)
Otochilus porrectus Lindl.	South and Southeast Asia	WP	Used as a tonic, against sinusitis and rheumatism	Pant (2013)
Panisea uniflora (Lindl.) Lindl	East, South, and Southeast Asia	LF	Used to treat pus-forming wounds	Rahamtulla et al. (2020)

TABLE 20.1 *(Continued)*

Epiphytic orchids	Distribution	Parts used	Ethnomedicinal uses	References
Papilionanthe teres (Roxb.) Schltr.	East, South, and Southeast Asia		Used to treat dislocated bones	Simmler et al. (2011)
Phalaenopsis mannii Rchb.f	South Asia	FL	Used for hair growth	Rahamtulla et al. (2020)
Phragmipedium pearcei (Rchb.f.) Rauh & Senghas	South America	WP	Used to treat stomach ache	Kong et al. (2003)
Pholidota articulata Lindl.	East, South, and Southeast Asia	LF, WP	Used to treat the bone fracture and dislocation	Jalal et al. (2008); Joshi et al. (2009); Rahamtulla et al. (2020)
Pholidota chinensis Lindl.	East and South Asia	PSB	Used to treat scrofula, toothache, stomach ache, chronic bronchitis, and duodenal ulcer	Wang et al. (2006)
Pholidota imbricata Lindl.	East, South, and Southeast Asia	PSB	Used to treat fever, expelling spines, and used as a tonic	Hossain (2009); Shanavaskhan et al. (2012)
Pholidota pallida Lindl.	East, South, and Southeast Asia	RH, PSB	Used to treat fever, sleep apnea, stomach pain, navel pain, intestinal worms and rheumatism, finger abscess	Rajendran et al. (1997); Hossain (2011); Subedi et al. (2013)
Pinalia spicata (D.Don) S.C.Chen & J.J.Wood	East, South, and Southeast Asia	PSB	Used to treat stomach aches and headaches.	Tsering et al. (2017)
Pinalia stricta (Lindl.) Kuntze	East, South, and Southeast Asia	WP	Used to reduce muscular pains	Rahamtulla et al. (2020)
Pleione humilis (Sm.) D.Don	South Asia	PSB	Used to treat cuts and wounds	Pyakurel and Gurung (2008)
Pleione maculate (Lindl.) Lindl.	East, South, and Southeast Asia	RH	Used to treat liver and stomach problems	Pant (2013)

TABLE 20.1 *(Continued)*

Epiphytic orchids	Distribution	Parts used	Ethnomedicinal uses	References
Pleione praecox (Sm.) D. Don	East, South, and Southeast Asia	PSB	Used to treat cuts and wounds	Thakur et al. (2010)
Polystachya ottoniana Rchb.f.	Africa		Used to treat diarrhea and teething babies	Chinsamy et al. (2011)
Renanthera imschootiana Rolfe.	India	LF	To treat dermatological problems	Nongdam (2014)
Rhynchostylis retusa (L.) Blume	East, South, and Southeast Asia	RT, WP	Used to treat rheumatism, asthma, tuberculosis, nervous twitching, cramps, infantile epilepsy, vertigo, palpitation, kidney stone, and menstrual disorders, induce vomiting, blood dysentery, wounds, malarial fever, and throat inflammation	Medhi and Chakrabarti (2009); Nongdam (2014); Rahamtulla et al. (2020)
Scaphyglottis livida (Lindl.) Schltr.	Central and South America	WP	Used as an analgesic and anti-inflammatory agent	Déciga-Campos et al. (2007a, b)
Smitinandia micrantha (Lindl.) Holttum	East, South, and Southeast Asia	WP	Used as a tonic, and has antibacterial property	Pant (2013)
Thunia alba (Lindl.) Rchb. F.	East, South, and Southeast Asia	WP	Used to treat dislocated bones	Pant (2013)
Tropidia curculigoides Lindl.	East, South, and Southeast Asia		Used to treat diarrhea and Malaria	Ormerod (2018)
Vanda coerulea Griff. Ex Lindl.	South Asia	LF, FL	Used to treat blindness, cataract, glaucoma and used as an expectorant	Rahamtulla et al. (2020); Nongdam (2014)
Vanda cristata Wall. ex Lindl.	South Asia	LF	Used to treat skin cuts, boils, and dislocated bones	Pyakurel and Gurung (2008); Rahamtulla et al. (2020)

TABLE 20.1 *(Continued)*

Epiphytic orchids	Distribution	Parts used	Ethnomedicinal uses	References
Vanda roxburgii R.Br.	South Asia	RT, LF, FL	To treat otitis, rheumatism, fever, and bronchitis.	Nongdam (2014)
Vanda tessellata (Roxb. f.) Hook. Ex D. Don	South Asia	RT, LF	Used to treat gout, edema, ulcer, dyspnea, colic pain, obstinate abdominal diseases including ascites, lowers blood pressure rheumatism, syphilis and otitis, scorpion sting, high fever, sexually transmitted diseases, nervous disorder, earache, muscle sprains, lumbago, back pain, fever, rheumatism, bronchitis, inflammation, hiccups, piles, boils on the scalp and used as an aphrodisiac, analgesic, nervine tonic alexiteric, antipyretic, sexual stimulant	Rajendran et al. (1997); Singh and Duggal (2009); Rahamtulla et al. (2020)
Vanda testacea (Lindl.) Rchb.f.	South Asia		Used to treat broken bones of cattle, asthma, cuts and wounds, malaria, rheumatism, and nervous disorders	Tiwari et al. (2012)
*Vanilla planifoli*a Jacks. ex Andrews	Central America and Southeast Asia	FR, SH	Used to treat fever, rheumatism, hysteria, increase energy and muscular system	Shanmugavalli and Umashankar (2009)

Dendrobium, Luisia, and *Pleione*. The prevailing climatic conditions with heavy rainfall during monsoon countered by dry season in the isolated islands and slopes of Southeast Asia (Brunei, Burma, East Timor, Indonesia, Kampuchea Cambodia, Laos, Malaysia, Myanmar, Philippines, Singapore, Southeast China, Thailand, and Vietnam) has favored to the diversity of epiphytic orchids up to 8% of Asia with dominance of genera *Aerides, Bulbophyllum Dendrobium, Phalaenopsis*, and *Vanda* (Teoh, 2016).

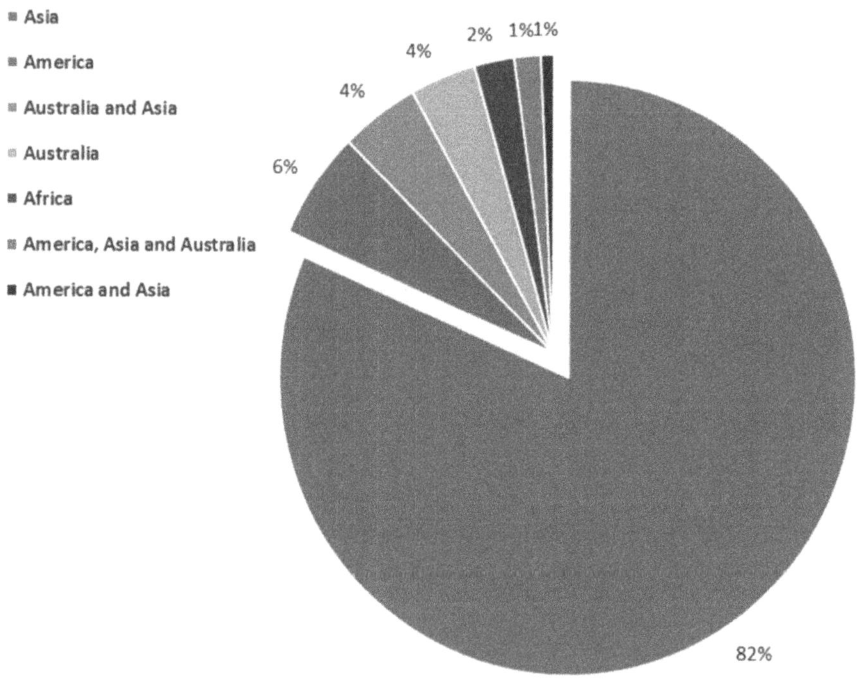

FIGURE 20.1 Distribution pattern of medicinally valued epiphytic orchids.

In America, about 5.9% of ethnomedicinal epiphytic orchids are used to cure various ailments. The diverse habitat and the high humidity found in the Caribbean region, primarily the mainland of the USA have favored the prevalence of many epiphytic orchids. Orchids of Mexico generally grow in dry periods and they are capable of withstanding prolonged dry periods with their pseudobulbs (Aguirre-Leon, 1992; Ng and Hew, 2000). The unique ecosystem present in the east side of the Andes Mountain has contributed to a greater diversity with most common genera like *Phragmipedium* and *Masdevallia*. The warm and humid conditions of the tropic has favored up to

3.7% of epiphytic orchids in Australia. *Cymbidium, Dendrobium, Grammatophyllum*, and *Liparis* are some of the common genera of this region (Smith, 2008). Majority of these epiphytes are found in the northeastern Queensland, however *Sarcochilus australis* is the only epiphyte found in Tasmania.

Around 2.2% of epiphytic orchids are known from Africa with different ecological regions in the Saharan Desert in the north, the Kalahari Desert in the south, while the tropical forest in the canter, and in the west coast with distinct dry and wet seasons provide appropriate environmental conditions for the epiphytic orchids to flourish. The genus *Aerangis, Angraecum, Ansellia, Bulbophyllum, Chamaengis, Podangis*, and *Polystachya* are commonly found in Central Africa. Madagascar has many endemic orchids with *Cymbidiella, Bulbophyllum*, and *Polystachya* as major genera (Biedinger and Fischer 1996; Cribb and Hermans, 2007).

It will be of great interest to note that some of the ethnomedicinal epiphytic orchid genera distributed in more than one continents showing the disjunct distribution and they are being used by aboriginals residing in a different part of the world as a potential source of ethnic medicine. About 0.7% of the epiphytic orchids is present in America and Asia, while 4.4% in Australia and Asia, 1.5% in America, Asia, and Australia.

20.3 ETHNOMEDICINAL IMPORTANCE

Dependence on plants as a source of medicine is an age old traditional practice of natives as well as tribals (Raghunathan, 1995). The ethnic group has its plantlore passed from one generation to another, which has paved way toward the discovery of pharmaceutically valuable bioactive principles. The genus *Bulbophyllum, Cymbidium, Dendrobium*, and *Vanda* are the most predominant epiphytic orchids used in the preparation of ethnic medicine. Medicinal values of the orchids have been found either in whole plants or in different parts (Figure 20.2). For example, whole plant (*Bulbophyllum odoratissimum, Cymbidium devonianum*, and *Phragmipedium pearcei*), roots (*Acampe papillosa* and *Eulophia speciosa)*, stem (*Dendrobium officinale* and *Eriopsis biloba*), leaves (*Renanthera imschootiana, Vanda cristata)*, pseudobulbs (*Bulbophyllum neilgherrense* and *Pholidota chinensis)*, tubers (*Oberonia caulescens*) and flowers (*Phalaenopsis mannii, Vanda roxburgii*) are used. The fruit and sheath of *Vanilla planifolia* are useful to treat fever and rheumatism (Shanmugavalli and Umashankar, 2009). Paste prepared from the bulbs of *Grammatophyllum scriptum* is applied externally to expel worms and the rhizome of *Pleione maculate* is used to relieve liver and stomach problems

(Yonzone et al., 2012; Pant, 2013). The seeds of *Cymbidium hookerianum* are exploited to treat cuts on the body (Yonzone et al., 2012).

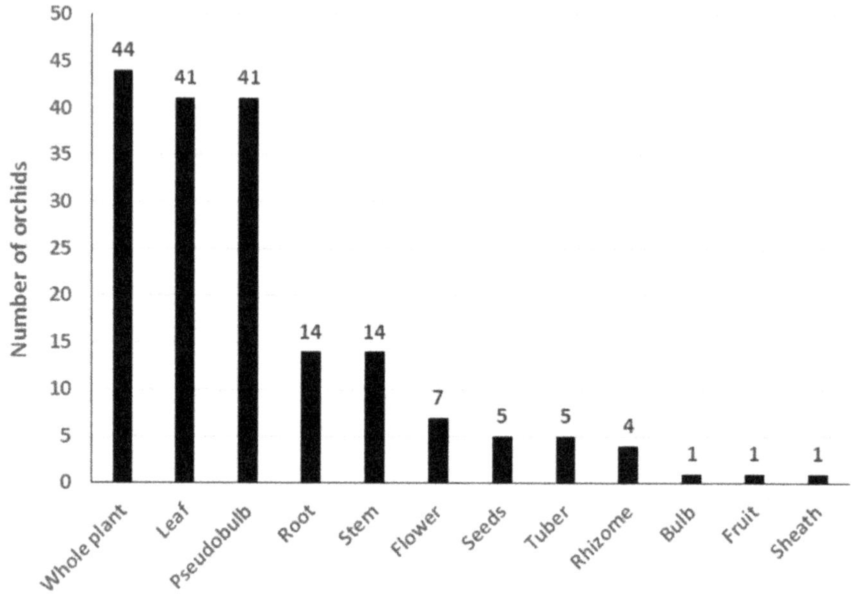

FIGURE 20.2 Different parts of epiphytic orchids used for medicinal purpose.

Use of orchids in the preparation of indigenous medicines has been in practice for ages and the first documentation was found in China. The Chinese pharmacopeia Shen-Nung Pen-Tsao Ching (200 BC) mentions the use of *Dendrobium* for the preparation of tonic, anti-inflammatory substance, analgesic, and astringent. Later the Han dynasty (200 BC–200 AD) to date, *Dendrobium* and *Flickingeria* species are used for the preparation of tonic to cure impotence, stomach ailments in China, Taiwan, Korea, and Japan (Chen et al., 1994). Fresh or dried stem of *Dendrobium* (*D. candidum, D. noibile* and *D. fimbriatum*) popularly known as *Shi Hu* in China, which is used in the preparation as strengthening tonic to the lower back, improves vision, cures stomach-, kidney- and lung-related ailments (Jaime et al., 2017). *Bulbophyllum kwangtungense* is useful in the preparation of *Yin Tonic* (Yi et al., 2005).

In India, species of the genus *Dendrobium, Cymbidium*, and *Vanda* are commonly exploited for medicinal purposes. The whole plant of *Coelogyne ovalis* is used to cure cough, urinary infections, and eye disorders in the western and southern parts of India (Singh and Duggal, 2009). Paste prepared out of the pseudobulb and leaves of *Bulbophyllum neilgherrense* is used in the southern part of India to treat leukoderma (Rajendran et al., 1997). *Koya* tribe uses a paste made up of aerial roots of *Cymbidium aloifolium* to plaster around the fractured bone, while *Kadars* people use rhizome paste of *Pholidota pallida* to cure finger abscess (Rajendran et al., 1997). Leaf extract of *Vanda tessellata* is useful in treating skin diseases by the *Jatapu* tribe (Rajendran et al., 1997). A preparation made from the leaves of *Vanda roxburgii* is externally applied to treat ear ache as well as to treat rheumatism (Nongdam, 2014). *Acampe papillosa, A. praemorsa, Luisia tristis, Pholidota imbricate*, and *Rhynchostylis retusa* are useful to treat various ailments in Bangladesh (Hossain, 2009). In Nepal, the *Lama* (Priests), *Amji* (Tibetan medicine men), *Jhankri* (healers), *Guraun* (Tharu priests), *Vaidya,* and *Guyaju* (Newar medicine men) use epiphytic orchids in the preparation of traditional medicine to cure the ailments of the local people (Gewali and Awale, 2008). The paste from *Coelogyne flaccida* is used to treat indigestion, while *Cymbidium aloifolium* is used to treat diarrhea, fever and inflammations, paralysis, otitis, dislocation, fracture, and it also acts as a hemostatic agent (Rajendran et al., 1997; Manandhar, 2002; Gewali and Awale, 2008; Nongdam, 2014; Rahamtulla et al., 2020).

People from America are using *V. planifolia* since the 15th century to treat fever, hysteria, impotence, and rheumatism. In the book, *Badiano Codex* by Martin de la Cruz—Aztec Physician in 1552 was the first American book mentioning the use of epiphytic orchids in medicine such as *Encyclia citrina* to treat wounds, *Stanhopea hernandezii* for sun-stroke and *Laelia autumnalis* to treat cough, while *Arpophyllum spicatum* and *Epidendrum pastoris* used to treat dysentery. In Mexico, tea prepared from the whole orchid *Masdevallia uniflora* facilitates to treat urination in pregnant women and reduce bladder inflammation (Kong et al., 2003). The early settlers and aboriginal tribes of Australia used epiphytic orchids as a source of food as well as medicine, while bulbs of *Dendrobium speciosum* served as food (Bulpitt, 2005). *Dendrobium aurantiacum* leaves were used in the preparation of decoction and as remedy against diabetes (Yang et al., 2005). Chewing of pseudobulb of *Cymbidium madidum* was practiced as a remedy against dysentery, while the seeds served as oral contraceptive (Yonzone et al., 2012). *Cymbidium canaliculatum, Dendrobium discolour*, and *D. teratifolium* are reportedly been used by aboriginals in treating dysentery, control ringworm, and relieving pain.

The *Zulu*, one of the largest ethnic groups of South Africa uses the stem of *Ansellia africana* (*A. gigantea*) as an aphrodisiac (Watt and Brandwijk 1962; Chinsamy et al. 2011). This orchid is endemic to Africa and used in different regions for therapeutic purposes. The people of Mpika and

Zambia use the infusion of the stem and leaves to treat madness (Gelfland et al., 1985), infusion of root is administered as an emetic in other regions (Gerstner, 1941), infusion of leaves and the smoke of burnt roots were also used to avoid bad dreams (Hutchings, 1996). *Ansellia africana* is useful to protect charm and serve as aphrodisiac in women of Zimbabwe (Gelfland et al., 1985). Berliocchi and Griffiths (2000) reported that the paste prepared from leaves and pseudobulbs of *A. africana* is useful as a short-term contraceptive in young men. In 1988, Cunningham (1988) reported use of *Aerangis mystacidii* in traditional medicine as an aphrodisiac. Pseudobulbs of *Bulbophyllum maximum* are used to treat madness and the leaf extract is used to protect against sorcery. People of Morobe of Papua New Guinea administered stem infusion of *Galeola foliate* to treat infections (Khan and Omoloso, 2004). Other epiphytic orchids especially *Eulophia cucullata* are used to treat impotence and infertility, while *E. cucullata* along with *Crytorchis arcuate* is useful to treat the skin infection as well as diabetes (Bryant, 1966; Pant, 2013).

20.4 BIOACTIVE PRINCIPLES

The undesirable side effects by the synthetic drugs and constantly increasing drug-resistant pathogens is a major concern and demands alternative source to combat several threatening diseases. The scope for detailed study in the field of natural products and their chemistry has greater potential in countries with rich biodiversity. The application of orchids in ancient medicines has paved the way for deeper insight into the effective bioactive secondary metabolites. The knowledge of medico-ethnobotany and ethnopharmacology along with proper scientific approach can aid in the discovery of newer bioactive principles those help saving lives. Research on profiling the phytochemicals, evaluating the efficacy and determining the bioactive principles from the ethnomedicinally important epiphytic orchids have resulted in the discovery of numerous compounds with pharmacological properties (Table 20.2).

By various solvents, a different class of secondary metabolites has been isolated from epiphytic orchids such as phenanthrenes, triterpenoids, stilbenoids, substituted bibenzyls, monocarboxylic acids, glycosides, pyrrolizidine alkaloids, phenolic compounds, phenanthraquinones, phenanthereneglycosides and others, which exhibits pharmacological properties mainly antioxidant, anticancer, spasmolytic, anti-inflammatory, anti-acetylcholinesterase, hypotensive, diuretic activities, hypoglycemic effect, and

TABLE 20.2 Bioactive Principles of Epiphytic Orchids and Their Pharmacological Significance.

Epiphytic orchids	Bioactive secondary metabolites identified	Pharmacological properties	References
Anoectochilus roxburghii (Wall.) Lindl.	Quercetin-7-*O*-β-D-[6″-*O*-(trans-feruloyl)] glucopyranoside, 8-C-*p*-hydroxybenzylquercetin, Isorhamnetin-7-*O*-β-D-glucopyranoside, Isorhamnetin-3-*O*-β-D-glucopyranoside, Kaempferol-3-*O*-β-D-glucopyranoside, kaempferol-7-*O*-β-D-glucopyranoside, 5-hydroxy-3′,4′,7-trimethoxyflavonol-3-*O*-β-D-rutinoside, and isorhamnetin-3-*O*-β-D-rutinoside	Antioxidant activity; Anticancer activity; Anti-inflammatory effect; Antihyperglycemic activity	He et al. (2006); Cui et al. (2013); Zhang et al. (2007a); Deng et al. (2020); Guo et al. (2019)
Bulbophyllum kwangtungense Schltr.	7,8-Dihydro-5-hydroxy-12,13-methylenedioxy-11-methoxyldibenz[b,f]oxepin, 7,8-dihydro-4-hydroxy-12,13-methylenedioxy-11-methoxyldibenz[b,f]oxepin, and 7,8-dihydro-3-hydroxy-12,13-methylenedioxy-11-methoxyldibenz[b,f]oxepin	Anticancer activity	Wu et al. (2006)
Bulbophyllum odoratissimum (Sm.) Lindl. ex Wall.	3,7-Dihydroxy-2,4,6-trimethoxyphenanthrene	Anticancer activity	Chen et al. (2007)
Bulbophullum leopardium	Bulbophyllanthrin	NE	Majumder et al. (1985)
Bulbophyllum triste	Tristin	NE	Majumder and Pal (1993)
Camaridium densum (Lindl.) M.A.Blanco.	2,5-Dihidroxi-3,4-dimetoxifenantreno, Eriantridina, Fimbriol-A, Gimnopusina, Nudol, Gigantol	Spasmolytic activity	Estrada et al. (1999); Radice et al. (2020); Estrada et al. (2004)
Catasetum barbatum (Lindl.) Lindl.	2, 7-Dihydroxy-3, 4, 8-trimethoxyphenanthrene, 2, 7-dihydroxy-3, 4-dimethoxyphenanthrene	Anti-inflammatory	Shimizu et al. (1988)
Coelogyne ochracea Lindl.	Ochrone-A	NE	Shimura et al. (2007)
Coelogyne ovalis	Bibenzyl, 3′-*O*-methylbatatasin.	NE	Sachdev and Kulshreshtha (1986)

TABLE 20.2 *(Continued)*

Epiphytic orchids	Bioactive secondary metabolites identified	Pharmacological properties	References
Cymbidium aloifolium (L.) Sw.	Aloifol I, Aloifol II, 6-*O*-methylcoelonin, Batatasin III, Coelonin, Gigantol,1-(4′-hydroxy-3′,5′-dimethoxyphenyl)-2-(3″-hydroxyphenyl) ethane,1-(4′-hydroxy-3′,5′-dimethoxyphenyl)-2-(4″-hydroxy-3″-methoxyphenyl)ethane,2,7-dihydroxy-4,6-dimethoxy-9,10-dihydrophenanthrene, Cymbinodin-A, Cymbinodin B	NE	Juneja et al. (1987) Barua et al. (1990)
Cymbidium goeringii (Rchb.f.) Rchb.f.	β-Sitosterol, Daucosterol, Ergosterol, Gigantol, Cymbidine A	Hypotensive, diuretic activities, Anti-inflammatory activity, Anticancer activity	Lee et al. (2005); Won et al. (2006); Watanabe et al. (2007)
Dendrobium amoenum Wall. ex Lindl.	Amotin, Amoenin, Amoenumin, Amoenylin, Isoamoenylin, 3,4′-dihydroxy-5-methoxybibenzyl, 4,4′-dihydroxy-3,3′,5-trimethoxybibenzyl (Moscatilin)	NE	Dahmén and Leander, (1978); Majumder et al. (1999)
Dendrobium aphyllum (Roxb.) C.E.C. Fisch	Flavanthrin, coelonin, iusianthridin, moscatin, gigantol, batatasin III, dibutyl phthalate, diisobutyl phthalate, *p*-hydroxyphenylpropionic methyl ester	NE	Lam et al. (2015)
Dendrobium candidum Wall.ex Landl.	(−)-Loliolide, (−)-Secoisolariciresinol, (−) Syringaresinol, (+)-Lyoniresinol-3a-*O*-β -D-glucopyranoside, (+)-Syringaresinol-4-D-monoglucoside, (10R)-10-(4-hydroxy-3,5-dimethoxylphenyl) propan-10-ol 4-*O* -D-glucopyranoside, (E)-*p*-Hydroxycinnamic acid, 2,4,7-trihydroxy-9,10-dihydrophenanthrene, 2-methoxyphenol-*O*-β -L-apiofuromosyl-(1→2)-β -D-glucopyranoside, 3,4-dihydroxy-5,4′-dimethoxybibenzyl, 3-*O*-methylgigantol,	NE	Li et al. (2008); Li et al. (2009); Guan et al. (2009); Wang et al. (2010)

TABLE 20.2 *(Continued)*

Epiphytic orchids	Bioactive secondary metabolites identified	Pharmacological properties	References
	4,4′-dihydroxy-3,5-dimethoxybibenzyl, 4′,5-dihydroxy-3,3′-dimethoxybibenzyl, 4-allyl-2,6-dimethoxyphenylglucoside		
Dendrobium chryseum Rolfe	Araxerol, Coumarin, Moscatilin, Chrysotobibenzyl, Chrysotoxin, Gigantol, Kaempferol, *cis*-Melilotoside, Defuscin, Dendroflorin, Dengibsin, Dihydromelilotoside, Naringenin, *n*-Octacosyl Ferulate, *trans*-Melilotoside	Antioxidant activity	Yang et al. (2006a, b); Yang et al. (2007)
Dendrobium chrysanthum Wall. ex Lindl.	(2S)-*N*-*cis*-cinnamoyl-2-oxopropyrrolidine, (2S)-*N*-trans-cinnamoyl-2-oxopropyrrolidine, (þ)-lyoniresinol, 2,5-dihydroxy-4,9-dimethoxylphenanthrene, 4,4′-dihydroxy-3,3′,5-trimethoxybibenzyl, 7,7′-bis-(4-hydroxy-3,5-dimethoxyphenyl)-8,8′-dihydroxymethyl-tetrahydrofuran-4-D-glucoside, Chrysophanol, Chrysotobibenzyl, Chrysotobibenzyl, Chrysotoxin, Crepidatin, Crepidatin, Dehydrodiconiferyl Alcohol-4-β-D-glucoside, Denchrysans A, B, Denchryside A, Denchryside B, Dendrochrysanene, Dendroflorin, Dengibsin, Emodin, Gigantol, Moscatilin, Moscatin, Physcion, β-Sitosterol	NE	Min et al. (1987); Yang et al. (2005); Yang et al. (2006a, b)
Dendrobium crepidatum Lindl. & Paxton	Crepidine, Crepidamine, Dendrocrepine	NE	Majumder and Maiti (1988); Arditti (1992)
Dendrobium densiflorum Lindl.	Homoeridictyol, Scoparone, Bibenzyl, Densiflorol a, Phenanthrenedione, Densiflorol b, Dendroflorin, Dengibsin, Cypripedin, Gigantol, Moscatilin,	NE	Fan et al. (2001); Lam et al. (2015)

TABLE 20.2 *(Continued)*

Epiphytic orchids	Bioactive secondary metabolites identified	Pharmacological properties	References
	Tristin, Naringenin, Homoeriodictyol, Moscatin, 2,6-dihydroxy-1,5,7-trimethoxyphenanthrene, 4,7-dihydroxy-2-methoxy-9,10-dihydrophenanthrene, Scoparone, Scopoletin, Ayapin		
Dendrobium fimbriatum Hook.	2-hydroxyethyl caeate, Ayapin, Chrysophanol, Chrysotobibenzyl (I), Confusarin, Crepidatin, Defuscin, Denhydroshizukanolide, Fimbriatone, *n*-Dotriacontanoic acid, i-Octacosyl ferulate, *n*-Triacontyl cis-*p*-Coumarate, Physcion, Rhein, Scopolin methyl ether, β -Sitosterol	NE	Bi et al. (2001); Qing et al. (2009)
Dendrobium longicornu Lindl.	Jebantine, Jibantic acid	NE	Khory and Katarak (1993); Khasim and Rao (1999); Lam et al. (2015)
Dendrobium loddigesii Rolfe	Dendrophenol (4,4′-dihydroxy-3,3′,5-trimethoxybibenzyl), Loddigesiinols A-D, Moscatilin, Moscatilin diacetate, Moscatin, Shihunidine, Shihunine, Stilbenes	NE	Li et al. (1991); Ito et al. (2010)
Dendrobium moniliforme (L.) Sw.	Heptacosane, 3,4-dihydroxy-4′,5-dimethoxy bibenzyl, 3,4-dihydroxy-5,4′-dimethoxy bibenzyl, 4-methoxybenzaldehyde, 6-hydroxynobiline, alkyl 4′-hydroxy-cis-cinnamates, Alkyl ferulates, Daucosterol, Denbinobin, Denbinobin, Moniline	Hypoglycemic effect	Lin et al. (2000); Chen et al. (1994), Liu et al. (2007)
Dendrobium moschatum (Banks) Sw.	Moscatin, Moscatilin	NE	Majumder and Sen (1987)

TABLE 20.2 *(Continued)*

Epiphytic orchids	Bioactive secondary metabolites identified	Pharmacological properties	References
Dendrobium nobile Lindl.	Dendronobiline A, Dendronobilosides A, B, Dendronophenol A-B, Dendroside A, Dendroside E-G, Dendroxineo, Ephemeranthol A, Epheneranthol C, Erianthridin, Fimbriol-B, Flavanthridin, Gigantol, Hircinol, Lusianthridin, Moscatilin Moscatilin, Moscatin, Gigantol, Nobilin D-E, Nobilone, Nobilonine, Stigmasterol, B-Sitosterol, β-Sitosterol glucoside.	Anti-inflammatory activity, Antioxidant activity	Okamoto et al. (1972); Talapatra et al. (1982); Liu and Zhao (2003); Zhang et al. (2007b); Hwang et al. (2010)
Dendrobium officinale	Dl-2-Aminooctanoic Acid, Cyanidin, *O*-malonyl-malonylhexoside, Methylglutaric Acid, 2-Hydroxy-2-methyl butyric Acid, 5-Aminolevulinate, Phenylacetyl-l-glutamine, 4-Aminoindole, L-Glutamine, 8-Methyl-2-oxo-4-phenyl-2H-chromen-7-yl 4-(hexyloxy) benzoate, 5-methoxyindole-3-carbaldehyde, Biochanin A, Spermidine, Neochlorogenic acid, Naringenin chalcone, Butin, Eriodictyol, *O*-malonylhexoside	NE	Cao et al. (2019)
Dendrobium plicata	Ephemeranthoquinone	NE	Yamaki and Honda (1996); Arora et al. (2017)
Dendrobium primulinum Lindl.	Dendroprimine, Hygrine	NE	Luning and Leander (1965)
Dendrobium transparens Wall. ex Lindl.	Pentadecanal, 1,2-di-palmitin, 14-methyl-pentadecanoic acid methyl ester, 17-octadecynoic acid, 6-ethyl-3-trimethylsilyloxydecane, (Z)-13-docosenoic acid methyl ester, Cholesta-3,5-diene.	Anticancer activity	Joshi et al. (2020)

TABLE 20.2 *(Continued)*

Epiphytic orchids	Bioactive secondary metabolites identified	Pharmacological properties	References
Epidendrum rigidum Jacq.	2,3-Dimethoxy-9,10-dihydrophenathrene-4,7-diol, 24-methyl-9,19-cyclolanostane-25-en-3-ol, 3,4,9-trimethoxyphenanthrene-2,5-diol, Apigenin, Batatasin III, Gigantol, Isovitexin, Stilbenoids I–IV, Triterterpenoids	NE	Hernández-Romero et al. (2005)
Epidendrum strobiliferum Rchb.f.	24-Methylenecycloartanol, Campesterol, Pholidotin, Stigmasterol, β-Sitosterol	Analgesic activity	Ferreira et al. (2000)
Eria bambusifolia Lindl.	Bambusifolol	NE	Zhan et al. (2016)
Liparis nervosa (Thunb.) Lindl.	Nervosine VII	Anticancer activity	Huang et al. (2020)
Mycaranthes pannea (Lindl.) S.C.Chen & J.J.Wood	Acervatol, Acervatone, Flavanthridin, Flavanthrinin	Anti-inflammatory	Namsa et al. (2009)
Nidema boothii (Lindl.) Schltr.	1,5,7-Trimethoxy-9,10-dihydrophenanthrene-2,6-diol, 1,5,7-trimethoxyphenanthrene-2,6-diol, 2,4-dimethoxyphenanthrene-3,7-diol, Aloifol II, BatatasinIII,EphemerantholB,Ephemeranthoquinone, Gigantol, Lusianthridin, Nidemin, Nidemone	Spasmolytic activity	Estrada et al. (2002); Hernández-Romero et al. (2004)
Otochilus porrectus Lindl.	9,10-Dihydrophenanthropyran dimer, 9,10-dihydrophenanthropyran	NE	Shi et al. (2010)
Papilionanthe teres (Roxb.) Schltr.	Eucomic acid, Vandaterosides I–III	Anticancer activity	Simmler et al. (2011)
Pholidota articulata Lindl.	2,7-Dihydroxy-3,4,6-trimethoxyla 9, 10-dihydrophenanthrene flavidin, Coelonin, 9, 10-dihydrophenanthrenes, Coelogin, Coeloginin, Flavidin, Flavidinin, Oxoflavidinin	NE	Majumder et al. (1982)

TABLE 20.2 *(Continued)*

Epiphytic orchids	Bioactive secondary metabolites identified	Pharmacological properties	References
Pholidota chinensis Lindl.	Blestrianol A, Blestrin A, Bulbophylol B, Cannabi dihydrophenanthrene, Coelonin, Coelonin, Cyclopholidone, Cyclopholidone, Cyclopholidonol, Cyclopholidonol, Erianthridin, Eulophiol, Flavanthrin, Flavanthrin, Gymconpin C, Hircinol, Lusianthridin, Lusianthridin, Phochinenins A–F, Phochinenins G-L, Pholidotols A-B	Anti-inflammatory, Antioxidant activity, Anticancer activity	Wen et al. (1986); Wang et al. (2006); Wang et al. (2007); Wu et al. (2008)
Scaphyglottis livida (Lindl.) Schltr.	3,4′-dihydroxy-3′,5-dimethoxybibenzyl, 3,7-dihydroxy-2,4,8-trimethoxyphenanthrene, 3,7-dihydroxy-2,4-dimethoxyphenanthrene, 5-lanosta-24,24-dimethyl-9(11),25-dien-3-ol, Batatasin III, Coelonin, Gigantol, Nidemin	Anticancer activity, Spasmolytic activity	Estrada et al. (1999); Estrada et al. (2002); Déciga-Campos et al. (2007a, b)
Vanda cristata Wall. ex Lindl.	Palmitic acid, 9-methyl-octadecenoate, Linolelaidoyl chloride, 1,2–15,16-diepoxyhexadecane, Erucic acid methyl ester, Cyclohexane, Alpha-Bisabolol	Anticancer activity	Joshi et al. (2020)
Vanda tessellata (Roxb. f.) Hook. Ex D. Don	Oxotessallatin	NE	Anuradha et al. (2008)

analgesic effects (Shimizu et al., 1988; Estrada et al., 2004; Cui et al. 2013; Chinsamy et al., 2014; Huang et al., 2020). The ethanolic extract of roots, leaves, and stem of Ansellia Africana showed anti-acetylcholinesterase activity, which could be used to derive biomolecules useful to treat the Alzheimer's disease (Chinsamy et al., 2014). Several studies demonstrated that monocarboxylic acid (eucomic acid) and glycosides (vandaterosides I–III) isolated from *Papilionanthe teres*, phenantherene (3,7-dihydroxy-2,4,6-trimethoxyphenanthrene) derived from *Bulbophyllum odoratissimum* and saturated pyrrolizidine alkaloid (nervosine VII) from Liparis nervos showed antitumor activity (Chen et al., 2007; Simmler et al., 2011; Huang et al., 2020). The compound asperergoster A obtained from the filtrate of culture of *Anoectochilus roxburghii* is a potent inhibitor of NO, IL-1β, and TNF-α (Deng et al., 2020).

Topical application of the ethanol extract from the aerial parts of *Catasetum barbatum* exhibited anti-inflammatory effects and upon analyzing the chemical constituents, phenantherenes (2,7-dihydroxy-3,4,8-trimethoxyphenanthrene and 2,7-dihydroxy-3,4-dimethoxyphenanthrene) were identified (Shimizu et al., 1988). Triterpenoids and stilbenoids obtained from *Mycaranthes pannea* also showed similar activity (Namsa et al., 2009). The aqueous extract and polysaccharides isolated from *Anoectochilus roxburghii* have shown anti-inflammatory effects (Tang et al., 2008; Guo et al., 2019). The methanolic extract of roots of Ansellia Africana and aqueous extract of *A. roxburghii* exhibit antioxidant activity (Cui et al., 2013; Chinsamy et al., 2014). The 2-glucosyloxycinnamic acid derivaties, that is, *cis*-melilotoside, *trans*-melilotoside, and dihydromelilotoside isolated from *Dendrobium aurantiacum* also showed antioxidant potential (Yang et al., 2007). The chloroform-methanol extract of Maxillaria densa has shown a substantial spasmolytic effect, while the stilbenoids isolated from the same orchid showed lesser spasmolytic effect compared to the crude extract, but higher than the control treatment (papaverine). Phenanthrene derivatives isolated from the Maxillaria densa have showed similar effects. The chloroform–methanol extract from the whole orchid of *Nidema boothii* has significantly inhibited the spontaneous contractions, while the aromatic compounds isolated from *Scaphyglottis livida* showed a concentration-dependent spasmolytic impact (Estrada et al., 1999; Estrada et al., 2004; Hernández-Romero et al., 2004).

Watanabe et al. (2007) showed that cymbidine A (a monomeric peptidoglycan-related compound) isolated from *Cymbidium goeringii* exhibits both hypotensive and diuretic effects. Kinsenoside isolated from the leaves of *Anoectochilus roxburghii* was effective as antihyperglycemic on oral administertion in diabetic rats (dose, 15 mg/kg) (Zhang et al., 2007a; Cui et al., 2013). Polysaccharides isolated from *Dendrobium moniliforme* also showed a similar effect. The compound, 7-*O*-α-D-ribosyl-5-hydroxy-2-methyl-4H-chromen-4-one isolated from the culture filtrate of *Daldinia eschscholzii* an endophytic fungi of *Dendrobium chrysotoxum* showed prominent activity on glucose uptake (Hu et al., 2019). The methanolic extract of *Epidendrum moseii* and the triterpenes, pholidotin, and 24-methylene cycloartenol isolated from the same orchid showed antinociceptive properties (Ferreira et al., 2000). The kinsenoside, a glycoside isolated from the leaves of *A. roxburghii* is a potent immunosuppressive drug for the autoimmune hepatitis (Zhang et al., 2007a; Qin et al., 2019).

20.5 BIOACTIVE ENDOPHYTIC FUNGI

Fungi play a significant role at different stages of the orchid's life cycle at the time of germination to the adult plant in the form of mycorrhiza or as endophytes. At the time of seed germination, the mycorrhizal association facilitates to fetch the required nutrients to the tiny orchid seeds since they lack functional endosperm. Some of the endophytes aids in a good establishment of the plant on the phorophyte, some exhibit plant growth promotion activity and aid in bioregulation of plant during its vegetative phase, while others serve as bioprotants by defense mechanisms (Pant et al., 2017).

Endophytes are microorganism which live within plant tissues without causing any immediate or adverse effects. Petrini defined "all organisms inhabiting plant organs that at some time in their life can colonize internal plant tissue without causing apparent harm to the host" as endophytes. The association of fungal endophytes with the epiphytic orchids has been evaluated by many researchers for decades and detailed account is given in Table 20.3. A total of 85 different genera of fungi have been reported to inhabit the epiphytic orchids, those are predominantly belong to the phylum Ascomycota (86%) and a few from Basidiomycota (14%) (Figure 20.3). Among the reported fungal endophytes of Ascomycota, chief members are belong to the class Sordariomycetes (41.5%), Dothideomycetes (31.7%), Eurotiomycetes (9.8%), Leotiomycetes (2.4%), and Saccharomycetes (1.2%). In the phylum Basidiomycota, the isolated endophytes principally belong to the Class Agaricomycetes (9.8%), while the other members belong to the classes Cystobasidiomycetes, Pucciniomycetes, and Tremelloycetes (1.2% each).

TABLE 20.3 Diversity of Endophytic Fungi Associated with Epiphytic Orchids.

Epiphytic orchids	Mycoendophytic diversity	References
Acampe praemorsa (Roxb.) Blatt. & McCann	*Aspergillus terreus, Aspergillus tubingensis, Bissochlamys nivea, Diaporthe gloeosporioides, Diaporthe eucalyptorum, Endomelanconiopsis endophytica, Fusarium proliferatum, Lasiodiplodia pseudotheobromae, Lasiodiplodia theobromae, Neofusicoccum umdonicola, Nigrospora sphaerica, Nodulisporium* sp., *Trichoderma asperellum, Trichoderma harzianum,* and *Xylaria badia, Trichoderma atroviride*	Deepthi and Ray (2019)
Anoectochilus formosanus Hayata	*Rhizoctonia* sp.	Jiang et al. (2015)
Anoectochilus roxburghii (Wall.) Lindl.	*Mycena anoectochila, Aspergillus versicolor, Annulohypoxylon cf. stygium*	Guo et al. (2019); Deng et al., (2020)
Bulbophyllum neilgherrense	*Aspergillus flavus, Aspergillus niger, Penicillium* sp., *Aspergillus ochraceus, Aspergillus tamari, Gliocladium viride, Aspergillus* sp. 1, *Penicillium chrysogenum, Aspergillus oryzae, Penicillium italicum, Aspergillus* sp. 2, *Aspergillus carbonarius, Fusarium* sp., *Nigrospora* sp., *Colletotrichum* sp. 1, *Colletotrichum* sp. 2, *Cylindrocarpon* sp., *Daldinia eschscholzii, Fusarium* sp., *Phyllosticta* sp., *Nemania* sp., *Pestalotiopsis* sp.	Sudheep and Sridhar, (2012); Sawmya et al. (2013)
Bulbophyllum sterile (Lam.) Suresh	*Aspergillus carbonarius, Aspergillus flavus, Aspergillus niger, Aspergillus ochraceus, Aspergillus oryzae, Aspergillus* sp., *Aspergillus tamari, Gliocladium viride, Penicillium chrysogenum, Penicillium italicum, Penicillium* sp., *Fusarium* sp., *Nigrospora* sp.	Sudheep and Sridhar (2012)
Crepidium acuminatum (D. Don) Szlach.	*Tulasnella* sp., *Aspergillus* sp., *Penicillium* sp., *Rhizoctonia* sp., *Emericella* sp.	Thakur et al. (2010)
Cymbidium aloifolium (L.) Sw.	*Aspergillus japonicas, Curvularia lunata, Nigrospora* sp., *Colletotrichum gleosporidioides, Rhizoctonia* sp., *Xylaria* sp., *Trichoderma* sp., *Fusarium chlamydosporum, Penicillum citrinum, Helminthosporium* sp., *Curvularia* sp. *Aspergillus sydowii, Cladosporium* sp., *Aspergillus terreus, Alternaria alternata, Fusarium oxysporum, Penicillium chrysogenum, Colletotrichum truncatum, Bipolaris* sp., *Talaromyces rotundus, Penicillium purpurogenum, Cylindrocephalum* sp.	Shubha and Srinivas (2017); Jagannath et al. (2019)
Cymbidium ensifolium (L.) Sw.	*Colletotrichum gloeosporioides*	Chen et al. (2011)

TABLE 20.3 *(Continued)*

Epiphytic orchids	Mycoendophytic diversity	References
Cymbidium goeringii (Rchb.f.) Rchb.f.	*Chaetomium* sp., *Cryptosporiopsis ericae, Cylindrocarpon pauciseptatum, Exophiala salmonis, Fusarium oxysporum, Fusarium solani, Nigrospora sphaerica, Trichoderma spirale, Tulasnella calospora, Umbelopsis nana, Umbelopsis dimorpha,*	Wang et al. (2017)
Dendrobium aphyllum (Roxb.) C.E.C. Fisch	*Pseudopestalotiopsis theae, Tulasnella calospora, Trichoderma viride, Colletotrichum tropicicola, Fusarium keratoplasticum, Fusarium oxysporum, Fusarium solani, Xylaria curta, Xylaria grammica, Xylaria papulis, Xylaria arbuscula, Nemania bipapillata*	Zi et al. (2014); Sopalun and Lamtham (2020); Sarsaiya et al. (2020); Chen et al. (2011)
Dendrobium candidum Wall.ex Landl	*Acremonium* sp., *Alternaria* sp., *Ampelomyces* sp., *Arthrinium* sp., *Aureobasidium* sp., *Bionectria* sp., *Candida* sp., *Cercophora* sp., *Chaetomium* sp., *Chaetophoma* sp., *Fusarium* sp., *Glomerularia* sp., *Hyalodendron* sp., *Nigrospora* sp., *Periconiella* sp., *Sclerotium* sp.	Chen et al. (2011)
Dendrobium catenatum Lindl.	*Tulasnella* sp., *Leptosphaeria* sp., *Guignardia* sp., *Arthrinium* sp., *Coniochaeta* sp., *Fusarium* sp., *Neofusicoccum* sp., *Zopfiella* sp., *Alternaria* sp., *Bjerkandera* sp., *Cercophora* sp., *Nigrospora* sp., *Trichoderma* sp., *Colletotrichum boninense*	Wang et al. (2017)
Dendrobium chrysanthum Wall. ex Lindl.	*Trichoderma* sp., *Pestalotiopsis* sp., *Verticillium leptobactrum, Glomerella truncate, Fusarium soloni, Fusarium oxysporum, Fusarium proliferatum, Apiosporaceae* sp., *Colletotrichum gloeosporioides, Pochonia bulbillosa, Chloridium virescens var. chlamydosporum, Xylaria* sp., *Xylaria grammica, Phialophora* sp., *Phomopsis* sp., *Cylindrocarpon destructans, Nemania bipapillata, Xylaria arbuscula, Xylaria cruta, Diaporthe medusaea, Diaporthe amygdali, Phanerina mellea, Hypoxylon* sp, *Hypoxylon lenormandii, Trichoderma reesei, Chaetomium globosum, Penicillium solitum, Dactylonectria estremocensis, Phanerochaete* sp, *Trichoderma harzianum, Chaetomium brevipilium, Penicillium solitum, Periconia* sp, *Periconia digitata*	Chen et al. (2011)
Dendrobium chrysotoxum Lindl.	*Daldinia eschscholzii, Xylaria grammica, Xylaria feejeensis, Xylaria papulis, Xylaria venustula, Xylaria badia, Annulohypoxylon* sp.	Chen et al. (2011)

TABLE 20.3 *(Continued)*

Epiphytic orchids	Mycoendophytic diversity	References
Dendrobium crumenatum Sw.	*Cladosporium cladosporioides, Cladosporium sphaerospermum, Colletotrichum gloeosporioides, Colletotrichum* sp., *Curvularia brachyspora, Fusarium nivale, Fusarium solani, Pestalotiopsis* sp., *Scolecobasidium* sp., *Xylohypha* sp., *Phyllosticta capitalensis, Guignardia endophyllicola, Westerdikella* sp.	Mangunwardoyo et al. (2012)
Dendrobium devonianum	*Fusarium* sp., *Fusarium tricinctum, Leptosphaerulina chartarum, Leptosphaerulina* sp., *Phoma* sp., *Arthrinium* sp., *Glomerella cingulate, Pestlotiopsis microspore, Xylaria* sp., *Cladosporium cladosporioides, Acremonium* sp., *Pestalotiopsis photiniae, Rhizopus* sp., *Trichoderma* sp., *Trichoderma koningiopsis*	Xing et al. (2011)
Dendrobium fimbriatum Hook.	*Nemania bipapillata, Xylaria grammica, Xylaria feejeensis, Xylaria apoda, Xylaria papulis*	Chen et al. (2011)
Dendrobium heterocarpum Wall. ex Lindl.	*Alternaria alternata, Fusarium oxysporum* f. sp. *Dianthi, Fusarium babinda, Hypoxylon* sp., *Muscodor* sp., *Epicoccum* sp., *Nemania bipapillata, Diaporthe maritima*	Hajong and Kapoor (2020)
Dendrobium longicornu Lindl.	*Trichoderma koningiopsi, Clonostachys rosea, Trichoderma atroviride, Xylaria* sp., *Trichoderma paraviridescens, Epicoccum poae, Nemania bipapillata, Fusarium babinda, Alternaria alternate*	Hajong and Kapoor (2020)
Dendrobium loddigesii Rolfe	*Acremonium* sp., *Alternaria* sp., *Ampelomyces* sp., *Bionectria* sp., *Cercophora* sp., *Chaetomella* sp., *Cladosporium* sp., *Colletotrichum* sp., *Davidiella* sp., *Fusarium* sp., *Lasiodiplodia* sp., *Paraconiothyrium* sp., *Schizophyllum* sp., *Sirodesmium* sp., *Thielavia* sp., *Trichoderma* sp., *Verticillium* sp., *Xylaria* sp., *Pestalotiopsis trachicarpicola*	Chen et al. (2011)
Dendrobium moniliforme (L.) Sw.	*Acremonium* sp., *Bionectria* sp., *Chaetomella* sp., *Fusarium* sp., *Glomerularia* sp., *Schizophyllum* sp., *Trichoderma* sp., *Verticillium* sp.	Chen et al. (2011)
Dendrobium nobile Lindl.	*Acremonium* sp., *Alternaria* sp., *Ampelomyces* sp., *Bionectria* sp., *Cladosporium* sp., *Colletotrichum* sp., *Fusarium* sp., *Fusicoccum* sp., *Paraconiothyrium* sp., *Pezicula* sp., *Pleospora* sp., *Verticillium* sp., *Xylaria* sp., *Nemania bipapillata, Xylaria grammica, Xylaria arbuscula, Xylaria venisula, Xylaria amphithela, Colletotrichum tropicicola, Fusarium keratoplasticum, Fusarium oxysporum, Fusarium solani*, and *Trichoderma longibrachiatum*	Chen et al. (2011); Sarsaiya et al. (2020)

TABLE 20.3 *(Continued)*

Epiphytic orchids	Mycoendophytic diversity	References
Dendrobium officinale	*Fusarium oxysporum, Xylaria cubensis, Colletotrichum* sp., *Pestalotiopsis* sp.v, *Alternaria* sp., *Aspergillus niger, Aspergillus flavus, Trichoderma atroviride, Cochliobolus* sp., *Cystobasidium slooffiae, Aureobasidium pullulans, Epicoccum sorghinum,*	Jin et al. (2017)
Dendrobium thyrsiflorum	*Fusarium* sp., *Fusarium tricinctum, Leptosphaerulina chartarum, Alternaria* sp., *Colletotrichum* sp., *Colletotrichum gloeosporioides, Epicoccum nigrum, Phoma* sp., *Epicoccum* sp., *Glomerella acutata, Rhizopus* sp., *Xylaria* sp., *Arthrobotray* sp.	Xing et al. (2011)
Dendrobium transparens Wall. ex Lindl.	*Helminthosporium* sp., *Fusarium* sp.	Shrestha et al. (2018)
Grammatophyllum scriptum (L.) Blume	*Chaetomium cochliodes, Chaetomium cupreum, Curvularia* sp., *Fusarium* sp., *Pestalotiopsis* sp., *Achaetomium* sp.	Sour et al. (2015)
Nidema boothii (Lindl.) Schltr.	*Troposporella* sp.	Richardson (1993)
Pholidota pallida Lindl.	*Chaetomium* sp., *Colletotrichum gloeosporioides, Cylindrocarpon* sp., *Daldinia eschscholzii, Entonaema liquescens, Fusarium* sp., *Phyllosticta* sp., *Hypoxylon* sp., *Pestalotiopsis* sp., *Chaetomium* sp., *Phomopsis* sp., *Penicillium* sp.	Sawmya et al. (2013)
Vanda coerulea Griff. Ex Lindl.	*Rhizoctonia zeae*	Aggarwal et al. (2012)
Vanda cristata Wall. ex Lindl.	*Agaricus bisporus, Alternaria tenuissima, Fusarium tricinctum, Alternaria* sp., *Pseudochaetosphaeronema* sp, *Fusarium oxysporium, Fusarium solani, Fusarium* sp., *Aspergillus* sp., *Paraconiothyrium hawaiiense*	Chand et al. (2020)
Vanda Testacea (Lindl.) Rchb.f.	*Alternaria* sp., *Aspergillus candidus, Aspergillus carbonarius, Aspergillus flavus, Aspergillus niger, Aspergillus ochraceus, Aspergillus oryzae, Aspergillus* sp., *Aspergillus tamari, Fusarium oxysporum, Fusarium* sp., *Gliocladium* sp., *Gliocladium viride, Nigrospora* sp., *Nigrospora oryzae, Paecilomyces* sp., *Penicillium chrysogenum, Penicillium italicum, Penicillium* sp., *Agaricus* sp.	Sudheep and Sridhar (2012)
Vanilla planifolia Jacks. ex Andrews	*Fusarium oxysporum* f. sp. *loti, Fusarium oxysporum* f. sp. *melonis, Fusarium solani, Fusarium* sp., *Colletotrichum boninense*	Gamboa-Gaitán (2013)

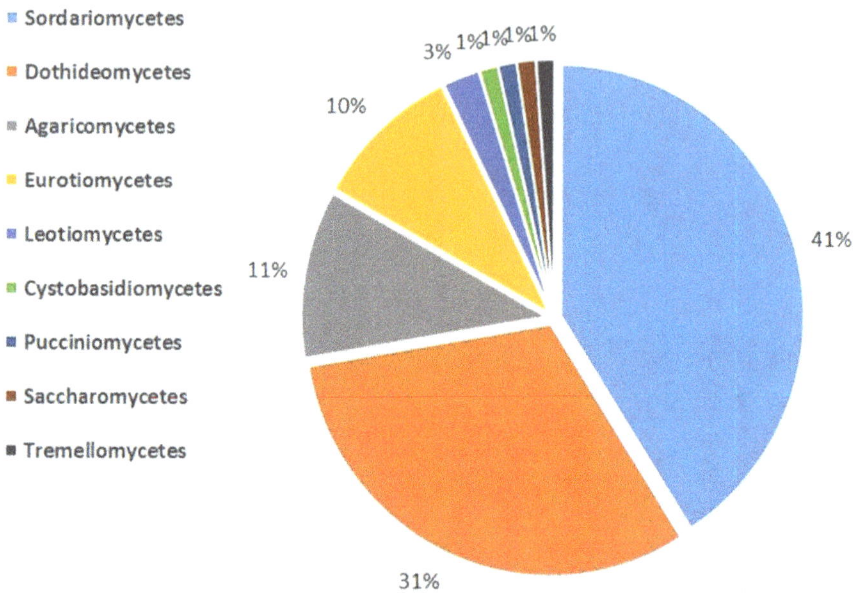

FIGURE 20.3 Endophytic fungal distribution in epiphytic orchids.

Mycoendophytes of some of the epiphytic orchids have been successfully isolated and investigated by various researchers. Some of the endophytes like *Colletotrichum tropicicola*, *Fusarium keratoplasticum*, *F. oxysporum*, *F. solani*, and *Trichoderma longibrachiatum* have been isolated from leaf segments of *Dendrobium nobile* (Sarsaiya et al., 2020). *Aspergillus tubingensis* has been isolated from *Acampe praemorsa* (Deepthi and Ray, 2019). It is reported that crude culture filtrate of *A. tubingensis* shows antibacterial property (Verma et al., 2014). Jin et al. (2017) reported *Aspergillus niger*, *Aureobasidium pullulans*, and *Fusarium oxysporum* occurring as endophytes in *Dendrobium officinale* showed broad-spectrum antimicrobial activity. *Fusarium nivale* endophyte of *Dendrobium crumenatum* has inhibited the growth of *Candida albicans* and *C. tropicalis* (Mangunwardoyo et al., 2012).

Metabolite profiling of organic extract of *C. alatae* from *Dendrobium moniliforme* revealed the presence of phenolic metabolites and essential oil (Shah et al., 2019). Shrestha et al., (2018) showed that the majority of the fungal endophytes isolated from *Dendrobium moniliforme* and *D. transparence* showed antibacterial activity against *S. epidermidis* as well as *E. coli*, while some of the species showed potent inhibition against *S. aureus*. Endophytic fungal inhabitants (*Phoma* sp., *Epicoccum nigrum* and *Fusarium* sp.) in *Dendrobium devonianum* and *D. thyrsiflorum* exhibited a strong inhibitory activity against six pathogenic microbes (Xing et al., 2011). Several compounds have been isolated from the culture extract of fungal endophyte *Daldinia eschscholzii* from the epiphytic orchid *D. chrysotoxum.* Compounds such as 3-hydroxy-1-(2,6-dihydroxyphenyl)butan-1-one and 2,3-dihydro-5-hydroxy-2-methylchromen-4-one showed photodynamic antibacterial activity against bacteria *Bacillus subtilis* and *Escherichia coli*, respectively. Similarly, the compound 7-*O*-α-D-ribosyl2,3-dihydro-5-hydroxy-2-methyl-chromen-4-one was effective antibacterial against against *Staphylococcus aureus* (Hu et al., 2019). Diketopiperazine (Chaetocochin C) isolated from the cultures of *Chaetomium* sp. and *Cymbidium goeringii* was a potent antitumor compound possessing the ability to arrest the cell cycle as well as arrest and activates caspase 3 leading to apoptosis (Wang et al., 2017).

20.6 CONCLUSIONS

Epiphytic orchids with their unique physiological lifestyles serve as an important source for various pharmacologically active natural products along with the their endophytic fungal partrners. A huge number of epiphytic orchids have been explored for their ethnomedicinal significance from different ethnic groups across the globe. Although epiphytic orchids are used as one of the major herbal medicinal sources, there is a knowledge gap in detailed information on the pharmacologically active substances. In addition to epiphytic orchids, their endophytic fungal inhabitants play a key role in production of secondary metabolites. One of the important questions to be answered in future is whether the active princples isolated from the epiphytic orchids is derived exclusively from the host or from the fungal endophyte or from both host and endophyte.

KEYWORDS

- **diversity**
- **distribution**
- **biological activity**
- **secondary metabolites**
- **pharmacological properties**

REFERENCES

Aggarwal, S.; Chongtham, N.; Beri, S.; Rastogi, S; Adholeya, A. In vitro symbiotic seed germination and molecular characterization of associated endophytic fungi in a commercially important and endangered Indian orchid *Vanda coerulea* Griff. ex Lindl. *Eur. J. Environ. Sci.* **2012**, *2*: 33–42.

Aguirre-Leon, E. Vascular Epiphytes of Mexico: A Preliminary Inventory. *Selbyana*, 1992; pp 72–76.

Anuradha, V.; Rao, M. V. B.; Aswar, A. S. Oxo-Tessallatin, a Novel Phenanthrapyrone Isolated from *Vanda tessalata*. *Orient. J. Chem.* **2008,** *24*, 1119–1122.

Arditti, J. *Fundamentals of Orchid Biology*; John Wiley & Sons, 1992.

Arora, M.; Mahajan, A.; Sembi, J. K. A. Review on Phytochemical and Pharmacological Potential of Family Orchidaceae. *Int. Res. J. Pharm.* **2017,** *8*, 9–24.

Banarji, M. L. *Orchids of Nepal*; Today and Tomorrow's Publisher: New Delhi, 1978.

Baral, S. R.; Kurmi, P. P. *Compendium of Medicinal Plants in Nepal*; Rachana Sharma: Kathmandu, Nepal, 2006.

Barua, A.; Ghosh B.; Ray, S.; Patra, A. hattacharyya, P.; Cymbinodin-B, A Phenanthraquinone from *Cymbidium aloifolium*. *ChemInform* **1990,** *29*, 3046–3047.

Berliocchi, L.; Griffiths, M. *Orchid in Lore and Legend*; Timber Press: Portland, OR, 2000.

Bi, Z. M.; Wang, Z. T.; Xu, L. S.; Xu, G. J. Studies on the Chemical Constituents of *Dendrobium fimbriatum*. *Acta pharma. Sini.* **2003,** *38*, 526–529.

Bi, Z. M.; Yang, Y. S.; Wang, Z. T.; Gong, Y. Q.; He, J. X.; Tani, T. Chemical Constituents of *Dendrobium fimbriatum* Hook. (I). *J. Chi. Pharma Uni.* **2001,** *32*, 200–202.

Biedinger, N.; Fischer, E. Epiphytic Vegetation and Ecology in Central African Forests (Rwanda, Zaire). *Ecotropica* **1996,** *2*, 121–142.

Blinova, I. V. Peculiarities of Seasonal Development of Orchid Species North of the Arctic Circle. *Botanicheskiĭ Zhurnal* **2011,** *96* (3), 396–411.

Bryant, A. T. *Zulu Mmedicine and Medicine-Men*; C. Struik: Cape Twon, 1966.

Bulpitt C. The Uses and Misuses of Orchids in Medicine. *Qjm: An Int. J. Med.* **2005,** *98*, 625–631.

Cao, H.; Ji, Y.; Li, S.; Lu, L.; Tian, M. et al. Extensive Metabolic Profiles of Leaves and Stems from the Medicinal Plant *Dendrobium officinale* Kimura et Migo. *Metabolites* **2019,** *9*, 215.

Chand, K.; Shah, S.; Sharma, J.; Paudel, M. R; Pant, B. Isolation, characterization, and plant growth-promoting activities of endophytic fungi from a wild orchid *Vanda cristata*. *Pl. Signal. Behav.* **2020,** *15*: 1744294.

Chen, C. C.; Wu, L. G.; Ko, F. N.; Teng, C. M. Antiplatelet Aggregation Principles of *Dendrobium loddigesii*. *J. Nat. Prod.* **1994,** *57*, 1271–1274.

Chen, J.; Hu, K-X.; Hou, X-Q.; Guo, S-X. Endophytic Fungi Assemblages from 10 *Dendrobium* Medicinal Plants (Orchidaceae). *World J. Microbiol. Biotech.* **2011,** *27*, 1009–1016.

Chen, K. K.; Chen, A. L. The Alkaloid of Chin-shih-hu. *J. Bio. Chem.* **1935,** *111*, 653–658.

Chen, Y.; Xu, J.; Yu, H.; Qing, C.; Zhang, Y. et al. Cytotoxic Phenolics from *Bulbophyllum odoratissimum*. *Food Chem.* **2008,** *107*, 169–173.

Chen, Y. G.; Xu, J. J.; Yu, H.; Qing, C.; Zhang, Y. L. et al. 3, 7-Dihydroxy-2, 4, 6-trimethoxy-phenanthrene, a New Phenanthrene from *Bulbophyllum odoratissimum*. *J. Kor. Chem. Soc.* **2007,** *51*, 352–355.

Chinsamy, M.; Finnie, J. F.; Van Staden, J. Anti-Inflammatory, Antioxidant, Anti-Cholinesterase Activity and Mutagenicity of South African Medicinal Orchids. *South Afr. J. Bot.* **2014,** *91*, 88–98.

Chinsamy, M.; Finnie, J. F.; Van Staden, J. The Ethnobotany of South African Medicinal Orchids. *South Afr. J. Bot.* **2011,** *77*, 2–9.

Cribb, P.; Hermans, J. The Conservation of Madagascar's Orchids: A Model for an Integrated Conservation Project. *Lankesteriana* **2007,** *7*, 255–261.

Cui, S. C.; Yu, J.; Zhang, X. H.; Cheng, M. Z.; Yang, L. W.; Xu, J. Y. Antihyperglycemic and Antioxidant Activity of Water Extract from *Anoectochilus roxburghii* in Experimental Diabetes. *Exp. Toxicol. Pathol.* **2013,** *65*, 485–488.

Cunningham, A. B. An Investigation of the Herbal Medicine Trade in Natal/KwaZulu (No. 29). Institute of Natural Resources, University of Natal, Natal/KwaZulu, 1988.

Dahmén, J.; Leander, K. Amotin and Amoenin, Two Sesquiterpenes of the Picrotoxane Group from *Dendrobium amoenum. Phytochemistry* **1978,** *17*, 1949–1952.

Dash, P. K.; Sahoo, S.; Bal, S. Ethnobotanical Studies on Orchids of Niyamgiri Hill Ranges, Orissa, India. *Ethnobot. Leaflets* **2008,** *12*, 70–78.

De, L. C.; Medhi, R. P. Orchid—A Diversified Component of Farming Systems for Profitability and Livelihood Security of Small and Marginal Farmers. *J. Glob. Biosci.* **2015,** *4* (2), 1393–1406.

Déciga-Campos, M.; Palacios-Espinosa, J. F.; Reyes-Ramírez, A.; Mata, R. Antinociceptive and Anti-Inflammatory Effects of Compounds Isolated from *Scaphyglottis livida* and *Maxillaria densa. J. Ethnopharma* **2007a**, *114*, 161–168.

Déciga-Campos, M.; Rivero-Cruz, I.; Arriaga-Alba, M.; Castañeda-Corral, G.; Angeles-López, G. E. et al. Acute Toxicity and Mutagenic Activity of Mexican Plants Used in Traditional Medicine. *J. Ethnopharma* **2007b**, *110*, 334–342.

Deepthi, A. S.; Ray, J. G. Applications of Endophytic-Fungal-Isolates from Velamen Root of Wild Orchids in Floriculture. *Braz. J. Biol. Sci.* **2019,** *6*, 577–589.

Deng, M.; Liu, Y.; Huang, Y.; Yin, X.; Zhou, Y.; Duan, Y.; Xie, S.; Guo, Y.; Qiao, Y.; Shi, Z.; Tao, L.; Cao, Y.; Qi, C.; Zhang, Y. New bioactive secondary metabolites from the *Anoectochilus roxburghii* endophytic fungus *Aspergillus versicolor. Fitoterapia* **2020,** *143*: 104532.

Dunn, F. L. Traditional Asian Medicine and Cosmopolitan Medicine as Adaptive Systems. In *Asian Medical Systems: A Comparative Study*; Motilal Banarsidass Publishers Pvt. Ltd.: Delhi, 1976; pp 133–158.

Estrada, S.; Acevedo, L.; Rodriguez, M.; Toscano, R.; Mata, R. New Triterpenoids from the Orchids *Scaphyglottis livida* and *Nidema boothii. Nat. Prof. Let.*, **2002,** *16*, 81–86.

Estrada, S.; López-Guerrero, J. J.; Villalobos-Molina, R.; Mata, R. Spasmolytic Stilbenoids from *Maxillaria densa. Fitoterapia* **2004,** *75*, 690–695.

Estrada, S.; Rojas, A.; Mathison, Y.; Israel, A.; Mata, R. Nitric Oxide/cGMP Mediates the Spasmolytic Action of 3, 4′-dihydroxy-5, 5′-dimethoxybibenzyl from *Scaphyglottis livida. Pl. Med.* **1999,** *65*, 109–114.

Estrada, S.; Toscano, R. A.; Mata, R. New Phenanthrene Derivatives from *Maxillaria densa. J. Nat. Prd.* **1999,** *62*, 1175–1178.

Fan, C.; Wang, W.; Wang, Y.; Qin, G.; Zhao, W. Chemical Constituents from *Dendrobium densiflorum. Phytochem.* **2001,** *57*, 1255–1258.

Ferreira, J.; Floriani, A. E.; Filho, V. C.; Monache, F. D.; Yunes, R. A.; Calixto, J. B.; Santos, A.R. Antinociceptive properties of the methanolic extract and two triterpenes isolated from *Epidendrum mosenii* stems (Orchidaceae). *Life Sci.* **2000,** *66*: 791–802.

Freiberg, M. Spatial Distribution of Vascular Epiphytes on Three Emergent Canopy Trees in French Guiana. *Biotropica*, **1996,** *28*, 345–355.

Gamboa-Gaitán, M. Á. Colombian *Vanilla* and its microbiota - I. *Acta Bot. Hung.* **2013,** *55*: 239–245.

Gelfland, M.; Mavi, S.; Drummond, R. B.; Ndemera, B. *The Traditional Medical Practitioner in Zimbabwe: His Principles of Practice and Pharmacopoeia*; Mambo Press, Hardre: Zimbabwe, 1985; p 411.

Gerstner, J. A Preliminary Check List of Zulu Names of Plants: with Short Notes. *Bantu Stud.* **1941,** *15*, 277–301.

Gewali, M. B.; Awale, S. *Aspects of Traditional Medicine in Nepal. Japan. Institute of Natural Medicine*. University of Toyama: Japan, 2008; p 185.

Giesen, W.; Wulffraat, S.; Zieren, M.; Scholten, L. *Mangrove Guidebook for Southeast Asia*; Rap Publication: Bangkon, 2007; p. 769.

Guan, H.; Zhang, X.; Tu, F.; Yao, X. Chemical Components of *Dendrobium candidum. Zhongcaoyao* **2009,** *40*, 1873–1876.

Guo, Y.; Ye, Q.; Yang, S.; Wu, J.; Ye, B. et al. Therapeutic Effects of Polysaccharides from *Anoectochilus roxburghii* on Type II Collagen-Induced Arthritis in Rats. *Int. J. Biol. Macromol.* **2019,** *122*, 882–892.

Gurib-Fakim, A.; Brendler, T. *Medicinal and Aromatic Plants of Indian Ocean Islands: Madagascar, Comoros, Seychelles and Mascarenes*; Medpharm GmbH Scientific Publishers: Stuttgart, Germany, 2004; p 567.

Gutiérrez, R. M. P. Orchids: A Review of Uses in Traditional Medicine, Its Phytochemistry and Pharmacology. *J. Med. Pl. Res.* **2010,** *4*, 592–638.

Hágsater, E.; Dumont, V. *Orchids: Status Survey and Conservation Action Plan*; IUCN: Gland Switzerland and Cambridge, 1996; p 173.

Hajong, S.; Kapoor, R. An amalgam of pathogenic and beneficial endophytic fungi colonizing four *Dendrobium* species from Meghalaya, India. *J. Basic Microbiol.* **2020,** *60*: 415–423.

He, C. N.; Wang, C. L.; Guo, S. X.; Yang, J. S.; Xiao, P. G. A Novel Flavonoid Glucoside from *Anoectochilus roxburghii* (Wall.) Lindl. *J. Integr. Pl. Biol.* **2006,** *48*, 359–363.

Hernández-Romero, Y.; Acevedo, L.; Ángeles Sánchez, M. D. L.; Shier, W. T.; Abbas, H. K.; Mata, R. Phytotoxic Activity of Bibenzyl Derivatives from the Orchid *Epidendrum rigidum*. *J. Agric. Food Chem.* **2005,** *53*, 6276 6280.

Hernández-Romero, Y.; Rojas, J. I.; Castillo, R.; Rojas, A.; Mata, R. Spasmolytic Effects, Mode of Action, and Structure—Activity Relationships of Stilbenoids from *Nidema boothii*. *J. Nat. Prod.* **2004,** *67*, 160–167.

Heyne, K. De Nuttige Planten Van Indonesië. In *Twee Delene*—Deel I.; Uitgeverij, N. V., van Hoeve, W., Eds., 3rd ed.; 1950; p. 1450.

Ho, C-K.; Chen, C-C. Moscatilin from the Orchid *Dendrobrium loddigesii* Is a Potential Anticancer Agent. *Canc. Invest.* **2003,** *21*, 729–736.

Hossain, M. M. Therapeutic Orchids: Traditional Uses and Recent Advances—An Overview. *Fitoterapia* **2011,** *82*, 102–140.

Hossain, M. M. Traditional Therapeutic Uses of Some Indigenous Orchids of Bangladesh. *Med. Arom. Pl. Sci. Biotechnol.* **2009,** *42*, 101–106.

Hu, M.; Yang, X. Q.; Zhou, Q. Y.; Li, S. Q.; Wang, B. Y.; Ruan, B. H.; Yang, Y. B.; Zhang, Z. X; Zhou, H.; Ding, Z. T. Benzopyran derivatives from endophytic *Daldinia eschscholzii* JC-15 in *Dendrobium chrysotoxum* and their bioactivities. *Nat. Prod. Res.* **2019,** *33*: 1431–1435.

Huang, S.; Shuang-Mei, Z.; Lian-Hai, S.; Xian-Li, Z. Antitumor Activity of Nervosine VII, and the Crosstalk Between Apoptosis and Autophagy in HCT116 Human Colorectal Cancer Cells. *Chin. J. Nat. Med.* **2020,** *18*, 81–89.

Hutchings, A. *Zulu Medicinal Plants: An Inventory*; University of Natal Press: KwaZulu-Natal, 1996; p. 450.

Hwang, J. S.; Lee, S. A.; Hong, S. S.; Han, X. H.; Lee, C. et al. Phenanthrenes from *Dendrobium nobile* and Their Inhibition of the LPS-Induced Production of Nitric Oxide in Macrophage RAW 264.7 Cells. *Bioorg. Med. Chem. Lett.* **2010,** *20*, 3785–3787.

Ito, M.; Matsuzaki, K.; Wang, J.; Daikonya, A.; Wang, N. L. et al. New phenanthrenes and stilbenes from *Dendrobium loddigesii*. *Chem. Pharma Bull.* **2010,** *58*, 628–633.

Jagannath, S.; Konappa, N. M.; Alurappa, R.; Chowdappa, S. Production, Characterization of Indole Acetic Acid and Its Bioactive Potential from Endophytic Fungi of *Cymbidium aloifolium* L. *J. Biol. Act. Pro. Nat.* **2019,** *9*, 387–409.

Jaime, A.; Teixeira, S.; Tzi, B. N. The Medicinal and Pharmaceutical Importance of *Dendrobium* Species. *J. Appl. Microbiol. Biotechnol.* **2017,** *101*, 2227–2239.

Jalal, J. S.; Kumar, P.; Pangtey, Y. P. S. Ethnomedicinal Orchids of Uttarakhand, Western Himalaya. *Ethnobot Leaflets* **2008,** *12*, 1227–1230.

Jana, S. K.; Sinha, G. P.; Chauhan, A. S. Ethnobotanical Aspects of Orchids of Shikim. *J. Orchid Soc. India* **1997,** *11*, 79–84.

Jiang, J. H; Lee, Y. I; Cubeta, M. A; Chen, L. C. Characterization and colonization of endomycorrhizal *Rhizoctonia* fungi in the medicinal herb *Anoectochilus formosanus* (Orchidaceae). *Mycorrhiza* **2015,** *25*: 431–445.

Jin Z.; Li, D., Liu, T.; Yu, F.; Zhang, Z.; Su, C.; Wang, Y.; Guo, Q.; Liu, Z. Cultural endophytic fungi associated with *Dendrobium Officinale:* Identification, diversity estimation and their antimicrobial potential. *Curr. Sci.* **2017,** *112*: 1690–1697.

Joshi, G. C.; Tewari, L. M.; Lohani, N.; Upreti, K.; Jalal, J. S.; Tewari, G. Diversity of Orchids in Uttarakhand and Their Conservation Strategy with Special Reference to Their Medicinal Importance. *Rep. Opin.* **2009,** *1*, 47–52.

Joshi, N.; Dhakal, K. S.; Saud, D. S. Checklist of CITES Listed Flora of Nepal. Department of Plant Resources (DPR), Thapathali, Kathmandu, Nepal, 2017; p 92.

Joshi, P. R.; Paudel, M. R.; Chand, M. B.; Pradhan, S.; Pant, K. K. et al. Cytotoxic Effect of Selected Wild Orchids on Two Different Human Cancer Cell Lines. *Heliyon* **2020,** *6*, e03991.

Juneja, R. K.; Sharma, S. C.; Tandon, J. S. Two Substituted Bibenzyls and a Dihydrophenanthrene from *Cymbidium aloifolium*. *Phytochem.* **1987,** *26*, 1123–1125.

Karnick, C. R. *Pharmacology of Ayurvedic Medicinal Plants*; Sri Satguru Publications: Delhi, 1996; p 67.

Khan, M. R.; Omoloso, A. D. Antibacterial Activity of *Galeola foliata*. *Fitoterapia*, **2004,** *75*, 494–496.

Khasim, S.; Rao, P. M. Medicinal Importance of Orchids. *The Botanica* **1999,** *49*, 86–91.

Khory, R. N.; Katarak, N. N. *Materia Medica of India and Therapeutics*; Neeraj Publishing House: Delhi, **1993,** 462.

Kong, J. M.; Goh, N. K.; Chia, L. S.; Chia, T. F. Recent Advances in Traditional Plant Drugs and Orchids. *Acta Pharma Sin.* **2003,** *24*, 7–21.

Lam, Y.; Ng, T. B.; Yao, R. M.; Shi, J.; Xu, K. et al. Evaluation of chemical constituents and important mechanism of pharmacological biology in *Dendrobium* plants. *Evid. Based Comp. Alt. Med.* **2015,** ***2015***, 1–25.

Lassak, E. V.; McCarthy, T. *Australian Medicinal Plants*; North Ryde: Methuen Australia, 1983; p 240.

Lee, J. H.; Kim, D. H.; Bang, M. H.; Yang, H. J.; Bang, S. H. et al. Isolation of Sterols from the Methanol Extracts of *Cymbidium goeringii* Reichb. fil. *Appl. Biol. Chem.* **2005,** *48*, 263–266.

Li, M. F.; Hirata, Y.; Xu, G. J.; Niwa, M.; Wu, H. M. Studies on the Chemical Constituents of *Dendrobium loddigesii* Rolfe. Yao xue xue bao. *Acta pharma Sin.* **1991,** *26*, 307–310.

Li, Y.; Wang, C. L.; Guo, S. X.; Yang, J. S.; Xiao, P. G. Two New Compounds from *Dendrobium candidum. Chem. Pharma Bull.* **2008,** *56*, 1477–1479.

Li, Y.; Wang, C. L.; Wang, Y. J.; Guo, S. X.; Yang, J. S. et al. Three New Bibenzyl Derivatives from *Dendrobium candidum. Chem. Pharma Bull.* **2009,** *57*, 218–219.

Li, Y. M.; Wang, H. Y.; Liu, G. Q. Erianin Induces Apoptosis in Human Leukemia HL-60 Cells. *Acta Pharma Sin.* **2001,** *22*, 1018–1022.

Lin, T. H.; Chang, S. J.; Chen, C. C. Constituents from the Stems of *Dendrobium moniliforme. Chin. Pharma J.* **2000,** *52*, 251–259.

Liu, Q. F.; Zhao, W. A New Dedonbrine-Type Alkaloid from *Dendrobium nobile. Chin. Chem. Lett.* **2003,** *14*, 278–279.

Liu, W. H.; Hua, Y. F.; Zhan, Z. J. Moniline, a new alkaloid from *Dendrobium moniliforme. J. Chem. Res.* **2007,** *6*, 317–318.

Lo, S. F.; Mulabagal, V.; Chen, C. L.; Kuo, C. L.; Tsay, H. S. Bioguided Fractionation and Isolation of Free Radical Scavenging Components from In Vitro Propagated Chinese Medicinal Plants *Dendrobium tosaense* Makino and *Dendrobium moniliforme* SW. *J. Agric. Food Chem.* **2004,** *52*, 6916–6919.

Luning, B.; Leander, K. K. Studies on Orchidaceous Alkaloids III. *Acta Chem. Scand.* **1965,** *19,* 1607–1611.

Majumder, P. L.; Guha, S.; Sen, S. Bibenzyl Derivatives from the Orchid *Dendrobium amoenum. Phytochem.* **1999,** *52*, 1365–1369.

Majumder, P. L.; Kar, A.; Shoolery, J. N. Bulbophyllanthrin, a Phenanthrene of the Orchid *Bulbophyllum leopardium. Phytochem.* **1985,** *24*, 2083–2087.

Majumder, P. L.; Maiti, D. C. Flaccidin, a 9, 10-dihydrophenanthropyran Derivative from the Orchid *Coelogyne flaccida. Phytochem.* **1988,** *27*, 899–901.

Majumder, P. L.; Pal, S. Cumulatin and tristin, two bibenzyl derivatives from the orchids *Dendrobium cumulatum* and *Bulbophyllum triste. Phytochem.* **1993,** *32*, 1561–1565.

Majumder, P. L.; Sarkar, A. K.; Chakraborti, J. Isoflavidinin and iso-oxoflavidinin, Two 9, 10-Dihydrophenanthrenes from the Orchids *Pholidota articulata, Otochilus porecta* and *Otochilus fusca. Phytochem.* **1982,** *21*, 2713–2716.

Majumder, P. L.; Sen, R. C. Moscatilin, a Bibenzyl Derivative from the Orchid *Dendrobium moscatum. Phytochem.* **1987,** *26*, 2121–2124.

Majumder, P. L.; Sen, S.; Majumder, S. Phenanthrene Derivatives from the Orchid *Coelogyne cristata. Phytochem.* **2001,** *58*, 581–586.

Malla, B.; Gauchan, D. P.; Chhetri, R. B. An Ethnobotanical Study of Medicinal Plants Used by Ethnic People in Parbat District of Western Nepal. *J. Ethnopharma.* **2015,** *165*, 103–117.

Manandhar, N. P. *Plants and People of Nepal*; Timber Press: Portland, OR, 2002; p 599.

Mangunwardoyo, W.; Suciatmih, S.; Gandjar, I. Frequency of endophytic fungi isolated from *Dendrobium crumenatum* Sw. (Pigeon orchid) and antimicrobial activity. *Biodiversitas* **2012,** *13*: 34–39.

Medhi, R. P.; Chakrabarti, S. Traditional Knowledge of NE People on Conservation of Wild Orchids, 2009.

Medhi, R. P.; Chakraborti, M. Orchid Biodiversity in India: Conservation and Utilization. *Ind. J. Gen. Pl. Breed.* **2012,** *72*, 148–156.

Min, Z. D.; Tanaka, T.; Iinuma, M.; Mizuno, M. A New Dihydrostilbene in *Dendrobium chrysanthum*. *J. Nat. Prod.* **1987,** *50*, 1189–1189.

Namsa, N. D.; Tag, H.; Mandal, M.; Kalita, P.; Das, A. K. An Ethnobotanical Study of Traditional Anti-Inflammatory Plants Used by the Lohit Community of Arunachal Pradesh, India. *J. Ethnopharma* **2009,** *125*, 234–245.

Ng, C. K. Y.; Hew, C. S. Orchid Pseudobulbs–False' Bulbs with a Genuine Importance in Orchid Growth and Survival! *Sci. Horti.* **2000,** *83*, 165–172.

Nongdam, P. Ethno-Medicinal Uses of Some Orchids of Nagaland, North-East India. *Res. J. Med. Pl.* **2014,** *8*, 126–139.

Nurfadilah, S. Utilization of Orchids of Wallacea Region and Implication for Conservation. In *IOP Conference Series: Earth and Environmental Science*; IOP Publishing, **2020,** *473*, 012063.

Okamoto, T.; Natsume, M.; Onaka, T.; Uchimaru, F.; Shimizu, M. Further Studies on the Alkaloidal Constituents of *Dendrobium nobile* (Orchidaceae)-Structure Determination of 4-hydroxy-dendroxine and Nobilomethylene. *Chem Pharma Bull.* **1972,** *20*, 418–421.

Ormerod, P. Notes on *Asiatic Tropidia* (Orchidaceae: Tropidieae). *Harv. Pap. Bot.* **2018,** *23*, 77–83.

Ozturk, M.; Altay, V.; Hakeem, K. R.; Akçiçek, E. *Liquorice from Botany to Phytochemistry*; SpringerBriefs in Plant Science, 2017. https://doi.org/10.1007/978-3-319-74240-3

Ozturk, M.; Egamberdieva, D.; Milica, P. *Biodiversity and Biomedicine-Our Future*; Academic Press, Elsevier Inc.: UK, USA, 2020.

Ozturk, M.; Altay, V.; Efe, R. *Biodiversity, Conservation and Sustainability in Asia: Volume I: Prospects and Challenges in West Asia and Caucasus*; Springer Nature: Switzerland AG, 2021a. DOI: 10.1007/978-3-030-59928-7

Ozturk, M.; Khan, S. M.; Altay, V.; Efe, R.; Egamberdieva, D.; Khassanov, F. *Biodiversity, Conservation and Sustainability in Asia: Volume II: Prospects and Challenges in South and Middle Asia*; Springer Nature: Switzerland AG, 2021b. DOI: 10.1007/978-3-030-73943-0

Panda, A. K.; Mandal, D. The Folklore Medicinal Orchids of Sikkim. *Anc. Sci. Life* **2013,** *33*, 92–96.

Pant, B. Medicinal Orchids and Their Uses: Tissue Culture a Potential Alternative for Conservation. *Afr. J. pl. Sci.* **2013,** *7*, 448–467.

Pant, B.; Raskoti, B. B. *Medicinal Orchids of Nepal*; Himalayan Map House Pvt. Ltd.: Kathmandu, Nepal, 2013; p 104.

Pant, B.; Shah, S.; Shrestha, R.; Pandey, S.; Joshi, P. R. An Overview on Orchid Endophytes. In *Mycorrhiza-Nutrient Uptake, Biocontrol, Ecorestoration*; Verma, A., Prasad, R., Tuteja, N., Eds.; Springer International Publishing AG, 2017; pp 503–524.

Pillon, Y.; Chase, M. W. Taxonomic Exaggeration and Its Effects on Orchid Conservation. *Conserv. Biol.* **2007,** *21*, 263–265.

Pleskanovskaya, S. A.; Mamedova, M. A.; Ashıralıyeva, M. A. et al. *Glycyrrhiza glabra* (Liquorice) in Turkmenistan—Medicinal and Biological Aspects. In *Plant and Human Health,—Pharmacology and Therapeutic Uses*, Ozturk, M., Hakeem, K. R., Eds., Vol. 3, Chapter 2; Springer Nature Switzerland, 2019; pp 23–35.

Pramanick, D. D. Pharmacognostic Studies on the Pseudobulb of *Coelogyne cristata* Lindl. (Orchidaceae)—An Epiphytic Orchid of Ethno-Medicinal Importance. *J. Pharmacog. Phytochem.* **2016,** *5*, 120–123.

Pyakurel, D.; Gurung, K. Enumeration of Orchids and Estimation of Current Stock of Traded Orchids in Rolpa District. District Forest Office, Rolpa, Nepal, 2008.

Qin, J.; Zhang, W.; Ge, Z-W.; Zhang, S-B. Molecular Identifications Uncover Diverse Fungal Symbionts of *Pleione* (Orchidaceae). *Fungal Ecol.* **2019,** *37,* 19–29.

Qing, L. H.; Rui, L.; Xing, W. T.; Yuan, L. G. Isolation and Purification of Two Constitutes from *Dendrobium fimbriatum* Hook by High-Speed Counter-Current Chromatography Using Stepwise Elution. *Sep. Sci. Tech.* **2009,** *44*, 1218–1227.

Radice, M.; Scalvenzi, L.; Gutiérrez, D. Etnofarmacología, bioactividad y fitoquímica de *Maxillaria densa* Lindl. Revisión científica y biocomercio en el neotrópico. *Colombia Forestal* **2020,** *23*, 20–33.

Raghunathan, K. Medico-Ethno-Botanical Surveys and Their Role in Research in Ayurveda. In *A Manual of Ethnobotany*; Jain, S. K., Ed.; Scientific Publishers: Jodhpur, India, 1995; pp 86–101.

Rahamtulla, M.; Pradhan, U. C.; Roy, A. K.; Rampilla, V.; Khasim, S. M. Ethnomedicinal Aspects of Some Orchids from Darjeeling Himalaya, India. In *Orchid Biology: Recent Trends & Challenges*; Khasim, S. M., Hegde, S. N., Arnao, M. T. G., Thammasiri, K., Eds.; Springer Nature: Singapore Pte Ltd., 2020; pp 451–472.

Rajbhandari, K. R. Orchids of Nepal: Status, Threat and Conservation. Proc. Natl. Work. NTFP/MAPs Sect. Action Plant Dev. Orchid. Department of Plant Resources, Ministry of Forest and Soil Conservation and central Department of Botany; Tribhuvan University: Kathmandu, Nepal, 2014; pp 1–40.

Rajendran, A.; Rao, N. R.; Kumar, K. R.; Henry, A. N. Some Medicinal Orchids of Southern India. *Anc. Sci. Life* **1997,** *17*, 10–14.

Ramesh, T.; Koperuncholan, M.; Praveena, R.; Ganeshkumari, K.; Vanithamani, J.; Muruganantham, P.; Renganathan, P. Medicinal Properties of Some *Dendrobium* Orchids—A Review. *J. Appl. Adv. Res.* **2019,** *4*, 119–128.

Richardson, K. A. Endophytic Fungi from Costa Rican orchids. MS Dissertation, University of Alberta, Edmonton, Canada, 1993.

Sachdev, K.; Kulshreshtha, D. K. Phenolic Constituents of *Coelogyne ovalis*. *Phytochem.* **1986,** *25*, 499–502.

Sarsaiya, S.; Jain, A.; Jia, Q.; Fan, X.; Shu, F.; Chen, Z.; Zhou, Q.; Shi, J.; Chen, J. Molecular Identification of Endophytic Fungi and Their Pathogenicity Evaluation Against *Dendrobium nobile* and *Dendrobium officinale*. *Int. J. Mol. Sci.* **2020,** *21*. DOI: 10.3390/ijms21010316

Sawmya, K.; Vasudevanan, T. G.; Murali, T. S. Fungal endophytes from two orchid species - pointer toward organ specificity. *Czech Mycol.* **2013,** *65*: 89–101.

Shah, S.; Shrestha, R.; Maharjan, S.; Selosse, M-A.; Pant, B. Isolation and Characterization of Plant Growth-Promoting Endophytic Fungi from the Roots of *Dendrobium moniliforme*. *Plants* **2019,** *8*, 5. DOI: 10.3390/plants8010005

Shanavaskhan, A. E.; Sivadasan, M.; Alfarhan, A. H.; Thomas, J. Ethnomedicinal Aspects of Angiospermic Epiphytes and Parasites of Kerala, India. *Ind. J. Trad. Know.* **2012,** *11*, 250–258.

Shanmugavalli, N.; Umashankar, V. R. Antimicrobial Activity of *Vanilla planifolia*. *Indian J. Sci. Technol.* **2009,** *2*, 37–40.

Shi, X.; Li, Y.; Liu, Y.; Jiang, J.; Wang, L. et al. A New 9, 10-Dihydrophenanthropyran Dimer and a New Natural 9, 10-Dihydrophenanthropyran from *Otochilus porrectus*. *Biochem. System. Ecol.* **2010,** *38*, 842–845.

Shimizu, M.; Shogawa, H.; Hayashi, T.; Arisawa, M.; Suzuki, S. et al. Anti-Inflammatory Constituents of Topically Applied Crude Drugs. III. Constituents and Anti-Inflammatory Effect of Paraguayan Crude Drug "Tamandá cuná" (*Catasetum barbatum* LINDLE). *Chem. Pharms. Bull.* **1988,** *36*, 4447–4452.

Shimura, H.; Matsuura, M.; Takada, N.; Koda, Y. An Antifungal Compound Involved in Symbiotic Germination of *Cypripedium macranthos* var. *rebunense* (Orchidaceae). *Phytochem.* **2007,** *68*, 1442–1447.

Shrestha, R.; Shah, S.; Pant, B. Identification of Endophytic Fungi from Roots of Two *Dendrobium* Species and Evaluation of Their Antibacterial Property. *Afr. J. Microbiol. Res.* **2018,** *12*, 697–704.

Shu, W.; Fengjuan, W.; Yongping, C. Anti-Oxidation Activity In Vitro of Polysaccharides of *Dendrobium huoshanense* and *Dendrobium moniliforme*. *Agric. Sci. Technol.* **2009,** *10*, 121–124.

Shubha, J.; Srinivas, C. Diversity and Extracellular Enzymes of Endophytic Fungi Associated with *Cymbidium aloifolium* L. L. *Afr. J. Biotechnol.* **2017,** *16*, 2248–2258.

Shyur, L. F.; Chen, C. H.; Lo, C. P.; Wang, S. Y.; Kang, P. L. et al. Induction of Apoptosis in MCF-7 Human Breast Cancer Cells by Phytochemicals from *Anoectochilus formosanus*. *J. Biomed. Sci.* **2004,** *11*, 928–939.

Simmler, C.; Antheaume, C.; André, P.; Bonté, F.; Lobstein, A. Glucosyloxybenzyl Eucomate Derivatives from *Vanda teres* Stimulate HaCaT Cytochrome-C Oxidase. *J. Nat. Prod.* **2011,** *74*, 949–955.

Singh, A.; Duggal, S. Medicinal Orchids—An Overview. *Ethnobot. Leaflet.* **2009,** *13*, 361–363.

Singh, D. K. Morphological Diversity of the Orchids of Orissa. In *Orchids: Science and Commerce*; Misra, S., Ed.; Bishen Singh Mehendra Pal Singh: Dehra Dun, India, 2001; p 135.

Smith, T. J. New Ecological Findings for *Sarcochilus Australis*, a Unique Orchid in Tasmania. *Tasmanian Nat.* **2008,** *130*, 112–1234.

Steege, H. T.; Cornelissen, J. H. C. Distribution and Ecology of Vascular Epiphytes in Lowland Rain Forest of Guyana. *Biotropica* 1989; pp 331–339.

Stewart, S. L.; Zettler, L. W. Symbiotic Germination of Three Semi-Aquatic Rein Orchids (*Habenaria repens, H. quinquiseta, H. macroceratitis*) from Florida. *Aq. Bot.* **2002,** *72*, 25–35.

Sopalun, K.; Lamtham, S. Isolation and screening of extracellular enzymatic activity of endophytic fungi isolated from Thai orchids. *South Afr. J. Bot.* **2020,** *134*: 273–279.

Sour, V.; Phonpho, S.; Soytong, K. Isolation of endophytic fungi from some orchid varieties. *Int. J. Agric. Technol.* **2015,** 1243–1254.

Subedi, A. Orchids Around Pokhara Valley of Nepal. *Occasional Papers* **2002,** *1*, 42-46.

Subedi, A.; Kunwar, B.; Choi, Y.; Dai, Y.; van Andel, T.; Chaudhary, R. P., de Boer, H. J.; Gravendeel, B. Collection and trade of wild-harvested orchids in Nepal. *J. Ethnobiol. Ethnomed.* **2013,** *9*, 1–10.

Sudheep, N. M.; Sridhar, K. R. Non-Mycorrhizal Endophytic Fungi in Two Orchids of Kaiga Forest (Western Ghats), India. *J. For. Res. 23*, **2012,** 453–460.

Sulistiarini, D. *Acriopsis javanica* Reinw. ex Blume. In *Plant Resources of South-East Asia # 12: Medicinal and Poisonous Plants 3*.; Lemmens, R. H. M. J., Bunyapraphatsara, N., Eds.; Backhuys: Leiden, The Netherlands, 2003; pp. 33–34.

Talapatra, B.; Mukhopadhyay, P.; Chaudhury, P.; Talapatra, S. K. Denbinobin, a New Phenanthraquinone from *Dendrobium-nobile* lindl (Orchidaceae). *Ind. J. Chem. Sec B Org. Chem.* **1982,** *21*, 386–387.

Tang, H.; Zhao, T.; Sheng, Y.; Zheng, T.; Fu, L.; Zhang, Y. *Dendrobium officinale* Kimura et Migo: A Review on Its Ethnopharmacology, Phytochemistry, Pharmacology, and Industrialization. *Evid. Based Compl. Alt. Med.* **2017,** 7436259.

Tang, J.; Deng, Y. R.; Zhuo, Y. R. Advances in Pharmacological Activity of *Anoectochilus roxburghii*. *Strait Pharm J.* **2008,** *20*, 77–79.

Teoh, E. S. *Medicinal Orchids of Asia*; Springer, 2016; p 559.

Teoh, E. S. Medicinal Orchids of Thailand and Myanmar. In *Orchids as Aphrodisiac, Medicine or Food*; Teoh, E. S., Ed., Springer: Cham, 2019a; pp 245–254.

Teoh, E. S. Medicinal Orchids in the Malay Archipelago. In *Orchids as Aphrodisiac, Medicine or Food*; Teoh, E. S., Ed.; Springer: Cham, 2019b; pp 255–289.

Thakur, R. B.; Yadav, R. P.; Thakur, N. P. Enumerating the Status of Orchid Species of Makawanpur District. *Hamro Kalpabricha*, **2010,** *20*, 1–18.

Tiwari, A. P.; Joshi, B.; Ansari, A. A. Less Known Ethnomedicinal Uses of Some Orchids by the Tribal Inhabitants of Amarkantak Plateau, Madhya Pradesh, India. *Nat. Sci.* **2012,** *10*, 33–37.

Tsering, J.; Tam, N.; Tag, H.; Gogoi, B. J.; Apang, O. Medicinal Orchids of Arunachal Pradesh: A Review. *Bull. Arunachal For. Res.* **2017,** *32*, 1–16.

Vaidya, B.; Shrestha, M.; Joshee, N. Report on Nepalese Orchid Species with Medicinal Properties. In *The Himalayan Plants, Can They Save Us? Proceeding of Nepal-Japan Joint Symposium on Conservation and Utilization of Himalayan Medicinal Resources*, 2000; pp 146–152.

Venkateswarlu, S.; Raju, M. S.; Subbaraju, G. V. Synthesis and Biological Activity of Isoamoenylin, a Metabolite of *Dendrobium amoenum*. *Biosci. Biotech. Biochem.* **2002,** *66*, 2236–2238.

Verma, S. K.; Gond, S. K.; Mioshra, A.; Sjarmas, V. K.; Kumar, J.; Singhj, D. K.; Kumar, A.; Gouitam, J.; Kharwar, R. N. Impact of environmental variables on the isolation, diversity and antibacterial activity of endophytic fungal communities from *Madhuca indica* Gmel. at different locations in India. *Ann. Microbiol.* **2014,** *64*: 721–734.

Wang, F. F.; Li, Y.; Dong, H. L.; Guo, S. X.; Wang, C. L.; Yang, J. S. A New Compound from *Dendrobium candidum*. *Chin. Pharma J.* **2010,** *45*, 898–902.

Wang, J.; Matsuzaki, K.; Kitanaka, S. Stilbene Derivatives from *Pholidota chinensis* and Their Anti-Inflammatory Activity. *Chem Pharma Bull.* **2006,** *54*, 1216–1218.

Wang, J.; Wang, L.; Kitanaka, S. Stilbene and Dihydrophenanthrene Derivatives from *Pholidota chinensis* and Their Nitric Oxide Inhibitory and Radical-Scavenging Activities. *J. Nat. Med.* **2007,** *61*, 381–386.

Wang, S. Y.; Kuo, Y. H.; Chang, H. N.; Kang, P. L.; Tsay, H. S.; Lin, K. F., Yang, N. S.; Shyur, L. F. Profiling and Characterization Antioxidant Activities in *Anoectochilus formosanus* Hayata. *J. Agric. Food Chem.* **2002,** *50*, 1859–1865.

Wang, X.; Li, Y.; Song, X.; Meng, Q.; Zhu, J.; Zhao, Y.; Yu, W. Influence of Host Tree Species on Isolation and Communities of Mycorrhizal and Endophytic Fungi from Roots of a Tropical Epiphytic Orchid, *Dendrobium sinense* (Orchidaceae). *Mycorrhiza* **2017,** *27*, 709–718.

Wangchuk, P.; Yeshi, K.; Jamphel, K. Pharmacological, Ethnopharmacological, and Botanical Evaluation of Subtropical Medicinal Plants of Lower Kheng Region in Bhutan. *Int. Med. Res.***2017,** *6*, 372–387.

Watanabe, K.; Tanaka, R.; Sakurai, H.; Iguchi, K.; Yamada, Y.; Hsu, C. S.; Sakuma, C.; Kikuchi, H.; Shibayama, H.; Kawai, T. Structure of Cymbidine A, a Monomeric

Peptidoglycan-Related Compound with Hypotensive and Diuretic Activities, Isolated from a Higher Plant, *Cymbidium goeringii* (Orchidaceae). *Chem. Pharma Bull.* **2007,** *55,* 780–783.

Watt, J. M.; Brandwijk, M. G. *The Medicinal and Poisonous Plants of Southern and Eastern Africa*; E. & S. Livingstone Ltd: Edinburgh, 1962.

Webb, L. J. Some New Records of Medicinal Plants Used by the Aborigines of Tropical Queensland and New Guinea. *Proc. Royal Soc. Queensland* **1960,** *71,* 103–110.

Wen, L.; Weiming, C.; Zhi, X.; Xaotain, L. New Triterpenoids of *Pholidota chinensis. Planta Medica* **1986,** *52,* 4–6.

Wiart, C. *Ethnopharmacology of Medicinal Plants: Asia and the Pacific*; Humana Press, Inc.: Totowa, NJ, 2006; p 228.

Won, J. H.; Kim, J. Y.; Yun, K. J.; Lee, J. H.; Back, N. I. et al. Gigantol Isolated from the Whole Plants of *Cymbidium goeringii* Inhibits the LPS-Induced iNOS and COX-2 Expression via NF-κB Inactivation in RAW 264.7 Macrophages Cells. *Planta Medica* **2006,** *72,* 1181–1187.

Wu, B.; He, S.; Pan, Y. J. New Dihydrodibenzoxepins from *Bulbophyllum kwangtungense. Planta Medica* **2006,** *72,* 1244–1247.

Wu, B.; Qu, H.; Cheng, Y. Cytotoxicity of New Stilbenoids from *Pholidota chinensis* and Their Spin-Labeled Derivatives. *Chem. Biodivers.* **2008,** *5,* 1803–1810.

Xing, Y. M.; Chen, J.; Cui, J. L.; Chen, X. M.; Guo, S. X. Antimicrobial Activity and Biodiversity of Endophytic Fungi in *Dendrobium devonianum* and *Dendrobium thyrsiflorum* from Vietman. *Curr. Microbiol.* **2011,** *62,* 1218–1224.

Yamaki, M.; Honda, C. The Stilbenoids from *Dendrobium plicatile. Phytochem.* **1996,** *43,* 207–208.

Yang, L.; Han, H.; Nakamura, N.; Hattori, M.; Wang, Z.; Xu, L. Bio-Guided Isolation of Antioxidants from the Stems of *Dendrobium aurantiacum* var. *denneanum. Phytother. Res.: Int. J. Pharmacol. Toxicol. Eval. Nat. Prod. Deriv.* **2007,** *21,* 696–698.

Yang, L.; Wang, Z.; Xu, L. Phenols and a Triterpene from *Dendrobium aurantiacum* var. *denneanum* (Orchidaceae). *Biochem. System. Ecol.* **2006a**, *8,* 658–660.

Yang, L.; Wang, Z.; Xu, L. Simultaneous Determination of Phenols (Bibenzyl, Phenanthrene, and Fluorenone) in *Dendrobium* Species by High-Performance Liquid Chromatography with Diode Array Detection. *J. Chrom. A* **2006b**, *1104,* 230–237.

Yang, L.; Zhang, C.; Yang, H.; Zhang, M.; Wang, Z.; Xu, L. Two New Alkaloids from *Dendrobium chrysanthum. Heterocycles-Sendai Institute of Heterocyclic Chemistry* **2005,** *65,* 633–636.

Yi, Y. F.; Xing, F. W.; Huang, X. X.; Chen, H. F.; Wang, F. G. Medicinal Plants of *Bulbophyllum* Species in China. *J. Trop. Subtrop. Bot.* **2005,** *13,* 65–69.

Yonzone, R.; Kamran, A.; Bhujel, R. B. Orchids in Ethnobotany. In *Proceeding of the International Seminar on Multidisciplinary Approaches in Angiosperm Systematics*; University of Kalyani: West Bengal, India, 2012; pp 661–669.

Younessi-Hamzekhanlu, M.; Ozturk, M.; Altay, V. et al. Ethnopharmacological Study of Medicinal Plants from Khoy City of West Azerbaijan-Iran. *Indian J. Trad. Knowl.* **2020,** *19* (2), 251–267.

Zi, X. M.; Sheng, C. L.; Googale, U. M.; Shao, S. C.; Gao, J. Y. In situ seed baiting to isolate germination-enhancing fungi for an epiphytic orchid, *Dendrobium aphyllum* (Orchidaceae). *Mycorrhiza* **2014,** *24*: 487–299.

Zhan, R.; Zhang, Y.; Chen, L.; Chen, Y. A New (Propylphenyl) Bibenzyl from *Eria bambusifolia*. *Nat. Prod. Res.* **2016,** *30*, 1740–1745.

Zhang, L.; Chen, F.; Zhang, G. Q.; Zhang, Y. Q.; Niu, S. et al. Origin and Mechanism of Crassulacean Acid Metabolism in Orchids as Implied by Comparative Transcriptomics and Genomics of the Carbon Fixation Pathway. *Pl. J.* **2016,** 86, 175–185.

Zhang, S.; Yang, Y.; Li, J.; Qin, J.; Zhang, W. et al. Physiological Diversity of Orchids. *Pl. Divers.* **2018,** *40*, 196–208.

Zhang, X.; Xu, J. K.; Wang, J.; Wang, N. L.; Kurihara, H. et al. Bioactive Bibenzyl Derivatives and Fluorenones from *Dendrobium nobile*. *J. Nat. Prod.* **2007b,** *70*, 24–28.

Zhang, Y.; Cai, J.; Ruan, H.; Pi, H.; Wu, J. Antihyperglycemic Activity of Kinsenoside, a High Yielding Constituent from *Anoectochilus roxburghii* in Streptozotocin Diabetic Rats. *J. Ethnopharma* **2007a,** *114*, 141–145.

Index

J

Q

R

S

T

U

V

W

X

Z

For Product Safety Concerns and Information please contact our EU representative GPSR@taylorandfrancis.com
Taylor & Francis Verlag GmbH, Kaufingerstraße 24, 80331 München, Germany

www.ingramcontent.com/pod-product-compliance
Lightning Source LLC
LaVergne TN
LVHW010628300926
849162LV00001B/91
* 9 7 8 1 7 7 4 9 1 2 2 7 0 *